Third Edition

MANUAL OF PREOPERATIVE AND POSTOPERATIVE CARE

COMMITTEE ON PRE AND
POSTOPERATIVE CARE

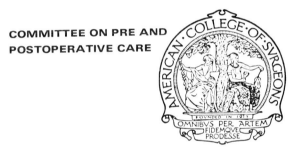

AMERICAN COLLEGE OF SURGEONS

Editorial Subcommittee

STANLEY J. DUDRICK, Chairman
ARTHUR E. BAUE
BEN EISEMAN
LLOYD D. MacLEAN
MARC I. ROWE
GEORGE F. SHELDON

W. B. SAUNDERS COMPANY • 1983

Philadelphia • London • Toronto • Mexico City • Rio de Janeiro • Sydney • Tokyo

W. B. Saunders Company: West Washington Square
Philadelphia, PA 19105

1 St. Anne's Road
Eastbourne, East Sussex BN21 3UN, England

1 Goldthorne Avenue
Toronto, Ontario M8Z 5T9, Canada

Apartado 26370—Cedro 512
Mexico 4, D.F., Mexico

Rua Coronel Cabrita, 8
Sao Cristovao Caixa Postal 21176
Rio de Janeiro, Brazil

9 Waltham Street
Artarmon, N.S.W. 2064, Australia

Ichibancho, Central Bldg., 22-1 Ichibancho
Chiyoda-Ku, Tokyo 102, Japan

Library of Congress Cataloging in Publication Data
Main entry under title:

Manual of preoperative and postoperative care.

    1. Therapeutics, Surgical.   2. Preoperative care.   3. Postoperative care.
I. Dudrick, Stanley J.   II. American College of Surgeons. Committee on Pre and
Postoperative Care. [DNLM: 1. Preoperative care.   2. Postoperative care. WO 178 M294]
RD49.M27   1982   617'.919   81-48095
ISBN 0-7216-1164-8   AACR2

Listed here is the latest translated edition of this book together with the language of the
translation and the publisher.

Italian — 2nd edition — Piccin Editore, Padova, Italy

Spanish — 2nd edition — NEISA, Mexico D.F., Mexico

Manual of Preoperative and Postoperative Care   ISBN   0-7216-1164-8

Last digit is the print number: 9   8   7   6   5   4   3   2   1

Committee
on Pre and
Postoperative Care

*DONALD S. GANN, *Chairman*
*RICHARD L. SIMMONS, *Vice Chairman*
JOHN R. BORDER
*MURRAY F. BRENNAN
FRANK B. CERRA
JOHN W. DUCKETT, JR.
C. McCOLLISTER EVARTS
JOSEF E. FISCHER
JOHN B. GATHRIGHT, JR.
HERBERT B. HECHTMAN
JOEL H. HOROVITZ
M. J. JURKIEWICZ
NICHOLAS T. KOUCHOUKOS

FRANK R. LEWIS, JR.
WILLIAM E. MATORY
JONATHAN L. MEAKINS
*RICHARD M. PETERS
ALBERT L. RHOTON, JR.
WILLIAM A. SCOVILL
HARRY M. SHIZGAL
JESSIE L. TERNBERG
DANIEL G. VAUGHAN
WALTER W. WHISLER
WILLIS H. WILLIAMS
*DOUGLAS W. WILMORE

SENIOR MEMBERS

J. WESLEY ALEXANDER
ARTHUR E. BAUE
CHARLES R. BAXTER
CHARLES E. BRACKETT
LARRY C. CAREY
CHARLES J. CARRICO
JOSEPH M. CIVETTA
JOHN A. COLLINS
P. WILLIAM CURRERI

STANLEY J. DUDRICK
JOHN H. DUFF
JAMES H. DUKE, JR.
RUBEN F. GITTES
LAZAR J. GREENFIELD
FRANK E. GUMP
E. JOHN HINCHEY
JOHN W. MADDEN
JOHN A. MANNICK

WILLIAM W. MONAFO, JR.
GERALD S. MOSS
JOHN M. PALMER
MARC I. ROWE
GEORGE F. SHELDON
ROGER T. SHERMAN
JOHN J. SKILLMAN
ROBY C. THOMPSON, JR.
HASTINGS K. WRIGHT

*Executive Committee members.

Contributors

J. WESLEY ALEXANDER, M.D., Sc.D.

Professor of Surgery, University of Cincinnati. Director of Research, Shriners' Burns Institute, Cincinnati Unit, Cincinnati, Ohio.

ROBERT W. BARNES, M.D.

David M. Hume Professor of Surgery, Medical College of Virginia/Virginia Commonwealth University. Attending Surgeon, Medical College of Virginia Hospitals. Chief of Vascular Surgery McGuire Veterans Administration Medical Center, Richmond, Virginia.

ARTHUR E. BAUE, M.D.

Donald Guthrie Professor and Chairman, Department of Surgery, Yale University School of Medicine. Chief of Surgery, Yale-New Haven Hospital, New Haven, Connecticut.

LESTER R. BRYANT, M.D., Sc.D.

Professor and Chairman, Department of Surgery, Quillen-Dishner College of Medicine, East Tennessee State University. Attending Surgeon, Johnson City Medical Center Hospital and Veterans Administration Medical Center, Johnson City, Tennessee.

LARRY C. CAREY, M.D.

Robert M. Zollinger Professor and Chairman, Department of Surgery, Ohio State University College of Medicine. Attending Surgeon, Ohio State University Hospitals; Consulting Surgeon, Columbus Children's Hospital, Grant Hospital, Columbus, Ohio.

HENRY CLEVELAND, M.D.

Clinical Professor of Surgery, University of Colorado Health Sciences Center, Denver, Colorado.

JOSEPH D. COHN, M.D., F.A.C.S.

Clinical Associate Professor of Surgery, College of Medicine and Dentistry of New Jersey. Attending Surgeon, St. Barnabas Medical Center, Livingston, New Jersey.

JOHN A. COLLINS, M.D.

Professor and Chairman, Department of Surgery, Stanford University School of Medicine, Stanford, California.

WILLIAM F. COLLINS, M.D.

Cushing Professor of Surgery (Neurosurgery), Yale University School of Medicine. Neurosurgeon-in-Chief, Yale-New Haven Hospital, New Haven, Connecticut.

WILLIAM T. CONNER, M.D.

Assistant Professor of Surgery, The University of Texas Medical School at Houston, Houston, Texas.

LEE H. COOPERMAN, M.D.

Professor of Anesthesia, University of Pennsylvania School of Medicine, Philadelphia, Pennsylvania.

EDWARD M. COPELAND, III, M.D.

Professor of Surgery, The University of Texas Medical School at Houston and The University of Texas System Cancer Center M. D. Anderson Hospital and Tumor Institute, Houston, Texas.

ARNOLD G. CORAN, M.D.

Head of Section of Pediatric Surgery and Professor of Surgery, University of Michigan Medical School. Chief of Pediatric Surgical Services, Mott Children's Hospital, Ann Arbor, Michigan.

MARVIN L. CORMAN, M.D., F.A.C.S.

Staff Surgeon, Department of Colon and Rectal Surgery Sansum Medical Clinic, Santa Barbara, California.

JOSEPH N. CORRIERE, Jr., M.D., F.A.C.S.

Professor and Director of Surgery (Urology), The University of Texas Medical School at Houston. Chief of Urology, Active Staff, Hermann Hospital, Houston, Texas.

JOHN M. DALY, M.D.

Associate Professor of Surgery, Cornell Medical School. Associate Attending Surgeon, Memorial Sloan-Kettering Cancer Center, New York, New York.

LOUIS R. M. DEL GUERCIO, M.D., F.A.C.S.

Professor and Chairman, Department of Surgery New York Medical College. Valhalla, New York.

STANLEY J. DUDRICK, M.D.

Professor of Surgery, The University of Texas System Cancer Center. Clinical Professor of Surgery, The University of Texas Medical School at Houston. Attending Surgeon, St. Luke's Episcopal Hospital and Texas Children's Hospital. Consultant in Surgery, M. D. Anderson Hospital and Tumor Institute and the Texas Institute for Rehabilitation and Research, Texas Medical Center, Houston, Texas.

JAMES H. DUKE, Jr., M.D., F.A.C.S.

Professor of Surgery, University of Texas Medical School at Houston, Medical Director, Emergency Center, Hermann Hospital, Houston, Texas.

CHARLES C. DUNCAN, M.D.

Associate Professor of Surgery (Neurosurgery) and Pediatrics, Yale University School of Medicine. Attending Neurosurgeon, Yale-New Haven Hospital, New Haven, Connecticut.

L. HENRY EDMUNDS, Jr., M.D.

W. M. Measey Professor of Surgery, University of Pennsylvania School of Medicine. Chief, Cardiothoracic Surgery, Hospital of the University of Pennsylvania, Philadelphia, Pennsylvania.

BEN EISEMAN, M.D.

Professor of Surgery, University of Colorado Health Sciences Center, Denver, Colorado.

E. CHRISTOPHER ELLISON, M.D.

Clinical Instructor in Surgery, Ohio State University College of Medicine, Columbus, Ohio.

ROBERT M. FILLER, M.D., F.A.C.S., F.R.C.S.(C.)

Professor of Surgery, University of Toronto. Surgeon-in-Chief, The Hospital for Sick Children, Toronto, Ontario, Canada.

LAZAR J. GREENFIELD, M.D.

Stuart McGuire Professor and Chairman, Department of Surgery, Medical College of Virginia/Virginia Commonwealth University, Richmond, Virginia.

WARD O. GRIFFEN, Jr., M.D., Ph.D.

Professor and Chairman, Department of Surgery, University of Kentucky Medical Center. Chief, University of Kentucky Hospital; Consultant, Veterans Administration Hospital, Lexington, Kentucky.

FRANK E. GUMP, M.D.

Professor of Surgery, College of Physicians & Surgeons of Columbia University. Attending Surgeon, Presbyterian Hospital, New York, New York.

TIMOTHY S. HARRISON, M.D., F.A.C.S.

Professor of Surgery and Physiology, Pennsylvania State University College of Medicine. Milton S. Hershey Medical Center, Hershey, Pennsylvania.

R. SCOTT JONES, M.D.

Stephen H. Watts Professor and Chairman, Department of Surgery, University of Virginia. Surgeon in Chief, University of Virginia Medical Center, Charlottesville, Virginia.

BARRY D. KAHAN, M.D.

Professor of Surgery, The University of Texas Medical School at Houston, Houston, Texas.

EDWIN L. KAPLAN, M.D.

Professor of Surgery, The University of Chicago Pritzker School of Medicine, Chicago, Illinois.

JOHN M. KINNEY, M.D.

Professor of Surgery, College of Physicians & Surgeons of Columbia University. Attending Surgeon, Presbyterian Hospital, New York, New York.

LARRY I. LIPSHULTZ, M.D., F.A.C.S.

Professor of Surgery (Urology), The University of Texas Medical School at Houston. Active Staff, Hermann Hospital, Houston, Texas.

LLOYD D. MacLEAN, M.D., F.R.C.S.(C), F.A.C.S.

Chairman, Department of Surgery, McGill University, Montreal. Surgeon-in-Chief, Royal Victoria Hospital, Montreal, Quebec, Canada.

JOHN W. MADDEN, M.D.

Clinical Professor in Orthopaedics, University of New Mexico School of Medicine. Staff Surgeon, St. Joseph's Hospital, Tucson, Arizona.

MICHAEL B. MARCHILDON, M.D.

Assistant Professor of Pediatric Surgery, University of Miami School of Medicine, Miami, Florida.

WILLIAM C. MEYERS, M.D.

Chief Resident, General and Thoracic Surgery, Department of Surgery, Duke University Medical Center, Durham, North Carolina.

JOHN J. MIKUTA, M.D.

Professor of Obstetrics and Gynecology, University of Pennsylvania Medical School. Director of Gynecologic Oncology, Hospital of the University of Pennsylvania, Philadelphia, Pennsylvania.

THOMAS A. MILLER, M.D., F.A.C.S.

Associate Professor of Surgery; Director of Academic Affairs and Resident Training, Department of Surgery, University of Texas Medical School. Attending Surgeon, Hermann Hospital, Houston, Texas.

WILLIAM J. MILLIKAN, Jr., M.D.

Associate Professor of Surgery, Emory University School of Medicine. Consulting Surgeon, Veterans Administration Hospital; Grady Memorial Hospital; Crawford W. Long Hospital; Atlanta, Georgia.

FRANCIS D. MOORE, M.D.

Moseley Professor of Surgery Emeritus, Harvard Medical School. Surgeon-in-Chief Emeritus, Peter Bent Brigham Hospital, Boston, Massachusetts.

JAMES A. O'NEILL, Jr., M.D.

Professor of Pediatric Surgery, University of Pennsylvania School of Medicine. Surgeon-in-Chief, Children's Hospital of Philadelphia, Philadelphia, Pennsylvania.

SAMUEL R. POWERS, Jr., M.D.*

Professor of Surgery, Albany Medical College. Attending Surgeon, Albany Medical Center Hospital; Consulting Surgeon, Veterans Administration Hospital, Albany, New York.
*Dr. Powers died on March 27, 1980.

BASIL A. PRUITT, Jr., M.D.

Commander and Director, U.S. Army Institute of Surgical Research, Fort Sam Houston, San Antonio, Texas.

HENRY THOMAS RANDALL, M.D., M.Sc.D., M.A.

Professor Emeritus of Medical Science, Brown University. Consultant in Surgery, Rhode Island Hospital, Providence, Rhode Island.

MARC I. ROWE, M.D.

Department of Surgery/Pediatrics, University of Miami School of Medicine, Miami, Florida.

EDWIN W. SALZMAN, M.D.

Professor of Surgery, Harvard Medical School. Associate Chief of Surgery, Beth Israel Hospital, Boston, Massachusetts.

SEYMOUR I. SCHWARTZ, M.D., F.A.C.S.

Professor of Surgery, University of Rochester School of Medicine and Dentistry. Senior Surgeon, Strong Memorial Hospital, Rochester, New York.

GEORGE F. SHELDON, M.D.

Professor of Surgery, University of California at San Francisco. Chief, Trauma and Hyperalimentation Services, San Francisco General Hospital, San Francisco, California.

JAMES C. THOMPSON, M.D., M.A.

Professor and Chairman, Department of Surgery, University of Texas Medical Branch. Surgeon-in-Chief, University Hospitals, University of Texas Medical Branch, Galveston, Texas.

M. DAVID TILSON, M.D.

Associate Professor of Surgery, Yale University School of Medicine. Attending Surgeon, Yale-New Haven Hospital, New Haven, Connecticut.

RICHARD C. TREAT, M.D.

Assistant Professor of Surgery, Medical College of Georgia, Augusta, Georgia.

DONALD D. TRUNKEY, M.D.

Professor of Surgery, University of California at San Franciso. Chief, Department of Surgery, San Francisco General Hospital, San Francisco, California.

RICHARD E. WARD, M.D.

Assistant Professor of Surgery, University of California, Davis. Attending Surgeon, University of California, Davis Medical Center, Sacramento, California.

G. DEAN WARREN, M.D.

Joseph P. Whitehead Professor and Chairman, Department of Surgery, Emory University School of Medicine. Chief of Surgery, Emory University Hospital, Atlanta, Georgia.

SAMUEL A. WELLS, Jr., M.D.

Professor of Surgery, Washington University School of Medicine. Surgeon-in-Chief, Barnes Hospital, St. Louis, Missouri.

HARRY WOLLMAN, M.D.

Robert Dunning Dripps Professor, Chairman, Department of Anesthesia, Professor of Pharmacology, University of Pennsylvania School of Medicine, Philadelphia, Pennsylvania.

H. K. WRIGHT, M.D.

Professor and Vice Chairman, Department of Surgery, Yale University School of Medicine. Assistant Chief, Department of Surgery, Yale-New Haven Medical Center, New Haven, Connecticut.

Preface
to the Third Edition

In response to its charge by the Board of Regents of the American College of Surgeons, the Committee on Pre- and Postoperative Care has attempted to revise and update clinical material that is relevant and useful in the preoperative and postoperative management of current surgical problems. The intent and purpose of the Manual remains essentially the same as stated in the Preface to the Second Edition. In each chapter, the authors have attempted to convey to the reader the manner in which they preoperatively and postoperatively treat their patients. Introductory remarks have been kept to a minimum and historical entries have been made only when they add to the understanding of specific points the authors wish to emphasize. Operative procedures have not been described or discussed except when such details have lent clarity to the rationale of the preoperative or postoperative management. Selected references have been added only when the authors thought that they led the reader to a valuable source of additional in-depth information on the subjects discussed. In no case have the authors intended to present merely an abridged version of a chapter they have written for a textbook.

The 58 contributors of the 40 chapters and the revised Appendix include 49 new authors for the Manual. This edition has been divided into four sections, entitled The Basics, The Pediatric Surgery Patient, The Organ Systems, and Special Patient Problems.

Several changes have been made in the Third Edition based upon the evolving interests and advancements that have occurred in the broad field of surgery during the past decade. In some areas material has been condensed, whereas in others the quantity and scope of the material presented has been expanded, reflecting the trends of the times. Although the total number of chapters has been increased from 31 in the Second Edition to 40 in the Third Edition, a net gain of 11 new chapters to the Manual has been achieved by consolidating some of the material presented previously in fewer chapters. The chapter on Surgical Nutrition has been expanded to two chapters entitled Enteral Nutrition and Parenteral Nutrition while the chapter on Problems in Infants and Children has been expanded to four chapters dealing with the specific problems of pediatric surgery patients. Other areas of special interest have been presented with the addition of the chapters on Preparation of the

Patient for Anesthesia, Multiple Systems Failure, The Urology Patient, The Patient with Neurologic Dysfunction, The Cancer Patient, The Extremities, and Physiologic Support Systems. The opening chapter on Preoperative Preparation adds a new and important dimension to this Manual.

The Editorial Subcommittee wishes to acknowledge the unusual and unselfish effort and time given cheerfully to the editing of this edition of the Manual by the following: Liz Blume, Homer C. Tolan, Jackie Shires Blain, Dr. Michael E. Miner, Terri Gammeter Jensen, Theresa Keen Dudrick, DeAnn Scott Englert, Dr. Malcolm B. Clague, and Dr. Joseph J. O'Donnell.

The Subcommittee also wishes to convey its particular appreciation to Dr. Edwin W. Gerrish and Claudia Delestowicz of the American College of Surgeons and to Albert E. Meier, Frank Polizzano, Lynne Mahan, Donna D. Ciccotelli, and Lorraine B. Kilmer of the W. B. Saunders Company for their encouragement, advice, and support. Finally, sincere gratitude is expressed to the many secretaries and others who have made significant but otherwise unacknowledged contributions to the preparation of this Manual.

Editorial Subcommittee
Stanley J. Dudrick, M.D., Chairman
Arthur E. Baue, M.D.
Ben Eiseman, M.D.
Lloyd D. MacLean, M.D.
Marc I. Rowe, M.D.
George F. Sheldon, M.D.

Preface
to the Second Edition

The purpose of this manual is to provide the busy clinical surgeon and surgical resident with quick and concise access to recent advances in surgical metabolism, nutrition, fluid and electrolyte balance, clotting disorders, infection and shock, together with cardiac, ventilatory and renal pathophysiology. It is intended to provide a useful outline of the modern management of problems of pre- and postoperative patients undergoing both elective and emergency operation. The authors have, in the latter chapters of this book, described the approaches to the handling of pre- and postoperative care of patients undergoing operation on particular body systems, including the management of related complications. Other chapters include the management of multiple injuries and the treatment of burns. The appendix includes a table of normal laboratory values, a list of selected tests of various organ systems and a brief discussion of acid-base balance.

The manual does not attempt to be a text, and so technical details of operations have usually been omitted in the interest of maintaining a volume of modest size and cost. References to standard texts and important articles will be found at the end of most chapters, and from them additional information can be obtained. It is hoped that such a manual may serve as a ready reference for the surgeon who lacks the time to read more extensive material on a given subject, or who might appreciate an abbreviated discussion prior to a more extensive review of the literature.

The manual has been prepared as an activity of the Committee on Pre- and Postoperative Care of the American College of Surgeons with the approval of the Regents of the College. Since the Committee's formation in 1959 under the chairmanship of Dr. Francis D. Moore of Boston, a major activity has been the sponsoring of teaching sessions in pre- and postoperative care. The manual is an outgrowth of the course in pre- and postoperative care given annually at the Clinical Congress of the American College of Surgeons.

The selection of the material for the second edition reflects certain changes from the previous volume. There are fewer chapters, of somewhat longer length, new illustrative material and additional references. This editorial committee does not contend that methods or approaches other than the ones presented in this volume may not be successful in the management of surgical patients. What we have endeavored to do is provide a useful guide for the management of surgical patients, based upon the description of the metabolic and physiologic principles that must underlie successful treatment.

We wish to acknowledge the unusual time and effort that was spent by the members of the first edition's editorial committee in translating the multiple wishes of the parent committee into initial book form. Our appreciation for this goes to Dr. Henry T. Randall, Chairman, Dr. James D. Hardy and Dr. Francis D. Moore. The success of the first edition confirmed the need for such a volume and contributed greatly to the preparation of this second edition.

Particular thanks are due to Dr. William Adams of the American College of Surgeons and Mr. Robert Rowan of W. B. Saunders Company for continuing advice and encouragement. In addition, we wish to thank the many secretaries whose patient and careful work contributed to the preparation of this volume.

RICHARD EGDAHL
GEORGE ZUIDEMA
JOHN M. KINNEY, *Chairman*
Editorial Subcommittee

Contents

II THE PEDIATRIC SURGERY PATIENT

III THE ORGAN SYSTEMS

I

The Basics

1

Aphorisms, Abjurations, and the Chemistry of Confidence

FRANCIS D. MOORE

"The most important thing before an operation —
is what I think about it the night before."

With this phrase a skilled senior surgeon of the older generation summarized his need for a careful consideration of every detail.

This brief account is intended to give the reader a mental checklist of concerns to cover before an operation and to outline a few of the salient points that concern the surgeon as he or she prepares the patient, the patient's family, the hospital entourage, and other physicians, as well as himself or herself, for the approaching operation. Details of microbiology, cardiology, nephrology, pharmacology, nutrition, blood coagulation, and pathology will not be covered, since they form the body of the rest of this text.

Our first aphorism, perhaps the most important, and surely the simplest to state is

"Avoid surprises."

Avoid things that surprise or alarm the patient. Prepare the patient with adequate advance knowledge so that there will be no large or unpleasant surprise that might destroy the chemistry of confidence.

Do not be surprised yourself by findings that you should have known about before the operation. Appropriate information should be communicated to the nurses, the operating room team, the radiology department, the patient's family, and the referring physician.

3

THE BODILY ECONOMY

ON ADMISSION AND THE DAY BEFORE OPERATION

History, Physical Examination, and Basic Work-Up

Be sure that all the things you ordered are not only in but also recorded and mentally digested, such as the electrocardiograms, roentgenogram readings, chemical values, and consultation; do not order any studies or tests unless you see the results and have them recorded before the operation. Encourage your colleagues to remind each other (or you) of items in the work-up data that you may have overlooked. Be sure that the necessary roentgenograms are on hand.

If there is a critical physical finding, such as a mass, a tender point, or an anatomic abnormality, that is critical to the operation itself or the placement of the incision, check it personally the day before and preferably the morning of the operation.

Nutrition

There is a persistent myth that a person cannot survive a weight loss of more than 40 per cent of his or her body weight, a myth exploded many times in our own experience with gastrointestinal cancer and inflammatory bowel disease. There is an accompanying myth that any weight loss at all, even of a few pounds, mysteriously and persistently interferes with immunology and wound healing.

These two views of nutritional assessment are both in error, because the weight loss itself is only one index of nutritional change.

The truth lies somewhere in between. Minor degrees of tissue loss, sometimes masked by edema, can be nutritionally very crippling in certain types of cancer and pulmonary disease. The rate and pathologic cause of the weight loss, macronutrient and micronutrient deficiencies, and water and salt changes, must all be evaluated. Most immunologic disorders arise from sources other than malnutrition alone. Obese persons can have a seriously disordered body cell mass hidden under all that fat. It is, therefore, wise to evaluate the patient's nutritional status in relation not only to the gain or loss of weight but also to signs observed by the physician, underlying pathologic conditions, and laboratory evidence of significant micronutrient or macronutrient starvation.

The signs to look for are cracks around the lips, smooth tongue, skin rash, loss of hair, peripheral edema, hyponatremia, hyperkalemia, hypoalbuminemia, weakness, and chronic cough. The nature and cause of weight loss often determine its degree of significant deficit. With mounting obstruction of the GI tract at any level, vitamin deficiency and trace mineral deficiency can be serious; voluntary weight loss of dietary origin under guidance rarely results in any debility. The late Philip Allison of Oxford advised his overweight patients with hiatus hernia to lose 20 to 40 pounds before operation. This did not produce any recognized immunologic, respiratory, or wound-healing disorder.

If you find that the patient does show "starvation with signs," remember the Humpty Dumpty aphorism:

> *"Preop reassembly is never complete.*
> *Start repair and avoid defeat."*

The objective of preoperative repletion is to accomplish as much of it as you can by mouth, to provide some calories and some protein precursors to reestablish normal glycogen in the liver, to provide substrates for muscle and viscera, to initiate protein synthesis, and to favor the normal metabolism of fat, thus eliminating blood ketones.

Most patients with gastrointestinal disease and weight loss suffer some degree of hypovitaminosis, which can also be corrected. These simple beginning objectives should be sought rather than total repair of the entire nutritional status of the patient.

If the patient has a serious nutritional problem and parenteral feeding is to be undertaken preoperatively, commit yourself, the patient, and the patient's family to a course of at least 7 to 16 days. Any period shorter than that is a waste of your time and the patient's money.

Body Water Changes

Distinguish between desiccation-dehydration — the loss of pure water as steam or vapor from the lungs, skin, or with renal disease producing high urine volumes with low electrolyte content — and its often confusing partner, desalting water loss. The former will be accompanied by an anomalously high sodium concentration. The latter will have a normal or low sodium concentration.

If the patient shows edema anywhere, determine the cause of this edema, whether venous obstruction, renal or hepatic failure, overadministration of fluid, or late starvation with hypoalbuminemia.

Red Flags

In the category of *avoid surprises*, there are certain things that keep recurring in the practice of surgery as "red flags" or "stop signs," meaning that the operation, if scheduled for the following day, should be canceled and more study should be carried out.

> *"All that is wrong cannot be righted.*
> *Be sure the wrongs are rightly sighted."*

First and foremost is unexpected occult blood in the feces. If this finding is not a part of the known disease process, the source and significance should be pinpointed before the operation.

Second is the unexpected occurrence of chronic obstructive pulmonary disease with an elevated carbon dioxide tension (PCO_2) in either arterial or venous blood. Don't forget that this is one place that venous gases can be useful, allowing for the approximately 5 mm Hg of allowable venous increase. Chronic pulmonary disease may be evidenced by chronic cough or cigarette stains on the fingers. This latter finding leads to suspicion, and when you find an accompanying elevation of bicarbonate, it indicates long-standing, partially compensated, chronic hypercapnia. Any arterial PCO_2 above 42 mm Hg or venous PCO_2 over 47 mm Hg requires further investigation, as it is dangerous if unexpected and untreated.

The unbuffered metabolic change in respiratory acidosis has been defined as 1.0 mM per liter elevation of bicarbonate per 10 mm Hg elevation of PCO_2. Anything greater than that suggests long duration of the respiratory acidosis and additional metabolic compensation by renal changes, adding to the plasma bicarbonate by the excretion of a urine of high titratable acidity and low pH.

By the same token, the "allowable" limits of respiratory compensation for metabolic acidosis have been defined: 1.5 mm Hg decrease in carbon dioxide tension per 1.0 mM per liter decrease in standard bicarbonate. These limits are interesting because changes beyond them suggest a search for other acid-base disorders.

Disordered Chemical Values

Plasma sodium and potassium concentrations move in opposite directions. Giving a large amount of sodium to an individual with a low sodium concentration in the plasma not only may be irrational (if the hyponatremia is due to overdilution) but also can produce severe hypokalemia, with resulting overdigitalization, as mentioned later. By contrast, remember that a rising plasma potassium concentration and acidosis tend to have a negative ionotropic effect on the heart, if it is not digitalized, and to dedigitalize it if the patient has heart disease under digitalis management.

The chemical "set" preoperatively may bias the postoperative acid-base change:

Postoperative alkalosis is common, usually harmless, usually transient, but beware if severe and prolonged, with a falling potassium level.

Low-flow acidosis is a pathologic change, always harmful; it indicates persistent hypoperfusion of tissues.

The best policy toward *post-traumatic alkalosis* is to prevent it and avoid it; give KCl or HCl.

The *treatment of low-flow acidosis* consists of the restoration of flow.

Preoperative alkalosis is a hazard, particularly when it occurs concomitantly with such diseases as acute pancreatitis and obstructed duodenal ulcer. This alkalosis may not be fully correctable in 24 to 36 hours, but the important thing is to have it on its way toward correction before anesthesia is induced.

If the patient has desalting water loss or true dehydration-desiccation, with a high sodium level, then remember the aphorism:

> *"Nudge the patient — do not kick.*
> *Just remember, he's quite sick."*

It is a mistake to infuse huge amounts of fluid just before an operation. If they are required by the disease process, try to avoid operation during rapid changes. The exception to this rule is hemorrhage.

Moderation is advised in all situations, especially when correcting metabolic defects: *Maybe you can't correct everything, but you can move the patient in the right direction.* In most cases, operation need not await total correction, and in fact the operation itself may be central to correction of the anomaly, particularly in low-flow states with undrained sepsis.

In acute hemorrhage, acute trauma, and shock with or without hemorrhage, operation itself is part of resuscitation.

> *"Massive blood loss seals his fate.*
> *Do not wait . . . Operate."*

Undrained sepsis has somewhat the same implications, though the rushed emergency is not as common today as it was in past years.

Drugs and Sleep the Night Before

Discuss the patient's normal sleeping habits and sleeping medications. Some patients have never taken a sleeping pill in their entire life. They will be upset and disturbed, "climbing the walls" with a drug to which they are unaccustomed. Other patients will want a large dose of the drug that they commonly take in a smaller dose. Do not introduce the patient to new sedatives or new hypnotics if the old ones work well.

Old Drugs

Do not be surprised by an adverse reaction traceable to your own ignorance about the patient's prior drug history. Many internists and family physicians have a bad habit of putting all their patients on some combination of the following: diuretics, antihypertensive medications, sedatives, hypnotics, and tranquilizers. Diazepam (Valium) withdrawal can produce delirium tremens. Chronic diuretic ingestion is widespread, often without adequate justification; it results in disordered electrolyte values, particularly with loss of potassium, often masked by a normal plasma potassium concentration. This makes the patient vulnerable to both hypokalemia and alkalosis. Antihypertensive medication is also widely used, often with inadequate study and justification, and it complicates matters for the anesthetist.

Alcoholism, smoking, and chronic salicylate ingestion are commonplace. Of all of these, a chronic smoking habit is the commonest and most ominous. As mentioned before, tobacco stains on the fingers suggest an elevated PCO_2. A "self-reproducing cough" indicates that the patient may not be telling you the truth about smoking habits or has some other underlying pulmonary disease. This test is easy to do. The patient is asked to cough hard. If that starts an uncontrollable paroxysm of coughing that the patient cannot stop, it suggests that there is more chronic bronchopulmonary disease than one might otherwise have expected. The extent of exercise tolerance is an excellent guide to cardiopulmonary function.

New Drugs

Do not start new medications just before operation if you can possibly avoid it. Remember that the anesthesiologist is about to produce coma by a huge dose of neuropharmacologic agents. The verbal concept of "sleep" in describing the events under deep anesthesia has been a bit of the wishful thinking mythology since 1846. As to deep anesthesia:

"It ain't sleep,
It's drug-doped coma, and it's really deep."

Don't complicate anesthetic management with new drugs started just before operation or with unusually high doses of drugs.

Beware of insulin and digitalis. If either of these potent substances is required, it is far safer for the patient to spend a day or two with gradual induction of a satisfactory level of insulin or digitalis with necessary cross-checks of function and chemistry and with stabilization before the operation, if the rest of the disease process will give you that time of grace. Rapid digitalization within 72 hours of the operation is a significant hazard in surgical patients. Rapid changes in insulin dosage can be extremely hazardous. Do not ever give insulin intravenously or as a bolus. If the infusion stops for any reason, the patient will have a very severe insulin reaction. Give insulin subcutaneously by the usual indices.

With digitalis, beware of the phenomenon of "toxicity on constant dose." This is most commonly seen in the patient in the early postoperative period who is becoming alkalotic or developing a low plasma potassium concentration, or both. Under these circumstances, severe digitalis toxicity, even including paroxysmal auricular tachycardia with block, can occur as a potentially lethal arrhythmia with no change in the dose.

ENROUTE TO THE OPERATING ROOM

*"Never operate on a patient who is getting
rapidly worse or rapidly better."*

This ancient aphorism is still true, particularly in cases of sepsis or pathologic intra-abdominal conditions. If the patient's status is changing rapidly, stop and find out why.

If the patient is suspected of having a subphrenic abscess but on the morning of operation suddenly seems much better with a lower temperature, white blood cell count, and easier breathing, then stop, look, and listen before resecting the rib.

If the patient is thought to have sepsis and just before the operation seems unaccountably and unexpectedly much worse, wait a bit, even if only for an hour, and obtain more data or roentgenograms in order to try to explain the sudden deterioration. Otherwise, you may be operating in the belly of a patient with an acute pneumothorax.

*"If you want a disaster of severe gravity,
Just try the wrong side or the wrong body cavity."*

Don't hesitate to do special contrast studies just before operation. Be prepared to do them during the operation if they might be of assistance.

However, in patients in the "rapidly worse" category, do not forget that if the patient is bleeding, immediate operation may be essential.

Gastric tubes are best inserted the morning of operation, prior to anesthesia, so the patient can swallow and avoid injury to the nasopharynx. Use plenty of lubricant and use a local anesthetic if the patient is especially frightened.

Examine the rectum digitally the morning of operation. It is an embarrassment to find the rectum full of unexcreted solids if it should have to be emptied.

A urinary catheter is best placed in the operating room when the patient is under anesthesia, using special sterile preparation and ideal lighting. In this way, it is possible to avoid the otherwise probable bladder infection.

AT THE OPERATING ROOM

Does the patient expect to see you in person before anesthesia is induced? The phenomenon of the hidden and mysterious surgeon is discussed later, but this is the place to ask yourself if it might not be wise to see the patient and chat a minute or two before the drugs are infused.

THE PATIENT AND THE FAMILY

SEEING THE PATIENT ALONE; SITTING AND TALKING

Do not make platoon rounds an unvaried habit. Do not always see the patient with a large group. If it is your custom to migrate through the hospital with a number of residents and students, with or without nurses, social workers, and secretaries, then be sure that on two or three occasions each week at least and surely once immediately prior to the operation, shake yourself loose from the rest of the group and sit down quietly with the patient for a personal talk, with the curtains pulled or the door closed. Only in this way can the patient express the real concerns about diagnosis, prognosis, business details, procedures, the family, fears and apprehensions, finances, and problems relevant to the doctor.

If you do not believe in this doctrine, try becoming a patient yourself. Try lying flat on your back and addressing a group of beings, all clad in white and standing around the bed. The situation chokes off open conversation, to say the least.

UNDERSTANDING AND CONSENT

The standard "consent form" is long on painful details but short on common sense. It is a relatively easy matter to tell a patient what to expect, what should be done, and what complications might arise. It is not easy to be certain that the patient will remember all you say or will understand the limitations of the operation itself, its potential sources of incompleteness, unfinished business, or mandates for further therapy. Especially for those many operations that require postoperative discipline on the part of the patient (stopping drinking, stopping overeating, stopping smoking, or not participating in sports for a few months), additional words are needed. Will the patient need prolonged treatment with steroids, chemotherapy, or insulin? Give the patient some warning of future expectations and limitations.

And then, always the pressing issue, what will it really be like? The consent form says nothing about how the patient will be anesthetized, how it will feel, who will be there, where the patient will awaken; will there be oxygen tubes, respiratory assistance, cardiac monitors, special nurses, intensive care? Tell the patient what to expect, and be sure the patient will see familiar faces on arousal from coma.

Be sensitive to the difference between the neophyte patient — taking the voyage for the first time — as contrasted with the "old pro." Some patients have been through so much so often that they know more about it than you do. A detailed account is only a source of humor. But others are wholly new to the hospital environment, frightened by it, by the doctors, nurses, and above all frightened by the prospect of the disease. It is almost impossible to be too detailed or too attentive in soliciting and answering questions from such a patient.

THE FAMILY

When the surgeon sits down to talk things over with the patient prior to operation, it is helpful if a spouse, parent, or child can be there. However, beware of unexpected family tensions. Sometimes the patient wants to be alone, or the family member on hand is the wrong one. Maybe the patient does not want any family members to share the knowledge or share his or her "secret." It can be the wrong sibling or child who has intruded into the situation to get the "lowdown" and tell all the relatives. Ask the patient which member of the family is really the closest and the one who should be there to share the details of planning.

If several others members of your staff, assistants, consultants, or residents are going to be importantly involved in the operation itself or in postoperative management, this is the time to tell the patient about the team approach, the single standard of care, and the fact that no matter who does what, the surgeon will be clearly in charge, knowledgeable, concerned, available, responsible, and accountable.

Don't hide behind an impenetrable wall of silence. Some surgeons disappear after an operation, and it is almost impossible to find them. No one will give out their phone number. It is my belief that this is unnecessary and only creates suspicion and distrust. There may be some cities where surgeons' numbers cannot be listed, but I think the "hiding place" approach is overdone. Silence after operation can interfere with the "chemistry of confidence." It is also extremely frustrating to other physicians, surgeons, or friends who are trying to find and talk to the person in charge.

If you are going to have to be away for a day or two after the operation, it is essential to tell the patient before you leave. Make it clear who will be in charge, where this person can be reached, and when you will return.

THE OTHER PHYSICIANS INVOLVED

DON'T WORK ALONE

Some surgeons make a lifetime habit of shielding their patients from the possibility of another opinion. This habit decreases the surgeon's stature in the eyes of the patient. More respect is granted to those surgeons who seek and welcome help and who discuss problems. Seek consultation even if it is not sure to help; *never be a lone wolf.*

Explain all this to the patient, including the role of the consultant, the pathologist, the radiologist, the internist, and the anesthetist, especially if the patient is going to see and talk with them, learn of their work, and if they will receive separate recognition, either in the case summary or in terms of a fiscal obligation.

THE DOCTOR BACK HOME

In most cases the clear relationship of the referring physician leaves little doubt as to who should be notified about the operation and the findings. But there are situations where embarrassment may result unless the patient is asked. The patient may actually have lost confidence in the home physician and may have sought other help intentionally; he or she may not wish to return to the original referring physician, who may have been postponing operation needlessly for many weeks or months. Ask the patient which physician at home is closest to the case.

Take a nurse into the patient's confidence, especially if malignancy is a possibility, if there must be a colostomy performed, or if some other aspect of the operation itself could arouse apprehension. Have the head nurse, charge nurse, or special nurse with you for at least a part of that conversation with the door closed. A competent nurse will be flattered and pleased to be involved, and it will help her or him interpret your findings to the patient.

INTERPRETING THE FINDINGS TO THE PATIENT

When the findings at operation are open to several possible interpretations, the surgical team should discuss among themselves and with the nurse and the anesthesiologist which interpretation is to be offered to the patient. This is not a conspiracy to withhold information but rather is a plan to avoid an early postoperative difference in wording that can only disturb the patient. *"What to do when doctors disagree"* is never a worse problem than in the hours when the patient first awakens from anesthesia. If there is an opportunity to discuss differences of opinion or interpretation, it is better to do it a day or two later.

THE SURGEON

Every patient is unique. Each anatomic problem is slightly different. Where should the incision be? What will the dissection involve? What roentgenograms should be taken during the operation, what special tests done, what pathology specimen examined? Our opening aphorism summarizes these aspects of self-preparation.

For the surgeon performing a large load of routine operations, four or five in a morning, such considerations might seem remarkable and unnecessary. And yet, at least one of those patients will present an unusual and unexpected problem or finding. Careful thought and conversation with the operative team before the operation will help to avoid surprises.

Should You Be the Surgeon?

Are you sure you are the right person for the job? This is sometimes a tough question for the surgeon and is probably not asked often enough. It is well to think of your practice experience as occupying a normal distribution curve with a peak or hump in the middle, including the diseases, pathologic processes, and anatomic situations most familiar to you. It is important to be self-conscious and acutely aware of when you might be approaching one or the other end of the normal distribution curve, faced with anatomic or pathologic findings unfamiliar to you. Intraoperative consultation is an important safeguard here. If the patient is told of this possibility first, it increases the confidence of the patient and eases the mind of the surgeon, rather than being interpreted as a sign of weakness or incompetence.

In Training and Fit

Surgery is an athletic event: "The surgeon is the captain of the health care team." His or her personal health, strength, and fitness play a more important role in the outcome than is true for most other fields of medicine.

What are the other conflicts of interest of a surgeon? None is more pressing than the conflict of all the demands on his time: "When I am carrying out a big, unusual, or difficult operation, I never plan anything later that day." In this way, a cardiovascular surgeon, regularly faced with long and difficult procedures, explained how he organized his week. He never wanted to be rushed or pressed to get out of the operating room by the demands of meetings, committees, appointments, travel, or office patients. With this leisure he could stay and be sure that hemostasis was perfect and homeostasis ideal. Wound closure and postoperative orders could be checked without hurry, and few of his patients needed to be rushed back to the operating room to have problems repaired or bleeders retied.

THE CHEMISTRY OF CONFIDENCE

In this book on preoperative and postoperative care, dealing with some of the most complicated chemistry and pathophysiology known to the life sciences, it might seem out of place to discuss these small, personal, and even emotional interactions. But it is the conviction of the author of this chapter that it is quite appropriate to do so.

Everything that we know about the endocrinology of stress and trauma emphasizes the importance of the neurotransmitters in the "set" of the patient's mind and endocrine system, the brain, and possibly his or her soul. Worry, nervousness, apprehension, uncertainty, despair, and lack of confidence all are stimuli to these neurotransmitters first described 100 years ago.

Whatever their chemistry or whatever their activation, when the patient can rest as serenely as preoperative circumstances permit, then these chemical mediators of stress, trouble, and difficulty will be at their minimum. The chemistry of confidence is the physiology of equanimity.

The preparation of the patient for operation is summarized with a final aphorism:

> *"For the body, homeostasis.*
> *For the mind, equanimity."*

2

The Metabolic Response to Injury

J. M. KINNEY
F. E. GUMP

Nearly two centuries ago, John Hunter described the reactions to injury as inducing "both the disposition and the means of cure." This idea that injury sets in motion a train of biochemical and physiologic responses that are not only the direct result of the injury but also the integrated mechanisms by which the body could cope favorably with the injury was a thought with far-reaching significance. The response to injury was originally thought of in terms of the local tissue response to physical injury — namely, local changes in vasoconstriction, coagulation, and vascular permeability. Later, cellular elements were attracted to the scene of the injury in order to provide host defense against bacteria, to assist in the breakdown and removal of necrotic tissue, and to initiate the successive biochemical changes of wound healing. However, it was not until Sir David Cuthbertson conducted his pioneering studies on the response of patients after long bone fracture that the response of the entire organism to local injury began to assume importance. Since that time, the outstanding contributions of Moore, Moyer, Randall, Shires, and many others have led the way in delineating the systemic changes in the metabolism of noninjured tissue following a major local injury.

Cuthbertson recognized that the early response to injury had different metabolic priorities than the later phases of convalescence; therefore, he divided the metabolic response to injury into an early "ebb," or shock phase, and a subsequent "flow" phase. The flow phase may be considered as the events following resuscitation and are usually initiated from 24 to 48 hours after the injury. The flow phase may be conveniently divided into the catabolic, or tissue breakdown, portion, and the anabolic, or tissue restoration, portion. The separation of events into the ebb and flow phases is useful in considering the local events at the site of the injury as well as the metabolic response of the whole body, although this chapter will be limited to the metabolic events involving the whole body.

The history of surgical metabolism has undergone an interesting transition from primary attention to fluid and electrolyte metabolism, first represented by the plasma volume, and then to the whole body, followed by an increasing interest in organic metabolism of the body and the interaction of the metabolism of foodstuffs with the special functions of tissues and organs. The development of total parenteral nutrition by Wretlind, Shuberth, and coworkers in Sweden and the dramatic demonstrations of hyperalimentation with glucose and amino acids by Dudrick, Wilmore, and coworkers have provided a giant stimulus to surgical metabolism, quite in addition to introducing a major improvement in patient care. Now, an understanding of the metabolic pathways of foodstuffs has moved from the area of academic interest to a matter of practical clinical importance.

The metabolic response to injury has often been considered as synonymous with the response to infection. The scope of this chapter does not permit a discussion of the metabolic aspects of infection per se; however, the authors will refer to selected areas in which there appears to be a unique metabolic influence exerted by infection, which differs from that of injury.

BODY COMPOSITION

Normal metabolism and the metabolic response to an abnormal situation, such as injury, must be based upon a knowledge of body composition in two ways: (1) in terms of organs and tissue and (2) in terms of chemical phases (Fig. 2–1). Only 12 to 15 per cent of body weight of an average adult male is made up of the vital organs and blood volume — the portion that occupies so much attention in the emergency ward and intensive care unit after major injury. Yet, if resuscitation is successful, the patient enters a phase of altered metabolism, in which the availability and appropriate responses of muscle (40 per cent of body weight) and adipose tissue (average of 25 per cent of body weight) are of critical importance for survival.

If one considers the average daily intake of water, sodium, potassium, fat, carbohydrates and protein in terms of the body content of each material in the average 70 kg male, some interesting relationships become evident (Fig. 2–2). The calorie reserve in adipose tissue is tremendous and hence, the average daily intake of fat is only approximately 0.5 per cent of the normal body content of fat. Crude body protein appears from indirect evidence to be approximately 15 per cent of the adult male body weight, and this may be arbitrarily divided into three

Body Composition of Adult Male

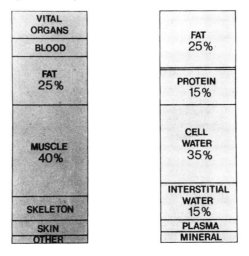

TISSUE ANATOMY   CHEMICAL ANATOMY

Figure 2–1. Average values for the body composition of a middle-aged, 70-kg male are presented in terms of tissue and organ anatomy and in terms of chemical phases.

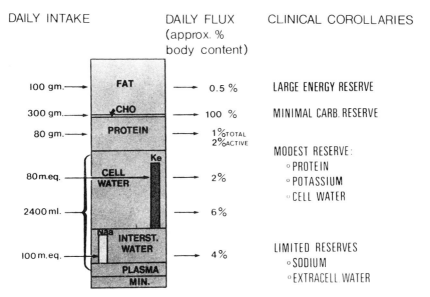

Figure 2–2. The average daily intakes of water, electrolytes, and foodstuffs are considered in terms of the normal body content of each material. See text for discussion.

parts: visceral and circulating protein (15 per cent), muscle protein (40 per cent), and connective tissue protein (45 per cent). The former includes proteins with the most rapid turnover rates and the latter those with very slow turnover rates. If one considers approximately 50 per cent of total crude body protein (visceral 10 per cent and muscle 40 per cent) as being active intracellular protein, then the daily intake would be approximately 2 per cent of this intracellular protein. This is similar to the situation with potassium, in which the average daily intake of 80 mEq represents 1.5 to 2.0 per cent of the total exchangeable potassium, which would average 3200 mEq per 70 kg. The intracellular constituents appear to have higher body content in relation to the normal daily intake than either sodium or water. The comparable considerations indicate that an average daily intake of 100 mEq of sodium is approximately 4 per cent of the total exchangeable sodium, while an average daily water intake is about 6 per cent of the average total body water. Therefore, a knowledge of body composition can help to explain why depletion of water and sodium from loss or decreased intake may have more serious early significance than depletion of nitrogen and potassium. However, carbohydrate is the one exception and plays a central role in the metabolic response to injury. Carbohydrate is of fundamental impor- tance as the substrate for tissues that depend upon carbohydrate for oxidation (such as the brain) or for glycolysis (such as blood cells). Note that an average daily intake of 300 gm of carbohydrate is approximately equal to the total body content of carbohydrate (extracellular glucose plus tissue glycogen). This, in contrast to other intracellular materials in which the daily intake is on the order of 0.5 to 2.0 per cent of the body content, the daily intake of carbohydrate is 100 per cent of the body stores. Therefore, it is not surprising that a central area of metabolic research over the past two decades has involved the mechanisms by which the body guarantees a continuing supply of glucose during starvation, when carbohydrate intake ceases, or after injury, when carbohydrate intake is reduced or absent together with an increased demand for glucose synthesis.

SHOCK OR EBB PHASE AFTER INJURY

WATER AND ELECTROLYTE METABOLISM

A direct qualitative relationship between plasma volume and the sodium content of the body was first discovered by Darrow and Yannet. Since then there has been ample confirmation of this relationship and great debate regarding its clinical implications. Exploration of this area is critical in any discussion of injury because reduction of plasma volume or loss of effective plasma volume constitutes a common denominator regardless of the nature of the injury. Plasma volume is inevitably threatened in the injured surgical patient, and maintenance of extracellular fluid volume continues to be the cornerstone of successful patient care.

Volume deficits encountered in the surgical patient may occur as a result of external losses or as a result of an internal redistribution of extracellular fluid into a compartment that is no longer in equilibrium with the circulating plasma volume. As a rule, both processes are involved, but internal redistribution of extracellular fluid in the injured patient has been more difficult to recognize. Sequestration of fluid into an area of injury represents an obvious example, while the immobilization of salts and water by devascularized injured tissue or the shift of sodium and water into the intracellular compartment has been more difficult to document.

Moyer has pointed out that in humans the surface area of extracellular collagen fibrils amounts to more than a million square meters. This extracellular material lying between the exchange vessels and the cells may be altered by injury so that additional water molecules and sodium ions will be absorbed upon the macromolecules making up this ground substance. In this fashion, the number of extracellular solvent molecules and ions will be reduced just as surely as if they had been lost externally by hemorrhage, vomiting, or diarrhea.

A similar end result would be expected if impairment of the energy-dependent sodium pump allowed the inflow of sodium into cells. It has been suggested by Shires that this takes place in skeletal muscle and that such cells represent the major site of fluid and electrolyte accumulation following severe hemorrhagic hypotension. Even though some potassium leaves the cell under these circumstances, its exchange with sodium is unequal, resulting in a net flow of water into the muscle cell. In this way, one can relate the decrease in extracellular water and sodium to the cellular swelling that has been shown to exist in experimental shock.

The relative importance of changes in the binding characteristics of connective tissue in contrast to failure of the sodium-potassium pump has yet to be defined to injured humans. However, the evidence that plasma and extracellular volume is threatened above and beyond external losses is clear cut, and it introduces a number of metabolic changes. Since exchangeable or total body sodium determines plasma volume, any tendency to volume reduction will stimulate the mechanisms responsible for sodium conservation. There is a sudden and massive increase in the production of renin from the juxtaglomerular cells of the kidney. Angiotensin appears in the periphery, and aldosterone secretion is greatly increased. Although the ACTH-adrenocortical response is less marked, it also represents a constant feature of this response.

Antidiuretic hormone is secreted in increased amounts following injury and results in excretion of urine of high osmolarity owing to increased distal tubular water reabsorption. In addition, there is a rapid response of the sympathetic nervous system mediated through the baroreceptor reflex. The resultant catecholamine release not only results in the classic hemodynamic responses but also influences nitrogen breakdown, gluconeogenesis, and fat oxidation.

Restitution of a decreased plasma volume starts promptly by means of transcapillary refill with the vigorous retention of sodium. In fact, the dramatic decrease in sodium excretion led early investigators to avoid the administration of solutions containing sodium in the early stages following injury. It was only after subsequent studies revealed a decrease in functional extracellular fluid that more vigorous infusion of sodium and water became commonplace. When the extracellular volume deficit associated with injury is corrected by administration of balanced saline solutions, sodium excretion again approaches normal. Extracellular fluid functions both to support plasma volume and to provide a proper aqueous environment for the cells. Injury appears to reduce the amount of extracellular fluid that is rapidly exchangeable and capable of fulfilling these two functions. Proper resuscitation restores this apparent loss, but this can only be achieved with an increase in total body water and sodium. The clinician observes this as a gain in body weight. Although a large gain in fluid may suggest overly vigorous intravenous fluid administration, some gain is actually the hallmark of proper resuscitation following injury. Monitoring of body weight changes is important in establishing the amount of additional fluid in the body and, even more important, how soon it is eventually excreted.

After volume restoration has been achieved, there is almost instantaneous cessation of the catecholamine and renin responses. The other neuroendocrine mechanisms brought into play to protect and restore plasma volume also abate, but the time needed for restoration of normal body composition may be quite variable. In a series of 12 consecutive severely injured patients who were resuscitated according to standard hemodynamic guidelines, some degree of weight gain was noted in every instance. This varied from 1.6 kg to as much as 4.9 kg. In eight of the patients, excretion of the additional fluid was complete within the first week, but a more variable course was evident in the remaining patients. The delay in excretion of the fluid load used in resuscitation may be due to a number of factors. At times fluid sequestration in an area of injury may persist beyond the first week, especially if the injury resulted in extensive tissue destruction. In some patients, the peritoneal cavity may be responsible, especially if there is persistent inflammation or bowel and mesenteric edema. The presence of infection with changes in capillary function and venous tone may result in expansion of the vascular bed and persistence of the hypovolemic response.

It has been suggested that nearly all the fluid and electrolyte changes seen in the successive phases after injury are in fact a response to the initial volume reduction. This would imply that volume reduction is fundamental to the endocrine and metabolic sequence that follows injury.

ORGANIC METABOLISM — ENERGY UTILIZATION

The metabolic response that follows injury-induced hypovolemia has obvious effects on the body's energy substrates. In this section, attention will be directed to the early changes following injury. Studies of alterations in plasma concentration of glucose and insulin secondary to injury have variously suggested both an increase and a reduction in insulin secretion, largely because the subjects were studied at different stages following injury. Glucose levels, on the other hand, have been consistently increased. Recent studies by Meguid and his associates and Giddings and his group have again documented the prompt rise in blood sugar levels following either accidental trauma or elective operation. In general, the rise in blood sugar parallels the severity of the injury and is associated with a sympathoadrenal discharge. Hyperglycemia occurs following injection of epinephrine in response to a complex series of events. First, there is a direct effect on the liver, resulting in glycolysis and simultaneously directing conversion of alanine, pyruvate, glycerol, and lactate into glucose (gluconeogenesis). Epinephrine also acts directly on skeletal muscle glycogen to produce lactic acid, which can then be converted into glucose in the liver (the Cori cycle). Finally, epinephrine has a direct effect on the pancreas that results in suppression of insulin release but stimulates the output of glucagon.

The role of insulin in this series of events has been somewhat controversial, probably because of species differences. However, in humans, a concentration of insulin inappropriately low for the corresponding level of blood sugar appears to be the usual early response to trauma. In a study by Meguid of 14 injured patients, the initial serum insulin levels were in the basal fasting range despite the fact that plasma glucose levels were greatly elevated. Plasma glucagon values were initially in the normal range in this group of patients although they began to rise within 12 hours after admission. The insulin-glucose (I:G) ratio thus remains normal and fails to indicate the severity of the catabolic state in these patients. Later in the course of the injury when glucagon levels are increased, insulin may also have risen, thus limiting any decrease in the I:G ratio. The popularity of the I:G ratio as a means for explaining a wide variety of metabolic events has decreased in recent years. However, the relative levels of the two hormones still appear to be intimately related to the handling of foodstuffs in the successive phases of injury. In diabetics the maximum catabolic effect of high glucagon levels appears when insulin is low or absent. Both insulin and glucagon levels have been more variable in surgical patients, but a similar situation may exist. Thus, the I:G ratio must be considered in relationship to the absolute level of circulating insulin.

Catecholamines have a pronounced effect on adipose tissue in that they rapidly mobilize fatty acids. The increase in free fatty acids has been repeatedly observed as one of the earliest responses to injury. While catecholamine release probably represents the major stimulus, glucagon may also increase during the ebb phase and contribute to the sustained free fatty acid rise. The low levels of insulin previously mentioned also play a role in potentiating the effect of catechols on adipose tissue. Thus, the bloodstream of the injured patient is rapidly flooded with the two major energy substrates: glucose and free fatty acids at a time when decreased tissue perfusion may be associated with impaired oxidation and heat production.

Amino acid changes in the early or ebb phase of the injury have not been as well defined as the responses involving glucose and fat. Insulin plays an important role not only in the incorporation of fatty acids into adipose tissue but also in uptake of amino acid for protein synthesis. Glucocorticoids are in opposition to insulin because they facilitate the mobilization of amino acids from muscle.

THE CELL IN SHOCK

The metabolic changes that have been described for the whole body and various organ systems can also be considered in terms of altered cell function. Abnormalities of metabolism of cells and subcellular organelles have usually been studied in experimental animals, but increasing application of these techniques to humans is under way. Since such studies are still in their infancy, most of our knowledge in this field is derived from basic science techniques carried out in vitro or in animals. These studies indicate that the initial effect of injury, provided it is severe enough to decrease perfusion, is to impair normal function of the cell membrane. Early workers described the results of this change when they noted cellular swelling. More recently it has been possible to quantify this abnormality by measuring the potential difference across the cell membrane. Shires and his group measured the transmembrane potential of a muscle cell and noted a change from -87 mv to values of -60 mv. This change in potential difference is consistent with the movement of sodium and water into the cell as has been previously postulated. However, the magnitude of water movement into the cells is probably not large, and Baue has estimated that such a change in membrane potential would involve less than 10 per cent of the extracellular fluid (ECF) volume. This would be far less than the changes in functioning ECF noted by Shires. Our own studies done in humans by means of a needle biopsy technique of muscle show a consistent increase in sodium while potassium falls only in severely catabolic patients. Most of the increased water in the muscle was extracellular.

Changes in membrane potential also have other effects that are probably of greater importance in the altered metabolism associated with injury. When the cell membrane allows increased amounts of sodium into the cell, the high-energy phosphate compound adenosine triphosphate (ATP) is used in increasing amounts in an effort to correct the situation. Eventually ATP levels in the cell fall, and this in turn leads to impairment of other intracellular functions. For instance, Chaudry and his associates have shown that skeletal muscle becomes resistant to the expected effect of insulin in promoting glucose uptake by muscle cells.

FLOW PHASE — CATABOLISM

Many forms of injury are followed by a convalescence that includes some degree of starvation; therefore, the metabolic response to starvation must be differentiated from the metabolic response to injury. In total starvation there is an early phase, lasting approximately three to five days, which is characterized by glycogenolysis, and a later phase of ketonemia, which achieves prominence during the second and third weeks of starvation and is fully evident by the fourth to sixth weeks. The early phase includes prompt diuresis, rapid weight loss, increased protein breakdown, and alanine release from muscle with a corresponding increase in hepatic uptake of alanine and gluconeogenesis. The latter, or ketonemic, phase of starvation is characterized by a decrease in both the resting energy expenditure and nitrogen excretion. These changes are associated with a decrease in protein breakdown and release of alanine from muscle, causing a decreased alanine uptake in the liver and gluconeogenesis reaching low levels in the liver while increasing in the kidney. The requirements for gluconeogenesis are reduced, as ketone utilization supplies up to 50 per cent of the fuel required by the brain.

There is general agreement that after an initial period of water retention the rate of weight loss parallels the extent of starvation or the severity of the injury. Various observers have reported that the rate and extent of nitrogen loss roughly parallel the rate of loss of body weight. Weight loss in the early postoperative period is often in the range of 300 to 400 gm per day after an initial tendency to water retention. More severe injury may have sustained losses of 400 to 800 gm per day. Sustained weight loss over two weeks or more can be assumed to be composed of protein, fat, and water. Recent studies of cumulative calorie and nitrogen balance in patients with major injury and infection have shown that the protein contribution to the weight loss over two to three weeks amounted to 10 to 14 per cent, while fat contributed 18 to 25 per cent of the weight loss. Analysis of data from studies of both total and partial starvation suggests that body protein represents a surprisingly reproducible portion of sustained weight loss regardless of the proportion of starvation or injury that caused the weight loss.

Successful resuscitation from the ebb phase is followed by the catabolism of the flow phase. At this time, the resting energy expenditure (REE) moves from low or low-normal values to varying elevations above normal, depending upon the type of injury and the sex, age, and body size of the individual. Elective, uncomplicated operations will be followed by increases that are usually less than 10 per cent above the preoperative values and last for only five to seven days. Multiple fractures usually show increases of 10 to 25 per cent above normal and remain elevated for 10 to 14 days. Major infections, such as peritonitis, may show elevations of 15 to 50 per cent as long as inflammation is present. Major third-degree burns usually have elevations of the REE of 40 to 100 per cent above normal, which remain elevated until the burn wound has been excised and grafted. Increases in urinary nitrogen loss after injury usually bear a rough correlation with increases in the REE. The young adult male who is heavily muscled and nutritionally sound will usually show the most marked metabolic response to injury, particularly in regard to the increases in both REE and urinary nitrogen loss. The female, the elderly, and the poorly nourished will exhibit smaller and more transient responses to injury than the normal adult male population.

Organic material (mainly protein and fat) makes up approximately 40 per cent of the body weight of an average adult male. The following discussion of catabolic events involves a general knowledge of the pathways that interconnect protein (arbitrarily separated into muscle and liver protein), carbohydrate, and fat (Figs. 2–3 and 2–4).

PROTEIN METABOLISM

The best-known feature of the metabolic response to injury is the increase in nitrogen loss. This rise in urinary nitrogen is associated with an increased excretion of sulfur, phosphorus, potassium, magnesium, and creatine. The cumulative nitrogen loss after an average elective operation usually reaches about 30 to 60 gm, while the massive catabolic response of major burns or multiple abscesses may reach losses of 250 to 300 gm. The sources of nitrogen and other intracellular constituents that are lost following injury have never been completely defined. However, the nitrogen-to-sulfur and nitrogen-to-potassium ratios of the urinary losses suggest that the nitrogen loss is mainly from muscle.

Moore and coworkers perfected a multiple isotope dilution technique for studying the changes in body composition of surgical patients. These changes emphasized that the catabolic process involves shrinkage of the body cell mass with an absolute or relative expansion of extracellular or supporting volume and its constituents.

The increase in nitrogen loss following injury has prompted various investigators to employ isotopic methods for the indirect measurement of protein synthesis and breakdown in the whole body. Studies in patients after both abdominal and orthopaedic procedures have indicated a decrease in the rate of protein synthesis with no change in the rate

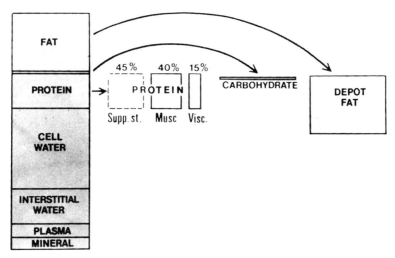

Figure 2-3. Crude body protein of a 70-kg male has been arbitrarily divided into visceral and circulating protein (15 per cent), muscle (40 per cent), and connective tissue (45 per cent). The relative amounts of these materials are compared with body stores of carbohydrate and fat.

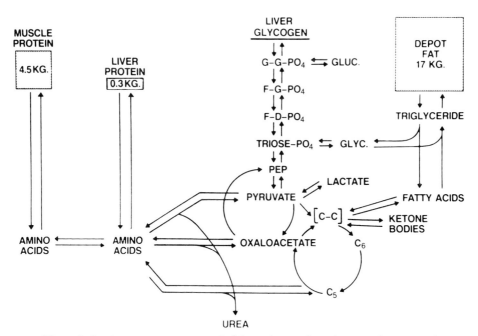

Figure 2-4. A summary is presented of the pathways that relate muscle, protein, liver protein, glycogen, and body fat. Note that extra carbohydrate intermediates can be readily converted to fatty acids, while an excess of fatty acids cannot yield an excess of carbohydrate intermediates.

of protein breakdown. This is in contrast to major surgical sepsis, in which there may be an increase in the rate of protein synthesis and an even greater increase in breakdown, hence a negative nitrogen balance.

A postinjury fall in albumin concentration and a rise in certain globulin fractions have been reported by many workers. It now appears that the albumin concentration decreases to reach a minimum by the third to the sixth day after injury and gradually returns to normal over many days to weeks. Fibrinogen levels rise to twice normal after skeletal injury and burns. The immunoglobulins IgG, IgA, and IgM seem not to change significantly after injury, unless there is a source of infection, as in burns, in which the increases can be considerable. An increased rate of catabolism of both albumin and IgG has been reported in burned patients, which appears to be proportional to the magnitude of increase in the resting energy expenditure.

Plasma amino acid nitrogen is reported to fall during the first 24 hours after operation if the patient has been in good preoperative health and nutrition. The plasma amino acid nitrogen is usually low in ill or malnourished patients, and operation causes no overt change. More recent studies have shown that most plasma amino acids decrease promptly after operation, and the nonessential amino acids continue to fall for several days while the essential amino acids have returned to normal or above normal levels. The branched chain amino acids are uniquely related to muscle metabolism and are not taken up by the liver. They have been reported to rise significantly in the plasma following bony and soft tissue injury. The changes in concentration of plasma amino acids are difficult to interpret without knowledge of the corresponding tissue levels, since a rise in plasma levels may indicate an increase in tissue release into plasma or a decrease in uptake of tissue, especially muscle.

About 80 per cent of free amino acids in the total body are found in skeletal muscle. A technique of percutaneous needle biopsy of skeletal muscle has been used by Bergstrom, Furst, and Vinnars to study postoperative patients. When receiving a form of total parenteral nutrition, no significant changes were seen in the plasma amino acid levels. However, the muscle amino acids revealed decreased nonessential amino acids with unchanged essential amino acids on the third postoperative day. These workers have also reported that in more severe surgical catabolism, the size of the essential free amino acid pool was reduced both in the plasma and the muscle. The total nonessential amino acids were further decreased in plasma but remained the same in muscle as in the postoperative patients. In plasma, all the essential amino acids were markedly decreased except for phenylalanine, which was increased. In muscle, phenylalanine was increased and lysine decreased. Percutaneous needle biopsy may offer an important means of separating the influence of trauma from that of starvation and of guiding the nutritional therapy of future patients in a more specific and rational manner.

CARBOHYDRATE METABOLISM

The increase in protein catabolism following injury was generally thought to be the result of increased fuel demands until it became evident that the energy contribution of the increased protein breakdown was relatively small compared with the caloric contribution of fatty acids mobilized from adipose tissue. Isotopic and regional studies have emphasized that the amino acid release from muscle protein breakdown is serving two important functions that are not directly involved in oxidation to yield energy. Amino acids from muscle can be deaminated and provide an important source of carbon for gluconeogenesis. Other amino acids from muscle can be taken up in viscera such as the liver and used for the synthesis of new protein. Both of these processes are represented in Figure 2–5 and are catabolic in terms of muscle protein but may be anabolic in terms of the liver. It is of particular interest that the acute-phase proteins, such as fibrinogen and complement whose manufacture in the liver is accelerated with injury or infection, are all glycoproteins. Thus gluconeogenesis in the liver may serve important synthetic functions beyond simply guaranteeing an adequate supply of circulating glucose.

Injury and infection are commonly associated with some degree of hyperglycemia and an abnormal glucose tolerance test. This has led to the concept of a "diabetes of injury," suggesting a relative or absolute

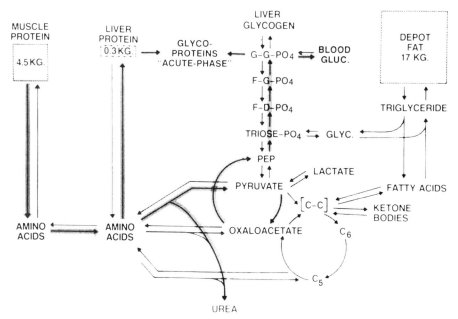

Figure 2–5. A major feature of catabolism is the breakdown of muscle protein to provide amino acids that can be deaminated for gluconeogenesis or taken up directly by viscera such as liver for synthesis of new protein.

lack of insulin and thus a decrease in the oxidation of glucose. This was shown not to be the case when isotopic studies demonstrated an increase in both the oxidation and turnover of glucose in injured and septic patients. An increased glucose output from the liver, despite a level of hyperglycemia that usually inhibited or abolished hepatic gluconeogenesis, was later shown in such patients. When the blood sugar is elevated during burn shock, the rate of passage through the expanded body glucose space is only slightly increased above normal. However, as the patient is resuscitated effectively and moves from the "ebb" to the "flow" phase, the glucose flow is increased as a result of increased hepatic production, apparently with no decrease in peripheral disappearance. The extent of the increase in the rate of glucose turnover appears to be related to the extent of the injury, but glucose turnover returns to normal with closure of the burn wound. As convalescence progresses, usually with some loss of body weight and tissue depletion, glucose dynamics approach those of the starved or semistarved man in association with the blood glucose level, which decreases to normal or low-normal ranges.

Allison has summarized glucose metabolism after injury as an acute stage where there is a catecholamine-mediated suppression of the insulin secretion associated with glucose intolerance and high plasma fatty acid levels. Subsequently there is a period of continuing glucose intolerance with high insulin levels, suggesting insulin resistance. These changes are related to the severity but not the type of injury or illness sustained. Allison and coworkers showed that in burned patients receiving a high protein, high calorie oral intake, the infusion of insulin and glucose could reduce the urea production and thus significantly reduce the breakdown of body protein. This group has since completed studies that suggest that any superiority of glucose over sorbitol-Intralipid for protein sparing is most evident in the severely catabolic patient and that exogenous insulin produces effects beyond those seen for glucose alone.

Wilmore and coworkers have noted that in burn patients the resting energy expenditure and glucose flow appear to change together with time following injury; however, this relationship was not the result of carbohydrate being the predominant fuel. Their patients commonly had respiratory quotients below 0.8, suggesting that fat was being oxidized as the primary tissue fuel. Thus, these workers have suggested that it may be the glucose flow from six to three carbons and back again, with the associated heat production, that plays an important role in convalescence.

Gram-negative sepsis in humans or endotoxin administration in animals inhibits hepatic gluconeogenesis, depletes glycogen stores, and may cause a falling blood sugar concentration, according to Wilmore. The patient with an extensive injury may have his or her accelerated glucose flow and hepatic glucose production reduced toward normal during a period of gram-negative bacteremia. Gluconeogenesis precursors increase in the blood, and alanine administration fails to cause a rise in serum glucose in injured patients with gram-negative bacteremia. Thus, the primary effect appears to be an endotoxin-mediated decrease in hepatic utilization of precursors for gluconeogenesis, and the response may linger after the bloodstream infection has been cleared.

FAT METABOLISM

Endogenous fatty acids are the primary source of energy for surgical patients not receiving large amounts of carbohydrate by enteric or intravenous routes. There is no conclusive evidence that the injured patient cannot oxidize fatty acids readily. However, the ready mobilization and oxidation of fatty acids should not obscure the fact that fatty acids cannot yield a net gain of glucose, glycogen, or carbohydrate intermediates for the synthesis of nonessential amino acids. Fat macroglobules formed by aggregation of lipid particles have been demonstrated in the blood after both injury and elective operation and are considered by some to be part of the general metabolic changes after injury. Serum triglycerides have been reported to increase in the early days after major fracture. However, Carlson has emphasized that there is usually a large early rise in the plasma free fatty acids of a burn patient that is proportional to the size of the burn and that occurs without comparable change in triglycerides. After being infused with an intravenous lipid emulsion, burn patients show only a slight increase in the plasma triglycerides, and the free fatty acid levels are decreased. The clearance from plasma of the lipid emulsion is accelerated in the presence of the burn injury and has been linked to the presence of increases in the resting energy expenditure.

Carlson and coworkers studied the possibility of "excessive" mobilization of free fatty acids in the injured animal or human. They infused norepinephrine for 24 hours into dogs so that free fatty acids were four to five times the normal level. This resulted in the appearance of fat droplets in the myocardium, skeletal muscle, kidney, lungs, and liver. The animals showed fever, tachypnea, increased oxygen consumption, and evidence of intravascular coagulation.

FLOW PHASE — ANABOLISM

The process of anabolism is often observed by surgeons as a matter of wound healing. Wound healing to full maturation is a long process that appears to continue for months after the wound occurs. However, the healing of the wound to a tensile strength that is satisfactory for patient ambulation, removal of sutures, and discharge to home will occur in normal fashion despite the fact that the nitrogen balance of the whole body might still be negative or just recently have become positive. A positive nitrogen balance is an important part of convalescence to restore muscle strength and function, not to allow a wound to heal. There is much interest in the question of whether high levels of nutritional intake, as in TPN, have any influence on the healing process in the previously normal and well-nourished patient. Thus far, the indications are that TPN is most important for the support of the convalescence that is threatened by *continued* tissue depletion after the initial loss of 4 to 8 per cent of body weight, which often occurs following routine elective operation.

Moore has pointed out that catabolic weight loss, with its excretion of nitrogen, potassium, and other intracellular materials, is largely a matter of cellular atrophy rather than cell death, except at the local site of an injury. With the onset of anabolism, there is an initial short-term weight gain that appears to be secondary to a rapid uptake of cell water, potassium, and nitrogen but at a high potassium:nitrogen ratio. This brief interval of early anabolism is probably associated with the restoration of tissue glycogen, followed by a slower weight gain in which the components of tissue gain (water, potassium, and nitrogen) approach that of normal muscle.

The body has only limited means to deal with a caloric intake that is greater than the caloric expenditure, except to store the excess calories as body fat. This is in contrast to an intake of nitrogen in excess of the rate of nitrogen excretion, in which the fate of the excess nitrogen can be either incorporation into new body protein or amino acid breakdown and extra nitrogen excretion. Many factors, such as fever, residual inflammation, inactivity, low-quality amino acid pattern of nitrogen intake, and inadequate calories, will tend to reduce the net gain in new protein with any given nitrogen intake and increase the loss via urinary nitrogen.

Early studies of body composition in surgical patients were interpreted to show that lean tissue restoration preceded the restoration of body fat. This seems unlikely in view of the above considerations, in which many factors may tend to limit the rate of lean tissue restoration while the restoration of fat is primarily a function of how aggressively the patient and physician achieve a positive calorie balance by oral, enteric, or intravenous routes. Balance studies have indicated that when patients are started on total parenteral nutrition after a period of significant weight loss, a positive nitrogen balance may be achieved for two or three days despite continued weight loss due to water excretion. However, any sustained gain in body weight in excess of 200 gm per day should be viewed with concern, for it will often include abnormal water retention, particularly for the first few weeks of anabolism. It sometimes seems as though the seriously depleted patient must reach a certain level of repletion before he or she can achieve a satisfactory water balance without the assistance of diuretics. Serial body weights are important in evaluating a patient's anabolic process. True gain of normal tissue without fluid retention is a slow process and requires understanding and patience on the part of the patient, family, and hospital staff.

NEUROENDOCRINE ASPECTS OF CATABOLISM AND ANABOLISM

INSULIN — WHAT IS INSULIN RESISTANCE?

Any discussion of the neuroendocrine aspects of the metabolic response to injury seems inevitably to start with insulin. The recent development of immunoassay techniques has greatly improved our understanding of the regulatory effects of this key hormone. It has been repeatedly stated that insulin is the principal anabolic hormone, but "fuel storage" hormone may be a better way to express this capacity. This is because insulin plays a key role in converting all the major body substrates into their storage form. The important corollary to this statement is that insulin deficiency will result in mobilization of stored fuels.

Insulin accelerates the clearance of glucose from the bloodstream into cells. The rate of glucose removal can be quantified by an intravenous bolus injection of glucose or by abrupt cessation of a constant glucose infusion. Serial blood glucose determinations can then be obtained in order to quantify the disappearance of glucose from the extracellular fluid. The slope of the disappearance curve (K value) serves to quantify glucose uptake into cells. K is a constant in normals but is decreased in diabetes and shock and varies during the successive phases of injury.

Hyperglycemia, decreased insulin levels, and a decreased K value are characteristic of the early or ebb phase of injury. The work of Allison, Hinton, and Chamberlain shows clearly that not only is the insulin response blunted during burn shock but also that there is impaired translocation of glucose into peripheral tissues, suggesting insulin resistance.

Glucose dynamics change somewhat during the flow stage, and the question of insulin resistance becomes more complex. Superficially, the ebb and flow phases appear to be similar in that hyperglycemia is present throughout and fasting blood sugar levels are generally elevated, depending on the severity of the injury. Terms such as the "diabetes of injury" have been used to describe such patients, and failure to clear glucose from the circulation has been assumed to be due to inadequate or ineffective insulin. On the other hand, our own studies done during the flow or postresuscitation stage showed an *increase* in both oxidative and nonoxidative dispersal of infused glucose. Wilmore's studies in burned patients during the flow phase (6 to 16 days following injury) showed the rate of glucose disappearance to be enhanced. The K value in these patients was similar to that obtained in normal individuals in spite of persistent hyperglycemia. In summarizing these studies, Wilmore suggested that the increase in blood glucose observed in these burned patients might be related to increased hepatic production of glucose rather than altered peripheral disappearance.

If one can equate insulin resistance with an abnormal decrease in the K value, it is clear that the question of insulin resistance following injury is more complex than had formerly been assumed. Normal glucose tolerance requires the coordination of three related processes. First, there must be increased secretion of insulin from the pancreas; second, there must be net uptake (not release) of glucose by the liver; and finally, there should be increased uptake of glucose by the peripheral tissues. Insulin is obviously involved in all three of these steps. Measurement of splanchnic insulin secretion has demonstrated an increase in insulin output following an intravenous injection of glucose. These studies were done during the flow phase and are consistent with numerous studies demonstrating that circulating insulin levels have risen from their initial depressed values by this time. Even when insulin levels are related to the simultaneous and usually elevated blood sugar values, the insulin response is comparable with that of normal subjects. The peripheral uptake of glucose as judged by the K value has been discussed previously, and no clearcut evidence of insulin resistance has emerged. This leaves only the response of the liver, and here definite abnormalities have been demonstrated. Hepatic vein catheterization of injured patients has shown not only increased basal hepatic glucose production but also a failure of inhibition of hepatic glucose uptake following injection of exogenous glucose. Increased gluconeogenesis, only partly responsive to the usual control mechanisms, has also been documented by isotopic techniques. Splanchnic insulin secretion was measured in some of these patients, and since it was found to be greater than normal, it appears that the hepatocyte response to insulin has been altered. Insulin resistance has traditionally implied impaired clearance of glucose from the extravascular compartment in the presence of normal quantities of insulin. The striking abnormality underlying the glucose intolerance of injury is an increased glucose flow associated with increased hepatic glucose production. Even though the liver may be "resistant" to the expected actions of insulin in these patients, it would probably be better not to apply the term "insulin resistance." Many other hormones affect hepatic glucose balance, and some of these will be considered next.

GLUCAGON

Glucagon has potent glycolytic and gluconeogenic effects on the liver, and it is clear that these properties are opposite to those of insulin.

Unger has formalized this reciprocal relationship by proposing that the molar insulin:glucagon (I:G) ratio be utilized in a quantitative and qualitative sense to describe hepatic glucose balance. Anabolism (fuel storage and nitrogen retention) takes place when insulin is increased relative to glucagon (I:G >5). When the ratio of insulin to glucagon falls below 3 one expects to see increased glycogenolysis and gluconeogenesis as well as increased excretion of urea and failure of protein synthesis.

Studies in injured patients have shown glucagon levels to be elevated even when hyperglycemia is present, but insulin levels have been more variable. As a result, I:G ratios have not always reflected the catabolic status of the patient. Since glucagon is thought to exert its effects only on the liver, the critical I:G ratio might be in portal blood rather than peripheral blood. It now appears that glucagon, either by itself or in terms of its molar ratio with insulin, can no longer be considered a definitive indicator of catabolism. This point has been well illustrated in a recent study of intravenous feeding with fat as the calorie source. Even though the I:G ratio fell below 3 because insulin levels were low, the patients were in positive nitrogen balance. The fact that glucagon fails to provide an infallible indicator of the patient's nutritional status does not alter the fact that it exerts a powerful influence on hepatic glucose balance. In fact, the failure of the liver to take up exogenous glucose and to turn off gluconeogenesis, mentioned in the section on insulin, may well be mediated by glucagon rather than a reflection of decreased hepatic sensitivity to insulin.

CATECHOLAMINES

Because of their widespread effects and the promptness and magnitude of their rise, catecholamines have been considered to be the primary stimulus in the neuroendocrine response to injury. While the primacy of catecholamines among the various hormones associated with the early stages of injury appears to be well substantiated, it is not certain that they exercise such a dominant role in the later stages of post-traumatic catabolism. It appears that no single hormone dominates the picture at that stage but rather certain hormones, such as glucagon and cortisol, combine with catecholamines to exert a strong catabolic effect.

Hyperglycemia is characteristic of catecholamine release, and while this is mediated in part through glucagon, there is also a direct effect on the liver and skeletal muscle. The hepatic effect results in the conversion of glycogen into glucose, while in the muscle glycogen is converted to lactic acid, which in turn is converted to glucose by the liver. Catecholamines also have calorigenic effects, and it may be that they play some role in the hypermetabolism associated with severe injury. Although epinephrine infusion has been shown to produce hypermetabolism in normal humans, the effect of heightened adrenergic activity in the injured patient is less well defined. It should be noted that urinary catecholamine excretion increases markedly in starvation, and yet metabolic expenditure is actually decreased in these subjects. At this time the role that catecholamines play in increasing heat production following operation or injury requires further study.

Catecholamines also affect fat mobilization. Sympathetic stimulation has a direct effect on fat deposits but is also potentiated by suppression of insulin release from the pancreatic beta cell. It is clear that catecholamine release plays a role in all the metabolic responses that characterize the severely injured patient. Catecholamines stimulate the supraoptic nuclei, resulting in ACTH release, and this in turn increases the output of cortisol from the adrenal cortex. At the same time, catecholamines mediate the pancreatic secretion of insulin and glucagon and also have a direct effect on the mobilization of fat. As long as the injury remains unhealed, the stimulus to the production of catecholamines continues, and the metabolic features of post-traumatic catabolism will continue.

ADRENAL CORTEX

The importance ascribed to glucocorticoids in the metabolic response to injury has varied greatly from Ingle, who felt that they were merely permissive, to Selye, who considered them the dominant mediators of the catabolic response. Some of the effects of glucocorticoids are clearly catabolic in that they promote gluconeogenesis, facilitate amino acid mobilization from skeletal muscle, and augment lipolysis. However, under certain conditions, adipose tissue is deposited rather than mobilized. Glucocorticoids thus appear to lyse body protein while building up fat stores.

Evidence that glucocorticoids are merely permissive has also been present. For instance, adrenalectomized animals maintained on a constant dose of glucocorticoids respond to injury in the expected manner. Furthermore, administration of glucocorticoids does not increase nitrogen excretion in fasting subjects. Such studies have probably tended to underestimate the importance of these hormones in post-traumatic metabolism. While they are clearly overshadowed by catecholamines during the early phase of injury, they now appear to play an important role in the later stages. During this period, glucocorticoids act in concert with glucagon and catecholamines to amplify and augment the specific metabolic features that are seen after·injury.

GROWTH HORMONE

Growth hormone stimulates the synthesis of protein and is recognized as a potent anabolic hormone. Its role in the altered metabolism that follows injury has not been as well defined as the hormones mentioned previously but it is secreted in increased amounts in the injured patient. It may be related to increased insulin levels since insulin-induced hypoglycemia has been used to test the capacity of the pituitary to release growth hormone. However, the fact that the injured patients are hyperglycemic rather than hypoglycemic makes it difficult to assess the importance of this stimulus. Growth hormone is also secreted in response to amino acid infusion, but it is not clear if this plays a role in injury. It is of value to note, however, that the hormonal response to both insulin hypoglycemia and arginine infusion is decreased in injured humans. Since growth hormone is anabolic, any decrease in its elaboration might add to the tissue breakdown associated with trauma.

Much of interest in growth hormone has been centered on its possible therapeutic application to ameliorate the catabolic effects of severe injury. Work in this area has been hampered by the fact that growth hormone appears to be rather species-specific, and only extremely limited supplies of human growth hormone have been made available. In animal studies the efficacy of growth hormone is clearly related to the level of caloric intake. When burned rats were treated with growth hormone, they actually lost more weight than the untreated burned controls unless an ample caloric intake was provided. Wilmore has been able to study the effects of growth hormone in a small number of burned patients and has found a similar dependence on the level of caloric intake.

CLINICAL RELEVANCE

The major elements of the metabolic response to injury have been examined in this chapter. After many years of uncertainty, it is now possible to present a unifying hypothesis explaining the metabolic sequence of events that follows injury. Catecholamines dominate the early events partly because of the rapidity with which their effects can be mediated. During the subsequent flow phase, other hormones whose metabolic manifestations develop more gradually assume equal or even greater importance. Finally, as the wounds heal, the various neuroendocrine mediators are turned off and convalescence proceeds.

At the present time, it appears that hypovolemia due to both external losses and internal shifts of extracellular fluid represents a logical starting point in the metabolic sequence. Not only are mechanisms designed to conserve salt and water brought into play, but in addition there is a rapid response to the sympathetic nervous system mediated through the baroreceptor reflex. Additional factors are probably involved in the release of catecholamines from the adrenal medulla and from sympathetic nerve endings throughout the body. Fear and apprehension by themselves constitute a stimulus, while tissue injury, hypoxia, and invasive infection add to the initiating factor of hypovolemia. It is clear that the magnitude of the catecholamine response is related to factors tied to the severity of the injury.

Catecholamines, in turn, stimulate ACTH production, thus increasing cortisol release from the adrenal cortex. While adrenal cortical secretion of mineralocorticoids takes place partly via the pituitary adrenal axis, local renal responses (renin and angiotensin) are also responsible for the retention of water and sodium. At the same time, the catecholamines inhibit insulin production from the pancreas and result in an increased glucagon release. When portal vein glucagon is elevated and insulin levels are low, rapid hepatic gluconeogenesis from amino acids follows. The deamination of amino acids results in the production of increased amounts of urea, which is excreted in the urine.

While high insulin levels favor the incorporation of amino acids into muscle protein, low levels have the opposite effect. Some of the amino acids lost from muscle provide the substrate for gluconeogenesis. Other amino acids may contribute to the maintenance of hepatic cell mass or the production of acute-phase proteins by the liver. In some way the muscle serves as an altruist by providing amino acids for glucose production, wound healing, and hepatic production of clotting factors and proteins to combat infection. While this may be of value in the immediate postinjury period, at some time the depletion of body protein becomes life-threatening, and protein stores must be replenished.

These facts are of critical concern to surgeons. Current techniques in surgical nutrition make it possible to administer amino acids to injured patients who are losing nitrogen at an accelerated rate. Both fat and carbohydrate are available to counter caloric deficits. Insulin, with and without the addition of glucose and potassium, has also been utilized to help these patients.

Unfortunately, there is a distinct danger that these important advances will distract surgeons from their primary responsibility, which is to deal with the components of injury so that the neuroendocrine stimulus will cease. Adequate resuscitation to shut off the hypovolemic stimulus is the obvious first step. After that has been done and the circulation has been stabilized, long-established principles of surgical care become of major metabolic significance. Once the patient turns from post-traumatic catabolism to uncomplicated starvation, foodstuffs are assimilated most avidly. Although our improved understanding of the complex sequence of events that follow injury suggests exciting possibilities for modifying the post-traumatic state, the surgeon's first goal should still be to drain the abscess, cover the wound, immobilize the fracture, or do whatever is needed to stop the continuing neuroendocrine stimulus associated with injury or infection.

REFERENCES

Allison, S. P., Hinton, P., Wollfson, A., and Heatley, R. V. C.: The importance of energy source and the significance of insulin in counteracting the catabolic response to injury. *In* Wilkinson, A. W., and Cuthbertson, D.: Metabolism and the Response to Injury. Kent, Pitman Medical Pub. 1976, p. 113.

Askanazi, J., Furst, P., Michelsen, C. B., et al.: Muscle and plasma amino acids after injury: Hypocaloric glucose vs. amino acid infusion. Ann. Surg., *191*:465–472, 1980.

Ballinger, W. F., Collins, J. A., Drucker, W. R., Dudrick, S. J., and Zeppa, R.: Manual of Surgical Nutrition. Philadelphia, W. B. Saunders Co., 1975.

Carlson, L. A.: Mobilization and utilization of lipids after trauma: Relation to caloric homeostasis. *In* Porter, R., and Knight, J. (eds.): Energy Metabolism in Trauma. London, J & A Churchill, 1970, p. 155.

Chaudry, I. H., and Baue, A. E.: Overview of hemorrhagic shock. *In* Cowley, R. A., and Trump, B. F. (eds.): Pathophysiology of Shock, Anoxia, and Ischemia. Baltimore/ London, Williams & Wilkins, 1982, p. 203.

Clowes, G. H. A., Jr.: Response to infection and injury. I. Physiology. Surg. Clin. North Am., *54*(4), 1976a.

Clowes, G. H. A., Jr.: Response to infection and injury. II. Metabolism. Surg. Clin. North Am., *56*(5), 1976b.

Kinney, J. M., and Felig, P.: The metabolic response to injury and infection. *In* DeGroot, L. J. (ed.): Endocrinology, Vol. 3. New York, Grune & Stratton, 1979, p. 1963.

Moore, F. D., Olesen, K. H., McMurrey, J. D., Parker, H. V., Ball, M. R., and Boyden, C. M.: The Body Cell Mass and Its Supporting Environment. Philadelphia, W. B. Saunders Co., 1963.

Moyer, C. A., and Butcher, H. R.: Burns, Shock and Plasma Volume Regulation. St. Louis, The C. V. Mosby Co., 1967.

Richards, J. R., and Kinney, J. M.: Nutritional Aspects of Care in the Critically Ill. Edinburgh, Churchill Livingstone, 1977.

Shires, T. G., Carrico, C. J., and Canizaro, P. C.: Shock. Philadelphia, W. B. Saunders Co., 1973.

Vinnars, E., Bergstrom, J., Furst, P.: Influence of postoperative state in the intracellular free amino acids in human muscle tissue. Ann. Surg., *182*:665, 1975.

Wilkinson, A. W., and Cuthbertson, D.: Metabolism and the Response to Injury. Kent, Pitman Medical Pub., 1976.

Wilmore, D. W.: The Metabolic Management of the Critically Ill. New York/London, Plenum Medical Pub., 1977.

Wilmore, D. W., Goodwin, C. W., Aulick, L. H., Powanda, M. C., Mason, A. R., Jr., and Pruitt, B. A., Jr.: Effect of injury and infection on visceral metabolism and circulation. Ann. Surg., *192*:491–504, 1980.

3

Fluid and Electrolyte Management

THOMAS A. MILLER
JAMES H. DUKE, JR.

Disorders in acid-base balance and fluid and electrolyte metabolism present some of the most challenging problems in the preoperative and postoperative care of surgical patients. Proper management of these disorders is impossible without a practical understanding of basic fluid physiology and a thorough appreciation of the types of problems encountered in the preoperative and postoperative periods. This chapter attempts to present in a concise yet complete fashion what we think is a rational approach to fluid and electrolyte therapy in the surgical patient. No attempt is made to provide an exhaustive treatise on water and electrolyte physiology or acid-base balance. Such information can be obtained, if needed, in textbooks on the subject or by consulting appropriate references listed at the end of this chapter.

COMPOSITION AND VOLUME OF THE BODY FLUIDS

A major portion of total body weight is water. The actual quantity of body water varies among individuals depending upon one's age, sex, and lean body mass, but in the average healthy adult male approximately 60 per cent of the total body weight is derived from water. Because women have a relatively greater amount of adipose tissue than do men, water contributes only about 50 per cent of total body weight in the female. Since fat is essentially water-free, the greater the body fat content, the less will be the water content. Hence, as lean tissue decreases with age, there is a relative increase in total body fat with a corresponding decrease in the percentage of body water.

Functionally, body water is divided into two main compartments. Water within body cells makes up the intracellular fluid compartment and constitutes about two-thirds of the total body water. On a weight basis, 40 per cent of the total body weight is intracellular. Water outside living cells makes up the extracellular fluid compartment, which constitutes about one-third of the total body water and 20 per cent of the total body weight. Approximately 25 per cent of the extracellular water (or five per cent of the body weight) is plasma, the fluid within the cardiovascular system. The interstitial fluid, which is essentially a gel between the capillary and the cell membrane, encompasses the other 75 per cent (or 15 per cent of the body weight). Several special fluids, including cerebrospinal fluid, synovial fluid, ocular fluid, and gastrointestinal secretions, occupy a small part of the extracelluar fluid compartment and normally constitute no more than 10 per cent of the interstitial fluid.

Each fluid compartment has its own unique electrolyte composition. The primary electrolyte components of the extracellular fluid compartment are *sodium* and *chloride* with small concentrations of potassium, magnesium, calcium, phosphate, bicarbonate, protein, and organic acids. The greater protein concentration of the plasma constitutes the only essential difference in elemental composition from that of the interstitial fluid. In contrast, the primary electrolytes of the intracellular fluid compartment are *potassium, magnesium,* and *phosphate* with relatively low concentrations of sodium and chloride. Proteins contribute significantly to the total intracellular concentration, but bicarbonate, calcium, and sulfate are relatively insignificant.

This difference in ionic composition between the intracellular and extracellular fluid compartments is due to the selective permeability of the cell wall. Although water freely diffuses through this semipermeable membrane, the passage of sodium and its salts intracellularly is restricted, while that of potassium and its salts is promoted. This ability of water to diffuse freely across the cell membrane means that the total solute concentration *(osmolality)* of all body fluid compartments is identical and that any change in concentration in one compartment will result in a corresponding movement of water until the concentration in all compartments has again become equal. If the number of solutes *(osmotic pressure)* in the extracellular fluid is greater than the number of solutes intracellularly, the resulting change in osmotic pressure will cause water to leave the cells and move toward the extracellular space to reestablish osmotic equilibrium. The inability of sodium to diffuse freely into the cell means that this ion is the principal solute of the extracellular fluid and that the osmolality of this compartment roughly parallels the sodium concentration. In actuality, sodium represents 90 to 92 per cent of all extracellular cations. Despite wide variations in one's individual intake of salt and water, the body attempts, through mechanisms of thirst and antidiuretic hormone secretion, to maintain the serum sodium concentration within narrow limits (i.e., 135 to 145 mEq per l). Therefore, measurement of this cation reflects rather accurately the osmolality of the body fluids and the water needs of the body. Accordingly, hyponatremia (serum sodium <135 mEq per l) would suggest either an excess of total body water or a deficit in total body sodium, while hypernatremia (serum sodium >145 mEq per l) would indicate an excess in total body sodium or a deficit in total body water. A rule of thumb that can be used to calculate extracellular osmolality is to multiply the serum sodium concentration by two and add 10. If the calculated value comes within five per cent of the normal serum osmolality (290 mOsm per l), a normal extracellular osmolality can be assumed to exist.

Maintenance of normal body fluid volume and electrolyte composition is primarily a function of the kidneys. Through processes of glomerular filtration and tubular reabsorption, sodium can be retained or excreted to match changes in the dietary intake. Similarly, water balance is regulated through changes in excretion or reabsorption in response to circulating levels of antidiuretic hormone. Although sodium and water losses also occur through the skin and stool, these are fixed losses and are generally small. The kidneys, on the other hand, can regulate losses in a finely balanced fashion so that volume and osmolality of body fluids remain unchanged in spite of wide variations in salt and water intake. Consequently, analysis of urinary volume and composition can provide valuable clues in the management of fluid and electrolyte disorders.

ACID-BASE BALANCE

During the course of daily metabolism, an enormous amount of acid is generated. As much as 15,000 to 20,000 mEq of volatile acid in the form of carbon dioxide are produced each day through oxidation of carbohydrates and fat. Another 60 to 70 mEq of fixed acid in nonvolatile form are produced daily from the breakdown of sulfur-containing amino acids and incompletely oxidized carbohydrates and fats. If efficient mechanisms were not available to buffer this acid and bring about its elimination, the pH of the body would quickly decline and death would rapidly ensue.

Under normal circumstances, this excessive hydrogen ion production has no net effect on the body pH because of a variety of internal buffer systems working in concert with pulmonary and renal mechanisms, which provide a defense against acid-base disturbances. Intracellularly, these buffers include phosphates and proteins. Extracellularly, they include hemoglobin, proteins, and the bicarbonate–carbonic acid system. Little is known about the mechanisms of intracellular acid-base balance, but extracellularly, the major buffer is the bicarbonate–carbonic acid system, and, from a practical standpoint, the one with which the physician must be concerned when dealing with acid-base disorders.

Normally the body regulates neutrality by attempting to maintain the ratio of bicarbonate (HCO_3^-) to carbonic acid (H_2CO_3) at 20 to 1. As long as this ratio is maintained, the pH of the extracellular fluid compartment will remain at its normal value of 7.4 (range 7.38 to 7.42). Deviations in this ratio will precipitate a corresponding disturbance in acid-base balance. Thus, an increase in this ratio will produce a state of *alkalosis* (an increase in pH), while a decrease in this ratio will produce *acidosis* (a decrease in pH).

From a purely chemical standpoint, the bicarbonate–carbonic acid buffer system is inefficient. However, judged biologically, it is quite efficient. This seeming inconsistency relates to the unusual property of carbonic acid to behave as an acid or as the neutral gas carbon dioxide (CO_2) and is expressed by the following equation:

$$CO_2 + H_2O \rightleftarrows H_2CO_3 \rightleftarrows H^+ + HCO_3^-$$

where formation of carbonic acid from carbon dioxide or reversion of carbonic acid to carbon dioxide will depend upon the acid-base status of the patient at any given time. When acid is added to this system, bicarbonate concentration will decrease (numerator of the ratio) with a corresponding drop in the bicarbonate–carbonic acid ratio below 20 to 1. To combat this state of acidosis, ventilation is increased, and the newly formed carbonic acid (denominator of the ratio) is quickly converted to CO_2 and "blown off" by the lungs, thereby reestablishing the ratio to near normal. Any compensation not immediately effected by the lungs will be ultimately mediated by the slower but more complete compensation of the kidneys through retention of bicarbonate or increased excretion of acid salts. Had alkali, rather than acid, been added to this buffer system initially, the reverse would have occurred, namely a retention of CO_2 (and hence carbonic acid) by the lungs through a decrease in ventilation and an increased excretion of bicarbonate by the kidneys.

Acid-base imbalance is common in disease and normally results from an excess or deficit in either carbonic acid or bicarbonate. Since the body attempts to maintain extracellular pH by balancing the ratio of this buffer pair, disturbances in acid-base balance can be divided conveniently into disorders of respiration or defects in normal body metabolism. If respiration is altered, elimination of carbon dioxide will be altered and will affect the carbonic acid side of this balance. In any state causing rapid or deep breathing (such as anxiety, hysteria, fever, and lack of oxygen), *respiratory alkalosis* will develop secondary to the carbonic acid depletion resulting from the excess carbon dioxide exhalation. This is reflected as an increase in pH of the blood due to an increase in the bicarbonate–carbonic acid ratio and a decrease in the alveolar

PCO_2 below 35 mm Hg. No change in the plasma bicarbonate is seen initially, but some degree of renal compensation almost always occurs through increased bicarbonate excretion in the urine to restore this ratio to normal. If monitored, the urinary pH is generally above 7 and the plasma bicarbonate is less than 25 mEq per l.

When normal respiration is depressed (such as in pneumonia, pleurisy, pneumothorax, asthma, emphysema, and pleural effusion), *respiratory acidosis* occurs. Excess retention of carbon dioxide develops with a consequent increase in the accumulation of carbonic acid. The PCO_2 is always about 45 mm Hg and often above 50 mm Hg. Owing to the decrease in the bicarbonate–carbonic acid ratio, the body pH drops. The kidneys attempt to compensate for this condition by increasing bicarbonate reabsorption and hyrogen ion excretion, but such compensation is usually inadequate. Thus, the fall in blood pH persists (usually below 7.36) despite a compensatory increase in the total plasma bicarbonate (generally above 30 mEq per l).

Disturbances in metabolism affect the bicarbonate side of this equation. In *metabolic alkalosis,* a state of excess bicarbonate exists. This condition develops in any situation in which chloride loss from the body is enhanced (such as in vomiting, prolonged nasogastric suction, and gastrocutaneous fistula). Since chloride and bicarbonate are both anions, which must equal the total number of cations in the extracellular fluid compartment, a loss of either anion will result in a compensatory increase in the other. Deficits in intracellular potassium may also give rise to this condition. As potassium escapes from the cell and is lost from the body, sodium and hydrogen ions move into the cell to reestablish intracellular ionic balance and integrity. This results in an extracellular alkalosis. Finally, excess administration of bicarbonate either orally or intravenously may also cause alkalosis.

Regardless of the cause, the ratio of bicarbonate to carbonic acid is increased in metabolic alkalosis. Consequently, the blood pH is increased (generally above 7.45 and frequently above 7.50), and the plasma bicarbonate concentration rises above 30 mEq per l. If chloride loss is the etiologic reason for this condition, plasma chloride levels may be 90 mEq per l or lower. In hypokalemic states, the serum potassium concentration is often below 3 mEq per l. Although some degree of respiratory compensation occurs (PCO_2 between 40 and 45), this is limited by the oxygen demands of the patient. Consequently, renal compensation becomes more important. Initially this is accomplished by an increased excretion of bicarbonate. However, as dehydration heightens, this compensatory mechanism eventually fails, and renal tubular reabsorption of sodium and bicarbonate increases, leading to a perpetuation of the alkalotic state and the paradoxical excretion of an acid urine.

In *metabolic acidosis*, a deficit in plasma bicarbonate exists. This occurs in diabetes (with excessive ketonic acid production), renal disease (with inadequate excretion of inorganic acids), and states of excessive bicarbonate loss from the body (such as diarrhea, pancreatic fistula, and enterocutaneous fistula). In this condition the blood pH is almost always below 7.35, the plasma bicarbonate concentration is below 25 mEq per l, and the urinary pH is below 6. The body attempts to correct the resulting decrease in the bicarbonate–carbonic acid ratio by increasing the elimination of carbonic acid (and hence CO_2) through the lungs. Usually successful initially in preventing a severely acidotic state, such compensation through pulmonary hyperventilation is always incomplete and will ultimately fail unless the underlying cause of this condition is corrected.

ANION-GAP

In any biologic system in which ions are present, electrical neutrality is maintained by balancing the total number of cations with the total number of anions. This principle can be utilized clinically in patients with suspected acid-base disorders by measuring the serum sodium, chloride, and bicarbonate concentrations. Normally the extracellular concentration of the cation sodium equals the sum of the extracellular concentrations of the anions, chloride and bicarbonate, plus a constant designated as delta (Δ). This is expressed by the equation,

$$mEq\ Na^+ = mEq\ HCO_3^- + mEq\ Cl^- + \Delta$$

where Δ equals 8 ± 4 mEq per l. If the relationship between the sum of these two anions plus Δ is less than the serum sodium concentration on repeated examinations, an "anion-gap" is said to exist.

Determination of the anion-gap may prove useful in assessing the etiology of metabolic acidosis. If one divides the acidoses of metabolic origin into two major groups, those in which hydrogen ion is retained in association with chloride (metabolic acidosis with hyperchloremia) and those in which hydrogen ion is retained in association with other anions (metabolic acidosis with an increase of unmeasured anions), the concentration of the other unmeasured anions can be estimated arbitrarily from the equation designated above by the number obtained for Δ. If Δ is normal or decreased, the acidosis can be assumed to be a hyperchloremic acidosis. When the acidosis arises from the addition of substantial amounts of another anion, Δ will be increased and one of the anion-gap acidoses will exist.

Metabolic acidosis with hyperchloremia most commonly occurs in surgical patients with prolonged or severe diarrhea (loss of HCO_3^- in stool) or the loss of intestinal contents through enterocutaneous fistulas. It may also occur in patients with renal tubular acidosis (decreased H^+ secretion by renal tubular cells), patients with ureteroenterostomy (loss of HCO_3^-, which exchanges for urinary Cl^- across the intestinal mucosa), and in states of excessive ammonium chloride ingestion. Metabolic acidosis accompanying an increase of unmeasured anions may occur in patients with renal insufficiency in which phosphate and sulfate as well as organic acid anions are retained, diabetic ketoacidosis in which ketogenic acids accumulate in the blood, in lactic acidosis as arises in hypoxia and hypoperfusion, and in states of intoxication with salicylates, methanol, paraldehyde, and ethylene glycol.

A RATIONAL APPROACH TO FLUID AND ELECTROLYTE THERAPY

From a practical standpoint, fluid therapy is basically an exercise in balancing the input and output of water and electrolytes. In the surgical patient, this is best accomplished by subdividing replacement needs into three general categories: (1) normal maintenance requirements, (2) abnormal losses resulting from the patient's underlying disease or its surgical treatment, and (3) correction of any existing deficits.

Regardless of the patient's disease or the type of operative procedure performed, water and salt losses occur daily through normal urinary output and evaporative losses from the skin and lungs. These *normal maintenance requirements* consist of both sensible and insensible losses depending upon whether they can be measured readily. Insensible losses (those not visible or readily measurable) occur from water losses through the lungs and evaporative losses from the skin. They usually amount to about 600 to 1000 ml daily in the nonactive, nonperspiring adult. Sensible losses (those that are visible and can be measured) include water losses in the feces and those due to excretion of urine. In the absence of diarrhea, water loss via the feces is essentially negligible and can be ignored. Urinary losses vary considerably depending upon the state of one's hydration, but generally a volume of water approaching 1000 to 1500 ml is required to excrete the daily solute load of the adult surgical patient in a urine concentration isosmotic with plasma. Depending upon the patient's age, sex, weight, and body surface area, daily maintenance requirements for both sensible and insensible losses will approach 1500 to 2500 ml. Since the electrolyte composition of these losses is low (particularly in the first 48 to 72 hours following operation), adequate replacement can be supplied under most circumstances with a five per cent dextrose and water solution. A rule of thumb that has been useful in estimating these needs is to multiply the patient's weight in kilograms times 30 ml per kg. A 70 kg male, therefore, would need approxmately 2100 ml of water daily to meet normal maintenance requirements.

Although urine and insensible losses are primarily water losses, it must be remembered that each of these sources contains sodium, potassium, and chloride, albeit in small amounts. For the patient requiring intravenous therapy for only short periods of time, replacement of these electrolyte losses is unimportant. In the individual requiring parenteral support for several days to a week or more, total body stores of these ions will eventually diminish if some replacement is not provided. This is particularly important for sodium, since a depletion of this ion can initiate an extracellular hypotonicity, resulting in a shift of water intracellularly and a state of water intoxication. Since exact determination of these electrolyte losses is neither practical nor necessary on a daily basis, replacement should be based on the usual requirements of most patients. For sodium, daily needs range from 50 to 125 mEq, while for potassium and chloride they approach 40 to 100 mEq. For practical purposes, however, usual replacement requirements for each of these ions is approximately 60 to 70 mEq daily. In meeting these needs, a second rule of thumb that can be used is to provide one mEq of each of these electrolytes daily for each kilogram of body weight. In a patient requiring 2 liters of fluid to meet normal maintenance needs, 1500 ml could be provided as dextrose and water, and the remaining 500 ml could be given as normal saline with the addition of potassium chloride in appropriate quantities.

Two notes of caution must be observed when supplying maintenance needs. First, potassium is usually unnecessary and may prove detrimental if given during the first 24 hours following operation. Endogenous release of intracellular potassium from tissue catabolism and operative trauma (and blood transfusions if given) generally provides sufficient quantities of this ion to warrant restriction during the early postoperative period. Second, the stress of operation, which stimulates the release of aldosterone and antidiuretic hormone with the accompanying retention of sodium, chloride, and water, may prove harmful to the patient with compromised renal or cardiac reserve if adjustments in fluid administration are not made. In these patients, only about two-thirds of the calculated maintenance volume should be infused for the first 72 hours following operation in order to keep the patient "dry" and to prevent circulatory overload.

Abnormal losses arising from the patient's underlying disease or its surgical treatment must also be replaced. By far, the most common source of these losses is the gastrointestinal tract. As with maintenance needs, proper replacement of these losses can also be accomplished if one remembers the basic composition of the gastrointestinal secretions and their relation to the composition of normal serum (Table 3–1). Generally, losses due to intestinal secretions, bile, or pancreatic juice can be replaced on a volume-for-volume basis with a neutral or slightly alkaline balanced salt solution, such as Ringer's lactate or normal saline, while losses from the actively secreting stomach are replaced with half-normal saline solution. To prevent hypokalemia, 15 to 20 mEq of potassium for every liter of fluid lost from any of these sites should also

Table 3–1. COMPOSITION OF GASTROINTESTINAL SECRETIONS

TYPE OF SECRETION	VOLUME (ml/24 hr)	Na (mEq/l)	K (mEq/l)	Cl (mEq/l)	HCO$_3$ (mEq/l)
Saliva	1000–1500	5–10	20–30	5–15	25–30
Stomach	1000–2000	60–90	10–15	100–130	
Pancreas	600–800	135–145	5–10	70–90	95–115
Bile	300–600	135–145	5–10	90–110	30–40
Small intestine	2000–3000	120–140	5–10	90–120	30–40

be given. Although replacement in this manner is only semiquantitative, problems are rarely encountered with electrolyte imbalance. If losses from the gastrointestinal tract exceed one liter daily for several days, an aliquot of the fluid (or fluids) lost should be sent to the laboratory for more specific electrolyte analysis in order that appropriate adjustments can be made to insure more precise replacement.

Abnormal losses may also arise from increased evaporation from the skin and respiratory tract. In states of hyperventilation, increased metabolism, or fever, losses (primarily electrolyte-free water) approaching 1000 ml daily may occur over and above normal insensible losses. The patient with a temperature between 38.4 and 39.4°C (101 to 103°F) or a respiratory rate of 35 respirations or more per minute may lose an additional 500 ml of water daily over that of usual insensible losses. In toxic states, in which body temperature is persistently above 39.5°C (103°F), as much as 1000 ml of body water may be lost daily. Consequently, in writing fluid orders, replacement of these losses must be included.

A unique fluid loss encountered in the postoperative patient is that brought about by *sequestration* at the site of operative trauma. This situation is created when interstitial fluid or plasma is sequestered in abnormal amounts in an area of tissue injury. Depending upon the magnitude of the operation, such losses may be small or exceedingly great. The several hundred milliliters of fluid lost in an inguinal hernia repair is generally of no physiologic significance. On the other hand, the extracellular fluid sequestered in a total proctocolectomy may be substantial. Since there is no way to measure these losses accurately, replacement must, at best, be based upon clinical approximation. Usually 500 to 750 ml of fluid is given in addition to maintenance needs for the first two to three postoperative days to compensate for these losses when a major operation has been performed in which tissue dissection was extensive or postoperative tissue weeping may be excessive. These losses are plasma-like, so that replacement with a balanced salt solution is indicated. The sequestered fluid, however, will eventually return to the intravascular compartment once normal capillary function is restored to the affected area (usually on the third to the fifth postoperative days).

In anticipation of the increase in circulating blood volume, restrictions in calculated fluid needs at this time may become necessary in order to prevent fluid overload.

Finally, *any existing solute or volume deficits* must be corrected. These most commonly occur in the preoperative patient (see section on preoperative preparation) and arise primarily from gastrointestinal tract losses due to vomiting, diarrhea, or sequestration of fluid as in bowel obstruction. The difficulty in correcting these deficits relates to the difficulty in quantifying their magnitude. Generally, a detailed history from the patient summarizing the duration of disease, the frequency and amount of fluid losses (such as in vomiting or diarrhea), and other pertinent information is helpful in assessing the magnitude of the underlying deficits. Coupled with a careful clinical evaluation of the patient's hydrational status, the degree of fluid depletion can be estimated, and appropriate replacement of calculated losses can be provided as clinically indicated.

Using the principles outlined in this discussion, a rational approach to fluid and electrolyte therapy can be formulated. Remembering that maintenance requirements will remain essentially unchanged from day to day, the major variables in daily intravenous rations will relate to the correction of any existing deficits of volume or composition and the replacement of ongoing losses. Although a wide variety of intravenous solutions are available to meet these needs (Table 3–2), it is unnecessary and impractical to be familiar with every intravenous solution marketed. Rather, each surgeon should familiarize himself or herself with a few selected parenteral solutions and should manage clinical problems by manipulating the appropriate proportions of each of these solutions for a given clinical situation. For most needs, five per cent dextrose and water, normal saline, and Ringer's lactate solution (or combinations thereof) are entirely satisfactory, with appropriate supplementation of

Table 3–2. COMPOSITION OF INTRAVENOUS SOLUTIONS

SOLUTIONS	GLUCOSE (gm/l)	Na	Cl	HCO₃	K	Ca	Mg	HPO₄	NH₄
					(mEq/l)				
Extracellular fluid	1000	140	102	27	4.2	5	3	3	0.3
5% dextrose and water	50								
10% dextrose and water	100								
0.9% sodium chloride (normal saline)		154	154						
0.45% sodium chloride (half-normal saline)		77	77						
0.21% sodium chloride (¹/₄ normal saline)		34	34						
3% sodium chloride (hypertonic saline)		513	513						
Lactated Ringer's solution		130	109	28°	4	2.7			
0.9% ammonium chloride			168						168

°Present in solution as lactate but is metabolized to bicarbonate.

potassium and other solutes (such as magnesium, phosphate, and calcium) as the clinical circumstances dictate.

It is essential to good patient care that the fluid requirements of each patient be reevaluated frequently. Intravenous orders should be rewritten at least every 24 hours, and more often if indicated by the clinical situation. In the first day or two following an operation, internal fluid shifts and the accompanying circulatory instability may necessitate frequent reassessment of the patient's fluid status if potentially detrimental effects on water and electrolyte balance are to be obviated. In patients undergoing major operative procedures (such as pancreatectomy, gastrectomy, and abdominoperineal resection), it is a good habit to reevaluate the patient's fluid needs on the day of operation as often as every four to six hours. In this way, corrections can be made as necessary to insure the maintenance of normal fluid and electrolyte equilibrium.

Each clinical circumstance will dictate the frequency with which serum electrolytes should be obtained. Serum electrolyte determinations are generally unnecessary for patients requiring intravenous support for only one or two days. However, for patients requiring such support for prolonged periods of time, sodium, potassium, chloride, and bicarbonate concentrations should be obtained every two to three days. If large fluid losses from nasogastric suction, gastrointestinal fistulas, or other drainage sites are encountered, such determinations may be necessary on a daily basis. Daily weights are often helpful in determining whether abrupt changes in fluid balance (fluid overload or fluid deficit) have occurred. Probably the most important single means of assessing the patient's fluid status is the maintenance of daily intake and output records. By carefully tabulating the composition and volume of intravenous solutions infused and comparing them with the patient's daily losses from drainage, insensible loss, and urinary sources, water or electrolyte abnormalities that may be developing insidiously can be detected before major imbalances occur.

ESTABLISHING FLUID BALANCE PRIOR TO OPERATION

Patients tolerate operations best when they are properly hydrated. For the majority of patients this poses no problem, as reflected in the absence of peripheral edema, the presence of normal vital signs, stable weight, adequate urine output, good skin turgor, moist mucous membranes, and normal serum electrolytes. Those patients suffering from varying degrees of dehydration or overhydration, however, will not tolerate operation as well. This relates to the potentially devastating effects that fluid and electrolyte imbalance may have on what otherwise should be an uneventful operation. The dehydrated patient, for example, is likely to develop hypotension at the time of induction of anesthesia, which may be aggravated further by the fluid losses encountered during the operation. Similarly, edematous tissues in the patient who is overhydrated are more difficult to dissect, heal less efficiently, and frequently will not hold stitches. It is for these reasons that the preoperative fluid and electrolyte status of all patients must be assessed carefully to identify those patients who will require special attention and management prior to undergoing operation.

Dehydration with accompanying salt loss, also called volume deficit, is the most frequent disorder encountered in the preoperative patient. Pathologic states that give rise to this condition include intestinal obstruction, vomiting secondary to pyloric outlet obstruction, diarrhea, various enterocutaneous fistulas, and sequestration of extracellular fluid into injured tissues. Depending upon the underlying disease process, the degree of fluid loss may be relatively easy to assess or extremely difficult to quantify. Fluid losses secondary to vomiting and diarrhea are apparent and are reflected as weight losses. Internal losses, though, are often not appreciated and may reach massive proportions despite minimal weight loss. These "third space" losses, as they are called, may result from the loss of fluid beneath a burn, losses into the bowel wall and lumen in states of intestinal obstruction, losses into tissues in massive trauma and fractures of long bones, losses into hypoxic damaged tissues following shock, and losses as ascitic fluid caused by cirrhosis of the liver or peritonitis.

Since exact quantification of these losses is virtually impossible, the degree of volume deficit must be based on a detailed history of the patient's disease coupled with a careful evaluation of the physical signs. The patient who has not eaten for four days while experiencing almost persistent diarrhea will be more volume depleted than the individual who presents to the emergency room with vomiting of only several hours' duration. Similarly, a patient with sunken eyes, loss of skin turgor, and a dry tongue is much more dehydrated than the patient without these findings. Of particular importance is an assessment of the cardiovascular status. Depressed blood pressure, rapid pulse, and low urinary output are all indices of significant volume depletion. Accompanying these findings are a hemoconcentrated serum, a urine of high specific gravity, and an elevated blood urea nitrogen. Depending upon the tonicity (osmolality) of the fluid losses, serum electrolytes may be normal or may reflect individual electrolyte abnormalities. In the patient with pyloric outlet obstruction, for example, there is a marked loss of chloride with smaller losses of sodium and potassium, while in the patient with small bowel obstruction, the fluid that is lost resembles interstitial fluid in electrolyte composition.

Clinically significant volume depletion usually does not become manifest until a loss of fluid approximating five per cent of the body weight has occurred. Under these circumstances, skin turgor is usually depressed, eyes may be sunken, mucous membranes have lost their moistness, and urine volume is decreased and hyperconcentrated. With severe degrees of volume loss (10 per cent or more), urine output is markedly depressed, tachycardia is almost always present and may be accompanied by shortness of breath, and blood pressure is quite labile. Based on these observations, a rough approximation of the volume deficit can be made. Thus, a 70 kg male who has lost five percent of his body weight (3.5 kg) will need about 3.5 liters of fluid to restore homeostasis.

It must be emphasized that in correcting existing deficits, no attempt should be made to replace all losses in a single 24-hour period. Since most deficits develop over a period of days (and sometimes weeks), the patient has usually adjusted quite well physiologically to the deficiency induced by the illness. In fact, rapid replacement of estimated losses may actually impose a greater risk than the primary illness. This is particularly true in the elderly patient with compromised cardiac reserve. If careful attention is not paid to volume replacement, inadvertent fluid overloading may rapidly supervene. It is for this reason that only one-half of the estimated deficits should be replaced in a 24-hour period (in addition to daily maintenance needs and other losses). Reassessment of the clinical situation is mandatory before giving more fluid. If additional fluid administration is needed, one-half of the remaining deficit is replaced in the next 24 hours and so on, until fluid equilibrium has been restored. An especially helpful guide to fluid balance is the hourly measurement of urine volume. In the absence of diuretics or glycosuria, an adult patient who excretes 40 to 50 ml of urine per hour is in satisfactory fluid equilibrium.

The only exception to this general approach is the patient with volume depletion who needs emergency surgery (such as the patient in shock secondary to peritonitis from a perforated duodenal ulcer). In this circumstance, rapid replacement of fluid deficits should be accomplished in one to three hours, following which exploratory laparotomy is performed. Usually, a liter or more of fluid is given per hour until fluid equilibrium has been reestablished and the risks of anesthesia have been minimized. Again, the measurement of hourly urine volumes will prove helpful in assessing fluid balance.

The type of fluid replaced will depend, in most cases, on the serum electrolyte profile. If electrolytes are relatively normal in the face of obvious volume depletion, losses can be assumed to have been isosmotic with plasma and should generally be replaced with a balanced salt solution, such as Ringer's lactate. In contrast, if chloride losses exceed sodium losses, as occurs with vomiting, isotonic saline or half-normal saline is generally the preferred replacement fluid. In hypernatremic states, as may occur with patients receiving tube feedings, water alone as five per cent dextrose in water is used for replacement. Hyponatremia, on the other hand, responds in most instances to water restriction but may necessitate on rare occasions the use of hypertonic saline (three per cent sodium chloride) for correction. Usually, however, administration of isotonic saline will be adequate to replace most volume deficits. If a hypertonic salt solution is required, extreme care must be exercised in its use to prevent fluid overload, compromise of cardiac function, and resulting pulmonary edema.

Since potassium losses often accompany losses of salt and water, especially in vomiting and diarrhea states, the resulting hypokalemia will likewise need correction. The patient who has lost 4 liters of gastric juice while vomiting for two days has an 80 mEq (roughly 15 to 20 mEq per l) deficit of potassium from the vomitus plus an additional 40 to 60 mEq daily deficit in the urine. The patient's estimated losses, therefore, would be about 160 to 200 mEq for the two-day period. To correct these deficits, about one-half of the estimated losses (80 to 100 mEq) plus the daily maintenance needs (about 70 mEq) for a total of 150 to 170 mEq of potassium should be given during the first 24 hours. Since a serum potassium concentration below 4 mEq per l may be associated with cardiac arrhythmias, replacement of potassium losses should be monitored frequently with assessment of serum potassium levels. If emergency surgery is anticipated, more rapid replacement of potassium deficits may become necessary. This can be accomplished by administering potassium as a continuous intravenous drip. This must be done cautiously, however, with electrocardiographic monitoring, and at no time should such infusion exceed 15 mEq per hour in order to avoid a potentially lethal hyperkalemia.

States of overhydration are also seen in the preoperative patient. Volume restriction with gentle removal of excess fluid by mild diuretics is all that is needed in most cases in preparation for operation. Pure water excess leading to symptoms of water intoxication is more difficult to control. This condition, which has been observed in patients with central nervous system lesions and burns, is thought to be due to an inappropriate secretion of antidiuretic hormone resulting in an excessive tubular reabsorption of water. Cessation of all water administration coupled with the use of solute diuretics, such as mannitol, is the treatment of choice. If these measures are nonproductive, the cautious administration of hypertonic salt solutions will usually assist in the diuresis of the excess water.

Alterations in acid-base balance may accompany fluid derangements but usually require no specific treatment. The alkalosis or acidosis arising from pulmonary dysfunction is usually corrected without difficulty by improving ventilation. Acid-base disorders of metabolic origin respond quite well to correction of electrolyte deficits and restoration of normal fluid volume. Rarely is it necessary to administer an acidifying agent such as ammonium chloride in the treatment of metabolic alkalosis if fluid and electrolyte equilibrium has been reestablished. Although lactic acidosis resulting from anaerobic metabolism in the presence of hypoxia may necessitate the vigorous intravenous infusion of alkaline solutions, most forms of metabolic acidosis will respond to volume replacement and correction of electrolyte deficits.

Finally, care must be exercised to insure that derangements in fluid balance are not iatrogenically created. The use of cathartics and enemas in preparation for colonic surgery may severely deplete the extracellular fluid volume, as may prolonged periods of fluid restriction in preparation for various radiologic examinations or other diagnostic procedures. These potential losses must be recognized and treated as they occur if complications during anesthesia induction and operation are to be prevented. In anticipation of these frequently unrecognized subtle losses, patients undergoing major abdominal surgery, such as abdomino-perineal resection, pancreatectomy, and gastrectomy, should be given a liter of balanced salt solution intravenously during the 12-hour period immediately preceding operation. This procedure insures adequate volume repletion at the time of induction of anesthesia and provides a margin of safety for excessive but unexpected losses encountered during the surgical procedure.

POSTOPERATIVE DISORDERS IN FLUID AND ELECTROLYTE BALANCE

Based on the principles outlined in this chapter, fluid and electrolyte balance can be accomplished easily in the vast majority of surgical patients. A wide variety of fluid abnormalities may occur in the postoperative period, but in general, these derangements can be classified into three basic patterns: (1) volume disorders, (2) composition disorders, and (3) acid-base balance disorders. Although two or possibly all three patterns may coexist in the same patient, one pattern usually predominates. For purposes of discussion, therefore, each disorder will be considered separately.

VOLUME DISORDERS

Volume Overload

By far, the most common clinical disorder we have observed in the postoperative period is *volume overload*. Characterized by an isotonic expansion of the extracellular fluid compartment, this condition occurs when fluids having the same tonicity as plasma (such as balanced salt solutions, including normal saline and Ringer's lactate solution) are infused intravenously in excess of body needs. Such solutions do not affect the osmolality of the extracellular space; hence, no net shifts in water between this compartment and the intracellular space occur. Therefore, intracellular volume remains unchanged, and any excess fluid infusion is reflected as an increase in the volume of the extracellular compartment alone. The greater the excess infusion, the greater will be the expansion of this compartment with a corresponding decrease in the concentration of hemoglobin, hematocrit, and protein, even though the sodium concentration remains unchanged.

This complication of fluid therapy can occur at any time postoperatively, but it is particularly common in the early postoperative period when the hormonal response of the patient having undergone the stress of operation is one that results in maximal retention of water and sodium. Frequently, large volumes of balanced salt solution are given during the operation to maintain a satisfactory urine output and to prevent circulatory instability. Thus, most patients entering the recovery room are either adequately volume repleted or possibly even overexpanded. The common tendency to continue to infuse large volumes of isotonic salt solutions around the clock during the first 24 to 48 hours after operation in an effort to maintain a large-volume urine output is not only unnecessary but also may prove quite detrimental to the patient. There is no physiologic evidence to support the hypothesis that an hourly urine volume of 100 ml is any better than 50 ml unless there is some concurrent pathologic renal process contributing to the overall clinical situation. As long as a urinary output of 30 to 50 ml per hour is maintained, renal perfusion is quite adequate and renal failure is most unlikely.

The misconception that excess salt water will be excreted by the kidneys automatically if the body has no use for it is fallacious. It is the change in tonicity of the extracellular fluid space that allows the kidney to retain or excrete water and electrolytes as needed. This fact becomes particularly important in dealing with elderly patients. The younger patient with a normal cardiovascular status can usually tolerate an acute overexpansion of the extracellular fluid compartment, but such excess fluid administration may prove detrimental to the elderly individual. Most of these patients have some degree of cardiac and renal dysfunction, and depending upon the degree of renal impairment, the kidneys may not be able to excrete the excess fluid load. Furthermore, the status of these patients may change quickly, in that a small excess in fluid retention may give rise to a rapid deterioration in cardiopulmonary reserve. These patients must be observed carefully and monitored frequently if pulmonary edema and its detrimental sequelae are to be prevented. Care must also be exercised in preventing excessive fluid overload in patients undergoing pneumonectomy or craniotomy. In both instances, fluid overload is not well tolerated. The increase in intracranial pressure in postcraniotomy patients accompanying the infusion of large volumes of isotonic salt solutions may have devastating effects upon recovery.

The earliest sign of fluid overload is an increase in body weight. The more prolonged the excessive infusion, the more pronounced will be the weight gain. This is a particularly important sign in the postoperative patient, since the normal catabolism during postoperative recovery and convalescence usually results in a weight loss of ¼ to ½ pound per day.

It is for this reason that meticulous attention to daily weights and water balance in any patient receiving intravenous therapy is absolutely essential.

Depending upon the extent of fluid expansion, peripheral edema may be present. This clinical situation is usually accompanied by an increase in central venous pressure, a high pulse pressure representing an increase in cardiac output, swollen eyelids, hoarseness, and occasionally exertional dyspnea. If extracellular volume overload is allowed to continue, circulatory overload may ultimately occur, giving rise to pulmonary edema with the easily recognizable signs of dyspnea, coughing, neck vein distention, and occasionally cyanosis. Since this complication appears late and represents a rather massive fluid overload, it is totally preventable with careful attention to daily intake and output records.

Depending upon the degree of fluid overload, treatment may be relatively simple or exceedingly complex. When detected early, volume restriction, which consists of withholding all fluids until excess water and electrolytes have been excreted, may suffice to restore balance. Usually though, diuretic supplementation will be necessary. If cardiac reserve is compromised, digitalis must also be given. For most purposes, furosemide and ethacrynic acid, which inhibit the renal tubular reabsorption of sodium and water, prove entirely satisfactory. Care must be exercised in using these agents, however, since a brisk diuresis resulting in a rebound hypovolemia may ensue. Except in unusual situations, low doses (10 to 25 mg) given as single intravenous infusions are sufficient if normal renal function has been maintained. In the presence of renal impairment, some form of dialysis may be needed ultimately if fluid restriction and diuretic therapy are not effective.

Volume Deficit

In contrast to volume overload, volume deficits are not encountered as commonly in the postoperative patient as they were a decade ago. This phemonenon relates primarily to the emphasis in recent years on maintaining adequate volume repletion to insure satisfactory urinary output. If volume depletion does develop, it usually results from gastrointestinal losses due to nasogastric suction, enterostomies, entercutaneous fistulas, and diarrhea or sequestered losses that occur at the site of traumatized tissues or in disease states such as pancreatitis, peritonitis, ileus, and multiple trauma.

Like volume overload, volume depletion primarily affects the extracellular fluid compartment since losses are generally isosmotic with plasma. As plasma volume decreases, interstitial fluid slowly moves into the vascular space to support the depleted circulation, resulting in an overall deficit in the volume of the extravascular extracellular fluid compartment. Since red cell mass remains essentially unchanged, except in instances of widespread tissue injury or hemorrhage, a rise in hematocrit and hemoglobin occur. Similarly, total protein concentration increases unless significant amounts of albumin were also lost, as may occur in peritonitis, bowel obstruction, and pancreatitis. Because losses are isosmotic with plasma, there is usually no change in the serum sodium concentration.

The clinical manifestations of volume depletion include weight loss, tachycardia, and, if sufficiently severe, hypotension, particularly of the orthostatic variety. Some degree of oliguria almost always accompanies these findings, even in the absence of significant hypotension. If the urinary sodium concentration is measured, it frequently is 10 mEq per l or less owing to the action of aldosterone on the renal tubule to maintain extracellular osmolality and intravascular volume. Because renal perfusion is diminished in the presence of a decrease in circulating blood volume resulting in a decrease in daily urinary production, the urine is hyperconcentrated (specific gravity is usually greater than 1.020), and some elevation of the blood urea nitrogen (BUN) and creatinine is almost always present. This prerenal azotemia due to volume depletion can be distinguished from acute tubular necrosis, in that the former is associated with a disproportionate rise in BUN as compared to creatinine (frequently 20 to 1 or greater), whereas in renal failure this ratio remains close to its normal value of 10 to 1.

The treatment of volume depletion will depend to a large extent on the composition of the fluid lost. In most instances, replacement with a balanced salt solution will prove satisfactory. If large amounts of protein have been lost, plasma or an albumin-containing solution should be administered in conjunction with the salt solution. For gastrointestinal losses below the pyloric sphincter, either Ringer's lactate solution or normal saline will usually suffice. For pure gastric losses, replacement with half-normal saline solution is usually appropriate unless sodium losses are excessive, in which case normal saline should be used. In either circumstance, appropriate amounts of potassium must also be administered.

Although the degree of volume deficit often can be assessed by carefully reviewing the intake and output records and determining the change that has occurred in body weight, exact quantification is frequently difficult. Consequently, in deciding whether adequate replacement has been given, the best guide to follow is the adequacy of urinary output. In the absence of underlying renal disease, glycosuria, or diuretic administraton, a urine output of 30 to 50 ml per hour with a specific gravity of 1.015 or less suggests satisfactory repletion of volume deficits. Reversion of hemoglobin and hematocrit to normal levels is also a helpful indicator of adequate volume replacement, but this clinical method has not proved to be as reliable as the measurement of urinary volume. In severely traumatized patients, replacement of deficient red cell mass is frequently the most significant factor in restoring cardiovascular equilibrium and securing adequate tissue perfusion and nourishment.

COMPOSITION DISORDERS

Hyponatremia

With the emphasis in recent years on giving adequate volumes of isotonic salt solutions both intraoperatively and in the immediate postoperative period to prevent circulatory instability and to maintain satisfactory urinary output, deficits in serum sodium concentration are not commonly encountered. If hyponatremia should occur, it usually develops in the early postoperative days when water retention is maximal secondary to the stress of operation.

The underlying pathophysiology of this condition is the abnormal expansion of all body fluids owing to excess water. In contrast to excess infusion of salt solutions in which volume increases but tonicity of the extracellular compartment remains unchanged, *water alone* not only increases the volume of this compartment but correspondingly decreases the concentration of the extracellular ions. The resulting hypotonicity of the extracellular space relative to the tonicity of the intracellular compartment causes a net diffusion of water into the cells until both compartments are isosmotic. Thus, an increase in volume occurs in both the extracellular and intracellular compartments at the expense of a decrease in ionic concentrations. Hyponatremia then ensues even though the total body content of sodium may be normal or even increased.

At least three clinical situations either separately or in concert may give rise to hyponatremia. The first is the inappropriate replacement of body salt losses by infusing water alone. This common error most frequently occurs in patients who are losing large amounts of electrolyte-rich fluids via vomiting, diarrhea, or prolonged nasogastric suction. Rather than receiving solutions containing adequate amounts of sodium and chloride, patients are given either some hypotonic salt solution or water in the form of five per cent dextrose solution. Although five per cent dextrose in water is virtually isotonic with plasma at the time of administration, the carbohydrate is rapidly metabolized, leaving the remaining free water to dilute and expand both the extracellular and intracellular fluid compartments.

Hyponatremia may also occur in the patient with head injury or preexisting renal disease. The hyponatremia associated with head injury is probably due to an inappropriate secretion of antidiuretic hormone with excessive water retention, while the defect in the patient with renal disease is due to a renal tubular dysfunction resulting in an inability to concentrate the excreted urine appropriately. Although uncommon in the young and middle-aged adult, this salt-losing nephropathy is frequently seen in the elderly patient and may present a difficult management problem if not suspected. Often the usual indices of renal function (i.e., blood urea nitrogen or creatinine) are normal even though the urine of these patients may contain large amounts of sodium (100 to 150 mEq per l). Since little or no sodium is excreted in the urine of patients with normal renal function and hyponatremia, the diagnosis of hypotonic volume expansion should be entertained in the elderly patient receiving what appears to be adequate amounts of balanced salt solution but who also has symptoms of hyponatremia (see below). Salt restriction, which is commonly imposed on the geriatric patient because of apparent cardiovascular disease, may severely aggravate this condition.

Finally, hyponatremia may occur from one of two metabolic processes: the water of oxidation from utilization of nutrient fuel and mobilization of water from cellular catabolism. More than one liter of salt-free water may be produced from the oxidation of 1 kg of fat, while 750 ml of cellular water may be mobilized following the oxidation of 1 kg of lean body mass. Hydrated living protein contains between 73 and 82 per cent water. As many as 750 gm of tissue may be catabolized daily following a major operation and thereby produce approximately 500 ml of endogenous water. If adequate caloric intake is not maintained, excessive quantities of cellular water may ensue, decreasing the requirements via exogenous infusion.

Although hyponatremia is the laboratory hallmark of hypotonic volume expansion, the detrimental aspect of this condition is not the low sodium concentration per se. Rather, it is the volume increase in the intracellular fluid compartment. As water moves intracellularly, the cells swell. For most cells this poses no particular problem, but when brain cells swell, an increase in intracranial pressure will eventually ensue. This occurs because the brain is enclosed in a confined space with a relatively fixed capacity. As excess water accumulates, the volume of the intracellular space likewise increases, producing a state of severe *water intoxication*. Clinically, this state may manifest itself by a variety of signs and symptoms, including confusion, apathy, weakness, nausea, and vomiting. If not corrected, the water excess may ultimately progress to a state of severe muscle twitching, convulsions, stupor, and even death. Because fluid intake is greater than fluid output, weight gain is always present. Blood pressure is usually normal but may be elevated if a significant increase in intracranial pressure occurs.

In patients with normal renal function, symptomatic hyponatremia does not commonly occur even though the serum sodium concentration may fall as low as 120 mEq per l. In this circumstance, simple restriction of water intake may be all that is needed to correct the abnormality, as the insensible daily water loss will raise the sodium concentration and reverse the fluid derangements in the intracellular and extracellular compartments. In situations in which hypotonic volume expansion is sufficient to cause clinical symptoms or in which the serum sodium level is severely decreased, water restriction alone may not suffice, and efforts should be employed to raise the serum sodium concentration to 130 mEq per l or above. Because this condition develops slowly, correction toward normal should be deliberate, cautious, and without haste. Since normal saline is hypertonic to a patient with hyponatremia, it will usually suffice in correcting this sodium abnormality. Nevertheless, hypertonic saline (three per cent) should not be withheld if it is required. When employed, it should be administered in small amounts of a few hundred ml at a time. Except in very unusual circumstances, this solution should not be given to patients with marginal cardiac reserve.

Hypernatremia

In contrast to hyponatremia, hypernatremia is encountered less commonly in the postoperative surgical patient. When it does occur, it is always accompanied by a decrease in the volume of the intracellular fluid compartment owing to the increased osmolality of the extracellular space, which tends to draw water from the cells until an isosmotic equilibrium has been established between the intracellular and extracellular compartments.

A variety of disorders may give rise to this condition, but a particularly common etiology in the postoperative period is fever in the septic patient. Depending upon the degree and duration of the temperature elevation, several liters of salt-free water may be lost daily through the evaporation of sweat. Patients with tracheostomies may also develop this problem, because if inspired air is not properly humidified, as many as 1.5 to 2 liters of water may be lost per day through insensible loss.

Patients with renal disease or those who have sustained injuries to the central nervous system or who have undergone intracranial surgery are also at high risk to develop hypernatremia. In both situations, extremely large volumes of solute-poor urine may be excreted daily. In the renal disease commonly encountered in the elderly patient, the basic defect is decreased responsiveness of the renal tubule to antidiuretic hormone, making it impossible to excrete a concentrated urine. This inability to reabsorb water by the renal tubule may also occur in the postoperative patient with renal failure, particularly high-output renal failure. In neurologic disease, a true diabetes insipidus exists since the defect in renal tubular water absorption results from a deficiency of circulating antidiuretic hormone.

In addition to these endogenous etiologies, a variety of iatrogenic causes of hypernatremia exist. Solute loading, for whatever reason, may give rise to hypernatremia. Tube feedings, if not diluted with adequate amounts of water, may precipitate a tremendous extracellular water loss through renal solute diuresis. Not only will a decrease in circulating blood volume result, but also a severe extracellular hypernatremia will ensue with its detrimental effects on the hydration of cells. A similar condition may develop if hypertonic saline is infused too rapidly to replace massive sodium losses or to promote the excretion of excess body fluids.

A particularly unique water loss syndrome not infrequently encountered in the postoperative patient is nonketotic hyperosmolar dehydration. Occasionally observed in the patient with moderate to severe diabetes alone but more commonly encountered in the individual receiving intravenous hyperalimentation, this syndrome is characterized by severe dehydration induced by the diuresis and glycosuria secondary to the high glucose concentrations in the serum. The biochemical profile is one of hyperglycemia, often with blood sugars as high as 1000 mg per 100 ml, and hypernatremia. The cerebral intracellular dehydration induced by the osmotic diuresis associated with glycosuria may precipitate a variety of neurologic symptoms, which often result in coma and death if not promptly corrected.

The clinical manifestations of free water loss depend upon the osmolality of the extracellular space and the accompanying intracellular dehydration. Because this condition often develops insidiously, symptoms may appear late. Some degree of thirst is usually present, but in the elderly patient even this finding may be absent. Irritability and restlessness are common. As the disease process continues, disorientation develops, which may eventually result in coma, convulsions, and even death. The pathogenesis of this sequence of events is at best only poorly understood but appears to be related to the decrease in volume of the cells of the central nervous system. As water diffuses from the brain cells to the hypertonic extracellular fluid compartment, the resultant decrease in intracellular volume causes a corresponding decrease in intracranial pressure. The surrounding intracranial vessels may then dilate and eventually tear or rupture. The observation that cerebral hemorrhage is a frequent finding in patients dying of hypernatremia supports this hypothesis.

Owing to the potentially dire outcome of hypernatremia, every effort should be made to correct this condition as soon as it is suspected. Serum sodium concentrations above 160 mEq per l are particularly dangerous and associated with a significant mortality. Tantamount to any effective treatment is correction of the underlying pathologic process. Thus, fever should be lysed, the tracheostomy properly humidified, insulin added to hypertonic glucose infusions, the tonicity of tube feedings decreased or supplemented with adequate amounts of water, and Pitressin injected for control of diabetes insipidus. To correct the hypertonicity of the body fluids, adequate volumes of water as five per cent glucose solution intravenously or water by mouth, if the patient can drink, should be administered to restore electrolyte concentrations to normal and to maintain adequate urine volumes. The rate of correction will depend on the rate at which water was initially lost. In most instances, one to two days of fluid administration will be required before the serum sodium concentration reverts to normal.

Potassium Abnormalities

In contrast to sodium metabolism, in which a variety of exquisite neurohumoral and renal mechanisms are initiated postoperatively to maintain normal body stores, the kidneys continue to excrete large amounts of potassium (30 to 60 mEq per l) daily in spite of inadequate replacement. In fact, during the stress imposed by a major surgical procedure, urinary losses of potassium are often greatly increased. It is not surprising, therefore, that the most common potassium abnormality encountered in the postoperative period is *hypokalemia*. In most instances, this potassium deficiency results from either the prolonged administration of potassium-free intravenous solutions or the inappropriate replacement of daily potassium losses, particularly those resulting from the gastrointestinal tract due to vomiting, diarrhea, or prolonged nasogastric suction. In rare situations, a potassium-losing nephropathy may lead to excessive potassium losses. This latter etiology is particularly important to remember in the patient who develops postoperative renal failure, as the diuretic phase of recovery from acute tubular necrosis is often characterized by renal wastage of the potassium ion.

Since adequate stores of body potassium are crucial for the maintenance of normal muscle (skeletal, smooth, and cardiac) contractility, every effort should be made to replace incurred daily losses. In this way, serious potassium depletion can be prevented. Only in the early postoperative period (day of operation and first postoperative day), when the trauma of operation has mobilized considerable amounts of intracellular potassium, is the exogenous replacement of this ion unwarranted. Subsequent to this high catabolic period, daily supplementation becomes necessary. If the kidneys are functioning normally, potassium should be administered in amounts of 60 to 100 mEq daily to replace the gastric and urinary losses and should be tapered accordingly as oral alimentation is resumed.

Patients with potassium deficiencies commonly exhibit neuromuscular and cardiac disturbances. Depending upon the duration of the deficiency, the level of the serum potassium, the extent of the intracellular potassium deficit, the rate at which the serum potassium has changed, and the associated acid-base imbalances (potassium tends to move into cells during alkalotic states), symptoms may range from mild muscular weakness and paresthesias to flaccid paralysis. Usually, however, manifestations rarely develop until the serum potassium concentration has fallen below 3.0 mEq per l.

Of particular note are the cardiovascular effects of potassium deficiency. Hypotension, bradycardia, and cardiac arrhythmias may all develop when intracellular potassium falls and are heralded by the electrocardiographic abnormalities of flat or inverted T waves, prominent U waves, and depressed S–T segments. Of special importance is the considerable enhancement of digitalis toxicity by even modest degrees of potassium deficiency in patients receiving this drug.

Once hypokalemia is diagnosed, care must be taken in correcting the potassium deficit since aggressive compensatory therapy always risks creating a hyperkalemic state. It is important to insure that renal function is adequate before administering potassium. Except in unusual circumstances (serum potassium less than 2.0 mEq per l), hypokalemia is not an emergency and can be corrected over a 24- to 48-hour period. Since administered potassium must traverse the tiny extracellular pool before replenishing the intracellular compartment, rapid correction is usually not possible. If possible, oral therapy is the desired approach. Dietary supplementation with potassium-rich foods (oranges, bananas, and other fruits) coupled with enteric coated potassium chloride (KC1) tablets, when necessary, usually suffices. If intravenous therapy is needed, potassium chloride should be used. The rate of administration is determined by the existing potassium deficit but in most instances should not exceed 150 to 200 mEq per day or 10 to 15 mEq per hour. During potassium replacement, continuous electrocardiographic monitoring and frequent serum potassium determinations are mandatory. Once the estimated deficits have been replaced and the serum potassium has returned to normal, maintenance replacement can be resumed.

In contrast to hypokalemia, *hyperkalemia* is distinctly uncommon in the postoperative period and usually indicates some degree of renal impairment. Although overaggressive potassium infusion and metabolic acidosis, for whatever reason, may give rise to mild degrees of hyperkalemia, prolonged and markedly elevated serum potassium levels suggest a concomitant abnormality in renal function. As with hypokalemia, the detrimental effect of elevated serum potassium is on myocardial function and may result in bradycardia, hypotension, ventricular fibrillation, and cardiac arrest. Characteristic electrocardiographic manifestations include peaked T waves, depressed S–T segments, prolonged P–R intervals, diminished P waves, and widened QRS complexes.

In contrast to hypokalemia, which seldom is an emergency, hyperkalemia, particularly when the serum potassium level is greater than 7 mEq per l, may prove fatal if not corrected rapidly. Treatment includes the abrupt cessation of all potassium intake with simultaneous correction of the underlying cause. If the potassium level is dangerously high, emergency measures may become necessary to correct the hyperkalemia. An intravenous infusion of hypertonic dextrose (50 ml of 50 per cent dextrose over 30 minutes) together with regular insulin (10 to 25 units) will lower the extracellular potassium temporarily by promoting its intracellular transport. If acidosis is a contributing etiologic factor, the infusion of sodium bicarbonate will rapidly lower the serum potassium level. Since calcium counteracts the toxic effects of hyperkalemia on the heart, the intravenous infusion of calcium gluconate (5 to 10 ml of 10 per cent solution over two minutes) may also prove helpful. However, if the patient is receiving digitalis, calcium should not be given, as the combination of these two drugs may instead accentuate the cardiotoxic effects of hyperkalemia.

A long-term means of controlling hyperkalemia is to administer a cation exchange resin orally or by enema. The resin binds potassium in the intestine in exchange for sodium. Combined with sorbitol, it enhances the rate of potassium excretion by inducing osmotic diarrhea. The most common resin currently used is sodium polystyrene sulfonate (Kayexalate) in a dose of 40 to 80 gm per day. Although these measures may initially prove satisfactory, some form of dialysis may ultimately become necessary if the hyperkalemia is a manifestation of renal failure.

DISORDERS OF ACID-BASE BALANCE

Acidosis

Acidosis is the most important acid-base disorder encountered in the postoperative period because of the potentially devastating effects that acidosis may have on the cardiovascular system. At least three distinct effects have been identified and include (1) decreased myocardial contractibility, causing a reduction in cardiac output; (2) decreased responsiveness of the peripheral vasculature to circulating catecholamines, which causes systemic hypotension; and (3) increased refractoriness of the fibrillating heart to defibrillation, making efforts at cardiac resuscitation unusually difficult. Although acidosis occurs in response to a wide variety of etiologic factors, the most common postoperative causes include pulmonary insufficiency, poor tissue perfusion leading to lactic acidosis, impairment of renal function, diabetes mellitus, and loss of alkali via gastrointestinal secretions.

Regardless of the magnitude of the operation, every effort should be made to insure satisfactory postoperative ventilation. Any factor that may predispose to depressed pulmonary ventilation, such as airway obstruction, atelectasis, hypoventilation due to incisional pain, pneumonia, pleural effusion, or restriction of diaphragmatic movement by abdominal distention, can lead to *respiratory acidosis* and should be corrected. At particular risk for development of this condition are patients with preexisting lung disease, such as emphysema, pulmonary fibrosis, chronic bronchitis, bronchiectasis, and chronic pulmonary hypertension. In these subjects, strict attention to tracheobronchial hygiene is mandatory. Deep breathing and coughing, suction of retained tracheobronchial secretions, humidification of air to prevent inspissation of secretions, and the avoidance of oversedation are all important measures to insure adequate ventilation.

Recognition of respiratory acidosis is often difficult, particularly in the early postoperative period. The common signs of irritability, twitching, hypertension, and tachycardia due to the increasing hypercapnia and inadequate ventilation are often attributed to the residual effects of anesthesia or postoperative pain. If treatment is not rendered expeditiously, precious time may be lost as the acidosis worsens and its detrimental effect on cardiac and vascular smooth muscle accrues. Thus, in any patient with the clinical findings mentioned before, a blood gas analysis should be obtained immediately to determine the pH, the arterial oxygen tension, and the presence or absence of arterial hypercapnia. In acute respiratory acidosis, the pH is usually 7.35 or less. As renal compensation occurs, however, bicarbonate is retained by the kidneys so that the pH may be relatively normal in the more chronic form. In either situation, the arterial PCO_2 is always elevated, indicating pulmonary hypoventilation. Whether the arterial PO_2 is depressed as well will depend upon the inspired oxygen concentration and the efficiency of gas exchange in the alveoli. Patients who become hypercapnic while breathing room air are always hypoxic, while those who are hypercapnic while receiving supplementary oxygen may have relatively normal arterial oxygen levels.

The treatment of respiratory acidosis consists of measures to improve alveolar ventilation. If the lungs are normal and the hypoventilation is due to accidental oversedation or accompanying head injury with depression of the respiratory center, temporary ventilatory support following endotracheal intubation may be all that is required. In patients with chronic pulmonary disease, long-term ventilatory support may prove helpful. If the pulmonary reserve is particularly compromised, elective tracheostomy may be especially beneficial at the time of operation to obviate difficulties with postoperative ventilation. In any case, the prevention and treatment of respiratory acidosis are the same, namely, an aggressive approach to pulmonary care to insure the optimal functioning of all available alveoli.

A variety of *metabolic* disorders may also lead to *acidosis*. Diabetes mellitus, not infrequently observed in the surgical patient, may produce a severe acidosis in the postoperative period if not recognized and not appropriately treated. This endocrine disorder, characterized by a defect in normal glucose metabolism, utilizes the body's own endogenous fat and protein to provide calories necessary for energy production. In the process of such catabolism, acidosis results from the accumulation of acid byproducts (ketone bodies), reducing both the plasma bicarbonate level and the blood pH. As the energy demands of the body increase, fat and protein are further catabolized and acidosis is compounded. Concomitantly, there is a rise in the blood sugar that ultimately spills over into the urine, causing osmotic diuresis and dehydration. If not corrected with adequate administration of insulin, bicarbonate, and fluid (usually hypotonic salt solutions), a severe extracellular fluid deficit may ensue, and the acidosis may approach lethal levels.

Renal impairment, if sufficiently severe, may result in metabolic acidosis. Since the kidneys normally play an important role in the maintenance of acid-base balance through resorption of bicarbonate and excretion of nitrogenous waste products and inorganic acids such as phosphate and sulfate, renal damage may result in a loss of these vital functions. Accumulation of these acids during renal failure results in acidosis, but in most instances, no specific therapy for the acidosis per se will be required. However, great care should be exercised to restrict potassium and volume replacement, since hyperkalemia and fluid overload are commonly encountered in states of renal dysfunction. If these relatively simple measures are not satisfactory, hemodialysis may prove necessary.

Loss of alkali from the gastrointestinal tract may cause acute or chronic metabolic acidosis. Although diarrhea is the most common etiology of metabolic acidosis in the preoperative period, small bowel obstruction, prolonged suction of gastrointestinal secretions from long intestinal tubes (such as Cantor or Miller-Abbott tubes), and biliary, pancreatic, and small bowel fistulas are the most frequently encountered causes in the postoperative patient. Correction of acidosis in these disorders is usually uncomplicated as long as fluid and electrolyte losses are replaced with adequate volumes of balanced salt solutions. Appropriate amounts of potassium and bicarbonate should be added to these intravenous solutions to replace potassium deficits and restore blood-buffering capacity to normal.

Lactic acidosis secondary to circulatory failure is a particularly common form of acidosis confronting the surgeon. Caused by inadequate tissue perfusion, this condition occurs in a variety of low-flow states of either cardiac, septic, or hemorrhagic origin. As tissues become hypoxic due to failure of peripheral perfusion, energy must be derived from anaerobic glycolysis rather than from normal aerobic metabolic pathways. During anaerobic metabolism, tissue lactic acid levels rise, resulting in a further decrease in blood pH. As lactate levels mount, a deteriorating clinical course of increasing acidosis, decreasing tissue perfusion due to the detrimental effects of acidosis on the cardiovascular system, and further hypoxia ensues. Cardiac arrest will ultimately result if adequate circulation is not restored.

The therapeutic approach to this devastating situation includes restoration of adequate tissue perfusion with proper volume replacement and correction of the acidosis. If the underlying cause of shock is hemorrhagic, appropriate blood replacement should be given. In addition, a balanced salt solution should also be infused to replace the extracellular fluid deficits. This is particularly important in patients in whom the etiology of the inadequate perfusion is due to some other cause. Ringer's lactate solution is especially useful for this purpose. As adequate tissue perfusion is restored with appropriate volumes of this solution, tissue lactate levels decrease (Ringer's solution does not accentuate the lactic acidosis). Although the blood pH also reverts toward normal, supplemental infusions of a buffering agent such as sodium bicarbonate may be needed to completely restore the blood bicarbonate to normal levels. Efforts should be made to maintain the plasma bicarbonate level at about 15 mEq per l. Since about 2 mEq of sodium bicarbonate per liter of extracellular fluid are required to raise the plasma bicarbonate by 1 mEq per l, a patient whose bicarbonate is 12 mEq per l and who weighs 70 kg will require about 84 mEq of sodium bicarbonate to restore the plasma bicarbonate concentration to 15 mEq per l ($70 \times 0.2 \times 3 \times 2 = 84$). However, restoration of the circulation must be the primary thrust of all efforts to treat the metabolic acidosis associated with shock.

Alkalosis

In contrast to the potentially lethal effects of acidosis, *alkalosis* is usually well tolerated and is, in fact, the most common acid-base abnormality encountered in the early postoperative period. This trend toward alkalosis results from the interaction of one or more of four etiologic components frequently present following operation. Post-traumatic aldosteronism, stimulated by volume reduction during operation, tends to produce extracellular alkalosis through renal inhibition of sodium bicarbonate excretion and excessive excretion of potassium. Nasogastric suction, frequently required to manage the ileus accompanying abdominal operation, adds to this alkalotic state by removing hydrogen ions. When large quantities of blood are transfused, the infused citrate is oxidized to bicarbonate, which further favors alkalosis. Finally, hyperventilation secondary to apprehension, pain, or respiratory therapy is frequently present postoperatively and is the most common cause of alkalosis.

In most instances, the mild alkalosis following operation is of trivial importance and requires no specific treatment. *Respiratory alkalosis* secondary to hyperventilation is usually short-lived and abates as the postoperative pain lessens and the anxiety and apprehension associated with the operation resolve. If postoperative ventilatory support is required, however, care must be employed to prevent a more severe form of this condition. Attempts to raise the PO_2 in the hypoxic patient by increasing the respiratory rate or delivering large minute volumes can significantly lower the arterial PCO_2. The resulting hypocapnia may produce a profound hypokalemia as the extracellular potassium moves intracellularly. The digitalized patient is particularly sensitive to this form of alkalosis, and a state of digitalis intoxication may ensue with accompanying cardiac arrhythmias. Severe central nervous system disorders, including coma, convulsions, and occasionally death, may result from the cerebral vasoconstriction induced by the hypocapnia. The patient with compromised cerebral perfusion due to obstructive arterial disease, such as carotid artery atherosclerosis, is especially at risk in this situation. Thus, the management of patients requiring mechanical ventilation should include frequent assessment of arterial blood gases and appropriate adjustment of the ventilatory pattern as needed. Under no circumstances should the arterial PCO_2 be allowed to fall below 30 mm Hg.

Alkalosis due to metabolic disorders may also arise in the postoperative period. Unintentional overadministration of buffering agents, such as sodium bicarbonate and sodium lactate, may elevate the plasma bicarbonate level and raise the blood pH. As previously mentioned, transfused blood may also initiate alkalosis through the metabolic conversion of citrate to bicarbonate. Except under unusual circumstances, these alkalotic conditions do not pose particular problems to the postoperative patient since they are corrected spontaneously if renal function is normal.

The loss of gastric juice through vomiting or nasogastric suction is a different matter. In this circumstance, the chloride deficit and alkalosis resulting from hydrogen ion loss are not easily corrected by the kidneys since the hormonally dependent sodium retention and increased renal potassium excretion override the ability of the kidneys to excrete bicarbonate and retain hydrogen ions to restore acid-base equilibrium. As gastric losses continue, the kidneys attempt to maintain intravascular volume and osmolality by further increasing the tubular reabsorption of sodium. This results in a selective excretion of potassium in the urine to promote more efficient reabsorption of sodium, compounding the loss of potassium already incurred by vomiting or nasogastric suction. Since bicarbonate is reabsorbed with the sodium, the existing alkalotic state is further aggravated. As gastric losses continue and volume loss becomes more pronounced, sodium reabsorption by the kidney becomes virtually complete as does bicarbonate reabsorption. In an attempt to neutralize the alkaline blood, potassium moves intracellularly in exchange for hydrogen ions. This, coupled with persistent loss of potassium in the urine, results in a severe extracellular depletion of this ion. To conserve whatever potassium is left, the kidneys now reabsorb sodium in exchange for hydrogen ions rather than potassium. Not only does this further aggravate the alkalotic state but also it results in the paradoxically acid urine often seen in patients with prolonged metabolic alkalosis.

As is true with most complications, the best therapy for hypochloremic, hypokalemic metabolic alkalosis is its prevention, but once established, it must be treated by both volume and electrolyte replacement. This is usually accomplished best with a sodium chloride solution. Lactated Ringer's solution should not be given, since an excess of bicarbonate (lactate is metabolically converted to bicarbonate) is already present in patients with this syndrome. In most circumstances, either normal or half-normal saline solution will adequately replace the volume and salt losses. When volume repletion has been achieved, tubular reabsorption of sodium will decrease, allowing the kidneys to excrete the excess bicarbonate. Since most patients with metabolic alkalosis are potassium depleted, supplementation of this ion is also needed. Potassium should be given as the chloride salt since potassium lactate or citrate (both of which are metabolized to bicarbonate) will aggravate alkalosis. Until normal stores of total body potassium have been replenished, as much as 150 to 250 mEq of this ion may be required daily.

REFERENCES

Kinney, J. M., and Moore, F. D.: Surgical metabolism in metabolism of body fluids. *In* Bland, J. H. (ed.): Clinical Metabolism of Body Water and Electrolytes. Philadelphia, W. B. Saunders Co., 1963, pp. 337–359.

Moore, F. D., Olesen, K. H., McMurrey, J. D., Parker, H. V., Ball, M. R., and Boyden, C. M.: Body Cell Mass and Its Supporting Environment: Body Composition in Health and Disease. Philadelphia, W. B. Saunders Co., 1963.

Randall, H. T.: Fluid, electrolyte and acid-base balance. Surg. Clin. North Am., 56:1019, 1976.

Shires, G. T., and Canizaro, P. C.: Fluid, electrolyte and nutritional management of the surgical patient. *In* Schwartz, S. I. (ed.): Principles of Surgery, 2nd ed. New York, McGraw-Hill Book Co., 1974, pp. 65–96.

Skillman, J. J.: Disturbances of body fluids, ions and acid-base balance. *In* Skillman, J. J. (ed.): Intensive Care. Boston, Little, Brown and Co., 1975, pp. 63–127.

Smithline, N., and Gardner, K. D.: Gaps — anionic and osmolal. J.A.M.A., 236:1594, 1976.

4

Enteral Nutrition

HENRY THOMAS RANDALL

The majority of hospitalized surgical patients receive most of their nutrition via the enteral route. This is the safest, most effective, and least expensive way to provide nutrition for all patients. When all or even a portion of the gastrointestinal tract is functional, it should be used!

The purpose of this chapter is to describe the importance of enteral nutrition for surgical patients, to define the kinds of patients who require particular attention to nutrition, and to illustrate how enteral nutrition can be used effectively alone or in sequence with parenteral nutrition, complementing, supplementing, and, as soon as possible, replacing the parenteral route.

Most well-nourished and reasonably healthy patients at all ages who are subjected to a single major operation or trauma without complications do well postoperatively. A relatively simple program of parenteral infusion provides water, electrolytes, and dextrose. This prevents dehydration and electrolyte imbalance, and the dextrose reduces body protein catabolism by sparing some of the protein otherwise required for gluconeogenesis during acute starvation.

Unless the abdomen has been opened surgically, postoperative recovery from anesthesia and acute wound pain is usually sufficient within 24 to 48 hours to permit oral intake, and shortly thereafter the patient can be encouraged to increase his or her intake sufficiently so that adequate amounts of calories, protein, minerals, and trace elements may be obtained. Some vitamin supplementation is frequently indicated, particularly in children and elderly patients.

Patients who undergo abdominal operations tend to progress more slowly, particularly those whose operations involve the upper abdomen or the retroperitoneal area. Postoperative ileus following uncomplicated abdominal surgery usually has a relatively short duration. Postoperatively, the stomach and the colon tend to be affected most, with reduced and ineffective peristalsis lasting for three or four days, while the small bowel resumes peristalsis quite rapidly and is usually capable of absorbing water, electrolytes, glucose, and amino acids within one or two days. In such patients, peripheral infusions of five per cent dextrose in water in varying volumes with the additions of appropriate amounts of sodium and potassium chloride are usually sufficient. The use of dilute mixtures of amino acids with dextrose and electrolytes given by peripheral vein may be indicated if significant delay in return of gastrointestinal tract function occurs.

With the return of peristaltic sounds and passage of flatus, enteral nutrition may be started. Usually, clear fluids of restricted volume are ordered initially, followed by liquid diets that often contain large amounts of milk. This must be modified if the patient has lactose intolerance. If the patient soon ingests solid foods somewhat comparable to his or her normal diet, satisfactory progress of enteral nutrition is assumed to have occurred.

Body reserves of fat and the expenditure of four to 10 per cent of metabolically active protein, largely from skeletal muscle, provide the energy reserve necessary to sustain most patients for a week to 10 days during the usual inadequate calorie and protein intake without demonstrably serious consequences. Loss of one-half to one pound of body weight per day of hospitalization is average for an adult patient. Adequate calorie and protein intake is seldom achieved before discharge. Convalescence at home with home-cooked foods and tender loving care, for those fortunate enough to return to such an environment, soon restores depleted protein and body strength. For others, convalescence is not as easy or as quick.

In contrast to the well-nourished and reasonably healthy patients who constitute the majority of civilian surgical practice, a significant minority of surgical patients require as much careful attention to their nutritional program as to their operative procedure. These patients are of two types: those who preoperatively are severely debilitated as the result of chronic or subacute disease or chronic malnutrition, and those who as the result of severe trauma, sepsis, or complications of surgery are unable or unwilling to eat adequately for a prolonged period of time. Examples of major preoperative debility include patients with severe inflammatory disease of the large or small bowel, carcinoma of the stomach or colon, chronic pancreatitis, chronic infection, or some forms of liver, kidney, or heart disease. All have in common a substantial weight loss with severe reductions in their skeletal muscle mass and total body protein. Most have an increase in the relative proportion of extracellular fluid and total sodium despite quite common hyponatremia (Moore et al., 1963).

More acute problems occur in patients with acute or subacute pancreatitis, unresolved peritonitis, small bowel fistulas, abdominal trauma, major wound sepsis, retroperitoneal hematoma, major burns, and particularly in those who have sustained severe multiple trauma, including long bone or pelvic fractures. Many of these patients were healthy and well-nourished before the onset of their acute problem, but because of the major catabolic response to trauma or sepsis and simultaneous partial starvation, the demands on fat and particularly protein are so great that available reserves are exhausted within two to four weeks. Death will occur as a result of muscle weakness, respiratory failure, or sepsis unless these nutritionally depleted individuals are provided with fuel in sufficient quantity and of proper quality to spare essential body cell mass.

EVALUATION OF NUTRITIONAL STATUS

Assessment of the nutritional status of surgical patients, preferably preoperatively, or whenever responsibility for management is assumed, is essential to proper treatment.

ACUTE FAILURE OF ADEQUATE NUTRITION — THE MOST COMMON PROBLEM IN SURGICAL PATIENTS

Patients with multiple trauma or burns and patients who develop postoperative complications interfering with resumption of oral intake within one week should receive particular consideration of their nutritional status. In the past, attention was focused primarily on the acute needs for resuscitation and wound management and not on the nutritional status of burn and trauma patients. Routine postoperative fluids and electrolytes, very low in calories and often without protein or amino acids, were administered to patients, who then developed severe complications. Recognizing now that burn and trauma patients lose significant amounts of essential body protein as the result of stress and semistarvation, vigorous and effective attention to their nutritional needs is required.

PATIENTS WITH SUBACUTE WEIGHT LOSS

Loss of weight in the absence of deliberate and controlled dieting is probably the most significant clinical sign of potentially depleted body cell mass in preoperative patients. Inadvertent weight loss of five to 10 per cent of body weight over the preceding three months may signify significant protein malnutrition. More than 10 per cent weight loss in that period is evidence of a major problem. A complete history should include a dietary history, preferably taken by a dietitian experienced in clinical nutrition. Members of the patient's family are often helpful in describing recent dietary habits.

Chronic Illness

Frequently, patients with chronic illnesses such as inflammatory bowel disease, pulmonary insufficiency, or congestive heart failure are substantially below normal weight for respective heights and ages and have a small body cell mass. Some of these patients may actually gain weight owing to sodium and water retention while the protein depletion process continues.

Muscle Atrophy — A Sign of Protein Malnutrition

Clinical evidence of body cell mass loss can be obtained by inspection. Temporalis muscle atrophy produces a characteristic depression of the skin above the zygomatic arch. Thenar and hypothenar eminences of the hands become flattened with intrinsic muscle mass loss. Perhaps most characteristic is the decreased size of the thighs and the legs as these large muscle masses are resorbed. The patient or spouse is a good source of information about such changes.

Anthropomorphic measurements are frequently used in assessing the nutritional status of populations and more recently have been applied to hospitalized patients (Blackburn et al., 1977). Of the series of evaluations proposed, height and weight for age and sex, rate of weight loss with time, creatinine excretion, hemoglobin, and serum albumin concentration are some of the most useful indices in our clinical experience.

A level of hemoglobin below 11.5 gm per cent in women and 12.5 gm per cent in men in the absence of evidence of external blood loss may indicate malnutrition. Iron and iron-binding capacity or plasma transferrin measurements are useful if hemoglobin values are low. Hemoglobin tends to fall sooner than plasma albumin in patients with decreased protein synthesis or increased protein loss.

Plasma albumin of less than 3.5 gm per cent on two or more determinations indicates an abnormality, and liver function tests should be performed. Plasma albumin below 3.0 gm per cent indicates decreased protein synthesis, increased turnover or loss, or both.

Creatinine excretion in urine is a function of muscle mass and of its metabolism. We use 20 to 24 mg per kg per 24 hours as normal for males and 16 to 20 mg per kg per 24 hours for females. All that is required for this measurement is a carefully collected 24-hour urine sample. The total volume passed should be recorded accurately, and the patient should begin and end the 24-hour period with an empty bladder; a plasma creatinine determination should be drawn during this 24-hour period. With a normal plasma creatinine level, 24-hour excretion below the expected normal range indicates hypometabolism of muscle and suggests a diminished skeletal muscle mass. Creatinine clearance as a measure of renal function can be calculated from the same specimens. In the absence of sepsis, creatinine production and excretion are decreased with time in patients on total parenteral nutrition and on chemically defined diets. Creatinine excretion is, of course, markedly decreased in the presence of acute renal insufficiency.

Estimation of Nitrogen Balance

In seriously ill patients, estimates of caloric and protein intake and nitrogen loss are as important as conventional intake and output records of fluid balance.

Exact measurement of nitrogen balance is a highly complex procedure, and even in a well-organized metabolic unit the figures are subject to distressing cumulative variation. However, a clinically useful estimate of nitrogen balance can easily be obtained. For example, intake is precisely known if the patient is receiving total parenteral nutrition or a chemically defined diet. Additionally, precise information on the label of most commercially prepared liquid diets specifies nitrogen and protein content.

Hospital dietitians (R.D.) can make a quite accurate estimate of the total calorie, protein, fat, and carbohydrate intake of patients. Today, one or more registered dietitians are considered important members of nutrition teams or services in many hospitals.

Nitrogen loss can be estimated by measuring the *urine urea nitrogen* in carefully collected 24-hour urine specimens and adding to those measurements 3 gm per day for adult females and 4 gm per day for adult males (Blackburn et al., 1977). Exceptions are patients with diarrhea or bowel fistulas, for whom nitrogen content of large volumes of loss must also be measured.

Males: Urine urea N + 4 = N output.

Females: Urine urea N + 3 = N output.

A simple balance can be recorded as grams N intake minus grams N output.

With either parenteral or enteral nutrition, an objective is to keep net nitrogen loss below 6 to 8 gm a day at the peak of severe illness and to achieve a positive balance of about 4 gm a day as soon as possible. In our experience 45 to 50 kilocalories per kg body weight per day and 17 to 20 gm nitrogen as intravenous amino acids, or as enteral amino acids or protein, are necessary to achieve positive balance in seriously ill or septic patients. It may take several days to achieve these levels, either parenterally or through a combination of parenteral or enteral nutrition (Clowes et al., 1980). These levels can and should be sustained by enteral nutrition alone in most patients after a period of transition from TPN to enteral feeding.

The Metabolic Effects of Sepsis and Trauma

In Chapter 2, the metabolic response to injury and to sepsis is discussed in detail. The reader is referred to this chapter for a discussion of the importance of nutrition to survival in stressed patients.

In brief, trauma or sepsis induce the following changes:

1. An increase in energy requirements in an average adult male from a resting value of 1800 kilocalories per day to as high as 3500 kilocalories in sepsis and 4000 or more kilocalories in major burns;

2. elevation of blood glucose with a diabetic-type glucose tolerance curve and simultaneous elevated insulin levels with enhanced glucose utilization;

3. increased gluconeogenesis from protein, despite high insulin levels and blood glucose levels; accelerated loss of body cell mass above simple starvation; and

4. probable decreased protein synthesis, particularly with sepsis, including decreased immunocompetence.

These metabolic changes increase dramatically the necessity to provide optimal nutrition.

DISEASES AND CONDITIONS OF THE GASTROINTESTINAL TRACT AFFECTING ENTERAL NUTRITION

The common causes of dysfunction of the gastrointestinal tract in surgical patients are postoperative or post-traumatic ileus; intestinal obstruction at all levels; ileus accompanying sepsis, particularly intra-

Table 4–1. FACTORS AFFECTING INGESTION, DIGESTION, AND ABSORPTION

---

1. MECHANICAL
   Ill-fitting dentures and edentulous jaws
   Trauma to face
   Fracture of jaw
   Obstruction to upper gastrointestinal tract due to cancer, inflammation, or stricture
   Small- or large-bowel obstruction
   Ileus due to sepsis or trauma
   Fistulas

2. FAILURE OF DIGESTION AND ABSORPTION
   Lumenal: Hepatobiliary disease, pancreatic insufficiency, jejunal diverticulae, blind loop syndrome, scleroderma
   Mucosal Disease: Celiac disease, tropical sprue, acute radiation enteritis, gluten sensitivity, lactose deficiency, specific amino acid absorption defects, agammaglobulinemia, nonspecific malabsorption
   Bowel Wall Disease: Regional enteritis, amyloid disease
   Lymphatic Disease: Whipple's disease, lymphangiectasis, lymphoma of bowel
   Vascular Disease: Atheromatous or embolic obstruction of arterial blood flow, small vessel disease (diabetes), arterial or venous thrombosis, late-stage radiation enteritis
   Metabolic Diseases: Zollinger-Ellison syndrome, carcinoid, thyrotoxicosis, hypopituitarism, metabolic effect of cancer of GI tract

3. DISEASES WITH INCREASED LOSSES
   Ulcerative colitis
   Short-gut syndrome
   Dumping syndrome
   Vagotomy diarrhea, diarrhea due to bacteria or parasites
   Osmotic catharsis

---

abdominal sepsis; bleeding into the gastrointestinal tract; and gastrointestinal fistulas, either enteroenteric or enterocutaneous. However, a wide variety of diseases and conditions can exist that prevent or decrease the effectiveness of enteral nutrition. These are summarized in Table 4–1.

USING THE GUT

ORALLY INGESTED DIETS

Diets and food habits vary widely, by geographic area, ethnic group, education, and economic status. In addition, considerable variation exists among individuals within a given geographic area or cultural group. There is no single pattern of diet that is necessary to achieve or maintain good nutrition.

However, with hospitalized patients a basic principle in providing nutrition for those who receive all or a part of their energy requirements by mouth is that the foods provided should be as nearly compatible with the patient's normal dietary habits as his or her medical or surgical condition permits. The foods provided should be served as attractively as possible with careful attention given to appearance, odor, taste, and temperature. The timing of meals and supplements should correspond insofar as possible with the patient's normal eating habits.

Occasionally for children, the elderly, and some patients with religious or other dietary restrictions, home-cooked foods brought into the hospital by family may provide the stimulus to eat that is essential to recovery. Such practices interfere with hospital routine and are usually difficult to achieve, but they may occasionally be necessary.

REGULAR DIET

Hospital regular diet is based on the Recommended Daily Dietary Allowances of the Food and Nutrition Board, National Academy of Sciences–National Research Council. The 1980 revision is shown in Tables 4–2 and 4–3. These recommendations include energy (kilocalories), protein, fat- and water-soluble vitamins, and minerals for infants, children in 3 age groups, and males and females separately by age groups from age 11 and for pregnant and lactating females. They are based on average height and weight for age and assume both a normal metabolic rate and average physical activity for well persons. The amount of protein recommended is probably well below the average protein intake. Most hospital regular diets provide 70 to 80 gm of protein, rather than 50 gm.

Most surgical patients for whom a regular diet is ordered are in the hospital for diagnostic evaluation or have undergone surgery on the extremities or body surface. A regular diet is inadequate in protein and calories for stressed patients, particularly those with burns and with fractures of long bones.

Table 4-2. FOOD AND NUTRITION BOARD, NATIONAL ACADEMY OF SCIENCES—NATIONAL RESEARCH COUNCIL RECOMMENDED DAILY DIETARY ALLOWANCES,[a] Revised 1980

Designed for the maintenance of good nutrition of practically all healthy people in the U.S.A.

	Age (years)	Weight (kg)	(lb)	Height (cm)	(in)	Protein (g)	Vita-min A (μg RE)[b]	Vita-min D (μg)[c]	Vita-min E (mg α-TE)[d]	Vita-min C (mg)	Thia-min (mg)	Ribo-flavin (mg)	Niacin (mg NE)[e]	Vita-min B6 (mg)	Fola-cin[f] (μg)	Vitamin B12 (μg)	Cal-cium (mg)	Phos-phorus (mg)	Mag-nesium (mg)	Iron (mg)	Zinc (mg)	Iodine (μg)
Infants	0.0–0.5	6	13	60	24	kg × 2.2	420	10	3	35	0.3	0.4	6	0.3	30	0.5[g]	360	240	50	10	3	40
	0.5–1.0	9	20	71	28	kg × 2.0	400	10	4	35	0.5	0.6	8	0.6	45	1.5	540	360	70	15	5	50
Children	1–3	13	29	90	35	23	400	10	5	45	0.7	0.8	9	0.9	100	2.0	800	800	150	15	10	70
	4–6	20	44	112	44	30	500	10	6	45	0.9	1.0	11	1.3	200	2.5	800	800	200	10	10	90
	7–10	28	62	132	52	34	700	10	7	45	1.2	1.4	16	1.6	300	3.0	800	800	250	10	10	120
Males	11–14	45	99	157	62	45	1000	10	8	50	1.4	1.6	18	1.8	400	3.0	1200	1200	350	18	15	150
	15–18	66	145	176	69	56	1000	10	10	60	1.4	1.7	18	2.0	400	3.0	1200	1200	400	18	15	150
	19–22	70	154	177	70	56	1000	7.5	10	60	1.5	1.7	19	2.2	400	3.0	800	800	350	10	15	150
	23–50	70	154	178	70	56	1000	5	10	60	1.4	1.6	18	2.2	400	3.0	800	800	350	10	15	150
	51+	70	154	178	70	56	1000	5	10	60	1.2	1.4	16	2.2	400	3.0	800	800	350	10	15	150
Females	11–14	46	101	157	62	46	800	10	8	50	1.1	1.3	15	1.8	400	3.0	1200	1200	300	18	15	150
	15–18	55	120	163	64	46	800	10	8	60	1.1	1.3	14	2.0	400	3.0	1200	1200	300	18	15	150
	19–22	55	120	163	64	44	800	7.5	8	60	1.1	1.3	14	2.0	400	3.0	800	800	300	18	15	150
	23–50	55	120	163	64	44	800	5	8	60	1.0	1.2	13	2.0	400	3.0	800	800	300	18	15	150
	51+	55	120	163	64	44	800	5	8	60	1.0	1.2	13	2.0	400	3.0	800	800	300	10	15	150
Pregnant						+30	+200	+5	+2	+20	+0.4	+0.3	+2	+0.6	+400	+1.0	+400	+400	+150	h	+5	+25
Lactating						+20	+400	+5	+3	+40	+0.5	+0.5	+5	+0.5	+100	+1.0	+400	+400	+150	h	+10	+50

[a] The allowances are intended to provide for individual variations among most normal persons as they live in the United States under usual environmental stresses. Diets should be based on a variety of common foods in order to provide other nutrients for which human requirements have been less well defined.

[b] Retinol equivalents. 1 retinol equivalent = 1 μg retinol or 6 μg β carotene.

[c] As cholecalciferol. 10 μg cholecalciferol = 400 IU of vitamin D.

[d] α-tocopherol equivalents. 1 mg d-α tocopherol = 1 α-TE.

[e] 1 NE (niacin equivalent) is equal to 1 mg of niacin or 60 mg of dietary tryptophan.

[f] The folacin allowances refer to dietary sources as determined by *Lactobacillus casei* assay after treatment with enzymes (conjugases) to make polyglutamyl forms of the vitamin available to the test organism.

[g] The recommended dietary allowance for vitamin B12 in infants is based on average concentration of the vitamin in human milk. The allowances after weaning are based on energy intake (as recommended by the American Academy of Pediatrics) and consideration of other factors, such as intestinal absorption.

[h] The increased requirement during pregnancy cannot be met by the iron content of habitual American diets nor by the existing iron stores of many women, therefore the use of 30-60 mg of supplemental iron is recommended. Iron needs during lactation are not substantially different from those of nonpregnant women, but continued supplementation of the mother for 2-3 months after parturition is advisable in order to replenish stores depleted by pregnancy.

Table 4–3. ESTIMATED SAFE AND ADEQUATE DAILY DIETARY
INTAKES OF SELECTED VITAMINS AND MINERALS[a]

		VITAMINS		
	AGE (YEARS)	Vitamin K (μg)	Biotin (μg)	Pantothenic Acid (mg)
Infants	0–0.5	12	35	2
	0.5–1	10–20	50	3
Children	1–3	15–30	65	3
and	4–6	20–40	85	3–4
adolescents	7–10	30–60	120	4–5
	11+	50–100	100–200	4–7
Adults		70–140	100–200	4–7

		TRACE ELEMENTS[b]					
	AGE (YEARS)	Copper (mg)	Manganese (mg)	Fluoride (mg)	Chromium (mg)	Selenium (mg)	Molybdenum (mg)
Infants	0–0.5	0.5–0.7	0.5–0.7	0.1–0.5	0.01–0.04	0.01–0.04	0.03–0.06
	0.5–1	0.7–1.0	0.7–1.0	0.2–1.0	0.02–0.06	0.02–0.06	0.04–0.08
Children	1–3	1.0–1.5	1.0–1.5	0.5–1.5	0.02–0.08	0.02–0.08	0.05–0.1
and	4–6	1.5–2.0	1.5–2.0	1.0–2.5	0.03–0.12	0.03–0.12	0.06–0.15
adolescents	7–10	2.0–2.5	2.0–3.0	1.5–2.5	0.05–0.2	0.05–0.2	0.10–0.3
	11+	2.0–3.0	2.5–5.0	1.5–2.5	0.05–0.2	0.05–0.2	0.15–0.5
Adults		2.0–3.0	2.5–5.0	1.5–4.0	0.05–0.2	0.05–0.2	0.15–0.5

		ELECTROLYTES		
	AGE (YEARS)	Sodium (mg)	Potassium (mg)	Chloride (mg)
Infants	0–0.5	115–350	350–925	275–700
	0.5–1	250–750	425–1275	400–1200
Children	1–3	325–975	550–1650	500–1500
and	4–6	450–1350	775–2325	700–2100
adolescents	7–10	600–1800	1000–3000	925–2775
	11+	900–2700	1525–4575	1400–4200
Adults		1100–3300	1875–5625	1700–5100

[a] Because there is less information on which to base allowances, these figures are not given in the main table of RDA and are provided here in the form of ranges of recommended intakes.

[b] Since the toxic levels for many trace elements may be only several times usual intakes, the upper levels for the trace elements given in this table should not be habitually exceeded.

Orders for a regular diet should include "mechanically soft" foods for patients who have difficulty in chewing because of inadequate dentition. Orders should include a notation regarding any existing food allergies. Large portions should be indicated for patients with a large body cell mass. Particular dietary habits and religious or other constraints should be noted, and dietary consultation should be requested to assist such patients to obtain adequate amounts of suitable foods. Patients should not be required to eat foods that they do not like or that give them discomfort, no matter how bland and seemingly innocuous the food may appear to be.

An example of the importance of an accurate dietary history for formulating a diet is lactose intolerance. Lactose deficiency in the mucosa of the small bowel results in failure to hydrolyze and absorb lactose, which is the normal sugar in milk. While five to 10 per cent of adults of Western European ancestry exhibit lactose intolerance, it occurs in 60 per cent of Ashkenazic Jews, 70 per cent of adult Negroes, and virtually all adult Orientals. Small amounts of lactose, 15 to 30 gm a day, are tolerated as milk in foods or beverages by most adults. This is the equivalent of one or two glasses of milk (up to 500 ml) a day. However, 50 gm of lactose a day acts as an osmotic cathartic in those persons who are lactose intolerant; bloating, gas, cramps, and diarrhea are frequent symptoms of intolerance. Children of lactose-sensitive groups develop intolerance early and cannot tolerate a high milk diet thereafter. The average American regular diet may contain as much as 50 gm of lactose (as one quart of milk) a day. Bland diets, high protein diets, blenderized tube feedings, and many full liquid diets contain whole milk, skim milk, or fat-free milk powder, all of which contain lactose. Some dietary supplements contain lactose; some commercially prepared liquid diets also contain lactose. Defined formula diets presently available do not contain lactose.

HIGH PROTEIN DIET

This diet is essentially a normal one supplemented to increase the protein intake to 100 to 125 gm per day. The caloric content of the diet also is increased in most instances as the result of the addition of drinks containing milk or fortified milk. For adults with lactose deficiency, other sources of protein, such as additional meat, fish, or eggs, may be required instead of milk drinks. Most patients requiring a high protein diet should receive vitamin supplementation and supplemental iron.

A high protein diet may be inappropriate for some debilitated patients, particularly those with some degree of liver disease.

Other oral diet modifications include bland diets; residue-restricted diets; low lactose diets; low fat diets; and high protein and fat, low carbohydrate diets. Other diets may have specific restrictions, such as low sodium, low calcium, or gluten free.

PROBLEMS IN ENTERAL NUTRITION OF HOSPITALIZED PATIENTS

A common mistake in the care of hospitalized patients is for the physician to assume that when an order for a particular diet is written, the patient actually eats what is ordered. A "bland diet in six feedings" provides about 2400 kilocalories, with 275 gm of carbohydrate, 95 gm of protein, and 110 gm of fat. This should provide most, if not all, of the protein and caloric needs of the average-sized adult patient, if he or she is not severely stressed. However, many patients fail to eat a substantial part of what is served. The necessary mass production of meals for bedside distribution in hospitals results in a rather bland type of "all-American" diet that is often a sharp contrast to the usual foods and individual dietary habits of the patient. Meals are served at times other than the patient's usual meal hours and, not infrequently, in an environment of sights, sounds, and odors hardly conducive to a good appetite. As a result, the frightened or somewhat disoriented patient does not eat very much.

Preoperatively, diagnostic procedures, such as radiographic examination of the gastrointestinal tract and even many blood tests, require that the patient fast. Multiple blood tests withdraw a considerable amount of red cells and plasma protein. Preoperative preparation for gastrointestinal surgery often involves giving the patient "clear fluids" that have minimal nutritional value for one to three days, and cathartics and enemas add their toll in abnormal losses of water and electrolytes.

Postoperatively, return to a regular diet or some modification thereof with some choice of foods for the patient usually coincides with discharge from the hospital for the majority of surgical patients. In patients whose illness or injury results in prolonged hospitalization, such as patients with lower extremity fractures, burns, major sepsis, or high-output intestinal fistulas, significant protein depletion and weight loss may develop rapidly unless a major effort is made to provide the enormously increased protein and caloric needs. Initially, deficits may be met by utilization of total parenteral nutrition techniques (Chap. 5).

LIQUID DIETS FOR TUBE FEEDING — LONG-TERM FULL LIQUID DIETS (SEE TABLE 4–4)

These diets are designed to provide full enteral nutrition for patients who require a liquid diet because they must be tube fed and for others who, for varying periods of time, are unable to chew or to swallow. Patients with an esophagostomy or pharyngostomy, unconscious patients, and patients requiring forced feeding beyond their voluntary intake are candidates for a liquid diet.

As with all mixed food preparations, great care must be used to

Table 4–4. Fat, Protein, Carbohydrate, and Caloric Contents, Initial Osmolality, and Electrolyte Content of Representative Diets for Tube Feeding

Diet	Fat (gm/l)	Protein (gm/l)	CHO (gm/l)	KCAL/ml	Initial mOsm/kg	Electrolytes mEq/l				
						Na	K	Mg	Cl	Pmm
Defined formula diets:										
Vivonex	1	21	226	1	550	20	30	18.3	20.4	17.9
Vivonex HN	1	42	210	1	844	23	30	10.87	23.1	10.7
Vital	10	42	185	1	450	17	30	22.3	18.8	21.5
Flexical	34	22.5	152	1	550	15.2	32	16.7	35.2	16.1
Vipep	25	25	176	1	520	32.6	21.8	16.9	47.9	19.4
Criticare	3	38	222	1.06	650	27.7	28.9	17.7	29.8	17.1
Low residue diets: low fat, whole protein										
Precision HN	1	42	206	1.05	557	42.6	23.3	11.7	33.6	11.3
Precision LR	1	24	223	1.1	492	30.3	22.2	19.3	31	18.7
Citrotein	1.8	42	128	0.7	496	32	19.3	37	27.5	35.5
Liquid whole foods:										
Isocal	44	34	133	1.04	300	21.7	33.0	17.3	30	16.8
Isocal HCN	91	75	225	2	NA	34.8	35.8	22	33.8	21.5
Ensure	36	36	136	1.04	450	30.4	35.5	17.2	28.2	16.8
Ensure Plus	52	52	188	1.5	600	46.1	48.6	26.4	44.9	20.3
Compleat B°	40	40	120	1	390	51.6	33.6	20.3	22.9	40.3
Sustacal	23	61	140	1	625	40.2	52.7	31.3	43.8	29.6
Sustacal HC	58	61	190	1.5	NA	32	33.3	29.6	35.9	23.8
Magnacal	80	70	250	2.0	520	43.5	32	33.3	26.8	32.3
Milk, whole†	34	34	47	0.75	277	21.8	39.5	12.8	NA	30.6

°Contains lactose
†Not a complete food for adults
NA = not available
These diets are a sampling of a wide spectrum of diets now commercially available in the United States. The list does not include a variety of dietary supplements available, nor special-purpose diets for particular metabolic problems such as hepatic or renal failure.
WHO, RDA requirements for vitamins and trace minerals for normal adults are met by 1500 to 3000 cc per day of these diets. Supplementation is advised for ill or depleted patients.
For more detail, see the Appendix in the Manual of Surgical Nutrition, Ballinger, W. F. (ed.): Chairman, Committee on Pre and Postoperative Care, American College of Surgeons, Philadelphia, W. B. Saunders Co., 1975. Also see Shils, M. E., Bloch, A. S., and Chernoff, R.: Liquid Formulas for Oral and Tube Feeding, 2nd ed. New York, Memorial Sloan-Kettering Cancer Center, 1979.
The assistance of Barbara Ryan, R.D. in preparation of these data is acknowledged with thanks.

insure aseptic preparation and storage. These preparations are potentially excellent culture media for bacteria and molds. Storing them at 4°C and discarding all remaining food 24 hours after preparation are essential steps for prevention of spoilage and potential food poisoning.

A number of commercial liquid diets are now available in sterile form in cans or jars. Most preparations are moderately priced and do not require the extensive preparation necessary if individual foods are used. Flavor is acceptable to most patients, so that liquids can be taken orally when possible. Odor and appearance, which are very important to patients who cannot taste what they are fed, are acceptable, though monotonous.

Most but not all preparations are lactose-free. The fat content of all preparations is fairly high, 40 to 55 gm per 1000 calories. All are slightly to moderately hyperosmolar at the usual concentration of 1000 calories per liter. All present a solute load that requires administration of additional fluids in order to prevent dehydration.

Commercial preparations contain protein as whole protein, either as solubilized casein or whole meat, milk, soy, or egg protein, and emulsified fats. They tend to coagulate or clot when they come in contact with gastrointestinal tract juices; therefore, careful rinsing of feeding tubes with water is required, and somewhat larger tubes than those used for defined formula diets are required.

Liquid diets may be fed as a bolus given over 15 to 20 minutes into the stomach through either a nasogastric feeding tube or a gastrostomy. For the adult who has adapted to this method, feedings of 300 to 500 ml may be given, but diluted feedings of 150 to 200 ml should be used initially, and three to five days are generally necessary for adaptation. Water other than that used to rinse the tube should be administered between feedings, and a total volume of at least one-half the volume of total tube feeding should be given daily. These procedures should help reduce the incidence of diarrhea and cramps. The use of codeine or diphenoxylate hydrochloride (Lomotil) to control diarrhea may also be helpful.

It is usually wise to feed by gravity, using a funnel or the barrel of a large syringe held a foot to 18 inches above the level of the stomach.

Conscious adult patients and older children are easily taught to feed themselves in this fashion. Usually six feedings a day, spaced at intervals of three hours, will permit administration of 2000 to 3000 calories with 1000 ml of additional water as a minimum. It is wise to omit a feeding at bedtime if there is a significant danger of regurgitation. When these diets are given to patients in bed, the head and thorax should be elevated at least 30 degrees from the horizontal plane during administration and for at least one hour after feeding if at all possible.

Liquid diets contain virtually no bulk, and some contain milk. Constipation is a common problem after adaptation, and stool softeners or cathartics, given via the tube, are usually necessary.

LIQUID DIETS CONTAINING INTACT PROTEIN OR PROTEIN ISOLATES, OLIGOSACCHARIDES, AND DEXTRINS, WITH VARYING AMOUNTS OF FAT

In Table 4–4, a series of these commercially prepared liquid diets is described. Most contain partially hydrolized starch, and most contain substantial amounts of fat. They are somewhat more expensive than the preceding diets. Mineral and trace element content is also quite variable. Table 4–4 should be consulted for the specific content of each diet.

These diets can be fed through smaller tubes than the preceding group, but the presence of intact protein still permits accumulation of a deposit on tube walls and coagulation at the tip. Thus, the tubes should be carefully cleansed.

An advantage of this liquid diet may be that hydrolysis of intact protein yields dipeptides and tripeptides, the absorption of which may be more efficient than absorption of isolated amino acids. A disadvantage of many preparations is a high fat content, which, in the presence of severe pancreatic insufficiency or a lack of bile salts, may promote diarrhea and steatorrhea.

DEFINED FORMULA (ELEMENTAL) DIETS

In 1969, Stephens and Randall reported results obtained by chemically feeding eight patients with severe malnutrition that was a consequence of gastrointestinal tract disease or sepsis. The chemically defined diet consisted of essential and nonessential amino acids, simple sugars, essential fat, minerals including trace elements, and vitamins. Since that time, many observers have reported the use of what are now officially called defined formula diets in the nutritional management of a wide variety of surgical and medical diseases. When there is sufficient jejunal length (usually 100 cm but with adaptation as little as 65 cm has proved adequate) and adequate small bowel function to permit absorption, the following types of patients have been successfully fed their total nutritional needs with defined formula diets.

1. Persons depleted of protein reserves as a result of disease of the gastrointestinal tract, including ulcerative colitis and acute granulomatous disease of the small and large bowel, chronic infection, carcinoma of the gastrointestinal tract (particularly the stomach and colon), intestinal atresia in infants, and malabsorption syndromes in infants and adults;

2. patients with partial function of the gastrointestinal tract, such as that resulting from esophageal, gastric, and duodenal fistulas with feeding distal to the fistula; small bowel and colonic fistulas with feeding into the stomach or high jejunum; pancreatitis after the ileus has cleared; and short-gut syndrome;

3. patients with accelerated metabolism from jaw fractures, fracture of a long bone of the lower extremity, or severe burns who cannot or will not eat adequately; and

4. patients with immunologic depression due to sepsis or cancer, patients who are undergoing diagnostic studies of the gastrointestinal tract or being prepared for gastrointestinal tract surgery, and patients with septicemia while on high-calorie intravenous feeding who have sufficient small bowel function to permit absorption.

Defined formula diets are usually tube fed if prolonged use is anticipated, since the food is relatively unpalatable, particularly if feedings are of large volume and frequently repeated. Complete solubility permits feeding through an 8 French silicone rubber or polyethylene tube in the adult and a 5 French tube in infants and small children. These tubes can be placed nasogastrically and are well tolerated for prolonged periods of time. An 8 French catheter has been used as a gastrostomy tube for more than five years for continuous infusion of high-nitrogen Vivonex at home at night to feed a patient with 65 cm of jejunum ending in a jejunostomy. Similarly, an 8 French catheter as a jejunostomy has permitted continuous intrajejunal feeding of defined formula diet with minimal difficulty over a period of seven months.

Recently, weighted tubes of small caliber have become available for nasogastric intestinal intubation that are easier to introduce and also have the advantage of a radiopaque marker for localization.*

Because of their high osmolality, defined formula diets are not well tolerated as bolus feedings intragastrically and particularly are not well tolerated when introduced in bulk amounts into the small bowel. Cramps, distention, and diarrhea follow too rapid introduction into the small bowel, while gastric retention, nausea, and vomiting result from rapid drinking or nasogastric tube feeding. It has been our experience that a volume adjustable pump that has a constant flow rate or a very accurate gravity drip is necessary to prevent overly rapid administration.

Diet should be prepared with careful aseptic technique for all utensils used. Warm sterile water makes solution of the powder form of most diets easier, but *water above 40°C should not be used and under no circumstances should the diet be heated on a burner or boiled* since the amino acids react unfavorably with sugars at high temperatures.

The prepared diet should be used within 24 hours. It should not be permitted to be at room temperature for more than six to eight hours, as it is an excellent culture medium for bacteria and fungi.

The sequence of concentration and volume changes used for intragastric and intrajejunal administration in adults and in children is shown in Table 4–5. *Strict adherence to the principle of starting slowly and with more dilute material is essential.*

COMPLICATIONS OF THE USE OF DEFINED FORMULA DIETS

Nausea, Vomiting, and Diarrhea. This means too much too fast. Slow down, or stop entirely and begin again 24 hours later. Codeine may be useful to control diarrhea, as may Lomotil.

---

*Dobbhoff (Entriflex) Enteric Feeding Tube, Biosearch Medical Products, Somerville, NJ; Keeofeed Tube, Hedeco, Mountain View, CA.

Table 4–5. Protocol for Administration of Defined Formula Diets

I. Adults of average size and weight
  A. Intragastric administration
    1. Check position of nasogastric tube, preferably by roentgenogram.
    2. Start with 1/2 strength diet, 0.5 calories per ml. Administer at 40 to 60 ml per hour for first 12 hours.
    3. Aspirate stomach for nausea and to check residual at 12 hours.
    4. Increase concentration first, then volume in stepwise fashion every 12 hours: to 0.6 calorie per ml, then 80 ml per hour, then 0.7 calorie per ml, then 100 ml per hour, then 0.8 calorie per ml, then to 120 ml per hour.
    5. If diet concentration of one calorie/ml or higher is given, additional water is necessary, either through the tube or as a peripheral IV to avoid hyperosmolar dehydration from solute retention.
    6. If diarrhea or nausea occur, slow down administration or stop, and start again at step 1.

  B. Intrajejunal or intraduodenal administration
    1. Check position of tube by roentgenogram. A small amount (10 to 20 ml) of water-soluble contrast medium assists in localization and in being certain there is no leak with a jejunostomy.
    2. Start with 10 per cent weight per volume, 0.4 calorie per ml solution. Be sure it is not cold. Administer at 40 to 60 ml per hour for at least 12 hours.
    3. Increase volume to 80 ml per hour, then increase concentration to 0.6 calorie per ml, then volume to 100 ml per hour, then concentration to 0.7 calorie per ml, etc. Expect to take four to five days to achieve 0.8 calorie per ml and 150 ml per hour without significant diarrhea.
    4. With severe cramps or diarrhea, stop and start again.
    5. Codeine or Lomotil is useful in control of diarrhea.
  Do not fail to reduce parenteral solutions as enteral volume increases to avoid overload.
  In some patients, parenteral supplementation, particularly of fat, water, and electrolytes, may be necessary if abnormal external losses are high.

II. Infants and small children
    1. Check position of tube carefully.
    2. Start with 7 per cent weight per volume solution, 0.3 calorie per ml slowly, supplemented with parenteral nutrition.
    3. Increase volume slowly, cutting back if diarrhea or distention occurs.
    4. Then increase concentration cautiously. Young infants will not tolerate greater than 0.4 calorie per ml, particularly intrajejunally. Older children respond more like adults.
    5. Remember that infants and small children will take oral feedings much more readily than adults.
    6. Large volumes per kg body weight are tolerated, if sufficient electrolyte is given to permit excretion of water at or slightly in excess of plasma osmolality.
    7. Monitor infants and small children more carefully than adults.

III. Monitoring
    1. An accurate intake and output record is essential. Body weight helps to assess accuracy.
    2. Check blood glucose before starting defined formula diet, and again at 12 hours and after each advance in concentration or volume.
    3. Urine glucose and acetone measurement is useful after steady state is reached.
    4. Check plasma electrolytes daily while inducing elemental diets and twice a week thereafter unless significant clinical change occurs.
    5. Use high nitrogen preparations for protein depletion patients with normal renal function. Expect some rise in BUN but not in creatinine.
    6. Stop intragastric feeding in elderly or very debilitated patients at night if they are to be placed supine. Slow for one hour first to avoid hypoglycemia.

Aspiration. This occurs particularly in elderly or very debilitated patients. Keep the patient's head elevated. Turn off the pump at night if the patient is being fed intragastrically and will be flat in bed.

Hyperglycemia; Hyperosmolar Nonketotic Coma. These are preventable by appropriate observation of blood glucose and electrolyte levels and by the judicious use of insulin, if necessary, to achieve caloric intake desired. A defined formula diet such as Flexical (Table 4–4) that contains 15 per cent fat may be advantageous in patients with high blood glucose, which is difficult to control, since the carbohydrate content is lower in such diets. However, fat is not as well handled as carbohydrate in patients with pancreatitis or short-gut syndrome and does not potentiate sodium and water absorption by the small bowel as does glucose.

Disturbances of Water Balance. Patients fed a high carbohydrate diet tend to retain water and sodium. In fasted and refed patients, a gain of as much as two to three per cent of body weight occurs within 48 hours after beginning either a defined formula diet or high calorie intravenous nutrition. This weight is lost when the high carbohydrate load is discontinued.

Hypoprothrombinemia. Diets are low or deficient in vitamin K, particularly for patients also on broad-spectrum antibiotics. Ten mg of an intramuscular preparation of vitamin K is usually given three times a week. One mg of folic acid is added to the diet daily.

Defined formula diets represent an intermediate step between high calorie intravenous nutrition and the oral ingestion or tube feeding of normal foods. The advantages are ease of administration, rapid absorption without the need of digestion, and minimal stimulation of biliary, pancreatic, and small bowel secretions. Disadvantages are the osmotic load, which until the patient has time to adapt is likely to produce gastric retention, nausea, vomiting, and diarrhea, the complications listed before, and the cost, which is substantially higher per 1000 calories than other forms of enteral nutrition. Cost of defined formula diets is about 20 per cent of the cost of total parenteral nutrition for equivalent caloric and protein intake.

Some Additional Useful Information

For patients with intestinal fistulas, feed low fistulas high, preferably intragastrically. Feed high fistulas below the fistula. A small Miller-Abbott tube can often be guided beyond the fistula, balloon deflated, and used for feeding. Also, a jejunostomy is very valuable for feeding patients with esophageal, gastric, or duodenal fistulas.

For patients who are likely to have prolonged upper gastrointestinal tract dysfunction, esophagectomy, gastric perforation, Whipple procedure, insecure duodenal stump, or acute pancreatitis if operated, a feeding jejunostomy at the time of operation is highly recommended. The method of Page et al. (1976) using a 24-inch #16 intravenous catheter and securing the jejunum to the abdominal wall at the point of exit appears to have excellent results.

In patients with high-output small bowel fistulas, the sodium concentration of the fistula drainage should fall significantly if glucose is introduced into the small bowel proximal to the fistula and if the bowel is capable of sodium and glucose transport.

SUMMARY

The gastrointestinal tract is the safest, most effective, and most economical means of providing not only calories, protein, carbohydrate, and fat for nutrition but also minerals, vitamins, and trace elements. Access to the gastrointestinal tract is important. Gastrostomy and jejunostomy, together with intraluminal tubes, provide means of using functional gut when normal oral intake is not possible or feasible.

A large variety of special diets is now available to permit maximal enteral nutritional support for many patients who previously were unable to gain or maintain an adequate nutritional status preoperatively or postoperatively or while recovering from other trauma or disease processes.

REFERENCES

Andrassy, R. J., Page, C. P., Feldtman, R. W., et al.: Continual catheter administration of an elemental diet in infants and children. Surgery, 82:205, 1977.

Blackburn, G. L., Bistrian, B. R., Maini, B. S., et al.: Nutritional and metabolic assessment of the hospitalized patient. J. Parent. Enter. Nutr., 1:11, 1977.

Clowes, G. H. A., Jr., Randall, H. T., and Cha, C-J. M.: Amino acid and energy metabolism in septic and traumatized patients. J. Parent. Enter. Nutr., 4:195, 1980.

Moore, F. D., Olsen, K. H., McMurrey, J. D., et al.: Body Cell Mass and Its Supporting Environment: Body Composition in Health and Disease. Philadelphia, W. B. Saunders Co., 1963.

Page, C. P., Ryan, J. A., Jr., and Haff, R. C.: Continual catheter administration of an elemental diet. Surg. Gynecol. Obstet., 142:184, 1976.

Stephens, R. V., and Randall, H. T.: Use of a concentrated, balanced, liquid elemental diet for nutritional management of catabolic states. Ann. Surg., 170:642, 1969.

5

Parenteral Nutrition

STANLEY J. DUDRICK

No pathophysiologic process can be expected to respond more favorably to specific therapeutic endeavors when the patient is in a state of malnutrition than when he or she is well nourished. Therefore, it is not only advisable but absolutely essential that all surgeons, regardless of their specialty or area of expertise, have a practical knowledge of both the identification and the most effective management of nutritional and metabolic problems that exist or may arise in their patients. This is especially important and apparent in seriously ill individuals in whom the provision of adequate enteral or parenteral nutrient substrates may be critical in minimizing morbidity and recovery time and maximizing survival, rehabilitation, and quality of life.

Until such time as optimal digestion, absorption, and assimilation can be maintained via the alimentary tracts of all patients under all conditions at all times, a comprehensive knowledge of parenteral nutrition is an essential tool in the armamentarium of the most enlightened and successful surgeons. Just as the master practitioners of the past and even the present had to gain expertise in anatomy, pathology, physiology, and pharmacology, surgeons of the present day and of the future must be proficient in their knowledge of biochemistry. From a practical point of view, parenteral nutrition represents the very basis of clinical biochemistry in that this feeding technique may be the only means by which the substrates that fuel and support all cellular processes can be provided to the patient.

Ever since the discovery of the circulation, surgeons have been increasingly able to provide nutrition by parenteral means to patients requiring this mode of therapy. Indeed, at this time, it is possible to provide a truly complete diet by vein. However, as sophisticated as current parenteral nutrition regimens may appear to be, they represent only a small step toward the ultimate goals of complete knowledge of the metabolic cellular derangements induced by all pathologic processes and of the ability to prevent or treat them specifically, be it by total or adjunctive parenteral means.

Initially, the impetus for development of parenteral therapy was merely to provide the water, electrolytes, and minimal calories essential to support life. As knowledge and experience accrued in this vital area, attempts were made to maintain homeostasis in all aspects of cellular nutrition, that is, water, electrolytes, amino acids, carbohydrates, fats, vitamins, and trace elements. Soon it became apparent that no single parenteral regimen could be ideal for all patients with a wide variety of pathologic processes, nor for all age groups, nor for the same patient during all aspects of a particular disorder. This had led to tailoring specific parenteral nutrient regimens to the patient and to the pathophysiologic process. Thus, there are now available a wide variety of maintenance and therapeutic formulas for pediatric and adult patients and for the adjunctive treatment of patients in renal or hepatic failure. Moreover, considerable efforts are under way and must continue in order for us to understand and define the specific nutrient requirements that accompany the various forms of· cancer, major trauma, extensive full-thickness burns, sepsis, immunologically related diseases, genetically mediated metabolic disorders, and even atherosclerotic cardiovascular and peripheral vascular diseases. Although current special substrate mixtures are crude at best, they represent a step in the right direction and are the harbingers of the specifically formulated parenteral nutrition therapy of the future.

For the well-nourished patient who has normal function of the gastrointestinal tract that has not been and will not be adversely affected by the primary pathophysiologic disorder and its therapy, adequate nutritional therapy is usually not a major problem, and this is the case in a majority of hospitalized patients. However, in patients who exhibit signs, symptoms, or a history of malnutrition prior to hospitalization or who are likely to develop them during hospitalization as a result of stressful periods of diagnosis and therapy, a significantly higher morbidity and mortality can be expected to result if adequate attention has not been paid to their nutritional maintenance or restitution.

INDICATIONS

When the patient is able to eat, he or she receives dietary consultation and special attention to nutritional requirements via the oral route. If the patient is unable to eat adequately or at all but if the gastrointestinal tract is functional, he or she is then fed by an intestinal tube placed preferentially through the nose or mouth but at times inserted at operation through the esophagus into the stomach or directly into the stomach or small bowel. If the patient cannot eat, should not eat, will not eat, or cannot eat enough or has a special metabolic problem such as renal failure or hepatic failure, it may be necessary to feed him or her entirely or to provide supplementation via parenteral nutrition techniques. Great progress has been made in the development of many feeding alternatives and substrates during the past decade, so that the surgeon now has the means to nourish virtually every patient adequately despite the pathophysiologic status. Indeed, not to nourish a patient adequately at this time reflects a positive decision to starve the patient or a passive decision to accept starvation as an inevitable result.

The primary indication for the use of total parenteral nutrition (TPN) is to provide adequate nutrition as long as necessary intravenously when use of the gastrointestinal tract is impractical, inadequate, ill-advised, or impossible. The most critical indications for prolonged TPN exist when adequate nutrition cannot be obtained by the alimentary tract in seriously ill patients suffering concomitantly from malnutrition, sepsis, or major surgical or accidental trauma.

The decisions to initiate and to maintain adequate TPN should be based upon the achievement of a specific, definable, and realistic goal in each patient. It must always be borne in mind that the ultimate aim of the technique is to prolong meaningful life and not merely to prolong the process of inevitable death. A primary general goal of intravenous feeding in an individual patient is to provide nutrients adequate in quality and quantity to meet the normal or increased metabolic requirements for (1) growth and development, (2) "regrowth" of a depleted adult to ideal weight, (3) restoration of function, (4) achievement of homeostasis, (5) achievement of positive nitrogen balance, (6) improved response to therapy, (7) repair of tissue, (8) recovery from stress, (9) restoration of immunocompetence, and (10) accelerated convalescence and rehabilitation.

Specific examples of patients in this category include the following:

1. Premature newborn infants with low birth weights, in the range of 400 to 1200 gm, in whom early adequate nutrition may be essential for survival or to insure development of maximal organ potential.

2. Newborn infants with catastrophic gastrointestinal anomalies, such as tracheoesophageal fistula, gastroschisis, omphalocele, or massive intestinal atresia.

3. Infants with cardiac or respiratory insufficiency secondary to congenital heart disease, hyaline membrane disease, diaphragmatic hernia, or cystic fibrosis.

4. Infants who fail to thrive nonspecifically or secondary to gastrointestinal insufficiency associated with the short-gut syndrome, malabsorption, enzyme deficiency, meconium ileus, or idiopathic diarrhea.

5. Adult patients with short bowel syndrome secondary to massive small bowel resection or enteroenteral, enterocolic, enterovesical, or enterocutaneous fistulas.

6. Patients with high alimentary tract obstructions secondary to

achalasia, stricture, or neoplasia of the esophagus, gastric malignancy, pyloric obstruction, mesenteric artery syndrome, or adhesive bands.

7. Surgical patients with prolonged paralytic ileus following major operations; patients with multiple injuries, or penetrating or blunt abdominal trauma, or patients with reflex ileus complicating various medical diseases.

8. Patients with a normal bowel length but malabsorption secondary to nontropical sprue, hypoproteinemia, enzyme deficiency, pancreatic or hepatic insufficiency, regional enteritis, ulcerative colitis, or pseudomembranous enterocolitis.

9. Adult patients with functional gastrointestinal disorders such as idiopathic diarrhea, psychogenic vomiting, anorexia nervosa, hyperemesis gravidarum, or esophageal dyskinesia following a cerebrovascular accident.

10. Patients with severe myocardial failure or respiratory insufficiency in whom appetite and ingested nutrients are reduced while energy requirements are increased.

11. Patients with inability to ingest adequate nutrients following a radical surgical procedure or major trauma to the head or neck.

12. Patients who cannot ingest food or who regurgitate and aspirate oral or tube feedings because of a depressed or obtunded sensorium following severe metabolic derangements, neurologic disorders, intracranial operation, or CNS trauma.

13. Patients with excessive metabolic requirements secondary to straightforward or complicated severe trauma such as extensive full-thickness burns, major or multiple fractures, or large soft tissue injuries or losses.

Another general indication or goal of TPN is to reduce mechanical or secretory activity of the alimentary tract to basal levels in order to achieve a state of bowel rest. By providing all nutrients parenterally, the bowel mucosa is not exposed to roughage, peristalsis is not induced by intraluminal bulk, and potent digestive secretions of the gastrointestinal tract are not stimulated to the usual degree. Thus, the bowel is physiologically "splinted" and is able to undergo repair and recovery from various pathologic processes without being further traumatized or stressed by the rigors of digestion, absorption, and excretion.

The combination of bowel rest and adequate nutrition by vein have proved valuable in the following specific conditions:

1. Granulomatous colitis, ulcerative colitis, tuberculous enteritis, and infectious or parasitic enterocolitis, in which major portions of the absorptive mucosa are diseased at a time when increased absorption is indicated to provide the nutrient substrates required for repair and restoration of normal function. Spontaneous remissions of regional enteritis and ulcerative colitis have occurred in many patients treated with TPN alone.

2. Fistulas from one portion of the alimentary tract to another, to the

skin, or to the urogenital tract. Significant reductions in the secretion and volume of fistulous drainage diminish the mechanical and chemical impediments to fistula closure and reduce the number of microorganisms that pass through the fistula and thereby impair healing. Pancreatic and small bowel fistulas have shown a reduction in volume output of 70 to 90 per cent within a few days of initiating TPN. The combination of adequate nutrients and decreased secretions has resulted in reduced autodigestion of the skin and underlying soft tissues and has accelerated healing of previously indolent fistulas and wounds.

3. In malnourished patients requiring prolonged periods of bowel preparation prior to diagnostic studies and major surgical procedures, TPN has allowed adequate nutrition while keeping the bowel free of particulate matter. Even without antibiotic administration, the colonic bacterial flora is greatly reduced by this regimen.

4. In paraplegics, quadriplegics, or debilitated patients with indolent decubitus ulcers in the pelvic area, soilage and fecal contamination of these wounds have been greatly reduced, thus promoting spontaneous healing or conditions favorable to split-thickness grafting or to full-thickness flap grafts. In several patients, this has obviated the necessity for a diverting colostomy, and the beneficial effects of a bypass colostomy are achieved medically.

A third general indication for TPN is to provide specially tailored diets by vein to improve nutritional status without aggravating the metabolic disorders precipitated by pathologic conditions affecting the kidneys or liver. Thus, intravenous diets of high biologic value can be administered for the nutritional benefit of the patient in renal or hepatic decompensation without significantly elevating the blood urea nitrogen or blood ammonia.

A fourth general indication is to reduce the urgency for surgical intervention in patients who might eventually require operation but in whom prolonged, progressive malnutrition has greatly increased the risk of operation. One can "buy" time for such malnourished patients in high-risk morbidity and mortality categories without further increasing their risks while nutritional status is improved with TPN.

A fifth general indication for TPN is to avoid, reduce, or correct protein deficiencies and the complications of hypoproteinemia. The surgeon is not merely attempting to promote muscle synthesis when infusing intravenous amino acids and calorie substrates. The general goal is to provide the protein moieties that are required both for repair and for restoration of injured tissues. The specific goals for protein repletion are to (1) increase resistance to blood loss, (2) decrease the susceptibility to shock, (3) restore serum and tissue proteins, (4) increase plasma and blood volume, (5) increase resistance to infection, (6) reduce edema both locally at the wound and generally, (7) accelerate wound healing, (8) restore digestive enzymes to normal, (9) reverse the protein deficiency of malabsorption, (10) improve metabolic rate, (11) improve cardiovascular function, (12) decrease weakness and lassitude, (13) reverse mental depression, (14) reduce morbidity and mortality, and (15) reduce time and expense of convalescence.

A sixth general indication is to achieve a steady, definable metabolic or nutritional state in order to study more precisely the physiologic, biochemical, and pharmacologic effects of various parenteral or enteral nutrients on metabolism, body composition, body function, and their interrelationships in disease.

Optimal results from surgical procedures, pharmacologic therapy, chemotherapy, radiotherapy, respiratory therapy, physical therapy, and other forms of patient care can be obtained only when the patient is simultaneously maintained in optimal nutritional condition. Therefore, it is incumbent upon the surgeon to provide optimal nutrition to all patients under all conditions at all times.

NUTRITIONAL ASSESSMENT

During the past 10 years, four indices of evaluation have proved valuable in making decisions to provide special forms of nutritional support: (1) history of an unintentional or unexplained weight loss of 10 pounds or 10 per cent body weight during the previous two months; (2) serum albumin concentration of less than 3.4 gm per 100 ml; (3) anergy to a battery of four or five standard skin test antigens; and (4) an abnormally low total lymphocyte count. If a patient manifests evidence of any one of these indices, he is malnourished to a mild degree; if he manifests any two of these indices, he is malnourished to a moderate degree; if he manifests any three of these indices, he is malnourished to a moderately severe degree; and if he manifests all four indices, he is severely malnourished. These are the basic clinical criteria by which decisions can be made to employ special techniques and substrates for nutritional support.

Evidence of malnutrition may not be apparent on casual clinical examination. However, an accurate evaluation of the nutritional status of the surgical patient can be obtained readily from a carefully directed history, physical examination, and series of clinical and laboratory studies. The data assembled may be very helpful in planning preoperative and postoperative nutritional regimens for each patient.

HISTORY

An accurate determination of the dietary intake of the patient is most important in evaluating the nutritional status, especially as it relates to the degree and time course of weight loss. A history consistent with malnutrition may include the presence of anorexia, diarrhea, dysphagia, nausea, vomiting, lethargy, loss of vitality, and a decreased sense of well-being. A pointed systemic review and past medical history may elicit other signs, symptoms, or causes of malnutrition. An idea of the social and economic status of the patient is essential in determining the quality and quantity of food he usually ingests. In some instances, the age of the patient is important in evaluating the dietary history, especially in the geriatric population.

PHYSICAL EXAMINATION

Although apparently well nourished, a patient may be in a state of negative nitrogen balance and relative malnutrition as a result of a recent or current catabolic pathologic process. Careful examination of a healthy-appearing person may show that his tissues are edematous as a result of hypoproteinemia. On the other hand, a severe case of malnutrition is easily recognized by the loose inelastic skin, loss of subcutaneous fat, atrophy of muscle mass, hepatomegaly, and massive peripheral edema. Diagnosis of specific vitamin or mineral deficiencies can often be made by recognition of characteristic signs on physical examination. In the hospitalized patient, however, nutritional depletion often develops subtly and become clinically significant before overt deficiencies are manifested. In such cases, clinical anthropometric measurements such as triceps skin-fold thickness, mid-arm circumference, mid-arm muscle circumference, and creatinine-height index may be helpful in the clinical assessment of nutritional status.

ANTHROPOMETRIC EVALUATION

Adipose tissue is the primary caloric reserve of the body and may be assessed by measuring the triceps skin-fold thickness, which includes the subcutaneous fat layer. This measurement is made with the Lange caliper at the midpoint of the upper arm between the tip of the olecranon process of the ulna and the acromion process of the scapula. The status of skeletal muscle mass or somatic protein can be estimated by determination of arm muscle circumference at the midpoint of the upper arm minus ($0.13 \times$ triceps skin-fold in mm). The creatinine-height index is a valid estimate of skeletal muscle mass because urinary levels of creatinine are dependent principally upon the extent of skeletal muscle catabolism, especially during protein depletion. It is expressed as the 24-hour creatinine excretion of the patient divided by the expected 24-hour creatinine excretion of a normal adult of the same height.

LABORATORY EXAMINATION

Biochemical and hematologic studies are usually helpful in accurately estimating the nutritional status of a patient. Determinations of the hemoglobin and hematocrit in correlation with deviations in hydration and body weight may be very useful, although both measurements can be misleading and inaccurate following recent blood loss. Routine urinalysis may show significant protein, sugar, or electrolyte losses. A fasting blood sugar or two-hour postprandial determination may indicate previously unsuspected diabetes mellitus. The blood urea nitrogen or nonprotein nitrogen, in addition to helping assess the renal status, may reflect a catabolic state or gastrointestinal bleeding. Detection of occult blood in the stool by guaiac or benzidine determinations may yield a clue to the etiology of a pathologic process that is adversely affecting nutritional status. Measurement of serum protein, albumin, and globulin levels should be obtained, although these determinations may be misleading at times. The total serum protein level alone is of questionable value because a high serum globulin may mask a significant decrease in the serum albumin level. Electrophoretic fractionation of serum proteins provides more complete and reliable data than the traditional salting-out methods. Dehydration may mask hypoproteinemia to some extent by producing hemoconcentration, but a prompt fall in the serum protein level is usually observed after adequate replacement of existing water and electrolyte deficits. The critical levels of serum proteins, below which there is obligatory edema formation, have been defined as 5.5 gm per 100 ml for total serum proteins and 3.0 gm per 100 ml for albumin, the latter fraction being responsible for most of the colloid osmotic pressure of plasma. It must be appreciated, however, that there is no specific protein level below which edema fluid suddenly appears; the tendency to increase interstitial water occurs progressively as the serum protein concentrations fall over a broad range. There is poor correlation between serum protein levels and deviations in body weight, the serum protein levels being maintained for a considerable period after initial weight loss, and then suddenly decreasing in the latter stages of protein depletion.

Total circulating plasma protein is a more sensitive indication of protein deficiency than is the serum protein concentration. The total circulating plasma protein can be readily determined if the serum protein concentration and the plasma volume are known. Another rapidly responding index of protein nutrition can be obtained by measuring serial fasting plasma amino acid levels. However, this rather tedious and expensive procedure is generally reserved for only the most complex nutritional problems.

In the presence of known or suspected hepatic disease, liver function studies should be performed, because the patient with liver insufficiency is peculiarly unable to compensate well for the metabolic stresses of surgical procedures. In selected patients, it can be helpful to determine the serum lipid profile, specific individual serum vitamin levels, and serum levels of most of the biologically active electrolytes in addition to assessment of acid-base balance. Other indices that have gained increasing importance and application in the serial evaluation of protein nutritional status include the serum transferrin, prealbumin, and retinal binding protein concentrations. These proteins have respectively shorter half-lives and accordingly respond more rapidly to protein depletion or repletion, indicating effectiveness of nutritional therapy.

IMMUNOLOGIC EVALUATION

Protein malnutrition is associated with impaired host defense mechanisms, particularly cell-mediated immunity, and loss of immunocompetence can be an indication of visceral protein depletion. Recall skin test antigens such as Dermatophytin, Candida, mumps, and intermediate-strength purified protein derivative (PPD) may be injected into the dermis of the volar aspect of the forearm to stimulate the immunologic response.

At 48 hours postinjection, failure of the delayed cutaneous response, or anergy, is a well-documented characteristic of malnutrition, and repletion of body cell mass is usually followed by restoration of skin reactivity. Recently the anergic state has identified postoperative and post-trauma patients at increased risk for sepsis and mortality and presaged these complications in patients studied preoperatively. Increases in sepsis and mortality rates in anergic patients are highly significant, and patients with questionable nutritional status should be skin-tested preoperatively whenever possible.

In anergic patients, the total lymphocyte count is often reduced by as much as one third, and such low levels are consistent with impaired cellular defense mechanisms and malnutrition. The total lymphocyte count is calculated as the percentage of lymphocytes multiplied by the white blood cell count and should number at least 1500 cells per cu mm. Although immunologic status can be affected by many factors, periodic evaluation of cell-mediated immunity can add significantly to the sequential clinical appraisal of nutritional status. Serial repetition and interpretation of a profile of nutritional assessment indices can provide useful objective guidelines for indicating, monitoring, and modifying nutritional therapy.

NUTRIENT SOLUTION PREPARATION

The basic nutrient mixture is a hypertonic solution about six times more concentrated (1800 to 2200 mOsm per liter) than blood and consists of approximately 20 to 25 per cent dextrose and 4 to 5 per cent crystalline amino acids. It provides about 6.5 to 8.0 gm of nitrogen, equivalent to about 40 to 50 gm of protein, and approximately 1000 calories per liter (Table 5–1).

Although the base solution contains various quantities of some of the essential minerals, the composition and concentrations of which differ significantly from one product to another, electrolyte additives must be made immediately prior to infusion in order to satisfy the nutrient and metabolic requirements of most patients. For the average adult patient with no significant renal, hepatic, or cardiovascular dysfunction, 40 to 50 mEq of sodium as the chloride and/or acetate, bicarbonate, or lactate salt and 30 to 40 mEq of potassium as the chloride and/or acetate, lactate, or acid phosphate salt are added to each liter of base solution. To base solutions prepared from crystalline amino acids, which may contain a combined total of 25 to 50 mEq of chloride and/or hydrochloride per liter, sodium should be added as the acetate, bicarbonate, or lactate, and not the chloride salt, in order to avoid production or aggravation of hyperchloremic acidosis. Fifteen to 18 mEq of magnesium sulfate are added to each liter of solution. Calcium is not administered in organic form, usually as the gluconate salt to avoid precipitation. Generally, 4 to 5 mEq of calcium are added per liter of the base solution. However, phosphorus, a major intracellular ion, must be added in dosages of 10 to 20 mM per liter as the potassium acid phosphate salt if significant hypophosphatemia and its attendant complications are to be

Table 5–1. ADULT INTRAVENOUS HYPERALIMENTATION SOLUTION

BASE SOLUTION	
40-50% dextrose in water	500 ml
8.5-10% crystalline amino acids	500 ml
ADDITIVES TO EACH UNIT	
Sodium chloride	40–50 mEq
Potassium chloride	20–30 mEq
Potassium acid phosphate (10–20 mM phosphorus)	15–30 mEq
Magnesium sulfate	15–18 mEq
ADDITIVES TO ANY ONE UNIT DAILY	
Calcium gluconate 10%	4.5 mEq
Multivitamin infusion (MVI-12)	10 ml
Zinc sulfate	5 mg
Copper sulfate	1–2 mg
Iron-dextran (Imferon)	0.1 ml
Chromium chloride	1.5 mcg
Manganese chloride	0.5 mg
Selenium (Na_2SeO_3)	60.0 mcg
ADDITIVE TO ANY ONE UNIT TWICE WEEKLY	
Vitamin K	10 mg
INTRAVENOUS FAT EMULSION 10% OR 20%	
500 ml 2–7 times weekly over 4–6 hr	50–100 gm
Carbohydrate calories	850 kcal/liter
Protein calories	150 kcal/liter
Fat calories	500–1000 kcal/liter
Nitrogen	6.5–8.0 gm/liter
Amino acids	40–50 gm/liter

avoided during anabolism. To only one bottle of solution daily is added an ampule of water- and fat-soluble vitamins in therapeutic dosages. Vitamin K, which is not present in intravenous vitamin mixtures, can be added to one bottle of the solution daily or given less frequently intravenously or intramuscularly as indicated in required dosages. Iron can be added to the solution daily or less frequently in appropriately calculated doses or given intramuscularly in depot form. In patients who are anemic, it is advisable to restore normal red cell volume by judicious transfusion of whole blood or packed erythrocytes upon initiation of TPN. Supplemental zinc and copper must be added to the nutrient mixtures of all patients on long-term TPN if significant deficiencies of these minerals are to be avoided. Trace elements, such as chromium, fluoride, iodine, manganese, molybdenum, and selenium, are present as contaminants in some parenteral solutions but usually must be added individually as required in patients on long-term TPN.

Modifications of the standard adult formula are required for treatment of patients with congestive heart failure, liver disease, or massive nutritional edema, in whom sodium administration is reduced. In elderly patients or in those with compromised renal function, potassium administration is reduced or temporarily omitted, and in patients with overt renal or hepatic dysfunction, racemic mixtures of crystalline amino acids are restricted. Special solutions for the treatment of acute or chronic renal failure contain nitrogen of the highest biologic value in the form of essential L-amino acids in 50 to 70 per cent dextrose, thus restricting water administration but providing adequate nutrition and promoting reduction of blood urea nitrogen and ammonia.

Modifications of the solution are often necessary following the initiation of TPN, depending upon the patient's metabolic response to the disease, trauma, operation, infection, or other intercurrent conditions. It is essential for the surgeon to recognize that no single intravenous nutrient solution can be ideal for all conditions in all patients at all times, or for the same patient during the various phases of his pathologic process. Individual metabolic requirements may be satisfied by appropriate alterations in the solution formulas.

NUTRIENT SOLUTION ADMINISTRATION AND MONITORING

The average daily ration of hypertonic nutrient solution contains about 25 to 30 per cent solute and should be infused continuously over 24 hours at a constant rate in order to allow maximal assimilation of the nutrients without exceeding the patient's capabilities for water, dextrose, amino acid, or mineral metabolism. Because the solution is hypertonic, it must be infused into the circulatory system through a large-diameter, high-flow blood vessel, preferably the superior vena cava. Starting at generally safe levels of water metabolism (2000 to 2500 ml per day in adults) and dextrose utilization (0.4 to 1.2 gm per kg per hour), the daily intravenous nutrient ration is gradually increased as indicated or tolerated (3000 to 4000 ml per day in adults).

Basic guidelines for safe total parenteral nutrition include accurate determinations of body weight daily; water balance every 4 to 8 hours; fractional urine sugar concentrations every 6 hours; serum electrolytes, blood sugar, and blood urea nitrogen daily until stable, then every 2 or 3 days thereafter; and complete blood count, serum proteins, calcium, phosphorus, and magnesium weekly. Hepatic and renal function tests should be evaluated initially and every 1 to 3 weeks during TPN. Intermittent measurements of serum osmolality; zinc, copper, and vitamin levels; and urine specific gravity, osmolality, and electrolytes may be helpful in monitoring certain patients. Periodic determinations of arterial and central venous pressures, blood gases, and pH may also be indicated in the management of critically ill patients with significant cardiovascular, respiratory, or metabolic derangements.

Adjustments of water volume, sugar concentration, protein source, or electrolyte content in the nutrient solution may be necessary during the treatment of a critically ill or traumatized patient. Relative glucose intolerance is most likely to be manifested at the initiation of TPN immediately following trauma, during operation, in the immediate postoperative period, in the aged, in patients with pancreatic disorders, or in the presence of shock or sepsis. To avoid excessive glycosuria, which may result in water and electrolyte imbalances, or hyperosmolar, hyperglycemic, nonketotic coma, the infusion is maintained at a rate that will not allow quantitative urinary glucose to exceed 1 gm per 100 ml (3+ nitroprusside reaction). Ideally, the patient will not excrete any sugar in his urine. However, tract amounts of glucose in the urine do not represent significant losses of the total sugar administered, and such small amounts of glycosuria will induce a mild diuresis that may actually be helpful in excreting any excess vehicular water, and in indicating that the limit of the patient's ability to metabolize glucose has been approached.

In all patients with diabetes mellitus, crystalline insulin is equally distributed in the intravenous solution. At times in nondiabetic patients with relative glucose intolerance, crystalline insulin is added to nutrient solution in amounts of 5 to 50 units per 1000 calories. Addition of insulin is indicated in the presence of an elevated blood sugar in order to encourage more rapid and efficient glucose utilization and positive nutritional balance in elderly patients with dysfunction of the pancreas, in the early postoperative period, and in criticaly ill, nutritionally depleted patients whose survival appears to depend upon the expeditious achievement of positive caloric and nitrogen balance.

Albumin or blood is usually given early in the course of TPN to restore normal colloid osmotic pressure and red blood cell mass in patients with marked hypoproteinemia or anemia. In patients with borderline serum protein concentrations, administration of the nutrient solution alone is sufficient to correct the deficiencies.

Because fat has a high caloric density of 9 calories per gram, it can be an efficient energy substrate for intravenous feeding in man. The 10 per cent fat emulsions contribute little to osmotic pressure and yield approximately 1000 to 2000 calories per liter. Their use can also provide essential fatty acids, allowing parenteral nutrition regimens to be truly complete. Moreoever, fat emulsions can be given together with slightly hypertonic nutrient solutions by peripheral vein for relatively short periods of time with good results in minimally stressed patients and in normal man. An obvious advantage of the 20 per cent emulsion is that a large number of calories can be administered to a patient in whom water intake must be restricted. On the other hand, fat emulsions should be administered cautiously or avoided in patients with hyperlipidemias, acute pancreatitis, pulmonary insufficiency, and some forms of renal and hepatic failure.

Controversy still exists, however, as to the indications and efficacy of intravenous fat emulsions in the early management of moderately and severely stressed patients. As additional clinical experience is gained with the currently available soybean oil and safflower oil emulsions, the optimal role of intravenous fat in total parenteral nutrition will undoubtedly be better defined.

CENTRAL VENOUS CATHETERIZATION

PERCUTANEOUS TECHNIQUE

The preferred method of infusion of hypertonic total parenteral nutrition solutions is via the subclavian route. It consists of the percutaneous introduction of an 8 inch long polyvinyl, Teflon, or silicone rubber catheter, having an external diameter of 1 to 2 mm, into the superior vena cava via one of the subclavian veins. The catheterization can be accomplished safely and effectively if the following principles are conscientiously observed. The patient is placed in bed supine with his head 15 degrees lower than his feet, to allow maximal filling and dilatation of the subclavian vein to a diameter of 1 to 2 cm, thus making it a fairly large target. The shoulders are extended backward, and the head is turned to the opposite side, thus allowing the ipsilateral subclavian vein to become easily accessible for percutaneous puncture. The skin of the lower neck, shoulder, and upper chest is shaved, cleansed with acetone or Freon to remove skin oil, and prepared with povidone-iodine solution in a manner identical to skin preparation prior to major operation. With strict aseptic technique, including sterile gloves and surgical instruments, the prepared area of skin is draped with sterile towels, and local anesthetic solution is infiltrated into the skin, subcutaneous tissue, and periosteum at the inferior surface of the midpoint of the clavicle. A needle 2 inches long and 2.5 mm in diameter, attached to a 2-ml syringe, is inserted beneath the clavicle in a horizontal plane, with its tip aimed at the posterior aspect of the sternal notch. When the needle enters the subclavian vein, blood can easily be withdrawn from the vein into the syringe. The syringe is then disconnected from the needle, the bevel of which is directed caudally, and the catheter is introduced its full length into the subclavian vein and down into the superior vena cava. If any difficulty is encountered in advancing the catheter, both the needle and the catheter should be withdrawn together as a unit and another venipuncture attempted. Withdrawal of the catheter alone with the needle in place may result in transection of the catheter and embolism of the distal segment. During the time that the needle is detached from the syringe, the patient is asked to hold his breath or manual pressure is applied to his abdomen to minimize the risk of air embolism. The needle is then withdrawn its full length, with approximately 5½ inches of catheter left within the central venous system, its tip lying in the midportion of the superior vena cava. The catheter is secured firmly with a suture, and broad-spectrum antibiotic-antifungal ointment or antiseptic ointment is applied around the catheter exit site from the skin. A sterile gauze dressing is then applied and fixed in place with tincture of benzoin and adhesive tape. Intravenous administration tubing is connected to the hub of the catheter, and an infusion is begun with an isotonic solution. After a roentgenogram has been obtained to confirm that the catheter is correctly positioned, infusion of the concentrated nutrient solution can begin.

If a catheter is malpositioned in a vein other than the superior vena cava, it can be redirected by withdrawing it 2 to 3 inches, inserting a J wire through the catheter aseptically into the superior vena cava, and then advancing the catheter again over the wire. Malfunctioning central venous feeding catheters can also be replaced by inserting the J wire into the catheter, removing the defective catheter, and then advancing a new catheter over the wire.

IMPLANTED CATHETER TECHNIQUE

For patients on prolonged or permanent home TPN, a catheter is inserted operatively into the central vein and implanted into a subcutaneous tunnel. Access to the patient's central venous system is accomplished by insertion of a 90 cm long, barium-impregnated, silicone rubber catheter having a Dacron velour cuff 30 cm from the catheter hub. Catheter implantation is accomplished in the operating room with the patient under light general anesthesia. The catheter is tunneled subcutaneously from a small stab wound in the skin of the anterior upper abdominal wall inferior and lateral to the xyphoid to a second incision in close proximity to the vein to be cannulated. Accessible veins that may be catheterized include the pectoral, cephalic, subclavian, thyroid, facial, internal jugular, or external jugular veins. When the external or internal jugular vein is catheterized, an incision is made over the posterior border of the sternocleidomastoid muscle in its midportion, and the catheter must be tunneled the additional distance from the abdominal incision to the neck incision. The proposed length of the intravascular segment of the catheter is determined, the catheter is transected at its appropriate length, and the catheter is filled with sodium heparin solution containing 100 units per ml. After distal ligation of the target vein, a small transverse venotomy is made and the catheter is directed into the vein and advanced centrally until the catheter tip is situated in the superior vena cava. Roentgenographic examination precludes the possibility of catheter misplacement into the right atrium or elsewhere in the venous system. The venotomy skin wound is closed, the catheter is sutured to the skin at the exit site, and two small sterile occlusive dressings are applied. Three to five days after insertion, all sutures are removed and the sterile dressing at the catheter exit site is affixed to the skin to minimize bacterial or fungal contamination of the catheter and adjacent skin.

An alternative technique has recently been developed using a large pervenous pacemaker lead introducer, which has greatly simplified this procedure. A 19-gauge, 2 inch long needle on a syringe is directed into the subclavian vein through a 1 to 2 cm incision in the skin and subcutaneous tissue under the clavicle. The J wire is introduced through the needle into the superior vena cava. The large introducer, consisting of an internal obdurator and an external splittable cannula, is advanced over the J wire into the central vein. The catheter is then implanted into its subcutaneous tunnel via a Raimondi ventriculoperitoneal shunt passer and cut to appropriate length. The obdurator and J wire are then removed and the end of the catheter is inserted into the cannula. The cannula is then split apart and backed out of the vein as the catheter position is maintained in the superior vena cava. Much less dissection is required with this catheterization technique, which can be accomplished much more simply and rapidly and with local rather than general anesthesia. This technique has been used in children as well as adults and has also been successful in catheterization of the inferior vena cava via the femoral veins.

INFUSION TECHNIQUES

Standard intravenous solution bottles or plastic bags and infusion sets are used to deliver the nutrient solution at a constant rate. Rolling intravenous poles allow the mobility and exercise that are essential for optimal nutrition and rehabilitation. Use of closed, filtered infusion systems provides maximal protection against the ever-present airborne microorganisms that may gain entry into the solution or tubing. Portable lightweight AC-DC pumps, attached to the intravenous pole or directly to the patient, can be used to insure a constant rate of infusion while allowing considerable freedom of position and activity of the patient.

A specially tailored patient vest has been developed for total or supplemental intravenous feeding on an ambulatory basis. The vest is made of sturdy, lightweight fishnet polyester; is comfortable, attractive, and practical; and can be concealed if desired under loose-fitting clothing. A plastic nutrient bag is suspended from each shoulder area anteriorly. A miniature infusion pump, weighing less then 350 gm and powered by two encapsulated nickel-cadmium rechargeable batteries, propels the infusate through specially constructed Y-intravenous tubing inserted into the hub of the central venous feeding catheter. The ambulatory home TPN vest is custom-fitted for each patient, with several options as to the size, number, and location of pockets to accommodate the nutrient bags (50, 250, 500, or 1000 ml); the position of the pump pocket; and the location of the zipper or Velcro fasteners.

COMPLICATIONS

Prevention of infection or sepsis is of paramount importance to the success of long-term TPN. The occurrence of infection is very rare if the aseptic and antiseptic principles previously discussed are conscientiously observed in the insertion and maintenance of the central venous catheters. Because hypertonic nutrient solutions are excellent culture media for many species of bacteria and fungi, meticulous asepsis must also be maintained during solution preparation, additive injection, and long-term administration if infection is to be minimized. If fever should occur in a patient receiving TPN, the physician must immediately attempt to define its source in the ears, nose or throat, chest, urinary tract, gastrointestinal tract, or wound. If the etiology of the fever cannot be determined readily, the nutrient solution and tubing must be replaced empirically and promptly, and specimens of the blood and solution must be cultured for bacteria and fungi. Should the fever persist after replacement of the solution and administration apparatus, the infusion must be terminated immediately. The indwelling central venous catheter must be removed, and the distal tip of the catheter must be cultured for bacteria and fungi. Depending upon the clinical situation, another central venous feeding catheter may be inserted into the opposite subclavian vein, or administration of isotonic dextrose solution may be started via a peripheral vein to insure against postinfusion hypoglycemia. Systemic broad-spectrum antibiotic therapy or antifungal therapy is rarely required. However, if desired, or if the patient shows persistent signs of sepsis, an antimicrobial regimen may be instituted at this time and modified appropriately when specific sensitivity testing has been completed.

Fever or evidence of sepsis prior to institution of total parenteral nutrition does not necessarily contraindicate the use of the technique. In a traumatized, burned, debilitated, or critically ill patient, sepsis often accompanies the primary problem and accentuates the nutritional requirements. Specific antimicrobial therapy has already been instituted in most of such patients, and although seeding of the indwelling catheter by circulating microorganisms is a definite possibility, it has not proved to be an overwhelming clinical problem. Indeed, resolution of systemic infections has occurred regularly during periods of total parenteral nutrition. However, if the clinician suspects that the infectious course of the patient might be caused or aggravated by the central venous feeding catheter, it should be removed and cultured promptly. It is advisable to change central venous feeding catheters routinely from one site to another twice weekly in patients with major burns or sepsis from a known source in order to minimize the risk of metastasis of the microorganisms from their primary source to the catheter.

Although development of thrombophlebitis is always possible with the use of long-term indwelling central venous feeding catheters and infusion of hypertonic solutions, superior vena caval thrombosis has been observed clinically only rarely. Apparently, the high rate of blood flow in the large diameter vessel assures prompt dilution of the hypertonic fluid and prevents chemical phlebitis. Furthermore, attention to sterility has practically eliminated infectious thrombophlebitis. However, occasional incidences of thrombosis have occurred in patients when the catheter tips were misdirected into or malpositioned in a jugular, internal mammary, intercostal, or axillary vein. Other central venous catheter–related hazards, such as inadvertent air embolism or catheter embolism, can be avoided easily by adherence to principles and techniques of safe central venous catheterization. A thorough knowledge of anatomy combined with common sense and strict adherence to the principles and techniques of percutaneous central venous catheterization should minimize the potential hazards of accidental pneumothorax, hydrothorax, hemothorax, hydromediastinum, subclavian artery puncture, bleeding, arteriovenous fistula, endocarditis, injury to the thoracic duct, venobronchial fistula, injury to the brachial plexus or sympathetic chain, osteomyelitis of the clavicle, and even death (Table 5–2).

Hyperosmolar coma can be precipitated acutely by too rapid infusion of the hypertonic solution, causing marked osmotic diuresis, serum and urine electrolyte aberrations, dehydration, and malfunction of the central nervous system. A chronic form of this syndrome can occur surreptitiously when impaired glucose tolerance is not recognized, particularly in the presence of diabetes mellitus, after some extensive burns or major trauma, or after intracranial operations or trauma. Hy-

Table 5–2. POTENTIAL CATHETER COMPLICATIONS OF TOTAL
PARENTERAL NUTRITION

INFECTIOUS	TECHNICAL
Insertion-site contamination	Pneumothorax
Contamination during insertion	Tension pneumothorax
Contamination during routine care	Hemothorax
Catheter contamination	Hydrothorax
Improper technique of catheter insertion	Hydromediastinum
Administration of blood via feeding catheter	Cardiac tamponade
Use of catheter to measure central venous pressure	Brachial plexus injury
Use of catheter to obtain blood samples	Horner's syndrome
Use of catheter to administer medications	Phrenic nerve paralysis
Contaminated solution during preparation of additives	Carotid artery injury
Contaminated tubing via connections	Subclavian artery injury
Three-way stopcocks in system	Subclavian hematoma
Secondary contamination	Thrombosis, subclavian
Septicemia, bacterial or fungal	vein or superior vena
Septic emboli	cava
Osteomyelitis of clavicle	Arteriovenous fistula
Septic arthritis	Venobronchial fistula
Endocarditis	Air embolism
	Catheter embolism
	Thromboembolism
	Catheter misplacement
	Cardiac perforation
	Endocarditis
	Thoracic duct laceration
	Innominate or subclavian
	vein laceration

perosmolar coma is seldom seen with blood sugar levels below 400 mg per 100 ml, and in most instances the blood sugar concentration has been 600 mg per 100 ml or higher.

If blood and urine sugar levels are not conscientiously measured in such patients, hyperglycemia may occur with marked elevation of blood sugar, accompanied by weakness, listlessness, and coma. If the condition is not recognized and corrected promptly, permanent neurologic damage can ensue. Treatment of this syndrome consists of prompt infusion of isotonic or half-strength solutions of saline or glucose together with insulin, while frequent measurements of fluid losses, central venous pressure, electrolytes, and blood sugar are obtained. A thorough assessment and understanding of the patient's disease, his metabolic status, and the established principles of the technique of TPN will prevent the great majority of these complications (Table 5–3).

Table 5–3. POTENTIAL METABOLIC COMPLICATIONS OF TOTAL PARENTERAL NUTRITION

COMPLICATION	ETIOLOGY
Glucose Metabolism	
Hyperglycemic glycosuria, osmotic diuresis, nonketotic hyperosmolar dehydration, and coma	Excessive total dose or rate of infusion of dextrose; inadequate endogenous insulin; glucocorticoids; sepsis
Ketoacidosis of diabetes mellitus	Inadequate endogenous insulin response; inadequate exogenous insulin therapy
Postinfusion (rebound) hypoglycemia	Persistence of endogenous insulin production secondary to prolonged stimulation of islet cells by high-carbohydrate infusion
Respiratory acidosis with hypercarbia	Excessive dextrose administration
Amino Acid Metabolism	
Hyperchloremic metabolic acidosis	Excessive chloride and monohydrochloride content of crystalline amino acid solutions
Serum amino acid imbalance	Unphysiologic amino acid profile of the nutrient solution; different amino acid utilization with various disorders
Hyperammonemia	Excessive ammonia in protein hydrolysate solutions; deficiencies of arginine, ornithine, aspartic acid, and/or glutamic acid in crystalline amino acid solutions; primary hepatic disorder
Prerenal azotemia	Excessive total dose or rate of infusion of protein hydrolysate or amino acid solution
Lipid Metabolism	
Hyperlipidemia	Excessive total dose or rate of administration of fat emulsion
Hyperamylasemia	Lipoid pancreatitis
Hyperbilirubinemia	Excessive dose or rate of administration of fat emulsion
Hypoxia	Interstitial lipoid pneumonitis with alveolar-capillary block
Serum deficiencies of phospholipid linoleic and/or arachidonic acids; serum elevations of -5,8,11-eicosatrienoic acid	Inadequate essential fatty acid administration; inadequate vitamin E administration
Calcium and Phosphorus Metabolism	
Hypophosphatemia Decreased erythrocyte 2,3-diphosphoglycerate Increased affinity of hemoglobin for oxygen Aberrations of erythrocyte intermediary metabolites	Inadequate phosphorus administration; redistribution of serum phosphorus into cells and/or bone
Hypocalcemia	Inadequate calcium administration; reciprocal response to phosphorus repletion without simultaneous calcium infusion; hypoalbuminemia

Table continues

Table 5–3. POTENTIAL METABOLIC COMPLICATIONS OF TOTAL PARENTERAL NUTRITION (*Continued*)

COMPLICATION	ETIOLOGY
Hypercalcemia	Excessive calcium administration with or without high doses of albumin; excessive vitamin D administration
Vitamin D deficiency; hypervitaminosis D	Inadequate or excessive vitamin D administration
Miscellaneous	
Hypokalemia	Inadequate potassium intake relative to increased requirements for protein anabolism; diuresis
Hyperkalemia	Excessive potassium administration, especially in metabolic acidosis, renal decompensation
Hypomagnesemia	Inadequate magnesium administration relative to increased requirements for protein anabolism and glucose metabolism
Hypermagnesemia	Excessive magnesium administration; renal decompensation
Anemia	Iron deficiency; folic acid deficiency; vitamin B_{12} deficiency; copper deficiency; other deficiencies
Bleeding	Vitamin K deficiency
Hypervitaminosis A	Excessive vitamin A administration
Elevations in SGOT, SGPT, and serum alkaline phosphatase	Enzyme induction secondary to amino acid imbalance; excessive glycogen and/or fat deposition in the liver
Cholestatic hepatitis	Decreased water content of bile; amino acid and/or fatty acid imbalance

CONCLUSION

Current techniques of TPN are relatively safe and efficacious but will undoubtedly undergo changes and modifications as improved methods and materials become available. With judicious application of the technique as a clinical, therapeutic, and investigative tool, new indications for general and specific TPN will likely expand and extend into every medical discipline. The capability of providing all essential nutrients entirely by parenteral means, sufficient to support adequate growth, development, and maintenance for prolonged periods of time in both animals and man, is not only of great significance therapeutically to the practice of clinical medicine, but allows investigators to carry out basic and clinical research which has previously been impractical or impossible. It is in this latter area that discoveres and developments in physiology, immunology, cellular biology, biochemistry, and other disciplines will occur as a result of the thoughtful application of the technique of TPN to the solution of basic and clinical problems.

6

Infection, Host Resistance, and Antimicrobial Agents

J. WESLEY ALEXANDER

Between four and five per cent of all patients currently admitted to acute care hospitals in the United States develop a nosocomial infection. Of those who develop such infections, approximately one per cent die as a direct result, and infection contributes to the death of another 2.5 per cent. In surgical patients, the incidence varies between five and 15 per cent in reported series (averaging about seven per cent), and over one million of these infections occur yearly in surgical wounds at an estimated cost of $1.5 billion to $10 billion, depending upon whether only direct hospital cost or total economic losses are considered. In a recent study, wound infection was found approximately to double the expected direct costs of hospitalization regardless of the type of operation. In another large study, infectious complications contributed to one-third of all postoperative deaths. Taken together, these impressive figures demonstrate dramatically the need for improved methods of infection control. However, merely by applying current knowledge and techniques more strictly, it should be possible to reduce the incidence and cost of infections in surgical patients by 50 per cent or more. In this chapter, particular emphasis will be given to practical aspects of preoperative and postoperative care that could lead to reduction in the incidence of infection in surgical patients treated in virtually every type of hospital.

PREOPERATIVE CONSIDERATIONS

Much can be done during the preoperative period to protect patients from infection. This includes assessment of risk, correction of predispos-

106

ing factors, precise timing of operation, judicious use of antibiotics, and containment of contamination. The diagnosis of infection during the preoperative period is similar to that in the postoperative period and will be discussed subsequently.

PATIENT-RELATED FACTORS PREDISPOSING TO SURGICAL INFECTIONS

The status of the patient before operation significantly influences the incidence of infection during the postoperative period. A partial listing of factors having major impact upon predisposition to infection is shown in Table 6–1. Most of these factors are related to the severity of disease, and all are in some way related to host resistance (immunocompetence). Because of the recent ability to detect and qualify immunologic abnormalities, it is possible to analyze methods designed to improve immunologic functions in surgical patients. Research in this important area has already provided applications of practical value to the practicing surgeon.

At the present time, it appears that the most common and most important acquired immunologic deficiencies found in surgical patients are caused by malnutrition. While the interactions of various nutrients are still only partially understood, protein nutrition appears to be very important. Protein and protein-calorie malnutrition are not uncommon;

Table 6–1. FACTORS KNOWN TO INCREASE THE RISK OF INFECTION IN THE SURGICAL PATIENT

Malnutrition

Extremes of age (6 times greater infection rate age > 66 compared to age 1–14; Cruse, 1977)

Type and severity of underlying disease, e.g., trauma, diabetes mellitus, or advanced malignancy

Prolonged hospitalization (rate for > two-week preoperative stay three times greater for clean wounds and rate for one-week stay two times greater; Cruse, 1977)

Recurrent or remote infection

Recent antibiotic therapy

Immunosuppressive drugs

Anergy to skin tests

Poor tissue perfusion, whether from shock, vasoconstriction, or occlusive disease

Obesity

Indwelling catheters

some recent studies have indicated that as many as one-half of all surgical patients hospitalized for longer than one week are so affected. The immunologic abnormalities accompanying malnutrition that predispose patients to infection are both cellular and humoral. Prospective studies have shown that abnormalities of extracellular neutrophil function are the leading immunologic deficiencies contributing to bacterial infections in several types of high-risk surgical patients. Abnormalities of opsonic function have been identified in about one-half of the patients studied, and many episodes of bacteremia are preceded by defects of both phagocytic and opsonic function. Many patients with trauma and a variety of advanced diseases also have abnormalities of chemotaxis and delayed hypersensitivity responsiveness to skin tests. Also present in the serum of many patients are inhibitors of chemotaxis and of the responsiveness of lymphocytes to mitogens. The role of lymphocytic functions in antibacterial defense remains to be defined, but they appear to be much less important than the functions of phagocytic cells and serum opsonins. The acquired defects of immunologic function are generally not as severe as hereditary defects, but they are usually multiple and affect a much larger patient population.

High-risk patients having one or more of the first eight predisposing factors to infection shown in Table 6–1 should be assessed for immunocompetence (Table 6–2). Measurement of serum albumin and transferrin levels provides only a crude estimate of the nutritional status of an individual patient, as do measurements of arm muscle circumference and creatinine/height index. Skin testing with a battery of delayed hypersensitivity antigens will further identify high-risk patients, that is, those with complete or relative anergy. More refined but still simple measurements can be made to quantify serum levels of IgG, C3, and properdin by radial immunodiffusion. Direct measurements of the function of neutrophils and of serum opsonic activity are much better but are not yet routine tests in most hospitals.

Table 6–2. SIMPLE TESTS OF IMMUNOCOMPETENCE THAT HELP TO PREDICT SUSCEPTIBILITY TO INFECTION

Skin tests with delayed hypersensitivity antigens — reflects both cellular immunity and ability to develop an inflammatory response, the latter being more important

Serum levels of IgG, C3, and transferrin

Lymphocyte counts — depressed counts have many causes, often reflects poor nutritional status

Antibacterial function of neutrophils ⎫
                                                        ⎬ not available in most hospitals
Functional opsonic activity of serum ⎭

PREOPERATIVE CORRECTION OF FACTORS PREDISPOSING TO INFECTION

Patients who appear to be clinically malnourished, who have had recent weight loss of more than 10 per cent of their body weight, or who have low levels of serum albumin and transferrin can be assumed to have significant protein-calorie malnutrition and should not have an elective operation until they have received intensive nutritional support as described in Chapters 4 and 5. The enteral route is more efficient and preferred, but many of the immunologic abnormalities associated with malnutrition can be corrected by the parenteral route alone; it usually requires two to three weeks for complete restoration of adequate nutritional status. The amount and type of nutritional support must be determined by taking into account increased metabolic demands of the disease and external losses as well as existing deficits. It is likely that more than 15 per cent of the caloric intake should be provided as protein of high biologic value or as amino acids. However, the optimal protein-carbohydrate ratio has not yet been determined for stressed patients with surgical diseases, trauma, or both. Fats do not seem to play a very important role in improving resistance to infection.

The use of immunopotentiators to improve or restore immunologic function is now being evaluated in several medical centers. At this time, however, it is known only that they are useful in certain controlled animal experiments, and they are not available for routine clinical use. Those drugs and biologicals that currently appear to be the most promising are *Corynebacterium parvum*, pyran, levamisole, BCG, lithium, and muramyldipeptides. All of these cause direct or indirect activation of macrophages, and their effect on neutrophils is mediated via the activated macrophages.

PROPHYLACTIC SYSTEMIC ANTIBIOTICS

It has now been demonstrated amply that judicious use of prophylactic antibiotics significantly reduces the incidence of postoperative infections. Conversely, their use may be harmful because of toxic reactions, allergic responses, interference with normal immunologic defense mechanisms, overgrowth of resistant organisms in the individual patient, and population of the hospital environment with antibiotic-resistant organisms.

INDICATIONS AND CONTRAINDICATIONS

Systemic prophylactic antibiotics are of value in most operations in which significant bacterial contamination occurs. On the other hand, the adverse complications of systemic antibiotics appear to outweigh the

Table 6–3. CLASSIFICATION OF WOUNDS ACCORDING TO THE
DEGREE OF OPERATIVE CONTAMINATION
(FROM NATIONAL RESEARCH COUNCIL)

CLEAN
Surgical incisions made with no break in aseptic technique. Respiratory, alimentary, and genitourinary tracts not entered and no inflammation encountered.

CLEAN-CONTAMINATED
Gastrointestinal or respiratory tracts entered without significant spillage
Genitourinary or biliary tracts entered in absence of infected urine or bile
Vagina or oropharynx entered
Minor break in technique

CONTAMINATED
Gross spillage from gastrointestinal tract
Fresh traumatic wounds
Entrance into genitourinary or biliary tracts with infected urine or bile
Major break in technique

DIRTY OR INFECTED
Perforated viscus
Traumatic wound with delayed treatment, retained foreign body, or from dirty source
Acute bacterial inflammation encountered with or without pus

potential benefits when the expected incidence of infection is or should be less than two per cent. This includes nearly all clean operations and many clean-contaminated operations such as upper urinary tract or bladder operations without infected urine, elective cholecystectomy in patients less than 70 years of age, gastrectomy for peptic ulcer, and abdominal hysterectomy, among others (Table 6–3). Exceptions to this rule are made for operations for placement of permanent intravascular prostheses or major joint replacement because of the grave consequences of infections following such operations and for operations on individuals with recent or existing infections or who are known to be carriers of pathogenic bacteria. The use of prophylactic systemic antibiotics for patients who have compromised immunologic defenses against infection should follow the same guidelines used for immunologically normal patients.

Prophylactic systemic antibiotics are clearly contraindicated for the prevention of infections associated with indwelling intravascular or urinary catheters, intubation of the trachea, open wounds, and thermal injuries (with the possible exception of aqueous penicillin therapy during the first three postburn days as recommended by some authorities but opposed by others, including the author). In these situations, prophylactic antibiotics often lead to superinfections with resistant microorganisms.

The principal guidelines for the use of prophylactic systemic antibiotics in surgery are *(1) the duration of contamination must be limited to a brief period, usually only during the operative procedure, and (2) the anticipated degree of contamination should be sufficiently great to result in an expected incidence of infection greater than two per cent despite excellent surgical technique.* If an incidence of greater than two per cent occurs in clean cases, intensified efforts should be directed toward reduction of exogenous contamination during the operation rather than reliance on antibiotic therapy.

TIMING OF ADMINISTRATION

Experiments nearly two decades ago demonstrated that systemic antibiotics have value in preventing wound infection only when they are started before or very shortly after bacterial contamination. The best results are obtained when antibiotics are first given before operation; their effectiveness rapidly wanes when first given during or after operation and is lost by four to six hours postoperatively. In most elective operations, therefore, the first dose of antibiotic, when indicated, should be given with the preoperative medication, approximately one hour before induction of anesthesia. There is no evidence that

Table 6–4. MICROBIAL FLORA IN SELECTED ANATOMIC
LOCATIONS IN NORMAL AND DISEASED STATES

ANATOMIC SITE	EXPECTED ORGANISMS OF IMPORTANCE	RECOMMENDED SYSTEMIC ANTIBIOTICS FOR PREVENTING POSTOPERATIVE WOUND IN-FECTION° (AUTHOR'S CHOICE UNDERLINED)
Oropharynx	Postoperative infection nearly always mixed and synergistic.	
Normal	Large numbers of anaerobic bacteria, including *Fusobacterium, Bacteroides melaninogenicus,* and *B. oralis*	Penicillin alone
Debilitated state	Increased numbers of gram-negative aerobic rods, especially *E. coli, P. aeruginosa,* and other enteric pathogens	Penicillin or a cephalosporin plus gentamicin or tobramycin
Stomach		
Peptic ulcer disease	Sparse (about 10^2/ml), primarily anaerobic from oropharynx	None
Cancer or bleeding	Often large numbers of both oral anaerobes and gram-negative aerobic rods	Penicillin or a cephalosporin with or without tetracycline, gentamicin, or chloramphenicol
Small bowel		
Normal	Sparse ($< 10^4$/ml) at upper bowel, where anaerobic streptococci and lactobacilli predominate; increasing toward terminal ileum where colon flora predominate.	None
Obstruction	Marked increase in numbers	Same as for colon

°Alternative drugs may be found in Table 6–6.

Table 6–4. MICROBIAL FLORA IN SELECTED ANATOMIC LOCATIONS IN NORMAL AND DISEASED STATES (*Continued*)

ANATOMIC SITE	EXPECTED ORGANISMS OF IMPORTANCE	RECOMMENDED SYSTEMIC ANTIBIOTICS FOR PREVENTING POSTOPERATIVE WOUND IN- FECTION° (AUTHOR'S CHOICE UNDERLINED)
Colon	Large numbers, anaerobes outnumber aerobes 1000:1. Aerobes 10^2–10^5/gm; ana- erobes 10^9–10^{11}/gm. Post- operative infections almost always mixed and syner- gistic. Prophylactic therapy should be directed against *Bacteroides fragilis, Pepto- streptococcus, Peptococcus, Clostridium spp., Entero- coccus, E. coli, Klebsiella- Aerobacter* group.	Penicillin or a cephalosporin plus a tetracycline, gentamicin, or chloramphenicol
Biliary tract with stones	Gram-negative aerobic rods, primary *E. coli, Klebsiella, Aerobacter,* and *Proteus. Clostridium welchii* or other spp. in 10–30%. Occasion- ally *Peptostreptococcus.*	Penicillin or a cephalosporin plus a tetracycline, gentamicin, or chloramphenicol.
Vagina	Mixed aerobes and anaerobes, similar to colon but more anaerobic streptococci	Penicillin or a cephalosporin with or without an aminoglyco- side or chloramphenicol
Infected urinary tract	Predominantly *E. coli, P. aeruginosa,* or other gram- negative rod	Aminoglycoside and/or ampi- cillin or a cephalosporin
Traumatic wounds	Usually *Staphylococcus* or *Streptococcus.* Some wounds have *Clostridium* and/or gram-negative aerobic rods.	A cephalosporin, probably cephalothin because of better resistance to penicillinase

earlier administration of a prophylactic antibiotic provides better protection.

Traumatic wounds require special consideration since a significant amount of time may have elasped between injury and definitive therapy. In such instances, the surgeon should consider the rate of penetration of the antibiotic from the blood into the wound fluids in the selection of an antibiotic. Among the antibiotics with rapid tissue penetrance are ampicillin, aqueous penicillin, tetracycline, and the cephalosporins. Among those that penetrate more slowly are oxacillin, carbenicillin, erythromycin, gentamicin, and clindamycin. In all cases, the quickest way to achieve therapeutic levels of antibiotics in wound fluids is to inject a bolus intravenously. Prophylactic antibiotics should not be given for prevention of infection in simple lacerations. However, well-controlled studies have shown a beneficial effect of systemically administered prophylactic antibiotics in patients with compound fractures and penetrating wounds of the chest. Cephalosporins are the drugs used most for traumatic wounds because of their reasonably broad spectrum, which includes activity against penicillinase-producing staphylococci.

SELECTION ACCORDING TO OPERATIVE SITE

Knowledge of the usual bacterial flora in different parts of the body during both health and disease can aid materially in selection of an appropriate systemic antibiotic for either prophylactic or therapeutic use. Table 6–4 shows the expected flora and recommended prophylactic systemic antibiotics for selected areas. It is noteworthy that penicillin is a preferred drug not only for preventing streptococcal infections but also for preventing most anaerobic infections except those caused by *Bacteroides fragilis*. Gentamicin is an effective drug for preventing infection caused by most gram-negative aerobic organisms. However, when an aminoglycoside is to be used topically, it may be dangerous to use another aminoglycoside antibiotic systemically. Ampicillin penetrates well into tissue fluids and is preferred for many biliary and urinary tract procedures in which contamination is expected.

CONTAINMENT OF CONTAMINATION

Although contamination of the wound occurs almost exclusively during operation, several factors must be considered during the preoperative period. Patients with existing or recurrent infections should be treated aggressively before elective operations to eliminate infection whenever possible. Vectors of pathogenic bacteria, such as nasal carriers of *Staphylococcus aureus,* should also be treated to eliminate the organism if possible. Persistent carriers should be treated with prophylactic systemic antibiotics at the time of operation. Such individuals may also benefit from preoperative showers with antimicrobial soaps the evening before operation, but this practice has little demonstrated value for routine preparation.

SHAVING

Removal of hair from the operative site by shaving before operation clearly increases the incidence of infection and should not be done. The use of electric clippers to remove hair from the operative site, immediately prior to operation, has a significantly lower associated infection rate and is clearly superior to shaving. Depilatories to remove hair also may be used in preference to shaving.

BOWEL PREPARATION FOR COLON SURGERY

Considerable controversy exists regarding the potential benefit of preoperative antibiotic preparation in reducing the numbers of bacteria in the colon before surgery. Controlled trials have shown that oral neomycin-erythromycin base or oral neomycin-tetracycline with mechanical preparation is effective in reducing both aerobic and anaerobic bowel flora and postoperative wound infection. However, similar results can be obtained with prophylactic parenteral antibiotics alone without a marked disturbance of the ecology of the bowel flora. Many investigators feel that preoperative enemas are an important source for introduction of antibiotic-resistant organisms into the intestinal tracts of patients undergoing colon surgery.

THE OPERATIVE PERIOD

PREPARATION OF THE FIELD

Extreme variations exist in the methods by which the operative field is prepared, but all are directed essentially at decontamination of the skin and isolation from contact contamination. The time-honored practice of a 10-minute scrub for routine abdominal procedures has proven benefits. Whether shorter periods can be used depends upon the size of the field and the effectiveness of the decontaminating agent. Hexachlorophene, chlorhexidine, and povidone-iodine are all effective in reducing bacterial counts of the skin, and each has prolonged action. Of the three, povidone-iodine is probably the most popular and hexachlorophene is the least effective.

After mechanical cleansing, it is usually desirable to paint the skin with an antimicrobial agent. Again, a concentrated solution of one of the iodophors that slowly releases free iodine is effective and is widely used. If the patient is a carrier, has had recent remote infection, has furuncles, an open lesion on the body, an enteric or other fistula in the vicinity of the operative site, or is having an operation for implantation of a prosthesis, consideration should be given to painting the operative field with two per cent tincture of iodine since this agent is the most potent antiseptic available. Rarely a patient will develop a hypersensitivity reaction, and tincture of iodine can be irritating if left in skin creases for prolonged periods of time or after repeated use. However, the author has used tincture of iodine extensively for many years without ever observing a hypersensitivity reaction and feels that it should be used routinely wherever there is a high likelihood of wound contamination from the skin.

CONTAINMENT OF CONTAMINATION

Either paper or cloth materials are satisfactory for draping the operative field, provided they do not contain holes and are impervious to water. Protection of the operative wound from the skin may best be accomplished by applying cloth drapes to the skin edges. The use of adhesive plastic drapes to cover the operative field has not yet been proven to be effective in reducing the incidence of infection and increases the cost of the operation. The impermeable plastic drape, however, does have value in excluding contaminated areas such as colostomies or other stomas from the operation site. Newly designed incise drapes with an iodophor incorporated in the adhesive material have not been tested sufficiently to determine their beneficial role.

SURGICAL GARB

Preoperative preparation by the operative team should include a 10-minute scrub for the first operation of the day or for operations following contaminated procedures. A five-minute preparation is probably effective for second or third scrubs after clean operations during the same day. Either chlorhexidine or an iodophor may be used for the scrub to provide a residual antibacterial layer on the skin to restrict bacterial growth. Hexachlorophene may also be effective, but pregnant women are advised not to use the agent because of possible absorption through the intact skin. The presence of dermatitis, infected sites, or open lesions on the hands or forearms of a surgeon should exclude him or her from operating.

The front and sleeves of the surgical gown should be made of a material that is impervious to water, and the gowns should be designed so that they completely enclose the individual with a sterile wrap, that is, none of the back is contaminated. Headgear should cover all exposed hair since it has been demonstrated that some individuals shed bacteria from their hair. Paper masks are usually more effective bacterial filters than cloth masks. Gloves should be inspected for the presence of holes, both upon gloving and at intervals during the operation. If a hole is detected, the glove should be changed immediately since blood inside the glove provides a good pabulum for bacterial growth. Glove powder should never be allowed in the operating room for donning gloves because the particulate matter settles to the floor and other contaminated areas. These contaminated particles often become airborne with activity in the operative theater and can be carried into the sterile operative field.

Gross contamination of the gowns of the surgeon or scrub nurse occurs not infrequently by inadvertent contact of the gowned individual with the operating table during or immediately before draping. Subsequent contact of the contaminated gown with gloves or instruments will result in transfer of organisms to the operative wound.

Perhaps equally important is contamination of the operative field from dislodged lint and debris from the headgear of the operating surgeons when their heads come into contact over the open wound during attempts to gain better visualization. To avoid this problem, the surgeon and the assistant should wear sterile caps during lengthy, difficult, or high-risk operations.

AIR QUALITY IN THE OPERATING ROOM

Modern operating rooms have been designed with filtration systems to insure that the air is of good quality regarding bacterial contamination. It has been argued that laminar flow systems will decrease the incidence of infection in clean wounds into which major implants have been placed. However, this presumption has not been proved by rigorous clinical trial, nor has the use of the greenhouse type of enclosure. In most instances, these considerations are of secondary importance.

INTRAOPERATIVE USE OF ANTIBIOTICS

When there has been an indication for preoperative administration of systemic prophylactic antibiotics, this indication persists throughout the operative period, and an additional injection of the appropriate antibiotics should be made during the procedure to insure maintenance of an adequate blood level while the wound is open.

Equal consideration should be given to the use of topical antibiotics. For most contaminated wounds and some clean wounds in which the expected incidence of infection is greater than two per cent, such as vascular procedures involving the femoral area, a number of well-controlled studies have demonstrated that topical antibiotics can be effective in reducing the incidence of infections. This author believes that topical antibiotics should also be used routinely when the consequences of wound infection are especially serious, such as in immuno-depressed patients or in patients undergoing operation for implantation of prostheses. However, the use of topical antibiotics for irrigation of the peritoneal or pleural cavities may be harmful and should be reserved for very special circumstances because rapid absorption from these sites may result in toxic blood levels. Since early lodgment of bacteria in a wound may result in a protected environment for the bacteria and diminished effectiveness of topical as well as systemic antibiotics, they should be used one or more times during the procedure as well as at the time of closure. Several single drugs or combinations of drugs have been used effectively. In principle, a drug should be selected that is relatively nontoxic, has a broad spectrum of antibacterial activity, and is seldom used systemically. Kanamycin in a concentration of 1 gm per liter fulfills these criteria and has been used extensively by this author and many others without evidence of toxicity or injury to tissues. Other investigators have used combinations of neomycin, polymyxin, or others. While highly effective, these latter drugs are also more dangerous because of a much greater potential for absorption of toxic amounts. Particular concern regarding toxicity should be exercised when a patient is hypotensive or is given a systemic aminoglycoside or loop diuretic. Unfortunately, at the present time it has not been determined whether the use of a combination of systemic and topical antibiotics is more effective than either alone.

THE USE OF DRAINS

Numerous studies have now clearly demonstrated that rubber (Penrose) drains provide a two-way street, one for the egress of fluids and the other for the ingress of bacteria. Thus, wounds or operative sites drained with Penrose drains have a higher incidence of infection than those that are not drained at all. However, in wounds with a large potential dead space, the collection of fluids will greatly increase the incidence of infection. For wounds such as those associated with radical mastectomy, neck dissections, the perineal portion of an abdominoperineal resection, and abdominal incisions in obese individuals, closed suction drainage will provide for removal of fluids and apposition of the tissues while preventing retrograde contamination. Because of these considerations, it is recommended that Penrose drains be used *only* for the drainage of pus. Wounds and operative sites with a large potential dead space should be drained with closed suction catheters, and pancreatic operations or injuries should be drained with sump drains that have a bacterial filter on the air inlet to prevent contamination from airborne bacteria.

TISSUE CARE

It is surprising how few studies have been done to evaluate the influence of gentle tissue handling on subsequent wound infection, considering that this has long been acknowledged as the single most important factor influencing postoperative wound infection. However, compelling recent data from Cruse's surveillance studies (1977) indicate a rather striking difference in the incidence of wound infections among surgeons doing similar operations in the same hospital (Fig. 6–1). It has also been demonstrated amply in the laboratory that surgical wounds can be contaminated with relatively large numbers of bacteria, up to 10^6 staphylococci, without becoming infected, but in the presence of tissue damage, seromas, hematomas, or foreign bodies, the numbers required to cause an infection are markedly reduced. Débridement is absolutely

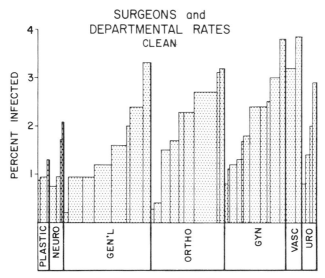

Figure 6–1. Clean wound infection rates for different surgeons at a single hospital. (From Cruse, P.: South. Med. J., 70(Suppl. 1):4–8, 1977. Reprinted by permission of the author.)

necessary to remove devitalized tissue and debris when present in traumatic wounds.

Traumatic wounds can usually be closed without infection if they contain fewer than 10^5 bacteria, as evidenced by absence of bacteria on gram stain; however, infection is common when wounds with greater numbers of bacteria are closed. Recent studies have shown that a pulsating jet lavage or high-pressure irrigation is more effective than conventional irrigation to remove surface bacteria and loose debris in contaminated wounds.

THE ROLE OF SUTURE MATERIAL

As early as 1957, Elek demonstrated in humans that a silk suture could decrease the size of a bacterial inoculum necessary to cause an infection in small wounds by a factor of 10,000. However, there are considerable differences among sutures in their abilities to potentiate wound infection. Multifilament suture materials are associated with increased infection compared with monofilament sutures of the same material, regardless of their composition. Monofilament polypropylene and monofilament nylon resist bacterial contamination better than other suture materials that have been tested, including monofilament wire. Since neither nylon nor polypropylene sutures extrude in the presence of infection, their use is strongly advocated for closure of virtually all contaminated wounds in which the risk of infection is a major consideration. Absorbable suture materials of any kind are metabolized more rapidly in the presence of infection and, therefore, should not be used for major fascial closures when the risk of infection is relatively great.

Many authorities also feel that the use of continuous sutures for fascial closure produces less necrosis at tension points where the sutures pass through the fascia, and, therefore, are less likely to become infected. However, this technical point has not been subjected to adequate experimental evaluation.

DELAYED PRIMARY CLOSURE

In heavily contaminated wounds, especially those associated with traumatic injury, delayed primary closure will significantly reduce the incidence of infection. Such wounds can withstand increasing amounts of bacterial colonization on their surface, on the order of a tenfold increase daily, until the fifth day, probably because of the progressive development of a reactive vascular network at the wound edges. Because of this, the optimal time for delayed primary closure is the fifth postoperative day.

POSTOPERATIVE CONSIDERATIONS

WOUND CARE

Postoperative wound infections most frequently result from intraoperative contamination. However, incisions can be, and often are, infected by postoperative contamination from the environment. Therefore, it is recommended that all incisions in areas that can be dressed be covered with sterile dressings during the postoperative period. Since the resistance of a wound to bacterial contamination increases progressively up to the fifth or sixth postoperative day, dressings are especially important during the first few days. It is equally important to keep the wound dry. Dressings moistened by blood or serous discharge should be changed as often as necessary to achieve a dry surface. Relatively light, air-permeable, and porous dressings are desirable. It is especially important to keep the incidence of stitch-related infections as low as possible in those wounds that might potentially require exploration because of postoperative complications. In such cases, the presence of small and even subclinical foci of infection around sutures markedly increases the incidence of postoperative infections. In the immunosuppressed patient, consideration should be given to excision of the entire wound, including the skin sutures, if reentry is indicated when skin sutures are still in place. The use of tape closure in lieu of suture closure or for support after very early suture removal also reduces the incidence of superficial infections.

Because sealing of the wound with a dry coagulum is critical to prevent exogenously induced infections, it is contraindicated to paint the wound surface and sutures with medicaments even though some of these may have antimicrobial action. The only possible exception to this is the use of tincture of iodine in the presence of superficial inflammation of localized foci of purulence. Topical antibiotics should never be used prophylactically on surgical incisions in an effort to prevent infection.

SYSTEMIC ANTIBIOTICS DURING THE POSTOPERATIVE PERIOD

Systemic antibiotics have several adverse effects. Perhaps the most important of these during the postoperative period is alteration of the microbial ecology of both the individual patient and the hospital environment. Because of this, administration of antibiotics should be restricted during the postoperative period. Several elegant studies have shown that the most effective antibiotic regimens are those that incorporate only three doses, one during the preoperative period, the second during the operation, and the third during the immediate postoperative period. In fact, one recent well-controlled study has demonstrated that a single dose of two antibiotics during the immediate preoperative period effectively reduced wound infections for operations classified as contaminated. In support, another controlled study on patients undergoing vaginal hysterectomy, performed to determine whether repeated doses of antibiotics during the postoperative period were more effective than a single dose, showed no difference in the incidence or severity of infections. Others have shown a slight but statistically insignificant increase in infections when antibiotics are continued past the immediate postoperative period. In general, prophylactic systemic antibiotics should be continued for no longer than six hours following an elective operation, and even this length of time is questionable. In contaminated wounds, such as penetrating wounds of the abdomen or other traumatic wounds in which contamination has occurred preoperatively, infection may already have become established, and administration of antibiotics for up to 72 hours or longer may be indicated.

URINARY TRACT INFECTIONS

The majority of postoperative urinary tract infections are related to bladder catheterization. There is clear evidence that the incidence of such infections increases with advancing age, is higher in females, occurs more often in patients with asymptomatic bacteriuria, increases with duration of catheterization, and is related to catheter care. Catheters should not be irrigated except in special circumstances to remove obstructing clots or debris, such as in the postoperative urologic patient. To and fro motion of the catheter will introduce bacteria into the urethra. Therefore, in the male, a bandage affixed to the catheter and the penile shaft is effective in preventing this motion and also protects the catheter-meatal junction from exogenous contamination. The application of an antimicrobial agent to the catheter-meatal junction is useless and in some patients actually increases the incidence of infection. Antibiotic irrigation of the bladder may delay the onset of infection by a few days, but when infections do occur, they are usually caused by antibiotic-resistant organisms, and thus this practice is not recommended. The use of systemic antibiotics to prevent catheter-related infection is totally contraindicated, not only because it is ineffective but also because antibiotic-resistant organisms cause the infections that do occur. The most important considerations in catheter care are use of a closed collection system and monitoring the urine for bacterial growth, by culturing samples obtained by needle aspiration from the catheter or tubing, since bacteriuria regularly precedes symptomatic infections. Catheters should be left in place for as short a time as possible because the duration of catheterization is directly related to the incidence of infection (see Chap. 33).

INFECTIONS ASSOCIATED WITH INTRAVENOUS CATHETERS

As with urinary catheters, the length of time that a catheter is left in a vein is directly related to the incidence of infection. This is especially true for small peripheral vein catheters, which should never remain at a single site for longer than 48 hours. During the postoperative period, plastic catheters should be avoided altogether in peripheral veins; instead, stainless steel needles of the butterfly type should be used since these are associated with a substantially lower incidence of infection. Even these should be changed every 72 hours. Central venous catheters can be left for a much longer period of time but require special attention. These catheters should be fixed by suture to the skin, placing the suture very near the catheter-skin junction to prevent to and fro motion. Antibiotic ointments at the entrance of central catheters have no proven benefit and are not recommended. Of more importance is to provide a dry environment, at the same time maintaining freedom from exogenous contamination. Inline bacterial filters can be used with central venous catheters for intravenous hyperalimentation, and the catheters should not be used for any other purposes.

POSTOPERATIVE PULMONARY INFECTIONS

These infections are often associated with contamination during intubation and endotracheal suctioning. Prolonged intubation or tracheostomy is associated with a high incidence of pulmonary infections, especially when performed for nonobstructive conditions. Careful daily monitoring of tracheal aspirates by Gram stain will help to differentiate between colonization and infection. When the pattern of scattered inflammatory cells changes to large numbers of inflammatory cells with intracellular and extracellular bacteria, a diagnosis of pulmonary infection can be made, and appropriate antibiotic therapy should be instituted. The onset of pulmonary infections in intubated patients can be delayed considerably by strict aseptic technique during tracheal aspiration and careful attention to the sterility of respiratory support equipment. The latter should be monitored routinely for the presence of bacterial contamination. Isolation procedures are particularly important in preventing respiratory tract infections in intensive care units.

NUTRITION IN THE POSTOPERATIVE PERIOD

Nutrition is considered extensively in other portions of this manual, but it is worthwhile to emphasize in this chapter that inadequate nutrition is probably next in importance to the degree of wound contamination in determining the incidence of serious postoperative infections. Therefore, patients who appear to be clinically malnourished should receive intensive nutritional support during the preoperative period. If this is not possible, intravenous hyperalimentation should be started during the first 24 hours after operation. Even well-nourished persons should be started on intravenous hyperalimentation to prevent associated abnormalities of immunologic function if they are unable to take enteral food five to six days postoperatively. Caloric requirements are often increased during the postoperative period, and the amount of calories and protein to be given should reflect both resting and hyper-metabolic demands as well as increased losses from the GI tract, fistulas, urine, or wounds. Depending upon the severity of injury and the presence or absence of infection, 500 to 1000 mg of vitamin C should be administered daily, and two to five times the recommended daily allowances of most of the other vitamins, except for vitamins E and K, which have no demonstrated increased requirement during stress. Details of such nutritional support are found in Chapters 4 and 5.

Hyperalimentation should not be delayed in the critically ill septic patient who does not respond promptly to antibiotic therapy. A central venous catheter should be placed early in such patients, and hyperalimentation should be started as soon as hemodynamic stability has been acquired since three to four days of poor nutrition in the face of stress and sepsis can often render a patient metabolically and immunologically destitute.

DIAGNOSIS OF SURGICAL INFECTIONS

The physiologic disturbances associated with infections in the surgical patient are like those in any other patient except that the cardinal signs of inflammation may be absent or modified because of postoperative pain, ileus, atelectasis, severity of disease, mental state, and therapeutic agents that interfere with inflammatory responses.

WOUND INFECTIONS

Infections of the surgical wound may occur from the first postoperative day to many months or even years following the procedure. They account for about 22 per cent of all nosocomial infections. The majority, perhaps 80 to 90 per cent, are detected within the first two weeks with a median time of nine to ten days. Both the time of clinical appearance of the infection and the type of operation performed are important clues as to the likely causative agents.

The sudden onset of a high spiking fever with accompanying toxicity within the first 24 to 48 hours following operation is not often thought to be related to wound infection. However, both acute clostridial wound infection and acute streptococcal wound infection can cause this clinical picture, and either of these can result in rapid demise of the patient if not diagnosed early and treated appropriately. Because these infections should be suspected by the clinical appearance of the wound, spiking fevers associated with clinical toxicity demand prompt inspection of the operative site.

Streptococcal infections characteristically cause swelling and redness of the normal tissues surrounding the incision with increased local skin temperature and tenderness. There may be a thin, watery, pinkish discharge that is characteristically odorless. Blisters, which are first serous and later hemorrhagic, often form about the wound. Gram stain of exudate or blister fluid will show numerous cocci that may or may not be in chains. By contrast, acute wound infections caused by clostridia are usually not erythematous and may not be painful. The wound is usually boggy and edematous with a brownish discharge that has a characteristic odor often described as sickeningly sweet. Crepitation is uncommon. Gram stain will reveal characteristic gram-positive rods in the exudate. The patient may be disproportionately toxic, and there is sometimes marked anemia and jaundice secondary to hemolysis caused by exotoxins. Acute clostridial wound infections may follow virtually any operation but are more often complications of biliary tract surgery, colon surgery, or contaminated wounds of violence.

Infections caused by *Staphylococcus aureus* frequently complicate accidental injury and are prominent following clean operative procedures. These infections usually become clinically manifest during the last part of the first postoperative week but may not make their appearance until weeks, months, or even years following the operation, especially when there has been purposeful implantation of a large foreign body. The cardinal signs of inflammation are usually present, especially in those making their appearance early, but any or all of the signs of inflammation may be absent. Staphylococcal organisms usually elicit the formation of pus, which may range in character from a serosanguineous discharge to a thick, creamy fluid. There is no diagnostic odor.

Infections caused by endogenous bacteria spilled into the wound intraoperatively are the most common cause of postoperative infections following gastrointestinal operations. Such infections are usually mixed and nearly always involve anaerobic species. Infections following head and neck operations when the mouth or pharynx is entered, for example, nearly always involve *Bacteroides melaninogenicus, B. oralis,* or *Fusobacterium,* and surgical wound infections following operations on the colon nearly always involve anaerobic streptococci, *B. fragilis,* and a variety of aerobic gram-negative organisms, usually together with *E. coli.* Often with such infections, the tissue appears necrotic, but there may be minimal signs of inflammation. The pus or purulent discharge almost always has a foul odor that is characteristic of the presence of anaerobic organisms. It is noteworthy that a high degree of accuracy can be achieved in predicting the infecting organism or organisms causing a wound infection simply by knowing the expected normal microbial flora at the start of operation (Table 6–4).

When wound infection is expected but cannot be proved by external examination, judicious needle aspiration is warranted to establish the diagnosis. Any fluid obtained should be cultured, and a smear should be made for Gram staining.

INTRA-ABDOMINAL INFECTIONS

Postoperative intra-abdominal infections are often exceptionally difficult to diagnose. However, accurate appraisal is essential because undrained collections of pus within the peritoneal cavity lead to progressive deterioration of the patient and may result in death. On the other hand, a mistaken diagnosis and an inappropriate operation may also jeopardize a patient's chances for recovery. Often, postoperative ileus and abdominal tenderness associated with the primary procedure make the assessment of physical findings difficult. In the patient who has undergone a recent abdominal procedure and has suggestive evidence of infection but no localized site, the old adage, "pus somewhere, pus nowhere, pus under the diaphragm," often holds true. Several diagnostic tests may be of aid. Introduction of barium into the gastrointestinal tract to demonstrate displacement of organs may be extremely helpful if the patient can tolerate such examinations. Often, disorganization of the mucosal pattern secondary to edema may lead to a correct diagnosis. Examination of the abdomen by ultrasonography has been used extensively in many hospitals and has been reported to be of help. However, the experience of others has been disappointing, and such tests may often be misleading. It is this writer's opinion that ultrasonography is rarely helpful in diagnosing intra-abdominal abscesses, although numerous specific exceptions have been documented. Gallium scans have also been used in recent years in many centers. Not only does this examination take a long time to perform, but also a sufficiently large number of false positives and false negatives make its value very limited and certainly not cost-effective. On the other hand, liver scans following the administration of appropriate radioisotopes have been of great value in diagnosing abscesses of the liver, and combined liver-lung scans have occasionally been helpful in diagnosing subdiaphragmatic abscesses. Clearly, the most useful of the recently devised tests for use adjunctive to the clinical diagnosis of intra-abdominal abscess is computerized tomography. It is now the diagnostic test of choice in the postoperative patient.

Retroperitoneal abscesses and infections can be diagnosed by similar means. In this regard, an inferior venacavogram followed by an intravenous pyelogram is often of value to demonstrate displacement by localized collections of pus. As above, CT scans remain the "gold standard."

SEPTICEMIA AND BACTEREMIA

The differentiation between bacteremia and septicemia is often clouded; the former is regarded as a transient release of bacteria into the bloodstream, whereas septicemia is considered to be a progressive growth of bacteria within the bloodstream. This is an artificial separation, however, and many authorities now use the more generic term bacteremia with modification regarding severity. Bacteremia is most often associated with a localized infection complicating an operation or with operative manipulation, such as instrumentation in the presence of urinary tract infection. The urinary tract is the primary site in 40 per cent of secondary nosocomial bacteremias. However, since most of the cases of "primary" bacteremia are associated with intravenous systems, one should not neglect the possibility that the infection is arising from contaminated intravenous fluids, contaminated intravenous catheters or arterial catheters, or that bacterial endocarditis has occurred. Thus, the most important consideration in the treatment of bacteremia is identification of the underlying cause or source. Like any infection, progressive bacteremia can result in hypothermia and diminished peripheral perfusion as the clinical state of frank septic shock is approached. The white blood cell count may be elevated, normal, or depressed, but there is virtually always a shift to the left that becomes accentuated with progression of the infection.

PNEUMONIAS

Lower respiratory tract infections are responsible for approximately 16 per cent of all nosocomial infections and are especially common following prolonged anesthesia. Postoperative pneumonias are usually easy to diagnose because they cause consolidation of pulmonary tissues evidenced by roentgenographic examination. However, the diagnosis may not be so easy when the patient has atelectasis or has just undergone pulmonary or cardiovascular surgery. When a patient is intubated, daily examination of a tracheal aspirate by Gram stain will determine when positive cultures become significant and when pneumonia first makes its appearance. When the pattern of the Gram stain changes from scattered inflammatory cells to dense numbers of neutrophils with bacteria, a diagnosis of significant infection can be made, and antibiotic therapy should be instituted. In patients who develop postoperative pneumonia who are not intubated, sputum cultures are virtually worthless except when taken from samples composed of marked inflammatory cell reaction associated with both intracellular and extracellular bacteria as proved by Gram stain. In patients who develop life-threatening pneumonias, transtracheal aspiration to obtain material for Gram stain and culture is usually mandatory if antibiotics are to be selected in a meaningful way. A negative transtracheal aspirate in a patient with an acute pulmonary infiltrate should lead one to suspect a diagnosis other than acute bacterial infection.

Nonbacterial opportunistic infections occasionally occur in the lung during the postoperative period. These usually occur in immunosuppressed patients who have been receiving immunosuppressive drugs for some time before operation. In such patients, when the transtracheal aspirate is negative, a transbronchial pulmonary biopsy may be indicated. If this is unsuccessful, consideration should be given to open lung biopsy because an etiologic diagnosis of the pulmonary infiltrate is usually important for appropriate management.

URINARY TRACT INFECTIONS

Infections of the urinary tract are relatively easy to diagnose because of the ready accessibility of urine for examination. The presence of bacteria on a Gram-stained smear of a properly collected, fresh, unspun specimen or colony counts greater than 100,000 per ml are felt by most clinicians to be diagnostic of urinary tract infection. The vast majority of such infections in both males and females are caused by gram-negative aerobic bacteria. In most patients, examination of a clean catch urine specimen is sufficient to establish a diagnosis. However, contamination from the perineum in females, especially when vaginitis is present, may prevent accurate interpretation of the urinary findings. In such patients, urine should be obtained by careful catheterization or suprapubic aspiration of the bladder. In the catheterized patient, urine can be monitored by daily aspiration with a fine-gauge needle from the catheter after iodine preparation. Most drainage systems are now equipped with an aspiration port so that urine sampling can be done repeatedly without contamination.

TREATMENT

SURGICAL DRAINAGE

Surgical drainage is the basis of therapy for most localized soft tissue infections in which pus is present. The type of incision to be made varies widely with the location of the abscess, but a cardinal rule is that adequate free drainage be obtained. In unusual situations, such as a deep brain abscess, needle aspiration may be the treatment of choice, but the clinical principle is always to remove localized pus since the normal bodily defenses against infections are not optimally effective in abscess cavities. In addition, antibiotics often penetrate poorly into collections of pus, and many of the antibiotics are rapidly degraded in this environment. Recently, percutaneous catheter drainage has been used successfully to drain localized abscesses without incision. Liver abscesses may be particularly amenable to this type of drainage, but results of catheter drainage of other intra-abdominal abscesses need to be compared carefully with those of surgical drainage before being accepted as a primary method of treatment.

Necrotizing infections should always be incised widely to allow exposure and excision of all the necrotic tissues whenever possible. Such infections include anaerobic streptococcal myositis, clostridial infections, necrotizing fasciitis, and mixed phlegmons. When adequate incision and débridement are not possible because of anatomic considerations or involvement of vital structures, consideration should be given to the use of supplemented hyperbaric oxygenation. With the exception of such anaerobic infections, it is doubtful that hyperbaric oxygen therapy has significant benefit in the management of surgical infections. However, it has been shown experimentally that hypoxia can inhibit the antibacterial function of phagocytic cells.

Certain localized infections, such as infected fracture sites or pyoarthrosis, are best treated by incision, débridement of devitalized tissues, placement of irrigation and drainage tubes, closure of the wound, and periodic irrigation of the infected site with topical antibiotics. This technique has sometimes been successful in the treatment of infected vascular grafts and foreign body implants, including total hip replacement prostheses. In such instances, it is necessary to use broad-spectrum antibiotics, most often a neomycin, polymyxin, and bacitracin mixture, to prevent the growth of potential contaminants during therapy. Depending on the condition, the course of therapy might last 7 to 14 days or even longer. The patient should be monitored not only with repeated cultures but also with sequential tests of kidney function and eighth nerve function to detect early damage caused by excessive absorption of these toxic antibiotics.

RADICAL DEBRIDEMENT OF THE PERITONEAL CAVITY

In 1975, Hudspeth described a technique of aggressive débridement of the peritoneal cavity in patients with peritonitis or localized infections of the peritoneal cavity associated with clinical deterioration on conservative therapy, often with a continuing source of infection from a perforation of the gastrointestinal tract. This procedure involves correction of underlying anatomic problems related to the gastrointestinal tract, including diversion or resection when necessary to prevent continued contamination, aggressive removal of all inflammatory exudate within the peritoneal cavity, extensive irrigation of the peritoneal cavity, the use of systemic antibiotics, and intensive supportive care. The results in a highly selected group of patients have been extremely impressive, and the technique is now being used in many centers. However, it must be emphasized that the vast majority of localized collections of pus in the abdomen should be drained by localized incision. The radical approach should be reserved for patients with generalized peritonitis and an anatomic defect such as a bowel perforation or for patients with multiple abscesses.

SELECTION OF ANTIBIOTICS

Initial antibiotic selection for treatment of established infections should be based upon the probable organism related to the anatomic site or surgical condition, coupled with inspection of Gram stain infectious material. With this very simply obtained information, better than 90 per cent accuracy can be achieved for selection of the appropriate antibiotic (Table 6–5). Whenever possible, the antibiotic spectrum should be broad enough to cover the range of suspected pathogens but restricted as much as possible to prevent overgrowth of antibiotic-resistant strains. When treating infections, the indications for antibiotic therapy should be reviewed no less frequently than every five days since one of the serious errors commonly made in most hospitals at the present time is continuation of antibiotics past their period of usefulness. This only aids the emergence of antibiotic-resistant strains. Table 6–6 outlines the characteristics of selected antibiotics with comments regarding their general usefulness and adverse reactions.

Table 6–5. INITIAL SELECTION OF ANTIBIOTIC THERAPY BASED UPON GRAM STAIN AND SOURCE*

TYPE OF BACTERIA FOUND ON GRAM STAIN	SOURCE	INITIAL CHOICE OF ANTIBIOTICS
Gram-positive cocci in pairs (pneumococci)	Lung or spinal fluid	Penicillin. Sometimes staphylococci may appear in pairs. When uncertain add nafcillin.
Gram-positive cocci in clumps (staphylococci)	Any source	Nafcillin
Gram-positive cocci in chains (streptococci)	Any source	Penicillin G
Gram-positive rods	Any source	Penicillin G plus a tetracycline or clindamycin
Gram-negative rods	Lower respiratory tract pneumonia	An aminoglycoside
	Lung abscess	Penicillin
	Urinary tract	Ampicillin with or without an aminoglycoside
	Surgical wound (abdomen)	Penicillin plus a tetracycline or chloramphenicol or ampicillin plus gentamicin
	Surgical wound (chest)	Ampicillin plus gentamicin
	Septicemia	Ampicillin or a cephalosporin plus an aminoglycoside. If anaerobic infection suspected, add clindamycin or chloramphenicol.
	Deep abscess	Same as septicemia
Mixed flora—gram-positive and gram-negative	Human bite	Penicillin and a tetracycline
	Septicemia	Penicillin and an aminoglycoside or penicillin and chloramphenicol or clindamycin and an aminoglycoside
	Severe cellulitis or peritonitis following intestinal surgery	Same as above

*See Table 6–6 for alternative drugs. (Modified from Altemeier, W. A., and Alexander, J. W.: Surgical infections and choice of antibiotics. *In* Sabiston, D. C., Jr. (ed.): Textbook of Surgery, 12th ed. Philadelphia, W. B. Saunders Co., 1981.)

Table 6–6. CHARACTERISTICS OF SELECTED ANTIBIOTICS*

ANTIBIOTIC	PRIMARY INDICATIONS	ALTERNATIVE AGENTS	MAJOR ADVERSE EFFECTS	COMMENTS
Penicillins Penicillin G	Agent of first choice for: S. pneumoniae (pneumococcus) Enterococcus (with streptomycin). Nonpenicillinase producing S. aureus	Erythromycin, vancomycin	Allergic reactions and anaphylaxis; CNS irritability and convulsions in high doses	Bactericidal. Inhibits cell wall synthesis. Requires growing cells for effects. Agent one of primary choice for prophylaxis against infections following GI tract surgery because of effect on anaerobic bacteria. Important for use in synergistic mixed aerobic and anaerobic infections for same reason. Has good rate of exchange from intravascular to wound fluid compartments.
	Streptococcus spp.	A cephalosporin, clindamycin, vancomycin, erythromycin		
	Peptococcus (anaerobic Staph.)	Erythromycin		
	Peptostreptococcus (anaerobic Strep.)	Erythromycin, clindamycin, chloramphenicol		
	Neisseria gonorrhoeae	Erythromycin, clindamycin, chloramphenicol		
	Neisseria meningitidis	Spectinomycin, a tetracycline		
	Clostridium spp.	Ampicillin, chloramphenicol		
	Bacillus anthracis	Clindamycin, chloramphenicol		
	Fusospirochetes	A tetracycline, erythromycin		
	Almost all other anaerobic bacteria except Bacteroides fragilis	Erythromycin, a tetracycline		
	Actinomyces israelii	Clindamycin, chloramphenicol, a tetracycline		
		A tetracycline		
Ampicillin	Agent of first choice for: Hemophilus influenzae	A tetracycline, trimethoprim-sulfa, chloramphenicol	Same as penicillin—allergic reactions higher where given by oral route	High biliary and urinary excretion make ampicillin useful for treatment of biliary tract and urinary tract infections, which are usually caused by sensitive organisms.
	Listeria monocytogenes	Penicillin		
	Shigella spp.	Trimethoprim-sulfa, chloramphenicol		
	Proteus mirabilis	A cephalosporin, an aminoglycoside		
Penicillinase-resistant penicillins	Agent of first choice for penicillinase-producing Staphylococcus aureus	Erythromycin, vancomycin, cephalosporins, clindamycin, an aminoglycoside	Same as penicillin plus interstitial nephritis, jaundice, and bone marrow depression	Nafcillin probably agent of choice for parenteral use—methicillin associated with increased risk of inter-

Drug	Combination	Clinical Uses	Side Effects	Comments
(continued)			Same as penicillin	stitial nephritis. Oxacillin exchanges slowly between serum and wound fluids. Dicloxacillin best absorbed from GI tract of the synthetic penicillins.
Carbenicillin, ticarcillin, piperacillin, and mezlocillin	An aminoglycoside	Variably useful for resistant *Pseudomonas aeruginosa*, *Providencia*, and many other gram-negative bacilli		High doses needed. Often combined with an aminoglycoside for resistant *P. aeruginosa* infections. Occasionally useful for other antibiotic-resistant gram-negative infections.
Cephalosporins	An aminoglycoside	Agent of first choice for *Klebsiella pneumoniae*	Allergic reactions. Approximately 10% of penicillin-allergic persons will be allergic to cephalosporins. Neutropenia rare. Nephrotoxicity and ototoxicity, especially in high doses or when given to patients in shock or to patients receiving furosemide or an aminoglycoside	Inhibits cell wall synthesis. Cephalosporins have proven effectiveness as prophylactic antibiotics for many indications. Appear to be useful in preventing mixed infections and penicillin-resistant staphylococcal infections. Cephalothin appears to be the cephalosporin most resistant to the effect of penicillinase. Several third-generation cephalosporins have recently been approved that have very broad antibacterial activity. Their use for specific indications has not been well established, but they probably should not be used as primary drugs.

Table 6–6. CHARACTERISTICS OF SELECTED ANTIBIOTICS* (*Continued*)

ANTIBIOTIC	PRIMARY INDICATIONS	ALTERNATIVE AGENTS	MAJOR ADVERSE EFFECTS	COMMENTS
Vancomycin	Secondary agent for resistant staphylococci. Appears to be agent of first choice for controlling pseudomembranous enterocolitis caused by antibiotic-resistant enterotoxin-producing strains of *clostridium*.	Erythromycin Metronidazole	Eighth cranial nerve damage	Inhibits cell wall synthesis
Aminoglycosides	Agent for first choice for most gram-negative aerobic enteric pathogens, especially *Enterobacter, Escherichia, Klebsiella, Proteus, Providentia, Pseudomonas,* and *Serratia*.	Wide variation depending on organism and resistance patterns	Ototoxicity and nephrotoxicity very frequent. Occasional peripheral neuropathies, allergic reactions, and blood dyscrasias.	Serial blood levels of all these drugs are important because of low toxic/therapeutic ratio. Amikacin resistant to most bacterial enzymes and should be reserved for treatment of organisms resistant to other aminoglycosides. Tobramycin slightly more effective than gentamicin against most strains of *P. aeruginosa*, but these drugs otherwise appear to be equivalent. Effective against *S. aureus* but not *Streptococcus*. Kanamycin useful as topical antibiotic in concentration of 1.0 gm/liter. All are bactericidal and inhibit protein synthesis by affecting 30s subunit of ribosome.

Drug	Clinical Use	Alternative Drugs	Toxicity/Side Effects	Comments
Chloramphenicol	Agent for first choice for *Salmonella spp.*	Ampicillin, amoxicillin, sulfatrimethoprim	Bone marrow depression. Occasional aplastic anemia. Parenteral route appears to be much safer since most cases of aplastic anemia have followed oral administration. Neuropathy.	Excellent drug for many anaerobic infections, including *Bacteroides fragilis*. Inhibits protein synthesis—affects 50s subunit of ribosomes.
Erythromycin	Agent of first choice for *Mycoplasma*	A tetracycline, chloramphenicol	GI and hepatic disturbances	Bacteriostatic. Inhibits 50s subunit. Good secondary agent for anaerobes and *Streptococcus pyogenes*.
Tetracyclines	Agent of first choice for: *Brucella sp.* *Pseudomonas peudomallei*	Chloramphenicol, sulfatrimethoprim Chloramphenicol	Catabolic. GI disturbances. Bone and tooth malformations in children. Hepatotoxicity, allergic reactions, blood dyscrasias.	Bacteriostatic. Inhibits protein synthesis (30s subunits). Useful with penicillin as a prophylactic antibiotic in bowel and biliary surgery. Varying effectiveness of the tetracyclines against anaerobic bacteria, especially *B. fragilis*.
Clindamycin	Agent of first choice for *Bacteroides fragilis*	Chloramphenicol, a tetracycline Metronidazole	Colitis Allergic reactions Hepatic disturbances	Bacteriostatic. Binds to 50s subunits of ribosomes. Antagonistic to erythromycin and chloramphenicol. Effective against a wide range of anaerobic bacteria. Ineffective against most aerobic gram-negative rods.
Amphotericin B	Agent of choice for all fungi	No good secondary drugs for most fungi. Hydroxystilbamidine useful for *Blastomyces*.	Highly nephrotoxic Liver damage, anemia, fever, shock	Must start with small dose.

°List and comments are not meant to be complete.

REFERENCES

Abramowicz: The choice of antimicrobial drugs. Medical Letter, 24:21–28, 1982.

Alexander, J. W.: Nosocomial infections. In Ravitch, M. M. (ed.): Current Problems in Surgery. Chicago, Year Book Medical Pub., 1973.

Alexander, J. W.: Life-threatening sepsis. In Condon, R. E., and DeCosse, J. J. (eds.): Surgical Care: A Physiologic Approach to Surgical Problems, Chap. 9. Lea and Febiger, 1980, pp. 302–313.

Alexander, J. W., and Good, R. A.: Fundamentals of Clinical Immunology. Philadelphia, W. B. Saunders Co., 1977.

Altemeier, W. A., and Alexander, J. W.: Surgical infections and choice of antibiotics. In Sabiston, D. C., Jr. (ed.): Davis-Christopher Textbook of Surgery, 11th ed., Chap. 17. Philadelphia, W. B. Saunders Co., 1977, pp. 340–362.

Altemeier, W. A., Burke, J. F., Pruitt, B. A., and Sandusky, W. R. (eds.): Manual on Control of Infection in Surgical Patients. Philadelphia, J. B. Lippincott, 1976.

Cruse, P.: Infection surveillance: Identifying the problems and the high risk patient. South. Med. J., 70 (Suppl. 1):4, 1977.

Edlich, R. F., Rodeheaver, G. T., Thacker, J. G., and Edgerton, M. T.: Fundamentals of wound management in surgery. Technical factors in wound management. South Plainfield, N.J., Chirurgecom, Inc., 1977.

Elek, S. D., and Cormen, P. E.: The virulence of Staphylococcus pyogenes for man: A study of the problems of wound infection. Br. J. Exp. Pathol., 38:573, 1957.

Green, J. W., and Wenzel, R. P.: Postoperative wound infection: A controlled study of the increased duration of hospital stay and direct cost of hospitalization. Ann. Surg., 185:264, 1977.

Hudspeth, A. S.: Radical surgical débridement in the treatment of advanced generalized bacterial peritonitis. Arch. Surg., 110:1233, 1975.

Patterson, H. R., Gustafson, E. A., and Sheridan, E.: Falconer's Current Drug Handbook 1980–1982. Philadelphia, W. B. Saunders Co., 1982.

7

Blood and Blood Products

JOHN A. COLLINS

The modern blood bank has become more than a place to store whole blood and crossmatch it for an intended recipient on demand. There have been great advances in blood banking in recent years, with potentially significant increases in safety, specificity, and efficacy for the patient. Unfortunately, there has not been a concomitant increase in educational activities (undergraduate, graduate, and postgraduate) designed to keep the practicing surgeon informed of these advances so he or she can take full advantage of them for the benefit of the patient. This chapter will review briefly what is available in a modern blood bank, the indications for transfusion of blood or its components, and the potential benefits and risks of various strategies of treatment. The coagulation factors and the use of nonblood fluids to treat hypovolemia will be discussed in Chapter 3.

PREPARATIONS, INDICATIONS, AND USE

RED BLOOD CELLS

Most whole blood in the United States is now stored at 4°C in citrate phosphate dextrose (CPD), a citrate-based liquid anticoagulant, in a ratio of 450 ml donor blood ± 10 per cent to 63 ml CPD, in plastic bags. There are significant changes from normal during storage, some of which are indicated in Table 7–1. CPD with adenine added has been approved for use by the FDA, and is beginning to be used in several blood centers because the longer storage facilitates the management of inventory. Blood stored in CPD adenine will have better post-transfusion survival of the red blood cells but more functional impairment of the hemoglobin early in storage and, of course, added adenine. Whole blood has been the standard product of the American blood bank, and it is the one against which most clinicians judge and compare the newer products. Much of

137

Table 7–1. CHANGES REPORTED IN HUMAN WHOLE BLOOD
STORED IN CPD AT 4°C IN PLASTIC BAGS

	1 WEEK	3 WEEKS
Acid load	15 mEq/l	30 mEq/l
Citrate	20 mEq/unit	20 mEq/unit
Phosphate	4–8 mg/dl	6–10 mg/dl
Ammonia	0.5 mg/dl	Up to 1 mg/dl
Particulate matter	Up to 1–2 gm/unit	Up to 2–4 gm/unit
Plasticizer	10 mg/unit	25 mg/unit
2,3-DPG	Nearly normal	Nearly 0
Factor V	About 50%	About 10%
Factor VIII	About 50%	About 15%

what is written in this chapter concerning risks and benefits relates to whole blood, except as noted.

"Packed red cells," now preferably called red cell concentrates, are simply whole blood with about two-thirds of the plasma component removed. Most of the time, the plasma is removed immediately after collection so that red cell concentrates are metabolically very similar to a unit of whole blood, except that there is one-third the amount of citrate, plasticizer, and plasma proteins, and a lesser reduction in antigenic debris, phosphate, plasma potassium, and negative thermal load.

Washed red cells offer a much "cleaner" form of red cells, in that usually at least 99 per cent of the plasma fraction is removed, depending on the method used for washing. This eliminates many of the potential disadvantages of the plasma fraction, probably decreases the level of immunization against non–red cell antigens, and probably significantly decreases the risk of transmitting disease via transfusion. The disadvantages are those of added cost, the loss of more red cells in the process of washing, and the necessity for administering red cells soon after washing. Electrolyte solutions that allow extended storage of red cells after washing are now being evaluated clinically in Sweden. These also contain adenine, and some contain mannitol, so the effect on the recipient can be complex if large volumes are used.

Frozen red cells retain the characteristics of the cells at the time of freezing. Thus, if frozen soon after collection, as is usual, they are functionally like freshly collected red cells even though they may have been stored for years. They must be washed before administration in order to remove the cryopreservative, and they share the disadvantages listed for washed red cells plus the added cost of initial processing and the cost of maintaining them frozen. It is possible to retrieve red blood cells from whole blood or red cell concentrates as the blood is about to lapse out of date (currently 21 days after collection), restore 2,3-DPG and ATP, freeze the cells, and thus convert cells that would have been lost from the system to cells that are functionally very similar to those freshly collected from a donor. This has obvious attractions despite the added costs.

The most common reason for using red blood cells is to treat anemia. Since blood carries with it significant risks, the decision to transfuse for anemia must be made carefully. The red blood cell mass of the patient represents the result of the balance between synthesis and destruction. It is not a static pool that transfused red cells will permanently increase. The effect of transfused cells will be obliterated within a few weeks by the dynamic equilibrium between production and destruction in the patient. Therefore, transfusion of red blood cells always has a temporary effect. Long-term correction of anemia requires correction of underlying disorders of production, destruction, or abnormal loss.

When is such temporary benefit warranted? This question is not easy to answer. Increasing the hematocrit increases the oxygen delivering capacity of the blood but also increases its intrinsic resistance to flow. The flow properties of blood in vivo are only beginning to be understood, however. Investigations in intact animals and in humans suggest that the optimal hematocrit for tolerating various stresses is near normal hematocrit levels. On the other hand, chronic stable anemia has been found to impair maximum aerobic work capacity to a surprisingly small degree. The ability of the body to increase the efficiency of hemoglobin as an oxygen delivering agent by decreasing its affinity for hemoglobin offsets much of the loss of mass of hemoglobin in anemia. This accommodation starts to occur within hours and is well developed in a few days. Restrictions of flow, however, especially in the coronary arteries, seem to greatly decrease the ability to accommodate to anemia. Some patients, for example, can quite accurately estimate their levels of anemia by the amount of anginal pain or claudication they experience with standard exercises. It is therefore probably wise to aim for a somewhat higher hematocrit in patients with restrictive arterial disease, limitations on cardiac output, or who are facing imminent stresses on the oxygen delivery system. Patients who are comfortable and stable and who are in the process of replenishing their own red cell mass should not be transfused. The important principle is that the decision to transfuse for anemia should be based on the condition of the patient; the patient, never a number, should be treated. This sounds rather trite, but a very large amount of blood is transfused in the United States because of an arbitrary hematocrit, not because careful analysis indicates that this patient needs more red blood cells at this time. If the latter were done, fewer patients would have transfusions.

PLATELETS

Platelet concentrates contain at least 5.5×10^{10} platelets stored in 30 to 50 ml plasma, all from the same donor. Platelets can currently be stored only for 72 hours and are usually used within 24 hours of collection. Whole blood that is kept over 24 hours in liquid storage should be considered as being without functioning platelets. Up to eight preparations are combined into a single pack for ease of administration. Ordinarily this means there are up to eight different donors in the pool. ABO compatibility is advisable. Matching donors and recipient for HLA type reduces immunization of the recipient and results in longer survival after infusion into previously immunized recipients. Using large numbers of platelets from a single HLA-matched donor, which can be done using techniques adapted from plasmapheresis, is the most elegant form of platelet therapy. It is advisable when infusions of platelets will be needed repeatedly over a prolonged period of time.

The proper dose of platelets depends on the starting level, the functional quality of the circulating platelets, and the condition of the patient. Accelerated destruction or utilization of administered platelets occurs commonly with fever, infection, prior immunization against platelets or HLA antigens, most forms of splenomegaly, disseminated intravascular coagulation, and large bleeding wounds. A suggested starting dose for adults is 0.1 unit per kg body weight. Postinfusion platelet counts are essential to evaluate the survival of transfused platelets, to detect the need for further infusions, and to find the proper dose.

The indications for the use of platelets are not sharply defined by available data. The platelet count alone is a rough guide. If thrombocytopenia is due to accelerated destruction and if production is intact, the resulting population of circulating platelets will be primarily young, large, and very effective. On the other hand, if thrombocytopenia is due to decreased production (such as following irradiation or cytotoxic chemotherapy), the circulating population of platelets will be old, small, and poorly functioning. Abnormal bleeding will occur at a much higher level of circulating platelets in the latter situation than in the former. With a normal population of platelets, there is good agreement between platelet counts and carefully done bleeding times. Prolongation of bleeding times occurs below a threshold of about 50,000 platelets per μl.

Platelets are used to treat active bleeding, spontaneous or posttraumatic, in which case there may be a clinical end point for effectiveness, or they may be given prophylactically, especially to prevent bleeding into the central nervous system. Many consider a platelet count below 10,000 per μl to be an indication for the latter, regardless of the functional quality of platelets, but some patients do not bleed spontaneously even at these low levels. Prophylactic use before operation requires special comment. Perhaps the most common such circumstance involves operating to remove a spleen that is the primary site of accelerated destruction of platelets. In most such instances, giving platelets before the spleen is removed is wasteful, as the infused platelets are rapidly sequestered in the spleen, which is then removed. Very often, giving the platelets after the spleen is removed is also unnecessary. If accelerated destruction is diminished, the improvement in hemostasis occurs very rapidly. If operative bleeding is not unusually great, it is preferable to wait and see what happens to the platelet count or bleeding time. Patients who are not bleeding spontaneously before splenectomy usually do not need platelets in the operative period if the splenectomy seems to be uneventful. On the other hand, if postoperative platelet counts reveal no favorable response to the splenectomy, then it is probably better to give platelets prophylactically at higher counts than would otherwise be done until the possibility of bleeding into the operative sites is passed (usually seven to 10 days if there are no complications). Meticulously performed bleeding times can be very helpful in deciding when to give platelets prophylactically.

LEUKOCYTES

The use of concentrates of leukocytes to help patients control infection is being evaluated in several centers. Most data so far suggest little beneficial effect unless the recipient is very neutropenic and the neutropenia is temporary. This material will probably have very limited usefulness, but further research could broaden the indications for use.

COAGULATION COMPONENTS

Disorders of coagulation are discussed in the next chapter. Only the characteristics of the products will be considered here. Much of the effect of more extensive use of component therapy in the United States has been to make more widely available various preparations containing coagulation factors. Table 7–2 lists some of the more common such preparations and some characteristics of each. Fibrinogen is a dangerous product with very limited indications for use, and the FDA has withdrawn the license for its manufacture in the United States. Cryoprecipitate provides sufficient fibrinogen in an acceptably small volume for most legitimate purposes at lower risk of transmitting hepatitis. Coagulation Factors V and VIII are important because they are consumed in the process of coagulation, are attacked by plasmin, and decline rather steadily during liquid storage. Factor V is present in normal concentrations in fresh frozen plasma (FFP). Factor VIII is similarly present in FFP and is present in more concentrated form in cryoprecipitate. Concentrates of coagulation factors are available for special purposes. Factor VIII concentrate contains mostly Factor VIII. Factor IX concentrate contains Factors II, VII, and X in addition. Use of either concentrate is likely to carry a high risk of hepatitis in recipients who have not been receiving blood products regularly. Use of some Factor IX concentrates has also been associated with dramatic and fatal incidences of

Table 7–2. Some Preparations Currently Available in Most Blood Banks

	Contents	Volume	Hepatitis	Storage
Whole blood	Whole blood, which changes during storage	450 ml blood plus 63 ml CPD	Single donor	21 days
Red cell concentrates	Same as whole blood but 2/3 non–red cell fraction removed	300 ml	Single donor (no less than whole blood)	21 days
Washed red cells	Red cells from either of above	Variable, resuspended in simple electrolyte	Probably reduced	24 hours after washing
Frozen, deglycerolized red cells	Red cells (see text)	Variable, resuspended in simple electrolyte	Probably reduced	Indefinite when frozen; 24 hours after thawing and washing
Platelets	5.5×10^{10} platelets, a few wbc and rbc, plasma	30–50 ml	Single donor	Up to 48 hours (most used in 24 hours)
Leukocytes	Wbc, some platelets, plasma	50–100 ml	Single donor	Up to 12 hours
Fresh frozen plasma	Citrated plasma, frozen soon after collection	250 ml	Single donor	1 year frozen; use quickly when thawed
Cryoprecipitate	I, VIII, XIII, von Willebrand's factor	10 ml	Single donor	1 year; use quickly when thawed
Fibrinogen	I	Lyophilized	Very high	Removed from market
AHG concentrate	VIII	Lyophilized	Very high	Dated
Factor IX concentrate	II, VII, IX, X	Lyophilized	Very high	Dated
Albumin	95% albumin	5%, 25% solution	None	Dated
PPF	60% + albumin, remainder α and β globulin	5% solution	None	Dated

intravascular coagulation. Until more data are available, FFP is preferred for rapidly reversing the coagulation defects of patients receiving warfarin (Coumadin). Theoretically, stored plasma should also be effective but is rarely available as such. Pooled plasma has been removed from the U.S. market because of the high risk of hepatitis and the availability of safer alternatives.

ALBUMIN AND PLASMA PROTEIN FRACTION (PPF)

These products are very similar, but there are a few significant differences. Both are used primarily to expand plasma volume or restore plasma-specific osmotic activity. Use of the concentrated form of albumin is more rational for the latter purpose. Products labelled "albumin" have at least 95 per cent of the protein content as albumin. PPF can have up to 35 per cent other proteins, usually alpha and beta globulins. Both products are stored at 60°C for 10 hours, which eliminates the risk of hepatitis.

There is evidence that PPF may contain vasoactive materials (or precursors or activators) that can cause paradoxical hypotension during rapid administration. This has been noted primarily intraoperatively or postoperatively. There is preliminary evidence implicating a prekallikrein activator, but this is not certain. If the cause can be found, the product can be made safer. Until then, it is not advisable to administer PPF rapidly.

There is generally poor appreciation of the factors determining the impact of administered albumin in the recipient. Although albumin generally stays in the vascular space early after administration, its final space of distribution is over twice the size of the plasma volume. This relationship is complicated by the fact that the extravascular "pools" of albumin act to buffer the intravascular pool. In the common situation of hypoalbuminemia, the true deficit of albumin is well over twice what would be calculated from the plasma volume and plasma concentration alone. The persistence of infused albumin is sometimes grossly underestimated. Under normal conditions, albumin has a half-life of about 11 days.

Calculating the effects of infused albumin on concentrations in the plasma is complicated by several other factors. Hypoalbuminemic patients often have abnormal losses into areas such as wounds, body cavities, the GI tract, and urine. It is widely assumed but not firmly established that albumin given to a catabolic patient will be more rapidly broken down for calories. Finally, a significant but variable amount of the albumin found in Albumin and PPF is in polymeric form. Dimers and polymers of albumin are cleared at accelerated rates and probably contribute very little to any of the usual functions of albumin. Better standardization of these products is required. It is small wonder then that the effect of administering albumin on the level in the recipient's plasma is usually much less than expected and that the proper dose is still best described as "enough."

If the correct dose is uncertain, so are the indications for use. When used for acute volume expansion, the therapeutic goals and indications of effect are usually reasonably well defined. When used to treat hypoalbuminemia, however, the indications and end points are rather vague. There are almost certainly levels of hypoalbuminemia below which pulmonary edema, impaired healing of wounds, and perhaps paralytic ileus occur. What those levels are is still a debated question. Administering concentrated albumin to a water-logged, hypoalbuminemic patient can paradoxically create a high risk of developing pulmonary edema during infusion, because interstitial fluid is drawn acutely into the intravascular space. A slow rate of infusion and adequate renal function are advisable.

The best way to restore albumin levels toward normal is to provide the patient with sufficient nutrition to accomplish this endogenously whenever possible.

COMPLICATIONS

HEPATITIS

Most blood products carry the risk of transmitting hepatitis to the recipient. Those products that can be treated at 60°C for 10 hours probably carry no risk. The amount of infected plasma sufficient to cause disease in a recipient is extremely small. Therefore, pooled products carry risks that are proportional to the number of donors forming the pool. It was hoped that hepatitis would be nearly eliminated as a complication of transfusion when methods were developed for detecting various markers of the hepatitis B virus. The transmission of hepatitis B by transfusion has been greatly reduced by the use of these assays, but hepatitis B has not been eliminated. More significantly, however, it has become apparent that most of the hepatitis transmitted by transfusion in the United States was not hepatitis B. Neither was it hepatitis A, cytomegalovirus, or Epstein-Barr virus. Probably 80 per cent of the hepatitis transmitted by transfusion remains undefined. It appears to be a variety of diseases, all probably viral, and now is called non-A, non-B hepatitis.

An accurate picture has not emerged of the risks of hepatitis after transfusion in the United States since the onset of widespread testing by radioimmunoassay for evidence of hepatitis B in donors. It appears that the mortality from hepatitis transmitted by transfusion has declined significantly but that the incidence has not declined greatly. This implies that hepatitis B may have been the most lethal form of hepatitis transmitted by transfusion.

The other approach to the control of hepatitis in blood products has been to promote the use of all-volunteer donors. The act of paying, of course, has nothing to do with hepatitis, but among those who sell their blood there are a higher number from the lowest socioeconomic groups, in whom the incidence of hepatitis is high. Such donors are also more likely to be less than candid or to be uninformed about their past medical problems. The effects of such programs will be hard to document because of the almost concurrent use of more sensitive testing for hepatitis B.

It is hoped that markers will be found for the other forms of hepatitis transmitted by transfusion, and much of the risk will thereby be removed. Serum alanine aminotransferase has shown some promise in this regard, but the results are preliminary and the implications for practice are unclear. Much more evaluation is needed. For the present, blood remains a potentially infecting form of treatment. The practicing surgeon should try to learn the risks of hepatitis from transfusion in his or her geographic area, as the incidence of hepatitis varies considerably among regions.

Other diseases are transmitted much less commonly by transfusion, at least as far as we now know. Considering the nature of blood, however, the potential for transmitting disease is very great.

IMMUNOLOGIC PROBLEMS

Every transfusion represents a graft of tissue from another individual, unless the patient is receiving his or her own blood or blood from an identical twin. Red cell antigens, specific platelet antigens, HLA antigens, and probably many others have the potential for inducing an immunologic reaction in the recipient, which will make subsequent transfusion more difficult. Whether this also makes subsequent grafting of other tissue more difficult is not certain.

A mistake in crossmatching or administering blood that results in random rather than matched administration (misidentifying the blood or the patient) has about one chance in three of resulting in a hemolytic transfusion reaction. Many such episodes are fatal. Great care must be exerted throughout the system to avoid mistakes in identification. Establishing proper identification is too often regarded as a red-tape bother or of secondary importance. With better control of hepatitis B, misidentification may now be the leading cause of death resulting from transfusion in the United States.

TRANSFUSION REACTIONS

1. Immediate hemolysis is usually the result of misidentification of blood, recipient, or specimen for crossmatch, as noted before. The clinical manifestations can include chills, fever, back pain, hypotension, or sudden generalized bleeding (especially if this occurs intraoperatively).

2. Delayed hemolysis usually occurs extravascularly days to several weeks after transfusion and is manifested by unexplained anemia, occasionally icterus, and, much less commonly, renal failure.

3. Reactions to leukocyte antigens are thought to be the cause of many or most urticarial reactions during and after transfusion. Although initially not severe, these can progress to anaphylactic-like reactions

with repeated transfusions. The usual urticarial reactions can be treated with an antihistamine and the transfusion can continue.

4. Reactions to transfused proteins, especially IgA, can be severe, resembling anaphylactic reactions, and can cause vascular collapse. Fortunately, they are unusual. Acutely increased pulmonary capillary permeability may also result from this class of reactions and can cause pulmonary edema during a single unit transfusion without circulatory overload.

5. Contaminated blood is fortunately rare but is a severe complication when it occurs. Vascular collapse is usually the manifestation. The organisms are usually gram-negative bacilli and may not grow in culture at 37°C. If this complication is suspected, a sample of blood from the patient and from the transfusion should be cultured aerobically and anaerobically at 37°C and at room temperature. Sometimes organisms can be seen on a stained smear of the blood used for transfusion. The organisms may no longer be viable at the time of transfusion. The limulus lysate test for endotoxin, if available, will help establish the diagnosis. The patient should be treated for severe gram-negative sepsis pending return of cultures if transfusion of contaminated blood is suspected. This should be a rare complication in a well-run transfusion service.

6. Platelet incompatibility can lead to specific platelet antibodies that may cause early or late thrombocytopenia. The late form is interesting in that it is very persistent and may respond to exchange transfusion or plasmapheresis.

There should be a general approach to suspected transfusion reactions that is established ahead of time in consultation with the transfusion service. The details may vary, but the following principles should be included:

1. Stop the transfusion, but keep the IV open. As noted, this is not necessary with most urticarial reactions but should be considered for all febrile or hypotensive reactions unless another cause is clearly operative.

2. Specimens of plasma and urine should be examined for the presence of hemoglobin (not red cells). Hemoglobin in either implies intravascular hemolysis.

3. The transfused blood must be saved for investigation. If multiple units were given, even the empty bags should be collected and returned. Specimens from the patient, the transfused blood, and the pilot tubes should be retested for ABO and Rh types, for compatibility, and the patient's blood by the direct Coombs' test.

4. All steps in identification should be back-checked, beginning with the labels on the transfused blood and on the patient. This one step often reveals the source of a major reaction.

5. If contaminated blood is suspected, the Gram stain and cultures discussed before should be performed.

6. If hemolysis or hypotension are features, renal function should be protected as much as is feasible by maintaining a full blood volume and good perfusion and by establishing a diuresis, if possible.

7. After hemolytic events it may be necessary to transfuse red cell concentrates, or preferably washed red cells, that have been carefully tested for compatibility.

8. If human error was involved, steps should be taken to minimize the chances of it happening again.

METABOLIC PROBLEMS

Stored blood differs from "normal" blood in many significant ways. When blood is transfused very rapidly and in large amounts into a bleeding patient, many of these differences can assume clinical significance. Citrate probably has the highest lethal potential of any of these. About one-third of the citrate in liquid-stored blood is in planned excess of that necessary to bind the ionized calcium. This citrate binds ionized calcium in the recipient's blood when infused and can cause death if infused rapidly enough. There are two protections against citrate: metabolic consumption, which occurs rather rapidly, and mobilization of calcium in response to release of parathyroid hormone. Renal excretion is variable. Supplemental calcium will prevent death from citrate but can itself be fatal if used in excess. A reasonably good guideline is that most normothermic adults can withstand an infusion of one unit of blood every five minutes without requiring supplemental calcium. If the patient is not responding as well as expected, it is usually because blood volume has not been sufficiently restored, but if this is thought not to be so, then supplemental calcium in an ionized form (calcium chloride) should be tried cautiously.

The functional properties of hemoglobin are progressively impaired after the first week of storage in CPD. The affinity of hemoglobin for oxygen increases because of depletion of 2,3-diphosphoglyceric acid (2,3-DPG) in the stored red cells. The effect on the recipient is not clear, but anyone bleeding massively is vulnerable to impairment of the oxygen delivering system. Various experimental studies yield conflicting evidence. It is probably wise to avoid anemia in patients whose red cells have been recently replaced by those stored several weeks in citrate, and it is probably best to use blood in the first week of storage in treating hemorrhage in patients with known or suspected coronary arterial insufficiency. The function of hemoglobin is restored to normal within about 24 hours after transfusion in most recipients.

A breakdown in the hemostatic mechanism in an extensively bleeding and transfused patient is a very distressing and somewhat common occurrence. The reasons for this are still debated, but most transfused blood must be considered as free of platelets and very low in Factors V and VIII. Therefore, supplemental use of FFP and platelets during extensive transfusion is reasonable. There are no precise guidelines, but FFP should be considered when one blood volume has been transfused, and platelets when two blood volumes have been transfused (perhaps much earlier). Objective testing with simple and widely available tests will help decide when supplementation is needed.

Stored blood is both acidic and hyperkalemic, yet these are uncommon complications of extensive transfusion. This illustrates the complexities of this clinical situation. The main acids are citrate and lactate, both normal intermediary metabolites that are rapidly consumed when perfusion is restored, which is the most important effect of the transfusion. Part of the citrate in the anticoagulant is in the form of sodium citrate, which on metabolic conversion yields sodium bicarbonate, so that many massively transfused patients become alkalotic. This in turn contributes to the low serum potassium, both seemingly paradoxical results.

Hypothermia, on the other hand, has much potential for causing trouble. Rapid infusion of refrigerated blood directly into a patient will both increase the patient's oxygen requirements at an inopportune time and will lower body temperature. The cold recipient is less able to handle lactate, citrate, and potassium, has a further shift of the function of hemoglobin in the wrong direction, and may have added interference with coagulation. Although minimally studied experimentally, hypothermia in the heavily transfused recipient is theoretically quite dangerous and should be avoided.

There are many other potential problems that are of uncertain significance. Plasticizers are certainly not helpful to the recipient, but it is not clear how harmful they are. The same can be said of the microaggregates that accumulate during storage. There is probably denaturation of some plasma proteins during storage but no clear evidence of significant clinical effects. As methods of preservation and of storage improve, these real and potential problems should become less important.

SPECIAL STRATEGIES

UNCROSSMATCHED BLOOD

Lives continue to be lost because of hesitancy to use uncrossmatched blood in an exsanguinating patient. Use of nonblood fluids for resuscitation is safe and effective up to a point, but as the remaining red cell mass gets progressively smaller, there may not be enough time to wait for crossmatched blood, especially if hemorrhage is continuing. In most such situations, one can learn the ABO and Rh type of the patient within minutes after arrival and can begin with type-specific blood. Rarely, type O blood must be given because there is not enough time for even that. Type-specific blood is safe for the vast majority of patients. The small added risk is well worth accepting if the alternative is incomplete, ineffective, or delayed resuscitation. A few minutes can mean the difference between success and failure in some rapidly bleeding patients. All the complications of hemorrhagic shock are time-dependent. Fear of legal liability should never be a factor in choosing essential treatment for a patient. In this situation ironically there may be more legal liability for not using it than for doing so when resuscitation is not progressing satisfactorily.

RED CELLS VERSUS WHOLE BLOOD

For the exsanguinating patient, whole blood is the most practical and best available treatment. For increasing red cell mass, that is, when transfusing for anemia, the cleanest available form of red cells is the best. As discussed previously, the plasma component of stored whole blood contains most of the metabolic abnormalities, most of the antigenic material, a variety of denatured and vasoactive proteins, and most of the transmissible diseases. Clearly, most patients would be better served by not getting whole blood. The trouble with red cell concentrates ("packed red cells") is that they are not clean red cells. This preparation contains about one-third of the original plasma component. This means only one-third the amount of the potentially harmful material, but probably the same risk of transmitting hepatitis because the amount of infected plasma required is so small. Red cell concentrates thus have less of the unwanted contents and represent the cheapest way of reducing those contents. They also free two-thirds of the collected non–red cell fraction for use in other patients. The platelets, Factor V, and Factor VIII would be lost during storage, even to the eventual recipient, if not harvested soon after collection. Red cell concentrates, while not perfect, are a step in the right direction. Use of whole blood for most patients represent unthinking, archaic therapy which is less than the best for the individual recipients and for the system.

FROZEN RED CELLS VERSUS LIQUID STORED RED CELLS

Use of frozen, deglycerolized red cells is a further step toward use of a clean preparation of red cells. In most methods, over 95 per cent of the plasma, leukocytes, and platelets are removed. There may be a significantly lower incidence of hepatitis because so much of the plasma is removed. The other advantages are the ability to preserve rare blood types or autologous red cells for prolonged periods, the preservation of the functional quality of the red cells, better management of inventory because of the indefinite duration of storage, and, we hope soon, the ability to restore and recover liquid stored red cells about to be lost from outdating, as discussed previously. The disadvantages are the significant increase in cost, the loss of more of the originally collected red cells in processing, and the current necessity for using the cells within 24 hours of thawing and washing.

FRESH BLOOD VERSUS OLD BLOOD

There are very few clinical situations in which the use of fresh blood is required. If platelets, labile coagulation factors, and red cells are needed for a patient and component therapy is not available, then fresh blood is required. Whenever component therapy is available, it is difficult to think of a situation justifying use of fresh blood. Most patients benefit from rational, individualized component therapy in which the needed components can usually be given in more concentrated and therefore more effective form. Use of fresh whole blood is too often based on anecdotal, desperate, or semimystical grounds. It represents a significant added burden on the blood banking system, and to be given truly fresh it must be administered before the various required tests are completed, the most important of which are the tests for hepatitis B.

AUTOTRANSFUSION

The safest form of blood for transfusion is the patient's own blood. With such blood there are no antigenic problems and no new transmitted diseases. There are two approaches to providing this. In elective autotransfusion, the blood is collected from the patient before some planned event, typically one or two weeks before an operation. The blood volume is quickly restored by the patient, erythropoiesis is stimulated before the operation, the reduction in red cell mass is functionally minimal, and very safe blood is available for use intraoperatively. This method should be used much more widely than it is because it is very beneficial to the individual patients, and it could relieve a lot of stresses on the blood banking system. More than one unit can be stored by starting well ahead of time and freezing the red cells (and the plasma, if desired) or by the more common liquid storage using a technique in which the previously collected blood is returned as additional units are collected ("piggy-backing"). Surgeons especially should be using these methods for the better care of their patients.

Emergency autotransfusion is very different. Shed blood is collected at the time of operation (or occasionally from chest tubes), promptly mixed with anticoagulant, and reinfused through various filters. This minimizes the use of homologous blood and makes blood immediately available when catastrophic and unexpected hemorrhage occurs. It is also very useful when there is difficulty obtaining compatible blood and operation cannot be deferred. It works best, of course, when the operative field is sterile and there is little other fluid or tissue mixed with the shed blood. Various strategies for anticoagulating the shed blood have been evaluated. There is a problem with either coagulation or with mechanical damage to the blood before reinfusion in most systems, so that if more than one blood volume is transfused, a significant coagulopathy might occur. The safest form for reinfusing shed blood is again the washed red cell preparations. This is quite safe but requires a significant delay between bleeding and reinfusing. There are situations in which this can be very useful, but it is not as appealing as the facile reinfusion of recently shed blood.

ANTI-RH₀ (D) IMMUNOGLOBULIN

Anti-Rh_0 (D) immunoglobulin is marketed for use in pregnant Rh negative women to prevent immunization against Rh_0 (D) antigen. This material is also effective when Rh_0 (D) positive blood or blood products likely to contain the antigen (such as platelet packs) have been given to Rh negative recipients. This may have been done deliberately if Rh negative material was not available, or it may have been done accidentally or unintentionally. If the recipient is a woman of childbearing potential, it is important to try to prevent immunization, and it is advisable in men because transfusion may be required in the future, and Rh negative blood might not be available. The recommended dosage is 300 μg of anti-Rh_0 (D) antibody for each 15 ml of Rh positive red blood cells transfused. The material should be given as soon as possible after the Rh positive cells are given, but it may be effective up to several weeks later if for some reason it was not given sooner.

SUMMARY

The ability to replace shed blood is one of the cornerstones of modern surgery and will remain so in the foreseeable future. Transfusion therapy has become more complex but also more specific and more effective. Methods are still under development that will further increase efficacy and perhaps safety of the products. Blood remains a complex, potentially life-saving, and potentially fatal form of treatment for which there are no apparent substitutes.

REFERENCES

Collins, J. A.: Massive transfusion. Clin. Haematol., 5:201, 1976.

Feinstone, S. M., and Purcell, R. O.: Non-A, non-B hepatitis. Ann. Rev. Med., 29:359, 1978.

Greenwatt, T. J., Finch, C. A., Pennell, R. B., Rath, C. E., Rosenfield, R. E., and Schmidt, P. J. (eds.): General Principles of Blood Transfusion, revised ed. Chicago, AMA, 1973.

Mollison, P. L.: Blood Transfusion in Clinical Medicine, 5th ed. London, Blackwell, 1972.

Myhre, B. A.: Blood Component Therapy: A Physician's Handbook, 2nd ed. Am. Assoc. Blood Banks, Washington, DC, 1975.

8

Hemorrhagic Disorders

EDWIN W. SALZMAN

Hemorrhagic complications are a frequent source of morbidity in surgical patients. In many cases, unexpected bleeding can be traced to a generalized defect in hemostasis. Recently there has been an explosive growth in the understanding of hemostatic processes. Hemorrhagic problems can be approached with confidence based on detailed knowledge of the pathways of fibrin formation and insight into the function of blood platelets. Precise diagnosis of bleeding disorders is the rule. Specific therapy is effective and has become widely available.

MECHANISM OF HEMOSTASIS

When a blood vessel is divided, it constricts, and platelet aggregation and plasma coagulation combine to stanch flow from the constricted orifice. At the cut end of the vessel, exposure of subendothelial connective tissue provides a surface to which platelets adhere and are activated. Interaction with collagen fibers causes them to secrete epinephrine, 5-hydroxytryptamine (serotonin), and adenine nucleotides, notably ATP and ADP, from storage sites in intracellular granules. The presence of these secreted compounds in plasma leads to aggregation of more platelets and the eventual development of a platelet plug, which in small vessels is sufficient to stop the flow of blood and provide provisional ("primary") hemostasis. At the same time, exposure of plasma to connective tissue activates plasma enzymes ("clotting factors") and sets off a series of reactions that result in the generation of thrombin and ultimately in the conversion of fibrinogen to a fibrin clot. Tough fibrin strands reinforce the friable platelet aggregate ("secondary hemostasis"), and platelets and fibrin together produce a resilient composite hemostatic plug that can withstand the force of arteriolar pressure when the constricted vessel eventually relaxes.

In parallel with hemostatic processes, initiation of coagulation leads also to the conversion of plasminogen, a plasma globulin, to its active

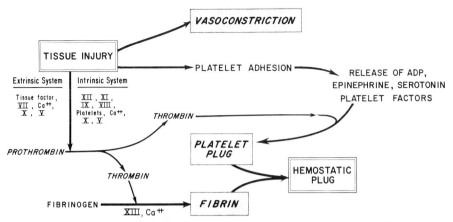

Figure 8–1. The mechanism of hemostasis. Vasoconstriction, platelet adhesion and aggregation, and the formation of fibrin cooperate to produce a hemostatic plug and arrest hemorrhage. Tissue injury causes the generation of thrombin and ultimately the formation of fibrin by provision of a clot promoting lipid tissue factor ("tissue thromboplastin") via the extrinsic clotting system, and by activation of plasma clotting factors through exposure of subendothelial connective tissue (intrinsic clotting system). Adhesion of platelets to connective tissue is followed by release of platelet constituents and aggregation of additional platelets. The release of biogenic amines from platelets is also induced by thrombin. Not shown are clotting factors prekellikinin and low molecular weight kininogen, which are involved in activation of the intrinsic system.

form, plasmin. The resultant proteolytic activity produces fibrinolysis. Although a natural defense against pathologic deposition of fibrin, activation of plasminogen is also a feature of certain disease states. It can also be induced deliberately for therapeutic dissolution of intravascular thrombi.

The mechanism of hemostasis is summarized in Figure 8–1.

ROUTINE EVALUATION OF SURGICAL PATIENTS

The existence of a hemorrhagic diathesis should be regarded as a possibility in the initial consideration of every patient who is to undergo an operation, for, if present, a bleeding tendency may convert an otherwise straightforward surgical procedure into a catastrophe. A lengthy battery of laboratory examinations is not required for routine evaluation. Most hemorrhagic disorders of significance can be detected by a careful history and physical examination, if particular attention is directed to episodes of bleeding as a complication of previous surgery, dental extraction, or trauma; hemorrhagic symptoms in other members of the family, especially if the pattern of inheritance follows the X-linked recessive pattern characteristic of hemophilia; unusual swelling of joints or soft tissue not recognized as bleeding; and the ingestion of medications known to influence hemostasis adversely, such as aspirin, oral anticoagulants, phenylbutazone, and indomethacin.

Preoperative evaluation of every surgical patient should also include assessment of the number of circulating platelets. Thrombocytopenia may develop de novo as a result of drug ingestion or infection or without known cause. If the patient has not been challenged by trauma or operation, the low platelet concentration may not be apparent to the examiner. Examination of a stained blood smear is sufficient for this determination; 6 to 10 platelets per high-power field are usually visible. A platelet count is not necessary for this evaluation.

The use of tests of coagulation for indiscriminate screening is not recommended. Laboratory tests that are inexpensive and readily available, such as whole blood clotting time, are so insensitive that they offer no security. For example, the whole blood clotting time is normal in classic hemophilia if the level of Factor VIII (antihemophilic factor) exceeds three to five per cent of the average normal plasma concentration, but a plasma level at least 30 per cent of normal is required for safe surgical hemostasis. Tests of sensitivity and reproducibility sufficient for demonstration of a bleeding disorder (such as partial thromboplastin time and one-stage prothrombin time) are more complicated and expensive. Their use for routine screening cannot be justified, but they should be obtained if there is any suggestion of a hemostatic defect. The bleeding time is a useful index of hemostatic competence in a patient suspected of ingesting a drug that affects platelet function. If the surgeon intends to administer prophylactically an antithrombotic drug for the prevention of venous thromboembolism, the preoperative assurance of hemostatic competence is particularly important, since the mild hemostatic defect induced by such agents will be exaggerated by any underlying bleeding tendency.

The touchstone should be a meticulously obtained history and thorough physical examination, which will suggest the presence of an underlying bleeding disorder in most patients whose hemorrhagic tendency is sufficiently severe to be of consequence. This suggestion should lead to hematologic consultation and precise diagnosis.

HEMORRHAGIC DISORDERS

Both congenital and acquired disorders affecting the various aspects of hemostasis will be described. They can be identified by appropriate laboratory tests, which are standard procedures performed with readily available commercial reagents.

Congenital Bleeding Disorders

Defects in Blood Coagulation. Inherited deficiencies of plasma clotting factor activities exist, either from absence of a particular protein

Table 8–1. Circulating Hemostatic Elements

OFFICIAL NAME	COMMON SYNONYMS	LIFE SPAN IN VIVO (HALF-LIFE)	FATE DURING COAGULATION	STABILITY IN ACID BANK BLOOD (4%)	AGENTS AVAILABLE FOR REPLACING DEFICIT	NORMAL LEVEL	LEVEL REQUIRED FOR SAFE HEMOSTASIS
Factor I	Fibrinogen	72 hours	Consumed	Very stable	Bank blood or plasma; concentrated fibrinogen	200–400 mg/100 ml	60–100 mg/100 ml
Factor II	Prothrombin	72 hours	Consumed	Stable	Bank blood or plasma; concentrated preparation	20 mg/100 ml (100%)	15–20%
Factor V	Proaccelerin, accelerator globulin, labile factor	36 hours	Consumed	Labile (40% at 1 week)	Fresh frozen plasma; blood under 7 days	100%	5–20%
Factor VII	Proconvertin, serum prothrombin conversion accelerator, SPCA, stable factor	5 hours	Survives	Stable	Bank blood or plasma; concentrated preparation	100%	5–30%
Factor VIII	Antihemophilic factor, AHF, antihemophilic globulin, AHG	6–12 hours	Consumed	Labile (20–40% at 1 week)	Fresh frozen plasma; concentrated AHF; cryoprecipitate	100% (50–150%)	30%

Factor	Synonyms	Half-life	In bank blood	Stability	Replacement source	Plasma level	Level for hemostasis
Factor IX	Christmas factor, plasma thrombo-plastin component, PTC, hemophilia B factor	24 hours	Survives	Stable	Fresh frozen plasma; bank blood; concentrated preparation	100%	20–30%
Factor X	Stuart-Prower factor	40 hours	Survives	Stable	Bank blood or plasma; concentrated preparation	100%	15–20%
Factor XI	Plasma thromboplastin antecedent, PTA	Probably 40–80 hours	Survives	Probably stable	Bank blood or plasma	100%	10%
Factor XII	Hageman factor	Unknown	Survives	Stable	Replacement not required	100%	Deficit produces no bleeding tendency
Factor XIII	Fibrinase, fibrin stabilizing factor, FSF	4–7 days	Survives	Stable	Bank blood or plasma	100%	Probably less than 1%
Platelets	—	8–11 days	Consumed	Very labile (40% at 24 hours; 0% at 48 hours)	Fresh blood or plasma; fresh platelet concentrates (*not* frozen plasma)	150,000–400,000/ mm³	60–100,000/ mm³

Roman numeral III was originally assigned to "Tissue Thromboplastin" and IV to ionized calcium. Factor VI proved to be an activated form of another clotting factor. These numerals are no longer used in the standard nomenclature of clotting factors.

or from the presence of an abnormal protein with impaired function. The most common of these is hemophilia, a deficiency of the activity of Factor VIII (antihemophilic factor). Hemophilia is inherited as an X-linked recessive trait, transmitted by the female but manifested only in the male. The disease occurs once in approximately 10,000 male births. The Factor VIII molecule is abnormal in hemophilia; the protein is present and can be identified immunologically by its cross-reactivity with an antibody to Factor VIII, but its function in coagulation is disordered.

Factor IX deficiency (hemophilia B, Christmas disease) is clinically indistinguishable from hemophilia and has a similar pattern of inheritance but involves a different clotting factor. The severity of the bleeding tendency in hemophilia and Factor IX deficiency is well correlated with the activity of the factor in question in clotting tests. Severely affected patients usually have less than one per cent of the normal activity. Patients with more than 30 to 40 per cent of normal are in most cases asymptomatic. At intermediate levels, spontaneous hemorrhage is rare, but serious hemorrhage may follow operation or trauma.

Inherited deficiencies of other plasma clotting factors have been described but are less common and, in most instances, less severe in their clinical effects than deficiencies of Factors VIII and IX.

Table 8–1 summarizes the important characteristics of the plasma coagulation factors.

Deficiencies of plasma clotting factors produce a defect in "secondary hemostasis." The initial arrest of bleeding by vasoconstriction and platelet aggregation is unimpaired, but the platelet plug that forms is not reinforced by fibrin and is unable to withstand the force of arteriolar pressure. When the protective effect of vasoconstriction abates, the flimsy platelet plug is likely to be dislodged and lead to delayed hemorrhage after hours or days. Tests of "primary hemostasis" such as the bleeding time and tourniquet test are normal in these conditions unless there is also a defect in platelet function, as in von Willebrand's disease. Diagnosis of inherited disorders of coagulation is summarized in Table 8–2.

Common clinical manifestations of congenital disorders of coagulation include bleeding into joints and soft tissues, occasionally into body cavities, and sometimes from the nose or the gastrointestinal or urinary tract. Affected patients rarely succumb to exsanguinating hemorrhage. The hypovolemic effects of blood loss are often overshadowed by the space-occupying nature of a hematoma, which predisposes to infection and ischemic necrosis of vital organs. Supportive measures, such as immobilization of hemarthroses, may be of value, but the mainstay of treatment is replacement of the deficient clotting factor activity by administration of blood, fresh or frozen plasma, or a relatively purified preparation concentrated from plasma. The level of the several clotting factors required for hemostasis, their biologic half-life, their stability on

Table 8–2. Diagnosis of Inherited Disorders of Coagulation

Deficient Factor	Partial Thromboplastin Time	One-Stage Prothrombin Time	Thrombin Time	Bleeding Time	Fibrinogen Level	Platelet Adhesiveness	Remarks
I (fibrinogen)	Long	Long	Long	Long or normal	Low	Normal or low	Corrected by stored or adsorbed plasma but not by serum
II (prothrombin)	Long	Long	Normal	Normal	Normal	Normal	Corrected by stored plasma
V	Long	Long	Normal	Normal	Normal	Normal	Corrected by adsorbed plasma
VII	Normal	Long	Normal	Normal	Normal	Normal	Corrected by stored plasma or serum
VIII	Long	Normal	Normal	Normal	Normal	Normal	Corrected by adsorbed plasma
IX	Long	Normal	Normal	Normal	Normal	Normal	Corrected by stored plasma or serum
X	Long	Long	Normal	Normal	Normal	Normal	Corrected by stored plasma or serum
XI	Long	Normal	Normal	Normal	Normal	Normal	Corrected by stored plasma or serum
XII	Long	Normal	Normal	Normal	Normal	Normal	Corrected by stored plasma or serum
XIII	Normal	Normal	Normal	Normal	Normal	Normal	Clot is soluble in 6M urea or 1% monoiodoacetic acid
Von Willebrand's disease	Long	Normal	Normal	Long	Normal	Low	Deficiency in Factor VIII; defective aggregation of platelets by the antibiotic ristocetin

Defects may be correctable by mixture of abnormal plasma with shelf-stored plasma (deficient in V and VIII), plasma adsorbed with BaSO₄ or Al(OH)₃ (deficient in II, VII, IX, and X), or serum (deficient in I, II, V, and VIII). Suspected defects can be confirmed by special assays for specific factors.

storage, and the materials available for replacement therapy vary with different clotting factors (Table 8–1).

Operation in a patient with a congenital coagulation disorder is a complicated undertaking. One must provide a safe blood level of the deficient clotting factor during the operation and the entire postoperative period until healing is complete. If the factor has a short half-life in the circulation (such as Factor VIII [antihemophilic factor], four to five hours) and is required in relatively high concentration for safe hemostasis (such as Factor VIII, 30 per cent of normal), infusions of two to three liters of plasma per day may be required. Circulatory overload is a hazard of such a program and can only be avoided through the use of concentrated preparations of the deficient factor with a low content of extraneous protein. Requirements for transfusion therapy increase with the magnitude of the surgical procedure and are also influenced by the size of the patient and his or her circulatory volume and by unusual metabolic demands, such as fever and infection.

The development of a natural anticoagulant inhibiting Factor VIII is a serious complication of transfusion therapy in a small fraction of patients with severe hemophilia. The plasma concentration of the inhibitor increases in response to infusion of the deficient clotting factor in such patients. The inhibitor neutralizes circulating Factor VIII and thus frustrates attempts at replacement therapy. Since transfusion raises the titer of the anticoagulant, administration of the deficient factor should be avoided except in an acute threat to life. In a desperate case, transient benefit may be obtained through the use of highly concentrated Factor VIII preparations of animal origin, by exchange transfusion, or by administration of a concentrate of the vitamin K–dependent clotting factors (VII, IX, X, and prothrombin), which also contains traces of activated factors and apparently bypasses the site of action of Factor VIII. Because of the attendant requirement for several weeks of effective replacement therapy, elective operation is absolutely contraindicated in patients with an acquired inhibitor of antihemophilic factor. Acquired anticoagulants directed toward the other clotting factors have also been described but are less frequent than in hemophilia. An acquired inhibitor to Factor VIII has also been recognized on occasion in elderly nonhemophilic male patients and less often in postpartum women, in whom it usually disappears with the passage of time. Other acquired anticoagulants are sometimes observed in leukemia and in disseminated lupus erythematosus.

Von Willebrand's disease is an inherited disorder of hemostasis transmitted as an autosomal dominant characteristic. It is the most common inherited coagulation disorder after hemophilia. The disease is characterized by a deficiency in Factor VIII and an associated decrease in platelet adhesiveness, resulting in a long bleeding time and simultaneous defects in primary and secondary hemostasis. In this condition the failure of platelets to be aggregated in vitro by the antibiotic ristocetin is helpful for diagnosis. The Factor VIII molecule, which is absent to a varying extent in this disorder, is related in some undefined way to a plasma factor ("von Willebrand's factor") required for adherence of platelets to surfaces. Transfusion of fresh plasma or cryoprecipitate leads to a transient correction of the abnormality in platelet function and to a more sustained rise in Factor VIII level, apparently augmented by synthesis of new Factor VIII from precursor material contained in the transfused plasma. Spontaneous correction of the characteristic defects has been observed late in pregnancy.

Inherited Disorders of Platelet Function. Thrombasthenia (Glanzmann's disease) is a rare hereditary bleeding tendency in which the platelets do not aggregate with ADP, epinephrine, or other agents. Plasma coagulation is normal, but platelet clumping is completely absent. Transfusion of fresh viable platelets is effective therapy.

In a more common qualitative disorder (Portsmouth syndrome, thrombocytopathia), the "release reaction" of platelets is impaired, and platelet aggregation is therefore deficient, although the platelets respond in normal fashion to exogenous ADP. The disorder may result from a flaw in storage of the contents of intracellular granules ("storage pool disease") or, less commonly, from an enzymatic defect in the secretion mechanism. In the latter case, the situation is in many respects analogous to that produced by aspirin. In severe cases, the bleeding time is prolonged, but in its more mild form the disorder can be diagnosed only by specialized tests of platelet function. Only recently recognized, this condition appears to be a frequent cause of hitherto unexplained mild bleeding tendencies. Transfusion of fresh viable platelets corrects the hemostatic defect.

ACQUIRED BLEEDING TENDENCIES

Many acquired disorders of hemostasis are complex and involve defects in several components of the hemostatic processes. An exception is the effect of administration of anticoagulant drugs, either heparin or derivatives of coumarin ("oral anticoagulants"). Heparin is a strongly anionic sulfated polysaccharide whose biologic activity is due to its ability to activate a natural plasma inhibitor of coagulation, antithrombin III (also called heparin cofactor). Antithrombin III inhibits coagulation by blocking the interaction of thrombin with fibrinogen and also by impairing the action of other proteolytic enzymes involved in the intrinsic clotting system, including the activated forms of Factors XII, XI, IX, and X (Fig. 8–1). The aggregation of platelets by thrombin is inhibited by heparin, but in conventional clinical dosage the drug does not impair other aspects of platelet function. Heparin is destroyed in the stomach and is not effective unless given parenterally. Its action is neutralized by protamine; 1 mg of protamine will reverse the effect of

100 units of heparin, on the average. One mg of heparin is required to contain at least 120 units of anticoagulant activity (defined in a standard bioassay).

Oral anticoagulants have no effect on coagulation in vitro. They inhibit the synthesis of vitamin K–dependent clotting factors (Factors VII, IX, X, and prothrombin [Factor II]) by the liver. Their pharmacologic effect is largely a function of their free blood level and is increased by a variety of other drugs, which may compete with coumarin derivatives for albumin binding sites and thus raise the free plasma level of the anticoagulant (such as phenylbutazone and sulfisoxazole), may reduce the rate of excretion by competition for degradative enzymes (such as tolbutamide and diphenylhydantoin), or may increase the affinity for the anticoagulant of enzyme receptor sites (such as quinidine and anabolic steroids) and thus reduce the dosage requirement for effective anticoagulation. The effect of coumarin derivatives is also subject to inhibition by drugs if they increase the activity of hepatic enzymes that degrade the coumarin (such as phenobarbital) and thereby reduce the effectiveness of the anticoagulant.

Administration of the oral anticoagulant blocks the synthesis of the four vulnerable clotting factors and is followed by a decline in their plasma concentration through natural processes of degradation. The initial effect is on Factor VII (half-life five hours). Factors IX and X disappear more slowly (half-life 24 hours and 40 hours, respectively), and prothrombin is even slower (half-life 72 hours). After discontinuation of the drug, restoration of plasma levels of these factors follows roughly the same course.

The bleeding tendency in anticoagulated patients is a direct function of the effect of the drugs on hemostasis, which increases in parallel with their antithrombotic effect. If a hemorrhagic complication is encountered when the level of anticoagulation is not excessive, an underlying lesion should be suspected. The propensity of unsuspected gastrointestinal neoplasms to bleed in anticoagulated patients is a classic example.

Important acquired disorders of platelets include thrombocytopenia and abnormalities of platelet function. A decrease in platelet number without a defect in coagulation may develop as an allergic reaction to drug ingestion (such as quinidine, thiazide diuretics, chloramphenicol, and anti-inflammatory agents), as a feature of leukemia, in association with marrow failure from metastasis or other causes, or by autoimmunization (idiopathic thrombocytopenic purpura). The gravity of the hemorrhagic state is a direct function of the platelet count. Hemorrhagic complications at operation are uncommon if the platelet count exceeds 60,000 to 100,000 per mm^3 unless there is also disordered platelet function. Spontaneous bleeding is seen at platelet counts less than 20,000 to 30,000 per $mm.^3$ Intracranial hemorrhage is a major hazard if the platelet count is less than 10,000 per mm.^{3} In idiopathic thrombocytopenic purpura, adrenal steroids often lead to a rise in platelet count. Splenectomy produces a remission in two-thirds of cases and will often increase the response to steroids, even in patients whose platelet count remains low after removal of the spleen. Replacement therapy requires viable platelets in fresh whole blood, platelet-rich plasma, or concentrated preparations. In idiopathic thrombocytopenic purpura, platelet destruction is accelerated by immune mechanisms, and the response to infused platelets is often evanescent. Platelets withstand storage poorly, especially in the cold; few survive reinfusion even into normal subjects after storage for 48 hours in ACD or CPD anticoagulant at refrigerator temperature, but if the blood is stored at room temperature, a useful rise in platelet count may be achieved with transfused materials three or four days old.

Acquired disorders of platelet function frequently result from ingestion of drugs that inhibit the "release reaction" of platelets and thus impair platelet aggregation. Aspirin is most commonly involved; it produces a profound effect after administration of only one or two tablets per day, the effect lasting four to six days. Many instances of otherwise unexplained faulty surgical hemostasis and diffuse wound bleeding appear to be the consequence of the use of aspirin by surgical patients. Other agents with a similar but less sustained effect include phenylbutazone, sulfinpyrazone, antihistamines, indomethacin, chlorpromazine, and many tranquilizers.

A functional platelet defect is also seen after the infusion of dextran of average molecular weight 70,000 or, to a lesser extent, 40,000. In patients who receive more than 1.5 gm dextran per kg as a single infusion, a clinically significant bleeding tendency is common, and increases in bleeding time and in operative blood loss are often seen.

The bleeding tendency of uremia is largely the result of abnormal platelet function. A qualitative platelet defect is a prominent feature of advanced renal failure. Defective platelet adhesiveness and impaired participation of platelet lipids in coagulation ("platelet factor 3") are characteristic. The gravity of the defect is roughly correlated with the degree of azotemia. Correction of the platelet abnormality has been described after dialysis and renal transplantation.

Mixed hemostatic defects involving both clotting factors and platelets occur in patients with liver disease. All the clotting factors whose source is known appear to be made in the liver, except for Factor VIII, which is apparently made by endothelial cells. Factors VII, IX, X, and II (prothrombin) require vitamin K for their synthesis; the others do not. Vitamin K is ingested in the diet and is produced by intestinal bacteria. A deficiency of this fat-soluble vitamin is seen in starvation, after the administration of broad-spectrum antibiotics with alteration of the gut flora, and is also observed following failure of absorption due to common bile duct obstruction or biliary fistula. In hepatic cirrhosis, these clotting factors and others synthesized in the liver are deficient. If present, portal hypertension with secondary splenomegaly often leads to thrombocytopenia. Failure of the cirrhotic liver to remove activators of plasminogen accounts for the coexistence of fibrinolysis, aggravated by a pathologic plasminogen activator produced by the diseased liver. The circulating products of fibrinolysis ("fibrinogen digestion products") are potent anticoagulants and also impair platelet aggregation. Consumption coagulopathy is occasionally present in patients with hepatic decompensation and may further embarrass hemostasis. Local causes of bleeding, such as esophageal varices, peptic ulcer, and gastritis, also play an important role.

Treatment of the hemorrhagic state accompanying hepatic failure is difficult because of the complicated nature of the hemostatic defect and in many instances because of inability to control the underlying disease process. Replacement therapy with fresh frozen plasma or concentrated preparations of the vitamin K–dependent clotting factors may be transiently effective, and platelet concentrates are sometimes of value. Epsilon aminocaproic acid (EACA), an inhibitor of plasminogen activation, has been employed to reverse the fibrinolytic state in these patients, but the results have been less encouraging than with fibrinolysis in other clinical settings.

A hemostatic defect accompanies extracorporeal circulation for cardiopulmonary bypass. A complex abnormality results from the invariable development of thrombocytopenia, the activation of fibrinolysis, the administration of heparin for anticoagulation during the period of cardiopulmonary bypass, occasionally from the initiation of intravascular coagulation, and probably from nonspecific denaturation of blood proteins at air interfaces. The problem may be compounded by faulty replacement of depleted clotting factors if cardiac failure with hepatic congestion has impaired synthetic mechanisms. Improvements in perfusion technique and meticulous attention to surgical hemostasis have reduced the frequency of this problem in patients after open heart surgery, but the solution awaits the development of nonthrombogenic surfaces for extracorporeal circuits.

Careful attention to neutralization of heparin with protamine eliminates the most frequent source of a generalized bleeding tendency after open heart operations. Protamine has anticoagulant activity itself, but its effect is trivial compared to heparin, and a modest excess of the drug is well tolerated. If evidence of a generalized hemostatic defect persists after an adequate dose of protamine, diagnostic studies should be performed as for any case of an acute bleeding state (see next section). The indiscriminate use of epsilon aminocaproic acid or other drugs is not recommended in the absence of specific diagnosis, but such agents may be useful if indicated by appropriate laboratory studies.

ACUTE TRANSIENT BLEEDING DISORDERS

A transient hemorrhagic tendency may develop de novo in a surgical patient as a complication of many disorders in which bleeding is not a primary feature. Such a phenomenon can arise through dilution of hemostatic elements by massive transfusion with stored blood, by consumption of plasma factors and platelets secondary to intravascular coagulation, and by destruction of hemostatic plugs through fibrinolysis.

Massive Transfusion. Replacement of blood loss with bank blood induces thrombocytopenia and a defect in plasma factors V and VIII because of the lability of these hemostatic components during shelf storage (Table 8–1). Neosynthesis or mobilization of clotting factors from body stores prevents major coagulation deficiencies in most massively transferred patients, except in those with severe liver disease or hemophilia. However, since the spare uncirculating pool of platelets is limited, thrombocytopenia is a frequent consequence of massive transfusion. If the volume of rapidly administered bank blood exceeds 8 to 10 pints, a platelet count less than 100,000 per mm^3 may be expected, and if the transfused volume exceeds 7 or 8 liters, a long bleeding time and a clinically significant hemorrhagic tendency are frequent. Treatment requires replacement of the deficient materials in the form of fresh blood or fresh platelet-rich plasma. Factors V and VIII may be supplied in frozen plasma, but this does not contain viable platelets. A practical preventive procedure is the administration of fresh blood or platelet-rich plasma or a platelet concentrate during the course of rapid transfusion. One fresh unit for each four or five banked units is usually sufficient to prevent the development of symptomatic dilutional thrombocytopenia.

Consumption Coagulopathy. At one time regarded as a curiosity, disseminated intravascular clotting has become recognized as a common mechanism of disease. A surprising variety of conditions are marked by entrance into the bloodstream of materials that induce blood coagulation and platelet aggregation. In some instances, as in bacteremia, malaria, amniotic fluid embolism, or snakebite, the procoagulant substance is a specific chemically defined agent peculiar to the disease. In other cases, as in massive soft tissue crush injury or disseminated malignancy, the offending substance may be a less well-characterized product of tissue destruction. Occasionally, as in hemolytic transfusion reactions or absorption of components of a retroplacental hematoma, the stimulus to intravascular clotting is a constituent of the blood itself. Sometimes, as in large hemangiomas or in the presence of gram-negative endotoxemia, a widespread vascular lesion may activate clotting and platelet alterations.

Disseminated coagulation within the circulation interferes with organ perfusion and may lead to a generalized hemorrhagic state, the consequence of a "consumption coagulopathy" due to consumption of labile hemostatic elements, including Factors V and VIII, prothrombin, fibrinogen, and platelets. Stable clotting factors, such as IX and X, may also be reduced, since once activated they are filtered from the circulation by the liver.

Diagnosis of consumption coagulopathy depends on demonstration of reduced levels of the labile clotting factors and of platelets (Table 8–3). Alterations in erythrocyte morphology are often present as a result of damage sustained by red cells in squeezing through fibrin clots. Products of fibrinolysis can usually be demonstrated, for activation of lytic mechanisms is a natural response to intravascular clotting. The common association of fibrinolysis with intravascular coagulation accounts for the failure to demonstrate occluding thrombi in autopsy material from patients who die with laboratory findings typical of consumption coagulopathy.

Treatment of disseminated intravascular clotting is most likely to be effective if the source of the stimulus to clotting can be removed, such as evacuation of the uterus in "obstetrical defibrination," drainage of abscesses and administration of appropriate antibiotics for bacteremia, and use of specific antivenins for snakebite. Replacement therapy is likely to be ineffective unless entrance of procoagulants into the bloodstream can be controlled. Heparin may be of value to block consumption of hemostatic elements; sometimes, as in disseminated malignancy, it may be the only therapy available. The required dose, best administered by continuous intravenous infusion, is that needed to produce an improvement in fibrinogen levels and prothrombin time. Replacement of the consumed hemostatic elements can then be carried out with fresh blood or fresh platelet-rich plasma. The use of concentrated fibrinogen is not recommended, since it lacks the other clotting factors likely to be deficient and since it is a major source of serum hepatitis, being prepared from pooled plasma. The role of inhibitors of platelet aggregation, such as aspirin and indomethacin, is at present under evaluation.

Fibrinolysis.   Activation of plasminogen to plasmin is a regular accompaniment of hemostasis, but fibrinolysis can also exist as a pathologic process and can lead to a severe bleeding diathesis. In addition to dissolution of fibrin clots, plasmin digests fibrinogen and other clotting factors. The products of fibrinolysis and fibrinogenolysis are polypeptides with potent anticoagulant activity. They block the further polymerization of fibrin and also impede platelet aggregation.

Most often fibrinolysis arises in the course of disseminated intravascular coagulation. Although fibrinolysis has been described as an isolated finding after resuscitation from cardiac arrest and occasionally in other circumstances, many authorities believe that activation of plasminogen occurs only in response to intravascular clotting and that primary fibrinolysis does not exist. Under these circumstances the administration of epsilon aminocaproic acid, an effective antidote to plasminogen

Table 8–3. ACUTE BLEEDING DISORDERS

	PLATELET COUNT	PROTHROMBIN TIME	THROMBIN TIME	FIBRINOGEN	FIBRINOLYSIS	REMARKS
Dilution (massive transfusion)	Low	Normal or long	Normal	Normal	Absent	—
Consumption coagulopathy	Low	Long	Long	Low	Absent or present	Clot lysis and euglobulin lysis time may or may not be abnormal; fibrinogen digestion products are usually demonstrable; abnormal erythrocyte morphology
Fibrinolysis	Normal	Normal or long	Normal or long	Normal or low	Present	Circulating plasmin demonstrable by clot lysis time, euglobulin lysis time, or fibrin plate
Circulating heparin	Normal	Normal or long	Long	Normal	Normal	Long thrombin time corrected by protamine
Underlying inherited coagulation disorder	Normal	Normal	Normal	Normal	Normal	Clinical evidence of generalized bleeding disorder but normal screening tests usually indicate preexisting hemorrhagic state involving coagulation, most often hemophilia

Simple rapid screening tests for working diagnosis of acute hemorrhagic states sufficient to guide therapy. Confirmation requires detailed evaluation.

activation, is hazardous, for inhibition of lysis may remove the patient's only defense against widespread thrombosis. Thrombotic catastrophes have followed the injudicious use of EACA. Unless one has laboratory evidence that fibrinolysis *does not* coexist with intravascular coagulation (in practice, this assurance requires a normal platelet count and fibrinogen level), EACA should probably not be used without the simultaneous administration of heparin.

Diagnosis of acute transient bleedng disorders is summarized in Table 8–3.

REFERENCES

Biggs, R.: Human Blood Coagulation, Haemostasis and Thrombosis, 2nd ed. Oxford, Blackwell Scientific Pub., 1976.

Brinkhous, K. M.: Hemophilia and New Hemorrhagic States — International Symposium. New York, Chapel Hill, The University of North Carolina Press, 1970.

Colman, R., Hirsh, J., Marder, V., and Salzman, E.: Thrombosis and Hemostasis. Philadelphia, J. B. Lippincott, 1982.

Damus, P. S., and Salzman, E. W.: Disseminated intravascular coagulation. Arch. Surg., *104*:262, 1972.

Poller, L.: Recent Advances in Blood Coagulation, Vol. 2. London, Churchill Livingstone, 1977.

Salzman, E. W.: Hemostatic disturbances and thrombosis. *In* Skillman, J. J. (ed.): Intensive Care. Boston, Little, Brown & Co., 1975, pp. 387–416.

Salzman, E. W.: Diagnosis of bleeding disorders. *In* Skillman, J. J. (ed.): Intensive Care. Boston, Little, Brown & Co., 1975, pp. 537–543.

Williams, W. J., Beutler, E., Erslev, A. J., and Rundles, R. W.: Hematology. New York, McGraw-Hill Co., 1972.

9

Wound Healing and Wound Care

JOHN W. MADDEN

The local response of tissues to injury determines the ultimate outcome of all surgical procedures. Disruption of tissue integrity by accidental trauma or the surgeon's knife initiates a series of striking morphologic, physiologic, biochemical, and physical changes leading to the rapid restoration of tissue integrity and strength. Within hours after an incised and sutured wound is closed, the wound space fills with an inflammatory exudate. The length of the acute inflammatory phase depends upon the extent of injury and the amount of foreign material present but rarely exceeds three weeks. By 48 hours, marginal epithelial cells have migrated down and across the wound surface, sealing the deeper structures from the external environment. By three days, fibroblasts in the local area have begun to proliferate and to invade the wound space. Budding capillaries follow, establishing a rich vascular network. Within seven days, invading fibroblasts begin synthesizing and depositing collagen fibers. Gradually, over a three- to four-week interval, the wound changes from a primarily cellular structure to a structure composed of dense connective tissue, the scar. Collagen fibers, the principal constituent of scar tissue, weld the disrupted tissues into a strong, functional unit. Strength changes, however, occur slowly. By three weeks, incised and sutured wounds have gained less than 15 per cent of their ultimate tensile strength. In most instances, scars continue to gain tensile strength for at least six months. In addition to the slow strength changes, wounds change their shape and color characteristics for years following the initial injury.

In normal individuals, provided the surgeon does not interfere excessively with normal processes, wound healing reactions produce a healthy scar quickly. The functional result is satisfactory to both patient and surgeon. Common sense and the application of a few simple principles prevent most wound complications from occurring. If compli-

169

cations do occur, applying the same principles leads to a satisfactory outcome in the majority of cases.

PRINCIPLES COMMON TO PREOPERATIVE AND POSTOPERATIVE CARE

Because wound healing reactions are local cellular events, scar formation depends upon the normal metabolism of local cells. Most wound complications are local problems. Hematomas, infected retained foreign bodies, and inadequate local perfusion with tissue necrosis are the most common complications. Sensible preoperative, operative, and postoperative care prevents the majority of these problems.

Although most complications are local, the general metabolic state of patients does play a role in wound healing. Healing wounds are parasitic to a certain extent, capable of utilizing the energy and products of general tissue breakdown to provide conditions necessary for effective scar formation. In spite of the wound's parasitic nature, however, improving the general metabolic state of debilitated patients preoperatively maximizes the rate of wound healing and minimizes complications. With the advent of hyperalimentation (Chap. 5), even severely debilitated patients can be improved physiologically prior to operation. The stronger the metabolic state of the patient preoperatively, the smoother the postoperative course.

In the past, some surgeons have stressed the importance of an adequate red cell mass for normal healing. Recent data suggest that hemoglobin, hematocrit, and red cell mass are less essential to normal wound healing than adequate tissue perfusion. Local tissue oxygen tension has a profound effect on all wound healing reactions. In relative hypovolemic states, blood flow to vital organs is maintained at the expense of decreasing perfusion to the cutaneous and muscular systems. Maintaining adequate blood volume and tissue perfusion preoperatively and postoperatively minimizes wound healing complications. Local as well as systemic perfusion deficits must be avoided. As an example, edematous, swollen tissues with poor perfusion in the lower extremities of patients with venous stasis disease heal much more quickly and effectively if the preoperative management includes elevation and rest to minimize local edema and increase tissue perfusion.

Specific nutritional deficits can also play a role in wound healing reactions and, if present, must be corrected preoperatively. Vitamin C deficiency (scurvy) interferes with normal wound healing significantly. Ascorbic acid is a necessary cofactor in the synthesis of collagen. Without adequate supplies of vitamin C, collagen synthesis slows or stops completely, scars gain strength slowly, and wounds disrupt easily. In patients with vitamin A deficiencies, the rate of epithelialization of open wounds decreases significantly. Finally, deficiencies in zinc, copper, magnesium, and other trace metals decrease the rate of scar formation. Unless individuals are taking odd or faddish diets or have long-standing chronic diseases affecting alimentation, significant vitamin deficiencies are a rarity in the United States. However, an adequate dietary history from all patients should be obtained prior to operation. If the history or physical examination indicates the possibility of vitamin or trace metal deficiencies, give supplemental vitamins and minerals preoperatively. Postoperatively, maintain adequate vitamin and trace mineral intake. Unfortunately, normal wound healing reactions cannot be accelerated by excessive amounts of vitamin C, vitamin A, or trace metals.

Physical and pharmacologic agents affect the wound healing process profoundly. High doses of radiant energy of short wavelength produce permanent adverse effects on local tissues. Excessive doses of radiation affect the fibroblast's ability to divide, migrate, and produce collagen. With time, small vessels in the irradiated area occlude and decrease local perfusion potentials. Because radiation effects last indefinitely, the surgeon should plan incisions to avoid areas of chronic radiation exposure, if at all possible. If patients must undergo radiation therapy as part of a postoperative care program, treatment should not begin until local fibroblast reactions are well established, approximately a week or so following local injury. Local infiltration of antimetabolic drugs produce the same chronic effects as local irradiation. Avoid making incisions in areas where antimetabolic drugs have been infiltrated inadvertently. Fortunately, systemic administration of antimetabolic drugs does not affect local wound healing significantly. The systemic administration of nitrogen mustard, thiotepa, 5-fluorouracil, doxorubicin (Adriamycin), and other antimetabolites rarely produces a tissue concentration high enough to influence fibroblast division, migration, and protein synthesis.

The administration of ACTH, cortisone, and the synthetic glucocorticoids affect the rate of wound healing significantly. Cortisone and its derivatives inhibit the normal inflammatory response, limit capillary budding, inhibit fibroblast proliferation, decrease the rate of epithelialization, and decrease the rate of protein synthesis. Although wounds will eventually heal in patients taking high doses of corticosteroids, production of scar tissue, gain in tensile strength, and maturation of scar tissue is extremely slow. When a history of chronic ingestion of corticosteroids exists, anticipate a slow gain in tensile strength and choose incisions and suture materials accordingly.

In summary, excellent preoperative and postoperative wound care requires providing and maintaining the best general metabolic status possible, excellent local tissue perfusion, and adequate supplies of the specific vitamins and trace elements necessary for normal wound healing. Avoid tissue injury by radiation or cytotoxic drugs. Anticipate specific wound problems in patients with old radiation injuries or with local antimetabolic drug injuries and in patients on high doses of corticosteroids.

PREOPERATIVE WOUND CARE

ELECTIVE INCISIONS

The object of preparing skin for elective incisions is to minimize infectious complications. Even in individuals with the best personal hygiene, loose hair, loose keratinized epithelial cells, and other foreign particles cover the skin surface. In certain areas of the body, where keratin layers are particularly thick (such as hands, feet, and elbows), foreign material can actually be imbedded in the surface layers. Introducing this foreign material into the depths of the wound increases the incidence of postoperative wound infection. Therefore, adequate preoperative preparation requires that the skin be shaved if hair growth is excessive and scrubbed thoroughly with soap or detergent solution to remove dead material. In addition, all skin has a resident bacterial population. Although most wound infections are caused by organisms introduced into the wound depths from the GI tract, from the surgeon's hands, or from the hospital environment, skin bacteria introduced during the surgical procedure cause a small percentage of infections. Applying bactericidal or bacteriostatic agents reduces the surface bacterial count significantly. The organic iodine complexes such as povidone-iodine (Betadine) are bactericidal agents that are particularly effective in reducing surface bacterial population. Careful mechanical preparation of the skin the night prior to operation in addition to careful preparation with organic iodine-containing soaps immediately prior to making the incision reduces infectious complications.

Mechanical preparation of the skin requires some common sense. Although intact skin supports a small bacterial population, open areas deprived of epidermal covering support bacterial growth much more effectively. Nicks and cuts in the skin are colonized rapidly by pathogenic organisms, particularly in the hospital environment. If the area to be operated upon is shaved the night prior to surgery, the skin should not be nicked or cut, leaving open wounds to be colonized over the ensuing 12 hours. A small stubble of hair present in the operative area with an intact epidermis provides a safer operative field than a closely shaved surface denuded of its epithelium. If time and personnel permit, scrub the operative area with a detergent solution containing a bactericidal agent the night prior to operation, but shave the area as close to the time of the operative incision as possible.

The preoperative use of antibiotics to prevent wound infection in elective incisions remains a controversial subject. The use of prophylactic antibiotics is discussed in Chapter 6.

PREPARATION OF RECENT TRAUMATIC WOUNDS FOR CLOSURE

In addition to the general principles of preoperative wound management described, the main objectives in the management of traumatic wounds are to prevent further contamination of the wound surface by pathologic bacteria, to maximize local tissue perfusion by proper position of the injured parts, to protect the exposed tissues from further injury by drying or contact with cytotoxic agents, and to remove major foreign contaminants quickly. Because most significant wound infections can be traced to the hospital personnel and the hospital environment, use aseptic technique with all open wounds from the moment the patient comes under medical management. In the rush to establish an airway, to prepare an intravenous access, and to begin therapy for hypovolemia and shock, do not forget the open wound. If the emergency area has an adequate staff, assign one individual to manage open wounds as life-saving emergency measures proceed. Use gloves and masks at all times. Adjust the position of the extremity or soft tissue parts to maximize local tissue perfusion. As bleeding from major vessels is being controlled, place injured parts in anatomic positions and remove large contaminating foreign objects gently with gloved fingers.

If trauma to the patient is so severe that several hours of fluid and respiratory preparation are required prior to surgical intervention, begin the wound toilet immediately. Gently irrigating open wounds with Ringer's lactate solution to remove clots and foreign materials minimizes the opportunity for bacterial colonization during the delay. In general, bactericidal agents should not be placed on tissues without an intact epithelium. A good rule of thumb: Never put anything in a wound that could not be placed in your own conjunctival sac! Although some studies indicate that organic iodine complexes can be applied to open tissues safely, simple mechanical flushing with tissue-compatible fluids is the safest and most effective method of early wound care. However, mechanically cleansing areas of skin with intact epidermis using the techniques described previously for elective incisions minimizes bacterial colonization from skin organisms. Following the careful flushing and débriding of gross contaminants, cover wounds with sterile materials and protect them from the hospital environment. Exposed tissues dry quickly, adding a desiccation injury to the initial insult. Keeping tissues moist and covered until they can be meticulously débrided in the operating room decreases secondary infectious complications significantly.

Because all open wounds are contaminated with bacteria, postoperative infectious complications can be minimized by administering broad-spectrum antibiotics systemically as soon as it is practical. High blood levels of the antibiotic preparation should be attained prior to surgical manipulation and débridement. Culture open wounds prior to the administration of the antibiotics. Early colonization of wound surfaces with pathologic bacteria is difficult to appreciate by inspection. In the occasional case in which infectious complications occur quickly in spite of broad-spectrum antibiotic coverage and meticulous débridement, prior wound cultures provide information necessary for sucessful secondary care.

CHRONICALLY OPEN WOUNDS

The major objective in the preoperative management of chronically open wounds is to prepare the wound surface for closure. In most cases, secondary closure will be accomplished with split-thickness skin grafting or delayed primary closure. If the initial injury exposes tissues with minimal intrinsic blood supply (bone and tendon), closure may be accomplished using pedicle flaps. Occasionally, smaller wounds can be allowed to close by epithelialization and contraction. Because the active contraction process produces a permanent contracture, avoid closure by contraction in areas adjacent to mobile joints or mobile surfaces.

Controlling local infection is the key to preparing open surfaces for closure. Open wounds begin the healing process normally. An inflammatory exudate collects on the surface; marginal epithelial cells mobilize, divide, and migrate down the edges; injured venules bud, forming capillary networks; and fibroblasts invade the injured area. Prior to the development of the inflammatory and vascular changes, pathologic bacteria invade exposed tissues easily. As the inflammatory process proceeds, however, local resistance to invasive infection increases. Careful bacteriologic investigations demonstrate that heavily contaminated wounds left open show a marked reduction in bacterial concentration during the first three to six days. Soft tissue wounds in noncritical areas that are heavily contaminated at the time the patient presents for care can be closed secondarily with minimal risk. During the three to six days when wounds remain open, keep tissues clean, protect them against the hospital environment with sterile dressings, and débride dead tissue fragments and foreign materials using fine forceps and scissors. If, at the end of three to six days, inspection of the wound reveals early clean healthy granulation tissue and quantitative studies indicate a minimal number of bacteria, wounds can be closed successfully. Secondary closure does create quantitatively large scars. In areas of the body where scar remodeling must produce gliding for injured parts to function (such as injured tendons in the hand and injured periarticular tissues), the extra scar produced by secondary closure limits function. When gliding structures are injured, close injured tissues as quickly as possible. In this instance, primary wound healing provides the best functional outcome.

In chronically exposed wounds, secondary closure produces a high incidence of secondary infectious complications. Therefore, delayed closure with split-thickness skin grafts or pedicle flaps is the technique of choice. The object is to prepare a wound surface that will accept the flap or graft without infectious complication. Obtain wound cultures immediately, and after the bacteria are identified and sensitivities are established, administer appropriate antibiotics systemically. Because dead tissue and foreign bodies support bacterial growth, débride local tissues of all dead and foreign materials meticulously. Maintain adequate tissue perfusion. If blood volume is low, correcting this deficit can improve local tissue appearance and resistance to infection. Determine the optimal time of closure by evaluating the gross appearance of the wound and analyzing quantitative wound culture data. Firm, flat, bright pink granulation tissue will usually support a graft immediately: exuberant, pale, or fiery red granulation tissue indicates significant bacterial colonization.

Débridement techniques vary depending upon the mechanical characteristics of the injured tissues. If dead fragments are large, débride the tissues using fine scissors and forceps with the patient under mild sedation or under anesthesia. If dead material is present in small pieces throughout the wound, dressing changes done properly can débride the wound effectively. Apply fine mesh gauze moistened with Ringer's lactate solution directly against the wound surface. Apply a dry or slightly moist gauze dressing over the fine mesh material. Allow the entire dressing to dry over a three- or four-hour interval. When the fine mesh gauze is removed from the wound surface without prior wetting, small bits and pieces of dead material adhere to the fabric and are thereby removed mechanically. Although large or chronically open wounds can sometimes be débrided with more comfort to the patient by immersion in physiologic solutions (such as Hubbard tanks and whirlpool baths), the chronic application of excessively wet dressings to open surfaces macerates tissue, encourages bacterial growth, makes patients uncomfortable, and contributes little to wound care. If thick wound secretions dry and crust, use slightly moistened dressings to remove this exudate and keep wound surfaces clean.

As a rule, open wounds accept split-thickness skin grafts when the wound surface supports epithelial migration. Epithelial cells will not spread on surfaces composed of dead material or tissues burdened with excessive numbers of bacteria. Unless the wound surface will support the spreading and growth of epithelial cells, split-thickness skin grafts will not adhere or revascularize. When careful inspection of the wound reveals that the epithelial cells at the edges are migrating across the wound surface, "showing a nice feathered edge," the wound will usually support a graft. When in doubt, apply a small trial split-thickness skin graft to the granulating surface. If the graft becomes adherent and revascularizes over a 24- to 48-hour period, proceed with definitive grafting.

Prepare wounds for coverage with pedicle flaps using the techniques outlined for split-thickness grafting. The type of definitive coverage necessary depends entirely on the characteristics of the local tissues. Exposed bone without periosteum or exposed tendon without paratenon will not support skin grafts adequately. The type of tissue exposed determines the coverage possibilities.

The preoperative care of large burn wound surfaces is a time-consuming and important task. Because of the special problems of the burned patient, the techniques of burn wound management are discussed in Chapter 38.

POSTOPERATIVE WOUND CARE

ELECTIVE INCISIONS

Within a few hours of incision, epidermal cells at the edges of the wound begin dividing, and daughter cells migrate down and across the wound surface. Gross inspection during the first 72 hours shows little change in the wound, but appearances are deceiving. By the end of this interval, histologic examination shows the epithelial covering to be intact, even in the depths of the incision. Therefore, for the first 48 to 72 hours, covering wounds with sterile dressings provides some protection from the hospital environment; after 72 hours, dressings provide little protection. In determining whether wounds should be covered after three days, the psychological attitude of the patient toward the incision and the social consequences of an exposed incision are the important factors. Some patients and their families are frightened of the exposed incision. Therefore, individual psychological and social factors should determine whether the wound remains dressed or is left exposed after three days.

The goals of postoperative incision management are to prevent secondary infectious complications, to prevent local tissue perfusion deficits, and to recognize complications early. Inspect wounds frequently. Because local inflammation alters small vessel permeability, all wounds become edematous. A suture initially encircling tissue under mild or slight tension may become a tight garrot, choking off all local blood flow as injured tissues swell. Remove tight sutures before local tissue perfusion is affected. Drain small collections of blood or serum quickly to avoid secondary bacterial contamination. Bacteria present in small abscesses around tight sutures can invade recently injured tissues rapidly. If sutures become the focus of small abscesses, remove them. Frequent inspection of abdominal wounds also helps prevent a potentially fatal complication, i.e., evisceration. Dehiscence of the deeper layers of an abdominal incision is almost always heralded by intraperitoneal fluid leaking through the skin incision. Dehiscence alone carries a low mortality. If thin brownish peritoneal fluid issues from the skin incision, palpate the wound carefully and determine the integrity of deeper structures. If a deep separation has occurred, protect the integrity of the skin incision with an external bandage and repair the disrupted deeper structures immediately.

The timing of suture removal requires common sense and an understanding of wound healing biology. Ideally, all skin sutures should be removed as quickly as possible. Any injury to the epithelial cell layer initiates cell division and migration. Skin epithelial cells migrate down suture tracts, causing inflammation and occasionally sterile abscesses. In addition, skin sutures left in place for long intervals injure underlying skin mechanically, creating additional scarring. On the other hand, skin sutures must remain in place until strength sufficient to resist local tissue tension and minor trauma develops. Although wound healing reactions begin quickly and scar formation is well underway by three weeks, wounds gain tensile strength slowly. Incised and sutured wounds have less than 15 per cent of their ultimate tensile strength by three weeks. Consider the kinetics of strength gain when planning the incision and choosing the type of suture material used.

Determining how much strength a suture must supply in each specific instance is difficult. The restoration of normal strength by wound closure is rarely necessary. The human body is overengineered. Dense connective tissues are much stronger than needed to absorb the stresses of everyday living. Even when disease states alter the physical properties of connective tissue significantly, such as in the Ehlers-Danlos syndrome, affected individuals do not fracture their tissues frequently. In most clinical situations, including the majority of abdominal incisions, 15 per cent of the ultimate tensile strength may be sufficient to resist all normal stress. One additional factor determines the magnitude of the strength required in each mechanical closure. Pain inhibits the full activity of most voluntary muscles. Therefore, injured tissues are splinted internally if normal pain mechanisms function. In the analgesic state immediately following an anesthetic, patients often produce tensions in the abdominal musculature of sufficient magnitude to rupture closures. Once the full pain mechanism is restored, however, the same mechanical repair resists stresses applied by the patient. Pain simply prevents the development of tensions high enough to disrupt tissues. Overengineering and the protective behavior following injury enable surgeons to close abdominal incisions and other stressed wounds successfully using a variety of materials.

Timing of skin suture removal varies widely and depends in part on the surgical technique used in closure. Placing permanently buried subcuticular sutures in the lowest portion of the dermis provides adequate strength to prevent wound spreading during the early phases of wound healing and during the prolonged remodeling phase. Additional suture line reinforcement can be obtained by using adhesive strips placed perpendicular to the cut surface. Finally, the timing of suture removal depends on the strength requirements of the wound. As an example, the tensions on a simple horizontal laceration of the upper eyelid are minimal. The strength attained during the first 24 hours by fibrin strands and epithelialization is usually sufficient to prevent dehiscence. In contrast, a vertical incision on the dorsal thorax may require three weeks to resist local tissue tension and the strain produced by bodily movements. The surgeon who always removes skin sutures on the same day in all areas and in all individuals will eventually have wound complications in his or her patients. When in doubt about the timing of suture removal or the strength of an individual wound, remove several sutures and test the wound gently with fingers.

Although the initial phases of wound healing are intense, dramatic, and rapid, wounds change shape and physical properties over prolonged intervals of time. Most scars become thicker, harder, and more unsightly for three months or more following incision. At three or four months, however, wounds slowly begin to change their physical properties toward a more natural and normal configuration. In most adults, physical properties and physical appearance of the wound attain a stable state within one year. In children, however, the process may take two years or longer. When considering revising an unsightly scar, be patient. Allow the wound to remodel completely before making the decision. Bulky prominent scars three months after injury may become smooth, flat, and inconspicuous by one year, eliminating the necessity of revision.

If superficial wound infections develop in spite of careful preoperative and postoperative management, wounds should be drained and cultured immediately. In the absence of significant cellulitis, draining the wound is usually sufficient to eradicate the infection. If significant cellulitis is present, initiate appropriate antibiotic therapy immediately. After the wound has been drained adequately, apply the techniques used to care for any open wound. Secondary closure can be accomplished using a delayed primary closure, epithelialization and contraction, or split-thickness skin grafting.

SKIN GRAFTS

Most split-thickness skin grafts placed on acceptable beds establish an adequate graft circulation within 72 to 96 hours. Unfortunately, at this point the strength of the interface between the graft and recipient bed is minimal. Several weeks must elapse before the scar at the interface gains sufficient strength to resist shearing forces. As a consequence, the objective during the immediate postoperative phase of skin graft care is to prevent all shearing movements between the graft undersurface and the bed. Shearing can be prevented by using tie-over bolus dressings to immobilize both the bed and the graft. Applying dressings carefully without the tie-over feature can be equally effective. The goal is simply to prevent relative motion between the graft and the recipient bed. If possible, avoid applying plaster casts or plaster splints immediately over soft tissue dressings. As soft tissue parts move under the rigid dressings, shearing occurs at the graft bed interface. If rigid immobilization is required, apply plaster splints away from the graft surface.

The resistance of skin grafts to destruction by invasive infection is minimal during the early phases of adherence. A small infected hematoma between the graft and the bed or a small suture abscess can produce an invasive infection, lifting the graft from the recipient surface and destroying the preparation. The timing of dressing changes should be altered accordingly. Grafts applied to clean, freshly excised surfaces, in which the risks of infection are minimal, can remain dressed for 10 days to two weeks without excessive risk. During this interval, tensile strength of the graft bed interface becomes sufficient to resist local stresses. Secondary dressing problems are minimal. On the other hand, when grafts are applied to chronically open surfaces or in areas where superficial infection is a possibility, dressings should be changed within three or four days. Débride small suture abscesses or contaminated collections occurring between the graft and bed immediately. Over the ensuing two weeks, apply dressings to protect the graft from shearing stresses. Inspect the wound frequently and care for local tissue contamination by local débridement and drainage.

In certain instances, skin grafts can be applied to open surfaces without occlusive dressings. In large open wounds, some wound areas will be ready to accept split-thickness coverage while others are still too contaminated to have grafts take successfully. Applying split-thickness skin grafts to the clean areas while continuing to prepare the contaminated areas for grafting produces earlier wound closure. In certain cases, the open skin grafting technique is mandatory. Applying dressings to skin grafts on the moving thoracic cage is impossible. In thoracic areas, a freshly cut split-thickness skin graft should be placed directly on the granulating surface. No sutures or dressings are utilized. If the graft bed is satisfactory, a plasma seal develops quickly and the skin grafts become adherent within hours. Protect grafts from external trauma at all times until the graft-recipient site interface becomes strong enough to resist shearing forces. Suspend bed linen over a frame. Protect the grafts from prying fingers. As small fluid collections develop, débride the area thoroughly. Small crusts and abscesses must be eliminated to prevent invasive infection. If crusting becomes a problem, apply a nonadherent gauze dressing adjacent to the graft surface and apply moist dressings to the surface of the nonadherent gauze. The moist gauze should be changed frequently, leaving the nonadherent gauze intact to protect the graft surface.

After two or three weeks, the interface between the graft and bed is strong enough to resist most minor trauma. Unfortunately, skin grafts cannot be ignored at this stage. During the first six to twelve months, grafted skin does not sweat. As a consequence, the epithelial surface of the graft dries and cracks unless covered once or twice a day with a thin coating of a greasy ointment. In addition, some grafts take a prolonged period of time to develop protective pigmentation. Sun exposure produces serious burns in the grafted surfaces and aids in the development of blotchy, unsightly pigmentation. For the best cosmetic results, protect skin grafts from direct sun exposure for at least six months. The recent development of PABA sunscreens has been a boon to graft care. Rather than wearing an occlusive dressing during sun exposure, patients can now coat the surface of the graft with a sunscreen agent, eliminating exposure problems. Finally, the new blood vessels formed between the graft-bed interface require at least six months to develop adequate pressure control regulating mechnisms. The walls of the interface vessels remain weak for prolonged intervals. The hydrostatic pressure created while standing can be enough to rupture new venules and capillaries in the graft-bed interface unless tissues are supported by external elastic bandages. To prevent hemorrhages, hematomas, and fluid collections from developing in the graft-bed interface months after successful graft application, provide a strong external elastic stocking support or Ace bandage support during the first four to six months following the application of skin grafts to lower extremities.

SKIN GRAFT DONOR SITES

After harvesting split-thickness skin grafts, the donor site is composed of a variable portion of the dermis and deep remnants of the epidermal appendages. Healing occurs by the spreading of epithelial cells from the epithelial appendages, reestablishing the epithelial covering. Dress donor sites with Scarlet Red gauze or Vaseline-impregnated fine mesh gauze immediately next to the raw surface. This gauze dressing should remain intact until the surface has epithelialized completely. External to this dressing, a soft sterile dressing can be applied for the patient's comfort. After a few hours, the gauze dressing immediately adjacent to the raw surface is adherent. By seven days, remove the external dressing and allow the patient to shower. Leave the adherent dressing intact. As the surface epithelializes, the adherent dressing is slowly liberated. The nonadherent edges can be trimmed with a pair of scissors to eliminate the nuisance of floppy dressings. By three weeks, donor sites should be reepithelialized. If infection develops or if reepithelialization is slow, use the principles outlined under the care of chronically open wounds.

FLAPS

Properly constructed pedicle flaps require a minimal amount of postoperative care. The objectives of flap care are to prevent infectious complications and to prevent circulatory insufficiency. In properly constructed flaps, circulatory problems are minimal. Inspect supporting dressings frequently to avoid kinking or distorting the flap. In some flaps, the slightest torsional or axial tension compromises venous return and arterial input, creating perfusion defects. Adjust the dressings to prevent this complication. Even the best of pedicle flaps shows slight diffuse duskiness and mild edema during the first 24 to 48 hours. Diffuse color changes rarely indicate significant problems. However, if a sharp line of color demarcation develops, measures must be taken immediately to improve circulatory dynamics or the flap will be lost. If certain skin sutures produce torsion or tension changes, remove them. If dressings produce positional abnormalities, change the dressings. If a sharp line of demarcation cannot be altered or removed by adjusting the dressings, removing selected sutures, or changing the position of the patient in bed, return the flap to its original bed as quickly as possible. The exposed recipient area should be dressed carefully and the flap monitored for 24 to 48 hours. If the flap survives, take the patient back to the operating room and reattach the flap. If the flap does not survive, a new flap should be designed or the old flap should be redesigned to produce adequate coverage.

During the two to four weeks required for the flap to develop an adequate parasitic blood supply from the recipient site, suture lines and open areas must be treated as discussed previously.

DRAINING SINUSES, FISTULAS, AND CHRONICALLY INFECTED WOUNDS

Draining sinuses, fistulas, and chronically infected wounds are usually the result of infected foreign bodies or intermittent spillage of gastrointestinal contents into the soft tissues. Definitive management requires the removal of the foreign body or the elimination of the gastrointestinal spillage. In the interim, protect intact tissues from corrosive drainage when at all possible. Use sumps, suction catheters, drainage bags, and other mechanical devices to keep intact tissues from becoming irritated and uncomfortable. Clinically, the analysis and treatment of the underlying defect is of critical importance. Manage wounds as discussed previously.

REFERENCES

Madden, J. W.: Wound healing: Biologic and clinical features. *In* Sabiston, D. C., Jr. (ed.): Davis-Christopher Textbook of Surgery, 11th ed. Philadelphia, W. B. Saunders Co., 1977.

Peacock, E. E., Jr., and Van Winkle, W.: Wound Repair, 2nd ed. Philadelphia, W. B. Saunders Co., 1976.

10

Organ Transplantation

BARRY D. KAHAN
WILLIAM T. CONNER

Organ transplantation, the phoenix of rebirth because it achieves restitution rather than destruction, is the refinement of the surgeon's craft. Functional loss of an organ rarely occurs as an isolated event; associated problems often develop in related systems. For example, liver failure is frequently accompanied by malnutrition, profound coagulation defects, and, occasionally, renal failure. Although end-stage renal disease patients usually achieve homeostasis with chronic hemodialysis treatment, this equilibrium is at neither a normal nor a totally stable level. Anemia, secondary hyperparathyroidism, and accelerated atherosclerosis are common problems. Thus, preparation for organ transplantation requires comprehensive evaluation of the entire patient as well as detailed study of each organ system by skilled clinicians and scientists.

Renal transplantation will be reviewed in detail, since it is a widely applied, relatively successful prototype of clinical organ transplantation. Dramatic advances have been made in renal replacement therapy during the past 25 years. Most patients with irreversible renal failure now have a realistic hope for survival, and those who qualify for transplantation may resume a normal life.

Selection of transplant recipients begins when renal failure is diagnosed. Federal regulations and good medical practice require that each patient with renal failure be educated regarding the disease state and given an opportunity to discuss alternative methods of treatment. Primary therapy by cadaveric or living donor transplantation is at least an equal alternative to hemodialysis.

EVALUATION OF THE PATIENT AS A TRANSPLANT RECIPIENT

Uncontrolled malignancy and infection are absolute contraindications to immunosuppressive therapy and, therefore, to transplantation.

The extremes of age pose special problems in management and may preclude organ replacement. Diseases that will recur in the transplanted organ may not be suitably treated by renal grafting, for example, persistent, active, rapidly progressive glomerulonephritis with circulating anti-glomerular basement membrane antibody, or focal sclerosing glomerulonephritis. However, most patients between the ages of 2 and 60 years with irreversible renal failure may be considered for transplantation, unless malignancy or infection is not controlled.

Prospective transplant recipients are admitted to a special hospital unit for intensive study. Every organ system is analyzed in detail. Evaluation includes not only medical and surgical problems but also social, psychological, and nutritional assessment by professional staff members familiar with the special problems of renal failure patients and the potential complications encountered during transplantation therapy.

A variety of relative considerations that may preclude transplantation include:

1. Cardiovascular Disease
   a. Myocardial infarction within six months
   b. Coronary insufficiency
   c. Significant valvular disease
   d. Arrhythmia
   e. Uncontrollable peripheral vascular disease
   f. Cerebrovascular accident with residual deficits
2. Neurologic Disease: Chronic and/or Progressive Disorders
3. Metabolic Diseases
   a. Diabetes mellitus
   b. Amyloidosis
   c. Oxalosis
   d. Other rare metabolic conditions
4. Liver Disease, including significant acute, subacute, or chronic disorders
5. Chronic Lung Diseases
6. Connective Tissue Diseases
   a. Systemic lupus erythematosus
   b. Scleroderma
   c. Periarteritis nodosa
   d. Rheumatoid arthritis
7. Urinary Tract Disease
   a. Uncontrollable lower urinary dysfunction
   b. Uncontrollable neuropathic bladder
8. Psychosocial Problems, particularly those that prevent compliance with postoperative care

Final acceptance of a prospective transplant recipient is made following presentation of all data to the Medical Review Board, an open meeting attended by the transplantation staff, nephrologists from dialysis centers, immunologists, a dietitian, social worker, and special consultants. The following items must be weighed in the decision:

1. Patient's general state of health
2. Objective evidence of complications of renal failure
3. Absence of absolute contraindications
4. Consideration of relative contraindications
5. Necessity for pretransplant surgery, particularly nephrectomy, splenectomy, vagotomy-pyloroplasty, or parathyroidectomy

Cases demanding transplantation exclusively (Class I) are rare compared with those wherein it is clearly preferable (Class II). There is little doubt that for children it is the primary mode of therapy. An increasing number of patients on dialysis for more than five years have hemodialysis access failure in spite of ingenious attempts to construct arteriovenous communications, frequently at the expense of limb ischemia. Individuals in the dialysis pool who are unsuitable for transplantation can be readily identified (Class III). Although these persons frequently tolerate hemodialysis poorly, the temptation to offer transplantation as a "definitive" treatment is usually ill-advised. Most patients who are good transplant candidates actually are suitable for either modality (Class IV), and the choice is left to the patient. The major consideration is whether the benefits of an improved lifestyle outweigh the potential risks of transplantation (particularly from a cadaveric donor). Because of improved mortality and morbidity rates, most patients choose transplantation.

If the patient is deemed a candidate, he is then assigned to a class of transplant treatment:

CLASS A: Transplant, living related donor
CLASS B: Transplant, on dialysis pending cadaver kidney availability
CLASS C: Transplant, on dialysis pending necessary operation or medical control
CLASS D: No transplant, permanent dialysis

TISSUE TYPING

The major cause of renal graft failure is host rejection. Rejection has been recognized as an immunologic phenomenon ever since demonstration of the "second-set" response: repeat grafts from the same donor are destroyed faster than the initial one.

When donor antigens are identical to those of the recipient, as in the case of identical twins, the immune system is not stimulated and rejection does not occur. Thus, "matching" of donor and recipient antigens such that there are no foreign factors on the graft is a compelling approach to averting rejection. Tissue typing is a procedure that identifies the transplantation antigens of any individual. Kidneys from human leukocyte antigen (HLA)–identical siblings display greater than 90 per cent two-year success rates compared with a 60 per cent overall success in unmatched family members.

Using humoral and cellular immune techniques, tissue typing procedures can identify several antigenic factors determined by gene sites within a single chromosomal region. This region, denoted as the major histocompatibility complex (MHC), includes the gene sites HLA-A, B, and C, each of which determine a peptide antigen provoking humoral antibody production, and HLA-D, which encodes an antigen stimulating cellular immune responses.

TISSUE TYPING WITH LYMPHOCYTOTOXIC ANTIBODIES (HLA-A,B,C)

The initial probes to recognize gene products of the MHC were lymphocytotoxic antibodies, so named because of their capacity to kill peripheral blood lymphocytes bearing antigens (HLA) foreign to the individual. HLA antibodies are now available to detect a large number of antigens for histocompatibility matching. Performance of HLA typing requires a purified lymphocyte preparation, prepared by depletion of a blood sample of erythrocytes, polymorphonuclear leukocytes, and monocytes. Under inverted phase-contrast microscopy, the percentage of viable cells, identified by their capacity to exclude eosin, as opposed to dead cells, which retain the dye and stain as dark droplets, are scored. Target cell death signifies that the patient bears the distinctive antigen.

Using this simple test one can identify as many as two HLA-A, two HLA-B, and two HLA-C antigens on lymphocytes in a peripheral blood sample. Although standardized reagents are available to detect HLA-A, B, and C antigens, clinical transplantation matching is primarily performed only with HLA-A and HLA-B factors.

The most outstanding application of HLA matching is to predict kidney transplant success from familial donors. HLA typing of family members identifies which individuals have inherited the same A6 chromosome. On the basis of probabilities, one of every four siblings should be HLA-identical to any given recipient. The HLA-identical individual is the ideal donor, with a 90 per cent chance of two-year graft survival. A kidney of intermediate match grade "D" with a one chromosome (or one haplotype) disparity has a 70 per cent chance of two-year graft survival. While the selection of the living donor is a difficult medical and ethical question, there is little doubt that the living donor not only affords HLA compatibility but also sharing of additional weak, non-HLA histocompatibility antigens.

On the other hand, selection of recipients for cadaveric kidneys based upon tissue typing for allelic factors at the HLA-A and HLA-B sites does not uniformly predict histocompatibility, and HLA typing appears to be of greater importance in patients who have previously rejected an allograft. Therefore, even with perfect matches for HLA-A and HLA-B antigens, graft success has not been assured, and numerous patients have well-functioning grafts in spite of obvious, multiple HLA antigenic differences.

TISSUE TYPING BY CELLULAR RESPONSES

Owing to the strong possibility that an important but as-yet-unknown transplantation antigen is determined by another site within the MHC on A6, a variety of immunologic techniques have been used to dissect gene products of this region. The admixture of peripheral blood lymphocytes from two individuals results in "transformation," that is, reversion of responding cells to blastic elements undergoing rapid cell division (mixed lymphocyte culture reaction, MLC). The degree of MLC response between family members correlates with the HLA match grade, suggesting that the antigens triggering cellular proliferation are located on A6. Thus, there has been increased attention to the possible role of antigens detected in MLC reactions for tissue matching for cadaver transplantation. Since the MLC reaction requires a five-day incubation in vitro, serologic techniques have been developed to recognize the distinctive antigens provoking the response. These factors, termed DRW antigens, can be detected using cytotoxic antibodies directed against B lymphocytes purified from peripheral blood. Compatibility for HLA-DRW antigens appears to be more important for successful cadaver kidney transplantation than compatibility for HLA-A or B factors. However, it is probable that another site within the major histocompatibility complex is the prime initiator of acute allograft rejection.

Until it is identified, a convenient practical rule is to transplant cadaver kidneys into well-matched patients when available. If a number of patients have two antigens in common with the donor, selection should be made for the recipient bearing the same haplotype, since these individuals may share other transplantation factors inherited in linkage with the HLA antigens. Due to the marked polymorphism of the factors currently identified, it is unlikely that tissue matching will prove to be the ultimate method for improving the success rate of cadaveric allografts.

PREPARATION FOR OPERATION

PREOPERATIVE CARE

The immediate preoperative care includes review of all data presented to the Medical Review Board, acquisition of interim history and laboratory work, and meticulous physical examination. The presence of an intercurrent infection or progression of a relative complication absolutely contraindicates transplantation. The procedure has a relatively low risk when there is strict adherence to ideal criteria.

DONOR MANAGEMENT

Living Related Donors

Patients with living related donors are maintained on chronic hemodialysis until the potential donor has been evaluated. The selection of a living related donor poses a difficult ethical decision even in the absence of medical, psychological, and immunologic contraindications. The mortality rate of living donors is less than 0.1 per cent, or about the risk of a general anesthetic. The suitably chosen donor is at no greater risk of death with one kidney than his age-matched counterpart with two kidneys. The morbidity of the procedure is modest; less than 10 per cent of donors experience complications such as urinary tract infection, pneumonia, thromboembolism, etc. Donors undergo medical evaluation and presentation to the Medical Review Board prior to angiography and final selection.

When a suitable living donor is available, the potential recipient is hospitalized for five days prior to operation in order to initiate immunosuppressive therapy, first with azathioprine (1-2 mg/kg) and then, 48 hours prior to operation, with prednisone (1 mg/kg). The living donor is admitted one day prior to operation, and is well hydrated with intravenous fluids the evening before donor nephrectomy.

Cadaveric Donors

Selection of Cadaveric Donors. Potential donors range in age from 18 months to under 60 years and must display normal renal function as defined by serum creatinine and creatinine clearance. Cadaveric donor candidacy is unequivocally contraindicated under the conditions of obvious sepsis, neoplastic disease, or primary renal disease. Additional important considerations in the selection of potential cadaveric donors include an absence of systemic disease with potential renal involvement, i.e., diabetes, collagen disease, and chronic or long-standing hypertension.

The renal function test battery routinely includes blood urea nitrogen (BUN), serum creatinine, six-hour creatinine clearance, and assessment of urinary sediment. Blood and urine cultures are repeated daily until transplantation. Candidacy is retained if all cultures remain negative.

Definition of Death. The patient must be pronounced dead by his attending physician, who determines the cerebral survival criteria at the time of death. The physician must be satisfied in his own conscience that the patient is dead; that is, he shows "irreversible cessation of total brain function according to the usual and customary standards of medicine." As prerequisites for the certification of brain death, there must be no induced hypothermia, no evidence of drug intoxication, and completion of all relevant diagnostic and therapeutic procedures. Consent for the utilization of organs from the potential cadaveric donor must be obtained from both the attending physician and the legal next of kin.

In order to make a judgment of brain death, the following neurologic criteria must be present consistently for at least 30 minutes, six hours after cerebral insult: no response to painful stimuli, particularly application of supraorbital pressure;. apnea; and absence of pupillary light response and of cephalic reflexes, including corneal, pharyngeal, endotracheal, and ocular response to passive head turning or to aural ice water irrigation. The electroencephalogram should fail to reveal electrical activity when performed at maximal gain for 30 minutes. Absence of cerebral blood flow should be ascertained by angiography if the examination is being done less than six hours after the cerebral insult, or if one or more criteria of brain death are indefinite or unable to be tested.

Optimal donor conditions prevail when the kidneys are perfused at satisfactory blood pressure and are functioning normally.

Donor Management. Kidneys are more resistant to injury if they are removed during diuresis. This is accomplished best preoperatively using a large dose of furosemide (80 mg) and 12.5 gm mannitol. In addition, it is important to preserve electrolyte balance, particularly avoiding hypernatremia, and to correct acidosis. If the donor appears edematous, concentrated salt-poor albumin should be used to correct or prevent hypovolemia. One gram of methylprednisolone is administered intravenously at least two and preferably six hours prior to operation.

CROSS-MATCH PROCEDURES FOR CLINICAL RENAL TRANSPLANTATION

Since the antigens triggering allograft immunity exist as a wide array of alternative factors at several gene sites, perfect matching of cadaveric grafts is impossible. Recognizing that foreign antigens must inevitably be introduced with the graft, it is mandatory that procedures be performed to exclude prior exposure to disparate factors on the donor (presensitization). An adequate crossmatch prior to transplantation includes tests to detect both humoral and cellular arms of the host response. In order to maximize the accuracy of the procedure, it should include not only current samples of recipient materials, but also previous samples obtained during documented alloimmune reactions, such as 7 to 50 days after previous transplant failure, after blood transfusions, etc. An accurate crossmatch affords no assurance of allograft success; however, it may preclude hyperacute and accelerated rejections that represent secondary immune reactions unresponsive to available immunosuppressants.

The incidence of hyperacute rejection and resultant allograft destruction within 48 hours of transplantation has been markedly reduced by the general application of the visual microlymphocytotoxicity crossmatch. Presumably, hyperacute rejection represents an in vivo correlate of the lymphocytotoxic reaction, with antibody deposition on glomerular and endothelial cells triggering complement activation, polymorphonuclear leukocyte chemotaxis, and fibrin and platelet deposition, resulting ultimately in arteriolar thrombosis. Once triggered, this cascade cannot be interrupted by available immunosuppressive agents.

False negative reactions have an extremely grave prognosis, since they would lead one to transplantation of a patient bearing low levels of cytotoxic antibody. Such a situation is frequently associated with hyperacute rejection because in vivo antibody performance may be considerably better than in vitro cytodestruction. In our experience, extended incubation periods have detected positive reactions not evident with the standard 30-minute incubation period. Antiglobulin reagents offer a more sensitive test: Following incubation of recipient serum and donor cells, a rabbit antihuman gamma globulin reagent is added to the washed lymphocytes. If recipient antibody has been fixed to the cell, the rabbit antihuman reagent is also deposited and thus increases the total immunoglobulin coating. Because of the increased number of antibody molecules now protruding from the cell, additional amounts of complement can be fixed and cell lysis is enhanced. A less specific method uses antilymphocyte serum, which cannot cause cell lysis itself but in the presence of patient antibody fixation can effect cell lysis.

While routine application of the microlymphocytotoxicity assay has averted the occurrence of hyperacute rejection, there has been increasing awareness of another form of host antidonor presensitization termed *accelerated rejection*. These reactions occur three to five days after transplantation and are characterized by a vigorous, rapid rejection response leading to graft destruction by day nine despite the administration of increased amounts of steroids and external irradiation. Accelerated rejection probably represents a secondary immune response reflecting preexistent host sensitization not detectable by the microlymphocytotoxicity assay owing to (1) insensitivity to low levels of cytotoxic antibody; (2) mediation by a vector other than humoral antibody; or (3) dependence upon co-factors other than complement to express its activity.

In order to address these problems, a multifaceted battery of in vitro assays is performed to detect cell-mediated lympholysis (CML), lymphocyte-dependent antibody (LDA), and low levels of complement-dependent antibody (CDA) based upon the release of ^{51}Cr from prelabeled donor cells, obtained from either the peripheral blood or, if the nephrectomy has already been performed, from lymph node cells. Preloading donor target cells with radionuclides amplifies cell death. Thousands of counts per minute of ^{51}Cr issuing from a destroyed cell are detected. The use of isotopes affords an objective, quantitative measure of the degree of cell destruction and facilitates the analysis of numerous serum samples.

Cell-mediated lympholysis has been recognized as a cause of early graft failure in patients. Circulating host lymphocytes react anamnestically upon the introduction of a graft bearing foreign histocompatibility antigens to which they are already sensitized. Since these cells are presensitized, they do not undergo the usual division cycle, which is suppressed by azathioprine, and thus are immediately available to attack the graft. In the CML test, potential recipient lymphocytes are used as effectors to kill ^{51}Cr-labeled donor targets in the absence of complement. This cytotoxic action is based upon the immunologic competence of peripheral blood T cells.

LDAs have been implicated in a number of immune phenomena, including allograft rejection, platelet transfusion reactions, tumor immunity, and chronic active hepatitis. In the LDA system, 7 S IgG antibody coated upon even a relatively few target cell surface sites binds and activates effector, medium-sized K (killer) lymphocytes. LDA is more sensitive than CDA for detecting alloantibodies, since it has the capacity to detect cell lysis upon binding relatively few antibody molecules. The LDA assay employs ^{51}Cr-labeled donor lymphocytes, recipient sera, and normal lymphocytes pooled from five unrelated individuals to serve as effectors. Following incubation of labeled target cells with recipient serum, effector lymphocytes from four or five donors are added for a four-hour further incubation.

Detection of complement-dependent antibody utilizing radiochromium techniques displays markedly enhanced sensitivity over the visual system. Release of greater than 15 per cent of the available ^{51}Cr from targets, particularly when reduced by absorption with donor platelets (bearing HLA-A, B, C) or with lymphocytes (bearing HLA-A, B, C, D, and other surface markers), is considered a positive result.

In summary, avoidance of allografting in the presence of CDA, CML, and LDA reactivity has practically eliminated accelerated graft loss at a price deemed to be meager, namely, disqualifying recipients with positive comprehensive crossmatches.

INTRAOPERATIVE MANAGEMENT

ANESTHETIC TECHNIQUE

Since the patient with renal failure presents novel challenges, most anesthesiologists appreciate guidance regarding aspects of management. Intravenous fluid management is maintained with 5 per cent dextrose/0.45 per cent normal saline via large-bore catheters at 50 to 100 ml/hr, depending on baseline urine output. With low urine output, fluid should be restricted. It can be useful to infuse a 250 ml fluid bolus one-half hour prior to revascularization, if the recipient is not overhydrated. Depolarizing agents (such as succinylcholine), which may raise serum potassium, should be avoided, except for a trace dosage for intubation; D-tubocurare is preferred for muscle relaxation. Gallamine is not recommended because of prolonged recirculation due to impaired renal excretion. Halothane inhalation anesthesia is usually preferred. At the beginning of the procedure, solumedrol 500 mg in 50 ml dextrose/0.45 per cent sodium chloride is infused over 30 minutes. At the time of vascular anastomosis, furosemide 80 mg and mannitol 12.5 gm are administered. The anesthesiologist should have on hand *but not give* the following: heparin 50 mg, in case of technical difficulties with the vascular anastomoses; sodium bicarbonate 3 amp, in case of hyperkalemia; and indigo carmine, to test the integrity of the urinary collecting system. The anesthesiologist should note when the kidney is available, when the vascular clamps are released, and when urine first appears. He should record urine flow every 30 minutes and notify the surgeon. Blood transfusions are generally avoided unless the hematocrit is less than 20 per cent. Albumisol (5 per cent albumin in saline) or salt-poor albumin is preferred for volume expansion. Blood pressure support for the vasodilator effects of halothane in the adequately hydrated patient is best provided by salt-poor albumin.

OPERATIVE TECHNIQUE

The allograft is usually placed retroperitoneally in either iliac fossa, although intra-abdominal placement may be required for children. The renal artery is anastomosed to either the internal or external iliac artery in adults — occasionally to the aorta in children. The venous anastomosis utilizes the external iliac vein in adults and the common iliac vein or inferior vena cava in children. The most reliable urinary reconstruction technique is the ureteroneocystostomy, using a submucosal tunnel and securely anchoring the ureter to the trigonal musculature. The bladder is closed in three layers. The transplant wound is irrigated with antibiotic solution and closed securely with nonabsorbable sutures without drainage other than a urethral catheter.

POSTOPERATIVE MANAGEMENT

The immediate postoperative management is determined by the renal function and preexisting problems in the recipient. With proper donor management, immediate allograft diuresis is the rule. Hourly urine volume is replaced, up to 250 ml, with an equal volume of 5 per cent dextrose/0.45 per cent sodium chloride solution. Potassium is added only when serum concentration falls below 3.0 mEq/l. Patients with acute tubular necrosis (ATN) require no more than 50 ml/hr of intravenous fluid and serial postoperative dialysis. Though ATN does not result in decreased graft survival, management is much more difficult in a patient with a nonfunctioning kidney.

From the recovery room, the patient is immediately transferred to the intensive care section of the Transplantation Center. Strict reverse isolation procedures are not necessary as long as the Transplantation Center is removed from the hospital traffic pattern and antisepsis is maintained. Prophylactic antibiotics are not used unless there is a proclivity toward bacterial infection (frequently staphylococcal); ongoing treatments, such as antituberculosis therapy, are continued.

During the week following renal transplantation, the patient is moved from the intensive to the intermediate care section of the Transplantation Center. Ambulation begins the day after operation; resumption of a normal diet is usual by the second postoperative day. On the fifth postoperative day, the urethral catheter is removed and a postvoiding scintiphotograph is obtained within one hour to facilitate prompt detection of urinary leakage.

THE RENAL TRANSPLANT DATA BASE

Laboratory tests include serum electrolytes, particularly to detect acidosis, hyperkalemia, and salt depletion, and urine electrolytes to monitor sodium and potassium losses. Determinations of blood urea nitrogen and serum and urine creatinine to estimate clearance provide a ready method to evaluate renal function. Microscopic examination of urine daily is critical to detect urinary tract infection, cellular allograft rejection, and/or glomerulitis. Crystalluria can be an important sign of potential stone formation. Rather sophisticated assessment of glomerular selectivity can be obtained by measuring urinary albumin and urinary immunoglobulin, and of tubular dysfunction by measuring urinary retinol binding globulin. Complete blood counts, reticulocyte counts and platelet counts are performed daily to monitor the bone marrow effects of azathioprine. Serum enzyme determinations are obtained twice weekly to detect evidence of hepatitis (due to azathioprine toxicity, infection, etc.). Serum calcium and phosphate alterations are common owing to suppression of parathormone secretion and improved intestinal absorption.

Radionuclide scanning has replaced intravenous contrast studies as the major technique for serial morphologic evaluation of the renal transplant. The study includes assessment of glomerular function with ^{99m}technetium-DTPA and of tubular function with ^{125}I-Hippuran. The renal handling of each radionuclide is determined by scintiphotographs of accumulated countings for 0.5 to 3.0 minutes and by digital and analog computer processing. The latter allows dynamic quantitative assessment or renal function and permits early detection of slight changes between serial studies. The initial images after injection of DTPA outline the iliac arteries and show allograft perfusion. Delayed images then reveal the distribution of blood flow and the glomerular phase of renal function. The Hippuran study shows the extent of tubular uptake, concentration, and excretion, both by scintiphotographs and by standard renogram curves, and the anatomy of the kidney, collecting system, and bladder are outlined. Postvoiding images assess residual urine and ureteral reflux. These studies are combined with serial blood levels to determine radionuclide clearances.

IMMUNOSUPPRESSIVE AGENTS

The success of transplantation depends upon dampening the host's response, for all allografts will undergo eventual rejection in the absence of immunosuppressive therapy. The regimen depends upon the judicious use of chemical, physical, and biologic reagents, all of which cause nonspecific suppression of the host response, that is, reducing reactivity not only to disparate donor antigens but also all foreign materials.

Four types of agents have acceptable ratios of efficacy to toxicity for use in human organ transplantation: corticosteroids, antiproliferative agents (azathioprine, cyclophosphamide or cyclosporin A), antilymphocyte serum, and external irradiation.

Until specific immunotherapeutic agents become available for prevention and treatment of allograft rejection, transplant physicians and surgeons will spend much of their time treating complications of the present broad-spectrum immunosuppressive drugs.

Corticosteroids

The key immunosuppressive agents are the corticosteroids, which exert anti-inflammatory and relatively nonspecific lymphopenic actions. Steroids are the critical agents, for all other drugs may be discontinued with a satisfactory result if the patient is maintained on steroids in adequate doses. All patients are maintained on prednisone from the time of the operation, generally starting at about 1.5 mg/kg/day and tapering relatively rapidly to a level of 60 mg/day and then to 40 mg/day by day 30. Once rejection is diagnosed, the dosage is increased. Steroid therapy may be given either as high-dose intravenous boluses of methylprednisolone, which may have the advantage of achieving high peak levels and of being rapidly excreted, or as oral prednisone to 3 mg per kg per day and tapering progressively thereafter. Oral steroids not only persist for a longer period of time but also are used in recycling of lower dosages.

Although the exact mechanism of steroid action is unknown, several effects may contribute to immunosuppression: (a) stabilization of membranes, thereby inhibiting the reactivity of cellular and lysosomal organelles, which occurs upon lymphocyte stimulation; (b) catabolic action on lymphoid cells, including diminution of RNA and protein synthesis; (c) impairment of degranulation and enzyme release from polymorphonuclear leukocytes; (d) inhibition of macrophage function, including phagocytosis; (e) interference with the complement system, and (f) dampening of the action of inflammatory mediators of rejection.

The side effects of corticosteroid therapy are well recognized. In the transplantation context, metabolic, immunologic, gastrointestinal, cardiovascular, and psychiatric actions are the major complications of therapy. The metabolic effects appearing with great frequency include (1) steroid-induced diabetes, which occasionally persists for several months in spite of reduction of steroid dosage below 15 mg prednisone per day; (2) myopathy, producing marked muscle wasting and the cushingoid habitus of truncal obesity with protuberant abdomen and thin extremities; (3) distinctive fat deposition leading to the buffalo hump; (4) cataracts; and (5) osteoporosis leading to demineralization and the not infrequent and somewhat independent complication of aseptic necrosis of the femoral heads.

The immunologic complication of sepsis due to overly aggressive steroid therapy is the most common cause of death, leading to 45 per cent of the fatalities after transplantation. The immunologic debilitation results from a profound depression of both the elements of nonspecific resistance, i.e., polymorphonuclear leukocytes (PMNs) and monocytes, and those of specific immunity, T and B cells. Since the PMNs are critical for disposing of bacteria through mechanisms of intracellular killing after antibody coating or inactivation through antibiotic therapy, paralysis of these essential functions produces the poor response of the septic transplant patient to overwhelming infection. Antibiotic therapy even with combinations of appropriate and specific agents frequently fails. Only vigorous nutritional repletion and granulocyte transfusion may provide the immunologic reconstitution necessary to salvage the patient. The effects of corticosteroids on the specific immune system of T and B lymphocytes produce immunodepression, permitting the growth of viral and fungal as well as more common bacterial pathogens. The immunodepressive actions are not rapidly reversible. Even rapid tapering of the dosage to physiologic levels (7.5 mg/day), a maneuver that may induce hypocorticalism in the septic patient, cannot be expected to ameliorate the cumulative depressant effects for many days.

Gastrointestinal disorders range from the relatively common symptoms of peptic ulcer disease, which may result in hemorrhage, one of the more common causes of death following transplantation, to the less common sequelae of cholestatic jaundice and pancreatitis. Cardiovascular effects of corticosteroids result from their mineralocorticoid actions of salt retention, producing hypertension and weight gain, and of an alpha receptor agonist effect. To minimize this complication, investigators have recommended the use of the diuretic spironolactone, an aldosterone antagonist, or use of oral methylprednisolone, a costly preparation claimed to have less mineralocorticoid effect. Steroid psychoses may occur after transplantation, particularly during periods of high dosage for the treatment of rejection. Although not all psychiatrists would agree, there appears to be an increased incidence of this complication in patients with a previous history of psychosis. Sedation with haloperidol may be useful on an acute basis. A variety of less severe syndromes of hallucination, seizure, and delirium may occur in patients with marginal graft function, presumably on an organic basis.

Antiproliferative Agents

Cyclosporin. A major advance in immunosuppressive therapy has been achieved by introduction of cyclosporin, a cyclic endecapeptide fungal product of novel chemical structure, which appears to selectively prevent the activation of T-helper cells and thereby abort antibody production and cell-mediated immunity. Since elements of nonspecific immunity are spared, bone marrow depression and bacterial infections are infrequent. However, the drug may induce dose-related hepato- and nephrotoxicity. The oral route of administration is clearly preferable, commencing at 14 mg/kg for one week, then 12 mg/kg for two weeks with dose adjustments thereafter guided to maintain rough serum levels determined by radioimmunoassay between 100 to 200 ng/ml or whole blood levels determined by high performance liquid chromatography between 200 to 300 ng/ml. In the presence of an ileus, 125 mg drug may be administered intravenously over two hours, each day unless serum levels reveal cyclosporin accumulation. Clinical studies clearly indicate that cyclosporin is the most effective drug to dampen immunocompetent host lymphocytes.

Azathioprine. The purine analog 6-mercaptopurine, conjugated with an imidazole side chain, interferes with proliferation of lymphocytes by competitively inhibiting the conversion of inosine monophosphate to adenosine and guanidine monophosphates. Inhibition of nucleic acid synthesis is most effective during the early phases of proliferation of small lymphocytes. The drug appears to have greater specificity for T lymphocytes than for B cells, possibly owing to specific metabolic characteristics of the former. Azathioprine therapy must be continued indefinitely to prevent development of new clones of immunocompetent cells. Therapy is generally initiated at 3 mg/kg/day and then reduced to 1 to 2 mg/kg/day as determined by toxicity, primarily bone marrow suppression. In the absence of allograft function the dose must be reduced to 0.5 to 1.0 mg/kg. While pancreatitis, febrile idiosyncratic responses, and alopecia occur rarely, granulocytopenia is a frequent complication of therapy. The dose-related effects of leukopenia and thrombocytopenia can be controlled by withholding the drug for short periods of time and reducing the maintenance dose. The total white blood count must be corrected for nucleated red blood cells to prevent overdosage. Frequently, initial evidence of bone marrow toxicity is demonstrated by falling platelet or reticulocyte, rather than leukocyte, counts. The authors withhold azathioprine if the white cell count is less than 4000 per cu mm or if the platelet count is less than 70,000 per cu mm. While leukopenia of less than 2500 per cu mm may be managed by reverse precautions, absolute granulocyte counts of less than 750 per cu mm are best treated by laminar flow isolation. Leukopenia unaccompanied by sepsis is generally not a serious complication. While the cytopenia is almost always the result of bone marrow depression, the occasional case of heretofore undetected hypersplenism demands bone marrow biopsy and/or spleen scan. Splenectomy is accompanied by increased hazard, but the benefits of the procedure in selected cases demand its consideration.

Total discontinuation of azathioprine for over five days frequently permits clonal proliferation and subsequent rejection crises. In some instances of stable, nonprogressive leukopenia, cyclophosphamide may be substituted with a synergistic immunosuppressive, but not marrow-toxic, action by interfering with lymphocyte division at a point after the azathioprine blockade. It should be noted that while the optimal azathioprine dose is assumed to be the maximal tolerable dose, it is probably much less than that amount in many cases. Mass spectrometry and high pressure liquid chromatography methods to determine blood levels of azathioprine and its metabolites may identify abnormal handling of the drug.

Cyclophosphamide. Cyclophosphamide therapy is usually reserved for patients unable to take azathioprine owing to progressive bone marrow toxicity, a history of hepatitis, or recent treatment with allopurinol, which interferes with azathioprine degradation. As an alkylating agent, cyclophosphamide forms stable covalent bonds crosslinking DNA and thus precludes cell division and lymphocyte proliferation. In addition to bone marrow toxicity, the metabolites of cyclophosphamide can cause hemorrhagic cystitis if not evacuated promptly from the bladder. Administration of the drug early in the morning with large volumes of water prevents this complication. The problems of azoospermia and alopecia are not as worrisome as the frequent chromosomal disruptions clearly implicated in the development of leukemia in some patients. Thus azathioprine is preferred to cyclophosphamide.

External Irradiation

Irradiation impairs immune function. Lymphocytes are sensitive to 50R, as opposed to the 1400R necessary to induce radiation nephritis. On each of three successive days, 150R are delivered to the allograft, particularly in patients displaying renomegaly. While from a theoretical standpoint three courses of irradiation might be delivered without exceeding the tolerable limit for renal cells, the uncertainty about dosage limits in individual cases suggests that restriction to two courses is prudent. Irradiation of the allograft prior to implantation in order to reduce the number of passenger donor lymphocytes in the graft has not been demonstrated to improve transplant survival.

Antilymphocyte Serum (ALS)

Since one of the primary vectors of host resistance to allografts is the T-lymphocyte, which mediates cellular immunity, reagents have been developed to inactivate this cell. Antilymphocyte sera bind to and coat lymphocytes, thereby making them susceptible to lysis via endogenous complement and macrophage digestion, particularly by hepatic Kupffer cells. Although the preparations in clinical use are produced from a variety of different sources — thymus (T-cell–rich) and/or lymphoblasts (primarily B-cell populations) — there is little apparent difference in their efficacy. While some investigators claim that rabbit antisera are most effective, others favor equine or goat hosts for immunization. The major reactions to the preparations, e.g., anaphylaxis, fever, chills, dyspnea, and/or tachypnea, can be avoided by (1) exclusion of patients with known allergy; (2) negative cutaneous hypersensitivity tests; (3) slow infusion through a high-flow vein such as an arteriovenous fistula; (4) extensive absorption of sera with human erythrocytes and platelets; and (5) careful pyrogenicity and endotoxin testing. Prophylactic therapy is generally administered at 7.5 to 15 mg/kg/day for the initial 14 days and on alternate days for an additional 7 to 14 days to avert a rapid rebound and rise in T-cells with a severe and frequently irreversible rejection response. Patients who benefit from the prophylactic regimen are those displaying strong T-cell immunity preoperatively. However, cyclosporine therapy achieves better success than ALS, with reduced incidence of viral infection. Recent studies indicate that ALS therapy can reverse steroid-resistant allograft rejection, thereby suggesting that combined ALS-steroid regimens may reduce the incidence of "rebound" re-rejection and produce improved one-year graft survival. Since allograft rejection in cyclosporine-treated patients tends to be mild and readily reversible, this combined regimen is not only unnecessary but also potentially causes over-immunosuppression.

IMMUNOLOGIC MONITORING

Since rejection is the major cause of graft failure, postoperative care of the transplant patient should include tests for evidence of immunologic activity against donor tissue. While it has not yet been proven that initiation of immunosuppressive chemotherapy at the earliest immunologic, but not clinical, sign of rejection improves the eventual result, there is no doubt that unequivocal evidence of an immune process can be useful in the differential diagnosis of the ill, febrile post-transplant patient. Furthermore, these tests may be used as a barometer to decrease immunosuppressive drug dosages in patients not displaying immune activity. Two types of immune activities are tested: nonspecific reactivity and specific host-antidonor immunity. The most common tests of the former variety are T-cell enumeration, nonspecific blastogenesis, and killer-cell activity; the latter variety includes mixed lymphocyte cultures, complement- and lymphocyte-dependent antibody, leukocyte aggregation, and cell-mediated lympholysis.

Nonspecific Assays of Immune Activation

The most rapid, flexible, and simple tool to assess host immune responsiveness following transplantation is serial estimation of the number of circulating thymus-derived (T) and bursa-equivalent (B) cells. Since acute allograft rejection directly reflects the activity of T cells more than B cells, T-cell monitoring is more useful. T-cell determinations can be performed by two methods. T cells bear receptors binding sheep erythrocytes to form rosettes. T cells can be fractionated based upon the speed at which the rosettes form into active T (short incubation) and total T (long incubation) populations. Decreases in the number of active T cells are associated with allograft rejection; successful treatment is associated with reversal of the fall. Secondly, T cells can be enumerated using monoclonal reagents that not only count the total number (pan T) but also discriminate the helper-inducer T cells from the suppressor-cytotoxic T cells. Obviously, T-cell determinations are of limited utility during periods of ALS administration, since these levels are used to determine dosages. Serial enumeration of B cells has no predictive or diagnostic value in transplantation. Estimation of the number of killer or K cells capable of mediating killing of antibody-coated targets, probably is not a useful index of specific antidonor immunity but rather reflects the intensity of the nonspecific immunosuppression.

Rapidly dividing lymphocytes appear in the peripheral blood coincident with allograft rejection. Spontaneous blastogenesis tests measure the amount of radioactive thymidine incorporation by whole blood incubated for a two-hour period. The test is an extremely simple and rapid clinical tool. An increase in spontaneous blastogenesis, particularly when accompanied by a fall in active T cells, correlates with the onset of cellular rejection reactions. While spontaneous blastogenesis is clouded by false positive reactions in cardiac transplantation, the problem has been rare in renal patients. Two situations produce false positive results: the presence of large numbers of immature myeloid cells in the circulation and the emergence of cell-mediated resistance to infection. However, as a daily estimate of host reactivity, total and active T cells and spontaneous blastogenesis afford rapid, flexible tools.

Specific Tests of Allograft Immunity

The critical issue in transplantation is not simply the presence of an active immunologic response, but one specifically directed against donor tissue. Unequivocal immunologic results documenting a moderate to severe immune reaction often precede clinical signs of rejection, which frequently appear only when there has been extensive tissue damage with alteration of renal function. Specific antidonor immunity may be measured in vitro by tests that detect four stages in the expression of the reaction: (1) adherence, (2) proliferation, (3) killing, and (4) release of lymphokinetic mediators. The leukocyte aggregation test measures recipient antidonor cell adherence. Separated peripheral blood leukocytes of the recipient are reacted with donor kidney cells grown in tissue culture. Adhesion of lymphocytes to donor targets produces clumps rather than a general distribution of cells. The response detected in the assay is purely a cellular one. In almost every case, it is capable of being reversed by administration of methylprednisolone, even when the drug is started after the appearance of clinical signs of rejection.

In order to avoid the need for tissue culture technology to grow donor kidney cells, and in view of the fact that transplantation antigens are shared by all nucleated cells, it is generally easier to utilize donor peripheral blood lymphocytes as targets for immunologic assays. At the time of donor nephrectomy, lymphocytes obtained from peripheral blood and from mesenteric lymph nodes are stored by freezing in dimethylsulfoxide at $-169°C$. At intervals after transplantation, aliquots are defrosted. Proliferation of recipient peripheral blood lymphocytes upon donor stimulation is measured in one-way mixed lymphocyte cultures (MLC). Although it may initially seem anachronous, a fall in the MLC response by peripheral blood lymphocytes reflects immune activation against donor histocompatibility antigens. The fall may be due to movement of immunoreactive cells out of the circulation and into the graft. The return of these cells into the circulation occurs with recovery. Specific killing is routinely measured by the capacity of immune elements to release radio-chromium from prelabeled donor target lymphocytes in three tests: cell-mediated lympholysis, lymphocyte-dependent antibody-mediated lympholysis, and complement-dependent antibody-mediated lympholysis. While lymphocyte-dependent, antibody-mediated, and cell-mediated reactions appear to be amenable to intensified corticosteroid therapy, pure antibody responses, detected as complement-dependent antibody, have a more serious prognosis. The presence of substantial antidonor reactivity, particularly if confirmed with appropriate control reactions performed against lymphocytes from unrelated individuals, affords unequivocal evidence of immune reactivity and strongly suggests that clinical evidence of impaired renal function is due to allograft rejection.

A final group of tests that are somewhat easier to perform but of less significance measures the release of lymphokinetic mediators by peripheral blood lymphocytes activated in vitro by exposure to donor target cells or their extracts. The most frequently used test estimates release of migration inhibition factor (MIF). In the direct test, peripheral blood leukocytes from the recipient are loaded into a capillary tube that has donor antigens placed at its tip. Contact of hypersensitive lymphocytes with the exciting foreign transplantation antigens activates production and/or release of MIF, which prevents monocytes in the host peripheral blood sample from migrating out of the capillary tube. In the direct assay, peripheral blood leukocytes are preincubated with donor tissue or extract. An aliquot of the supernatant of this interaction is added to a Petri dish or a capillary tube containing the third-party migrating population, which may be derived from normal individuals or, because MIF is not species-specific, from guinea pig peritoneal exudates. Failure of leukocyte migration or inhibition of migration by greater than 40 per cent constitutes cellular evidence of allograft rejection. At present immunologic monitoring is relatively crude, since the critical immune mechanisms of acute and chronic allograft rejection have not been identified. However, the concept of serial monitoring of the patient's immune mechanism is as critical as estimation of renal function for rational and judicious immunosuppressive therapy.

POSTOPERATIVE COMPLICATIONS

The combination of long-standing renal failure with its associated problems and implementation of immunosuppression following a major operation provides numerous opportunities for serious complications. While many problems can be averted by prophylactic correction of abnormalities detected during the pretransplant evaluation, careful postoperative monitoring, including thorough examination by the attending staff at least twice daily, is critical. Until specific immunotherapeutic agents become available for prevention and treatment of allograft rejection, transplant surgeons will spend much of their time treating complications of the present broad-spectrum immunosuppressive drugs.

SEPSIS

The most common signal of a complication in the postoperative period is fever. Minimal temperature elevations may reflect major problems in immunosuppressed patients. Swift, precise diagnosis is an absolute requirement for satisfactory clinical results. The most vexing problem is differentiating between signs of infection and those of rejection, a task that is essential although often difficult or impossible due to simultaneous events.

Infections, facilitated by immunosuppression, are the major cause of morbidity and mortality following transplantation. Even when the predominant organisms are common bacterial pathogens, as they frequently are in the first 60 days, diagnosis and treatment are considerably more difficult owing to depression of nonspecific immune elements that mediate the inflammatory expression of the usual clinical signs. Viral, mycobacterial, fungal, and protozoan pathogens occur frequently enough to require a comprehensive search whenever fever intervenes.

During the first postoperative days, pulmonary problems, especially atelectasis, frequently account for episodes of fever. The major cause of mortality in the first 30 days is bacterial pneumonia due to gram-negative organisms. Preventive measures of humidified oxygen, incentive spirometry, and vigorous pulmonary care are necessary. Intermittent positive-pressure breathing is avoided because of the hazards of gastric distention and of introduction of adventitious organisms. Atelectasis or pneumonia confirmed radiographically must be vigorously treated with chest physical therapy and endotracheal suctioning. Infections, detected by Gram stain and confirmed by culture, are treated with specific antimicrobial agents. Other causes of early fever include (1) rejection, a diagnosis that can be sustained only by a biopsy or a combination of unequivocal radionuclide and immunologic monitoring data; (2) urinary and wound infections, which tend to be caused by indigenous, chronic, low-grade processes; half of the patients with pyrexia of unknown origin are discovered to have wound infections; and (3) phlebitis, which is rare not only owing to the practice of prompt mobilization, but also to the relative thrombocytopenia induced by azathioprine and the hypocoagulable state of uremic patients. Because of the possibility of drug fever, any patient with a prolonged temperature elevation should have cyclophosphamide substituted for azathioprine to exclude an idiosyncratic reaction. Routinely, patients with temperatures greater than 100°F should have samples of blood, throat, sputum, urine, stool, and wound drainage sent for aerobic, anaerobic, mycobacterial, viral, and fungal cultures. Treatment of both the fever and its cause should begin as soon as a diagnosis is established. Initial specific broad-spectrum treatment with nafcillin, gentamicin, ticarcillin, and clindamycin may be essential for serious infections pending complete bacteriologic data. Body temperature should be kept below 100°F with oral or rectal acetaminophen, to reduce the concomitant tachycardia and systemic manifestations of fever that further stress the catabolic, steroid-treated patient.

Infections after the first two months are frequently due to unusual organisms, since cellular immunity mediates resistance to these invaders. Viral infections, particularly herpes and cytomegaloviruses, are most common and unfortunately most difficult to control. Herpes simplex virus (HSV) infections, ranging from the relatively trivial oral mucosal HSV-1 lesions to genital and cutaneous HSV-2 infestations to disseminated tissue infections such as hepatitis, occur in over one half the transplant recipients. While superficial lesions may be treated with Stoxil and conservative regimens, pulmonary, renal, or hepatic involvement documented by cultivation or histopathologic evidence in biopsy specimens demands systemic treatment with acyclovir dosage and rapid tapering of corticosteroids to maintenance levels. Herpes zoster infections are generally more benign and readily reversible. Cytomegalovirus (CMV) infection recurs in about 30 per cent of recipients, in many cases emanating from blood transfusions, and can be documented by complement-fixing antibodies or by cultivation of peripheral blood buffy coat leukocytes. Because CMV is frequently associated with febrile illnesses accompanied by altered renal function mimicking rejection, many patients are inadvertently treated with intensified immunosuppression. Immunologic assays failing to show alloimmunization can prevent fatal iatrogenic complications. Conservative treatment with steroid withdrawal is the only rational course. Isolated cases of disseminated varicella are usually fatal. It is probable that activation of latent agents such as adenoviruses occurs with chronic immunosuppression and may account for the debilitation occasionally seen in long-term recipients, or possibly the increased incidence of lymphomas. Furthermore, the secondary immunosuppression induced by viral agents further depresses the meager host resistance. The most commonly encountered protozoan infection is *Pneumocystis carinii,* which generally presents as hilar pulmonary infiltrates with marked hypoxia. The diagnosis may be established by methenamine silver staining of transtracheal or endobronchial specimens. Combination therapy with pentamidine and trimethoprim has markedly reduced the mortality from this complication. *Toxoplasmosis gondii* is a less frequent pathogen diagnosed in the patient with fever of unknown origin either by the Sabin-Feldman test or by complement fixation assays.

Fungal infections, usually presenting as pulmonic infiltrates or cavitations, may disseminate hematogenously to the brain. The infections vary in severity from the relatively benign *Nocardia asteroides,* which may be managed with oral sulfamethoxidol and trimethoprim, and actinomycosis treated with ampicillin or penicillin without reduction in immunosuppression, to *Aspergillus fumigatus,* which, in spite of reduction of steroids and aggressive treatment with amphotericin B, is frequently fatal. Mucocutaneous candidiasis, *Torulopsis glabrata* infection, coccidioidomycosis, blastomycosis, and mucormycosis are other pernicious conditions. Diagnosis depends upon a high index of suspicion and conscientious, comprehensive sampling of all body fluids, drainage and investigation of abnormal areas with Gram and Ziehl-Nielsen stains, cultures on appropriate media including Sabouraud's agar and guinea pig inoculation, and careful pretransplant assessment of documented and potential occult infections.

Host resistance against mycobacteria represents classic cell-mediated immunity. A documented past history of tuberculosis is rarely a contraindication to transplantation because of the availability of isoniazid and rifampin, which unfortunately are both hepatotoxins. However, a not uncommon problem is recrudescent infection in carriers. Unfortunately, a negative skin test in the chronic dialysis patient may reflect anergy rather than lack of exposure and offers no assurance of freedom from mycobacterial infection. The prevalence of atypical mycobacteria in urban areas presents a special challenge to diagnosis and therapy.

REJECTION

Four forms of host immune reactions against allografts are discernible: hyperacute, accelerated, acute, and chronic. The former two reactions are anamnestic responses reflecting host presensitization; the latter two, primary responses to the stimulus of foreign transplantation antigens. Of these four responses, only acute cellular rejection reactions are reliably reversed with available immunosuppressive agents.

Hyperacute rejection, mediated by preformed circulating antibody, may be due to major blood group ABO isoagglutinins, xenografting, high titers of cold agglutinins, or specific antidonor lymphocytotoxic antibodies. The last factor, which is the major cause of this complication, should not occur if a careful crossmatch has been performed. Hyperacute rejection occurs within the first 48 hours, indeed, often during the operative procedure. Deposition of antibody on vascular endothelium attracts polymorphonuclear leukocytes and platelets, subsequently leading to fibrin clot and thrombosis of the allograft, as documented by lack of perfusion on ^{99}Tc-DTPA scans. Nephrectomy of the infarcted black kidney is the only treatment.

Accelerated allograft rejection, presenting as an abrupt decline in renal function with associated clinical signs of rejection, occurs within the first postoperative week. Paradoxically, grafts suffering this fate often have excellent early function. The important considerations in the differential diagnosis, namely occlusion of the renal artery, vein, or ureter, can be excluded by radionuclide scanning, angiogram, retrograde pyelogram, and/or surgical exploration. The form of accelerated rejection primarily due to a cell-mediated immune mechanism may respond to bolus therapy with methylprednisolone, graft irradiation ($150R \times 4$ doses), and/or systemic heparin therapy. However, if humoral mechanisms are the predominant vectors, such as a secondary response to disparate HLA antigens, treatment is futile. Irreversible cases display vasculonecrotic histopathology with vessel disruption and interstitial hemorrhage producing a red kidney at exploration.

Acute cellular rejection reactions usually occur in patients during the first month. One or more of the following clinical signs and symptoms may accompany acute rejection: (1) allograft enlargement and/or tenderness, (2) oliguria, (3) malaise, (4) hypertension, and (5) weight gain. Most patients present with detectable changes in renal function: the creatinine clearance falls by at least 20 per cent, and the serum creatinine and blood urea nitrogen rise. Urinary examination reveals decreased sodium and osmolality, increased proteinuria of either the glomerular (poor prognosis) or the tubular (good prognosis) type, microscopic hematuria or lymphocyturia, and occasionally Type IV renal tubular acidosis. Radionuclide studies initially show retardation of the excretion slope of ^{125}I-Hippuran, followed later by an impaired concentration phase. There may be a patchy distribution of perfusion on ^{99m}Tc-DTPA scintiphotograph. Changes in radionuclide studies practically establish the diagnosis of rejection, particularly if spontaneous blastogenesis is increased and simultaneous active T-rosette–forming cells decrease. Vigorous acute reactions cause temporary and occasionally permanent loss of renal function.

Acute cellular rejection may be treated either with intravenous pulses of 500 to 1000 mg of methylprednisolone up to an absolute maximum total dose of 10 gm during the first postoperative month, or by recycling the oral steroids to 3 mg/kg, rapidly tapering to 1 mg/kg by 10 to 14 days. Based upon a kinetic analysis of the performance of peripheral blood lymphocytes from patients undergoing rejection in cellular immune assays, the authors recommend divided methylprednisolone doses of 500 mg initially every 8 hours thrice, followed by a recycling of oral steroids. Administration of methylprednisolone by rapid intravenous pulse has been accompanied by cardiac arrhythmia and death. In addition, the possibility of rebound rejection after intravenous steroid pulse therapy is reduced by recycling oral prednisone to 50 mg every six hours and rapidly tapering by 20 mg daily declinations in dosage over six days. A second rejection episode is not treated unless 50 per cent of the original or best function is regained. In any case, no more than two courses of steroids are given in the first 60 days after transplantation, because of the high incidence of septic complications of therapy. Graft irradiation with 150R each day for three days is also used. A disastrous complication of accelerated or acute rejection is allograft rupture, in which tissue pressure exceeds capsular pressure owing to engorgement. Pain, sudden graft enlargement, hypotension, and a tearing sensation may be noted. Nephrectomy reveals a fracture, usually along the cortical margin of the blue kidney produced by marked venous congestion and lymphocytic infiltration.

Chronic rejection reactions are produced by gradual occlusion of renal arterioles with ischemia of the corresponding segment and gradual decline in renal function, generally evident 60 or more days following transplantation. The clinical syndrome includes hypertension, moderate to severe proteinuria, microscopic hematuria, and graft shrinkage. Vascular occlusion is apparently mediated by humoral antibody deposition triggering endothelial cell swelling and proliferation. Chronic rejection is only modestly affected by the currently available methods of immunosuppressive therapy. Treatment consists of reducing prednisone dosage to the lowest tolerable limits, raising antiproliferative agents to maximal doses, and preparing for retransplantation. While chronic rejection occasionally follows a stormy course of incompletely resolved acute rejection reactions, it sometimes represents the initial and only evidence of host resistance. A white ischemic kidney is observed at allograft nephrectomy performed for relief of proteinuria, hypertension, or fever.

SURGICAL COMPLICATIONS

Vascular

Abrupt dehiscence of arterial or venous suture lines usually results in death or requires nephrectomy, while gradual occlusion or leakage leads to progressive damage to the allograft. Anastomotic disruption results from improper technique, faulty suture material, or adjacent infection, but rarely from diseased blood vessels. Although thrombosis and gradual stenosis of the renal artery may have a more varied genesis, they usually result from atheromatous disease. Endothelial injury from any cause may result in thrombosis during a low flow state due to hypotension, rejection, extrinsic compression, or venous hypertension. Endothelial injury may be induced by arterial stretching during donor nephrectomy, cannulation injury during the process of machine perfusion, toxic materials in perfusates, elevated perfusion pressures of over 60 mm of mercury, prolonged perfusion, atherosclerosis, immunologic injury, defective vascular clamps, or improper anastomotic technique. Immediate arterial occlusion in the operating room is treated by quickly washing out the kidney with cooled preservation fluid, which is a hypertonic solution mimicking intracellular fluid, and then proceeding with expeditious repair using surface cooling for hypothermia.

Renal artery stenosis, evident postoperatively and resulting in hyper-reninemia, hypertension, and an increasing femoral or transplant arterial bruit, should be repaired once renal dysfunction is evident. It should be noted that a femoral bruit due to increased flow is normal in the first few weeks following transplantation. Reconstruction of the stenotic artery is most reliably accomplished with a saphenous vein bypass graft, although excellent results have been obtained with an onlay patch at the stenotic area. The operative procedure for a given patient must be determined by precise angiographic demonstration of the anatomy, including oblique as well as anteroposterior radiographs. Percutaneous transluminal angioplasty utilizing a balloon catheter probably carries less risk than operative intervention.

Distal arterial occlusion may occur from embolization of atheromatous deposits in the aorta or iliac arteries, particularly after overzealous attempts at endarterectomy, or of a cardiac mural thrombus, or from atrial fibrillation. This event is heralded by hematuria, pain, hypertension, decreased renal function, and decreased perfusion of a renal segment during the initial phase of the ^{99m}Tc-DTPA scan. The treatment regimen depends upon the primary disease; intervention for renal infarction is necessary only if there is major parenchymal injury or a caliceal-cutaneous fistula.

Because of the predilection of chronic renal failure patients to the pernicious development of atherosclerosis, other vascular complications of transplantation are frequent, including cerebral vascular accidents, myocardial infarction, mesenteric occlusion leading to ischemic colitis (particularly when the left internal iliac artery has been utilized for the allograft), and testicular atrophy from spermatic artery thrombosis in the absence of adequate collaterals.

Renal vein thrombosis may result from endothelial injury during nephrectomy, venous compression, infection, rejection, or propagation of iliofemoral or intrarenal thrombosis. This complication is generally evidenced by massive proteinuria, graft tenderness, hematuria, oliguria, and hypertension. Systemic anticoagulation for at least six months is recommended in the absence of an underlying treatable problem. The relatively rapid normalization of the clotting mechanism of the uremic patient by successful transplantation produces an increased risk of ileofemoral thrombosis and occlusion of the arteriovenous fistula.

Lymphoceles, which are encapsulated collections of lymph issuing from divided lymphatics in the operative bed, occur in almost 10 per cent of transplant patients. Swelling of the ipsilateral thigh and leg is often the earliest clinical sign of this complication. Displacement of the ureter and bladder by relatively lucent areas may be visible on renal scans and readily demonstrable by excretory urography. Urinary collections (urinocele or urinomas) from ureteral or bladder dehiscence can frequently be excluded by contrast studies; lymphocele can be confirmed by lymphangiography. Treatment by internal drainage through a peritoneal window presents less risk of infection than external drainage. Thorough exploration is essential to avoid incomplete drainage of multilocular collections.

Urinary

Urinary infections are common following renal transplantation. Preexistent pyelonephritis demands nephrectomy of the host organs prior to transplantation; refluxing ureters must be totally excised to the vesicle level. Contamination of the bladder during insertion of the urethral catheters is particularly common in females with a history of recurrent cystitis, since the reservoir of infecting organisms may be the introitus. In males, the prostate is the bacterial reservoir of the lower urinary tract. Persistent or recurrent urinary infections in males should be thoroughly evaluated with fractional urine cultures. Meatal care to reduce colonization consists of removing the crusts and applying a water-insoluble ointment after withdrawing the catheter slightly from the meatus. The single most effective method of preventing bladder contamination during urethral catheter drainage is to establish and maintain a closed dependent drainage system. The catheter should never be disconnected from the drainage bag; urine samples may be obtained through the rubber puncture port. Using dependent closed drainage, most patients should maintain sterile bladder urine for four to seven days. Treatment of urinary infections is generally delayed until catheter removal, unless there is fever or pyelonephritis.

While the initial transplantation experience included a large percentage of urologic problems, refinement of organ removal and implantation techniques has significantly reduced the frequency of serious complications. While any part of the urinary collecting system may leak or become obstructed, most cases relate to the ureter. Devascularization may occur from arterial transection during donor nephrectomy and host implantation, or from thrombosis precipitated by reduced blood flow due to rejection or adjacent infection. When multiple donor renal arteries are present, protection of the ureteral blood supply during nephrectomy requires preservation of the lower polar arteries. Urine leakage is heralded by azotemia from peritoneal recycling of pooled material, urinary infection, fever, bladder displacement, and partial ureteral obstruction. The diagnosis is usually obtained from radionuclide scans, cystogram, intravenous excretory urogram, and/or retrograde ureteropyelogram. Effective treatment demands immediate exploration. Ureteral disruption may occasionally be remedied by repeat ureteroneocystostomy, if sufficient ureter length is available. Usually reconstruction depends upon using the ipsilateral or contralateral native ureteral segment for ureteropyelostomy, which may be protected with an indwelling Silastic stent either exteriorized through the renal parenchyma or left indwelling for later cystoscopic removal. A closed sterile drainage system must be constructed to minimize contamination.

In patients who have undergone bilateral nephroureterectomy, bladder advancement techniques to construct a vesicopyelostomy should be entertained only in the exceptional cases of total absence of immune reaction and reduction of immunosuppression to minimal levels. Permanent nephrostomy drainage represents a relatively unsatisfactory alternative, which offers the virtual certainty of continued pyelonephritis as an attendant, septic contraindication to simultaneous retransplantation.

Bladder dehiscence results from blockage of the urethral catheter, outlet obstruction due to prostatic hyperplasia or blood clot, devascularization by incisions parallel to those from previous surgery, or improper closure. Symptoms are similar to those of ureteral leakage. Closure of bladder dehiscences is more readily obtained than closure of ureteral leaks. Retrograde leakage along the ureteral tunnel may be controlled by one or two nonabsorbable sutures at the exterior vesical wall. Dehiscence of the vesical closure, usually accompanied by unsuspected bladder neck obstruction, requires thorough exploration, surgical correction of anatomic abnormalities, and three-layer reclosure followed by drainage per urethral catheter for 14 days. Short- or long-term drainage per cystostomy tube is generally ill-advised. Secondary urologic reconstructive procedures require wound drainage with soft tubes, and may be protected by omental pedicle grafts if the peritoneal cavity is violated. Although the majority of urinary fistulas can be handled without compromising graft success, persistent urinary infection with sepsis following unsuccessful reconstruction demands nephrectomy, aggressive antibiotic therapy, and wound closure by secondary intention.

Transient ureteral occlusion secondary to a blood clot presents as oliguria or anuria with or without hematuria. Radionuclide scans combined if necessary with excretory urogram or retrograde pyelograms may reveal the site of obstruction. Induction of a diuresis with furosemide is usually curative. Ureteral obstruction due to stone is unusual following transplantation, particularly if persistent hyperparathyroidism is surgically corrected.

MEDICAL COMPLICATIONS

Fluid and Electrolytes

Hyperkalemia is a serious threat before, during, and after renal transplantation. Corticosteroid treatment, depolarizing muscle relaxants, surgical trauma, allograft necrosis, potassium salts of drugs (e.g., potassium penicillin contains 1.7 mEq of potassium per million units), and blood transfusions may rapidly cause significant elevations of serum potassium levels. The best safeguards for patient care are prophylaxis by preoperative dialysis and frequent serum determinations. Kaliuresis accompanies the post-transplantation diuresis. However, the elevated total body potassium content of these patients demands that potassium never be administered unless the serum level is less than 3 mEq/l.

Treatment for hyperkalemia is determined by the rate of change of the serum level, the absolute concentration, and the presence of electrocardiographic changes. A rapid increase of 2 to 3 mEq/l to a level above 5.5 to 6 mEq/l requires immediate treatment with sodium bicarbonate (1 to 3 ampules of 44.6 mEq/l each) and hypertonic intravenous dextrose with or without intravenous insulin. Levels above 6.5 mEq/l are best managed by immediate hemodialysis. The transient effects of bicarbonate and dextrose therapy are augmented by furosemide diuresis and oral or rectal sodium polystyrene sulfonate (Kayexalate), an ion-exchange resin that removes 1 mEq of potassium per gram of resin under ideal circumstances. Oral doses of 30 to 70 gm are administered with 100 ml of 70 per cent sorbitol solution to prevent constipation. Enemas of a slurry, not a paste, of resin suspended in water or in 10 per cent dextrose are less efficient but must often be used in the immediate postoperative period. Sorbitol and sodium-containing solutions must not be used for dilution, since the former causes rectal mucosal injury and the latter prevents sodium-potassium exchange by the resin. Hyperkalemia may occur as a late complication due to steroid administration, dietary indiscretion, renal tubular dysfunction, or a smoldering interstitial rejection reaction. Diagnosis of the precipitating event requires urinary sodium, potassium, and pH determinations while the patient is on a controlled diet and renal biopsy. While thiazides have been recommended by some nephrologists, the authors prefer vigorous, intermittent furosemide therapy combined, when demonstrated to be appropriate by renal biopsy, with recycling of oral prednisone.

Hypercalcemia may occur in the early postoperative period owing to resumption of normal Vitamin D hydroxylation by the transplanted kidney, with consequent enhanced intestinal calcium absorption in the presence of an inappropriately elevated serum parathormone level. Calcium homeostasis usually returns spontaneously in the first month, unless the parathyroid tissue is functioning autonomously. Persistent hypercalcemia requires accurate diagnosis with urinary calcium and phosphorus and serum parathormone, calcium, phosphorus, and magnesium determinations. Autonomous parathyroid dysfunction leading to functional impairment of the allograft due to calcium deposition and acting synergistically with corticosteroids to produce bone destruction must be treated by resection of the adenoma or subtotal excision of glandular tissue. Hypophosphatemia, which results from a return of normal calcium homeostasis and the anabolic effects of improved nutrition in the patient depleted by long-term antacid binders, is treated with oral phosphate, since it can exacerbate steroid-induced myopathy and central nervous system disorders.

Metabolic acidosis, the usual acid-base disorder of uremia, is cured by restitution of renal function. Adjustment does not occur immediately, however, and treatment of metabolic acidosis with intravenous or oral sodium bicarbonate may be required for allografts displaying tubular dysfunction. Hyperkalemia due to egress of potassium in exchange for hydrogen ion occurs concomitant with severe acidemia and complicates the clinical picture. In addition, tissue hypoxia may develop from the combined effects of decreased myocardial contractility and responsiveness to catecholamines, as well as increased pulmonary vascular resistance. Emergency treatment requires intravenous sodium bicarbonate in sequential doses to partially correct the acidosis, until the pH is above 7.35 and the serum bicarbonate is over 20 mM/l. Administration of the total calculated dose necessary for correction of acidosis may lead to alkalosis with hypokalemia.

Other acid-base disorders are common but rarely lead to emergencies. Metabolic alkalosis, which seldom requires treatment, may result from the hypokalemia induced by furosemide diuresis or from corticosteroid drugs. Loss of hydrogen ion is unusual, since nasogastric suction is rarely required. Renal tubular acidosis of any type may occur transiently during the early phase of tubular recovery following transplantation or may be an early signal of rejection. Hyperchloremia and hyperkalemia should alert the transplant team to look for other evidence of rejection. Respiratory alkalosis and acidosis may be due to pulmonary abnormalities similar to those in other patients following major surgery.

Immediately after transplantation most grafts undergo a pronounced diuresis due to (1) arteriolar dilation following denervation, (2) host fluid overload, and (3) variable degrees of acute tubular necrosis. In spite of liberal fluid replacement, dehydration and hypotension may ensue. The typical weight loss during the first five days after successful transplantation is generally followed by progressive weight gain reflecting inefficient free water clearance by the recently transplanted kidney, as well as excessive sodium accumulation due to increased intake and corticosteroid therapy. Careful regulation of body weight and serum and urinary sodium are usually adequate for control, although some patients require furosemide diuresis.

Cardiovascular

Myocardial damage due to atherosclerosis, cardiomyopathy, and/or hypertension is preexistent in many patients. The superimposed stress of volume overload, hypotension, high-output failure from arteriovenous fistulas, and cardiac arrhythmias may lead to myocardial infarction, a highly fatal complication prior to and after renal transplantation. Significant valvular disease should be treated surgically prior to transplantation.

Preexistent renin-dependent hypertension should be remedied by host nephrectomy. Hypertension is a frequent malady in the postoperative period, due to hyper-reninemia from the allograft as a sign of ischemia or rejection, to hypercorticism, to renin release by host kidneys receiving less than normal blood flow or to volume expansion due to iatrogenically disturbed salt and water balance. The problem must be approached systematically to establish its pathogenesis. Anephric patients with high renin substrate concentrations may be very sensitive to normal renin production from the new kidney. Kidneys from cadaveric donors with the hepatorenal syndrome produce excessive quantities of renin. Mechanical obstruction of the afferent arterioles from any cause, including edema and microthrombosis during acute rejection reactions, may lead to increased production of renin. Later in the postoperative period, hypertension may result from renal artery stenosis, chronic rejection, or ureteral obstruction. Treatment is determined by the level of blood pressure and its cause.

Emergency management is essential if the diastolic pressure exceeds 130 mm Hg. Diazoxide (HyperStat), given rapidly as a 300-mg intravenous bolus, usually lowers the blood pressure within 5 minutes and controls hypertension for 1 to 12 hours. Repeat doses are often more effective than the initial dose, but treatment should not be maintained with diazoxide alone for more than 24 to 48 hours. Contraindications to its use include pheochromocytoma and compensatory hypertension due to aortic coarctation or an arteriovenous fistula. Other potent agents, nitroprusside and trimethaphan (Arfonad), are occasionally used for severe hypertension. When the situation is not emergent, alpha-methyldopa (Aldomet) is the agent of choice in most instances, starting at 250 mg every six hours and increasing to 500 mg every six hours, as necessary. In addition, some patients require prazosin (Minipres) at 4 to 12 mg daily and propranolol (Inderal) 40 mg daily for antirenin effect and 480 mg for full antihypertensive effect. Standing and supine blood pressures obtained every 6 hours afford an excellent guide to therapeutic efficacy. While almost half of the recipients require antihypertensives in the immediate postoperative period, most patients have only a short-term need for treatment. A requirement for therapy beyond six months or the onset of severe, unremittent hypertension demands estimation of plasma renin activity with differential venous sampling and arteriography.

Nutrition

Severe restriction of dietary protein is no longer practiced as a treatment for renal failure. Nevertheless, the diet required for maintenance of fluid balance and blood pressure, plus the anorectic effects of uremia, often leads to at least a modest degree of malnutrition. Following transplantation, patients usually acquire a hearty appetite and regain lean body mass despite the myopathic effects of corticosteroid treatment. Patients who develop complications requiring prolonged nasogastric intubation or displaying increased metabolic rates such as sepsis and fever should be treated with intravenous hyperalimentation either with essential amino acids or with ordinary mixtures as dictated by renal function.

Gastrointestinal

Surveillance for gastrointestinal complications in immunosuppressed patients requires frequent deliberate examination of the abdomen and awareness of the deceptive patterns of gastrointestinal disease under these conditions. The major signs of hemorrhage, obstruction, infarction, and perforation are often disguised by immunosuppressive drugs.

Common problems include oral and esophageal candidiasis, usually preventable with Mycostatin, which is used as a mouthwash and then swallowed. Active peptic ulcer disease, particularly with a history of bleeding, is usually treated surgically prior to transplantation. Postoperatively, all patients receive antacids every 6 hours until the prednisone dosage is below 20 mg daily. Symptoms of indigestion or evidence of gastric hypersecretion as minor manifestations of potential peptic ulcer disease are treated by intensification of the dietary and antacid regimen. Recent reports implicating cimetidine in the early irreversible rejection of allografts caution against its routine use.

Early detection of gastrointestinal bleeding is facilitated by stool examinations for occult blood three times weekly and a daily hemogram. Bleeding may occur from any point along the gastrointestinal tract, most commonly from hemorrhoids, peptic ulcer disease, diverticulosis, or polyps. Ischemic colitis, a rare cause of colonic bleeding, may occur soon after transplantation. Colonoscopy reveals friable ischemic mucosa. A proximal colostomy provides adequate treatment if transmural necrosis is not present. Eventual stenosis of the ischemic segment may require resection prior to colostomy closure. Severe proctitis may result from enemas of Kayexalate, particularly if sorbitol is inadvertently used. Perforated diverticulitis may be a lethal and frequently unrecognized complication. Lower abdominal tenderness may be modest, bowel sounds persistent, and fever only low grade. Occasionally the only sign of abdominal sepsis is multiple, small hepatic abscesses. Frequently, abdominal exploration, while appearing to be a radical treatment, actually represents the most conservative course.

Hepatic dysfunction has been reported in up to 15 per cent of renal transplant patients. Mild abnormalities of liver function tests are common and usually reverse with discontinuance of potentially hepatotoxic drugs, such as azathioprine, alpha-methyldopa, and isoniazid. More severe abnormalities, such as Australia antigen-positive or cytomegalovirus-associated hepatitis, demand reduction of immunosuppressive therapy, which rarely results in loss of the allograft. Active viral or idiopathic hepatitis carries a poor prognosis and must be distinguished from bacterial and mycobacterial causes that may be amenable to treatment.

Pancreatitis, a particularly lethal complication of transplantation, is fortunately not common. While most cases occur in the absence of an appropriate past history, hypercalcemia due to hyperparathyroidism and toxic reactions to azathioprine and corticosteroid treatment have been suspected. The diagnosis may be obscured by a high basal amylase level in the absence of adequate renal function, and by the concomitant presence of uremic parotiditis. Conservative treatment demands bowel rest, as is practiced for other forms of acute pancreatitis following major surgery, and careful vigil for complications of necrosis, hemorrhage, or pseudocyst. Immunosuppression should be discontinued in the presence of significant disease and the graft abandoned.

SUMMARY

Pre- and postoperative care of the renal transplant patient demands a coordinated effort of surgeon, nephrologist, nurse, immunologist, social worker, and special consultants. Patients frequently present with significant coexistent disease that contraindicates organ replacement and immunosuppression. Careful analysis of each patient's situation demands meticulous preoperative evaluation of not only the urinary tract, but also the gastrointestinal, cardiovascular, metabolic, pulmonary, and immunologic systems. HLA tissue typing is valuable in choosing living related, but not cadaveric, organ donors. Exclusion of donors bearing foreign antigens to which the host has been previously exposed by the use of crossmatch tests may avert early rejection, in spite of obvious antigenic incompatibility. Treatment of rejection reactions, the major cause of graft loss, engenders the enormous burden of multiple and destructive nonspecific effects of corticosteroids. Careful vigilance to maintain the balance of immunosuppression and avoid septic complications determines the final success of allotransplantation. For the surgeon, transplantation presents the challenging interface of clinical immunology with skilled surgical and medical care.

11

Preparation of the Patient for Anesthesia

LEE H. COOPERMAN
HARRY WOLLMAN

THE PREANESTHESIA VISIT AND ANESTHESIA PREMEDICATION

Traditionally, patients are visited the day before operation by their anesthesiologist. At this visit the physician obtains a pertinent history (previous anesthetics, current and past drug therapy, drug allergies and reactions), examines the patient (especially the head, neck, chest, back, and arms) and explains the anesthesia and operating room procedures. If the patient is to give some semblance of informed consent, the risks of anesthesia must be explained as well. Supportive statements will allay the patient's apprehension and provide some tranquility for what can be a most trying experience. Indeed, an informative and empathetic interview that concentrates on techniques of relaxation can decrease the need for postoperative narcotic analgesics.

The use of drugs as preanesthesia medication has a long history, dating back to ether anesthesia with its attendant excitement and profuse airway secretion during induction. Preanesthesia drugs were required to smooth a possibly stormy induction and inhibit secretions. With present-day anesthetic drugs and rapidly acting intravenous induction agents, the purpose of premedication has changed somewhat. Preoperative tranquility is now a major goal. A wide variety of drugs are available that can produce any desired degree of sedation. Which is chosen depends upon the age, condition, and requirements of the patient, the proposed operation and its urgency, the indicated route of administration for the premedicant and the preferences of the patient and anesthesiologist.

Narcotic analgesics are among the most widely used premedicant drugs because of their sedative and calming properties as well as their ability to relieve pain and supplement general anesthetics. These

213

desirable effects are counterbalanced by respiratory and cardiovascular depression, production of nausea and vomiting, and, on some occasions, biliary colic. The undesirable side effects can be reversed in part by naloxone, but the primary actions of the drug are antagonized as well. Morphine, meperidine, and fentanyl are probably the most widely used narcotics.

Various barbiturates, tranquilizers, and neuroleptic drugs are used alone or in combination, sometimes with the narcotic analgesics. In general, they have more benign side effects than do narcotics. Pentobarbital, secobarbital, droperidol, and diazepam are some of the more widely used premedicants in this group.

Anticholinergic drugs are often added to the premedication to reduce salivary and bronchial secretion and to ameliorate cardiac vagal reflexes. These effects are especially useful in children and before procedures involving the eye or pharynx or in peritoneal traction, when cardiac reflex slowing can be initiated. Though atropine (0.4 to 0.6 mg) is the usual drug used for these purposes, scopolamine has better drying properties as well as sedative and amnesic properties. Glycopyrolate, a new anticholinergic agent with a longer duration of action than atropine, may be of value in some situations.

APPROACH TO PATIENTS WITH SPECIAL PROBLEMS

THE PATIENT WITH CARDIOVASCULAR DISEASE

Hypertension. This is one of the most common cardiovascular problems presented to the anesthesiologist. It was formerly thought that antihypertensive drugs should be discontinued long before anesthesia, but it is now clear that hypertensive patients under good control have fewer and less marked changes in blood pressure and heart rate and rhythm in the perioperative period than do poorly controlled hypertensive patients. In fact, the cessation of antihypertensive therapy with propranolol or clonidine has been associated with hypertension and coronary accidents. A possible exception is occasionally a patient receiving MAO inhibitor drugs. Because of their sometimes unpredictable drug interactions and their serious side effects, a few people believe that they should be stopped several weeks before operation. A wise course is switching to another drug if possible. If this cannot be done, most anesthesiologists would still prefer to have the patient's disease controlled, and they do not discontinue the drug.

The degree of control that is desirable in a hypertensive patient is difficult to state categorically. This is true for both the newly discovered hypertensive patient as well as the hypertensive patient who is inadequately controlled. One notes not only the highest and lowest blood pressure measurements in the hospital but other signs as well, such as heart size, appearance of eye grounds, history of renal complications, and electrocardiograph and chest roentgenogram abnormalities. If there is little evidence of target organ involvement, then urgency for control is not so great, especially if the proposed operation is elective. Thus drug treatment is begun (or, in the case of the inadequately controlled patient, therapy is either changed or intensified) and stabilized for several days with any of the long-acting antihypertensive medications available.

In an emergency, rapidly acting antihypertensive agents such as diazoxide, nitroprusside, or trimethaphan can be used. Additionally, halogenated anesthetic agents that ordinarily depress blood pressure can be employed during operation to maintain systemic pressure in a desirable range.

Heart Failure. This problem certainly adds to the risk of anesthesia, although it is less worrisome if the failure is well compensated. In order to quantify the additional risk, useful signs of heart failure include distended neck veins, peripheral edema, rales, gallop rhythm, and prominent pulmonary vessels on chest roentgenograms. Response to exercise, another valuable test, is evaluated by walking with the patient up several flights of stairs while noting changes in heart and respiratory rate. Excessive increases in either of these vital signs suggest poor control of the heart failure.

If optimal reversal of heart failure cannot be obtained beforehand, acute left heart failure and pulmonary edema may occur during anesthesia when the patient is exposed to additional stress, fluids, and depressant drugs. If pulmonary edema occurs during anesthesia, it is treated in the standard manner with diuretics, oxygen by positive pressure, and perhaps inotropic agents. If central venous or pulmonary artery pressure is to be monitored during operation, it is valuable to place the catheters preoperatively in order to evaluate preoperative therapy and to obtain baseline measurements.

Coronary Artery Disease. The relationship of coronary artery disease to perioperative mortality has become increasingly clear. Several studies indicate that when anesthesia and operation occur within three months of myocardial infarction, reinfarction will occur intraoperatively or postoperatively in almost one-third of these patients. When anesthesia is delayed from three to six months, the reinfarction rate falls to 15 per cent, and after six months the rate levels off to about 5 per cent. Patients with coronary artery disease and angina pectoris but with no previous infarction are also at risk of having a myocardial infarction in the perioperative period. This is especially true if they have diabetes mellitus or hypertension. Unfortunately, the new drugs such as propranolol and vasodilators have not lowered the infarction rate associated with anesthesia. However, optimal therapy for the coronary artery disease is still best continued until the time of operation.

Arrhythmias. Older patients often display arrhythmias on routine physical and electrocardiographic examination. If digitalis, quinidine, procaine amide, or other antiarrhythmic drugs are being administered, they should be continued. The possibility of digitalis toxicity should be borne in mind. This is especially so with the changes in serum potassium levels that can be induced by diuretics, cathartics, and intensive intravenous fluid therapy as a patient is being prepared for operation.

There is some controversy about the continuation of propranolol before anesthesia, since this drug will reduce sympathetic response to cardiovascular depression caused by the anesthetic. The view that propranolol should be stopped at least two weeks preoperatively is extreme and outdated. Considering its short half-life in plasma (three hours), a more reasonable course of action is to administer propranolol up to six hours before operation.

Patients at risk of developing complete heart block can benefit from temporary insertion of a transvenous pacer. Examples include persons with Adams-Stokes disease and those with hemiblock involving two of the three fascicles.

Occasionally patients with intravenous or implanted external pacemakers require anesthesia. Care must be exercised when the pacer is external to insure that electrical currents are not conducted through the wires to the heart, thereby inducing ventricular fibrillation. All bare wires are covered, and monitoring and electrocautery devices are kept as remote as possible from the pacer.

The Patient with Respiratory Disease

Chronic Obstructive Pulmonary Disease (COPD). The patient with chronic lung disease can present numerous problems to the anesthesiologist. Evaluation is most important, especially when there is a history of repeated respiratory infection, smoking, sputum production, or diminished exercise tolerance. On examination, one should note increased anteroposterior diameter of the chest, use of accessory respiratory muscles, distant breath sounds, or widespread rhonchi. Changes in chest roentgenograms may also be indicative of recent disease and of correctable lesions.

With the multiplicity of pulmonary function tests available, evaluation of patients with COPD may seem complicated. In fact, just a few simple tests can be sufficient. Maximum expiratory flow rate and forced expiratory volume (one second) have been shown to be predictive of possible pulmonary complications postoperatively. They can be followed serially in the preparation of a patient for anesthesia. Short of formal pulmonary function tests, certain bedside maneuvers can be useful. The response to exercise and a marked increase in heart and respiratory rate have been mentioned. The ability to blow out a match placed several inches in front of the patient's open mouth can be tried. Vital capacity can be measured with a simple volumeter. Finally, preanesthesia arterial blood gas measurements indicate, in some measure, the degree of pulmonary dysfunction and provide baselines for comparison with postanesthesia values.

When examination indicates that a correctable pulmonary condition is present, operation should be delayed if possible. During this interval a course of intermittent positive pressure breathing (IPPB) with bronchodilators, chest physiotherapy, and postural drainage and antibiotics for culture-proven infection are indicated. Serial examinations and pulmonary function tests should indicate progress in preparing the patient for anesthesia and surgery. If the patient is a smoker who can be persuaded to stop smoking in the preoperative period, this too will be beneficial.

Asthma. An acute asthmatic attack during anesthesia is a dire though possibly preventable emergency. When time permits, the asthmatic patient should be stabilized on a bronchodilator program, and other correctable problems, such as infection, should be treated. Preanesthetic and anesthetic drugs that cause histamine release, such as narcotics and curare, are avoided. So too is instrumentation of the airway during light anesthesia because this may precipitate bronchoconstriction. If possible, the operation should be done under regional anesthesia. If general anesthesia is required, some advocate using only a face mask. The use of an endotracheal tube with general anesthesia will, however, provide an opportunity to clear the upper tracheobronchial tree of secretions.

Bronchodilators can be given during general anesthesia, though there is the hazard of producing cardiac arrhythmias, hypertension, or both with overdoses. Some prefer to use aminophyllin, whereas others prefer epinephrine or isoproterenol. Any of these drugs can be given by continuous infusion with careful monitoring of the ECG and blood pressure.

Airway Problems. A prime preanesthesia concern is the patency and size of the airway. If suspicions are aroused by the history (such as trauma or previous surgery in the neck) or pharyngeal examination (such as inability to open the mouth, deformity of the jaw, or a large goiter), then indirect laryngoscopy using a mirror or direct inspection with a fiberoptic laryngoscope will help in the evaluation. Lateral neck roentgenograms or xerograms can indicate rather clearly the size and configuration of the airway.

Preparation for anesthesia involves improvement if possible in the airway. When there is laryngeal edema, inhalational epinephrine and systemic corticosteroids may help. When tracheal intubation (via the nose or mouth) is difficult or impossible due to airway narrowing, and the proposed surgical procedure (such as laryngectomy and neck dissection) demands it, a tracheostomy, using local anesthesia, can be performed before inducing general anesthesia. Awake nasal or oral tracheal intubation either blindly or using visual methods (fiberoptic or standard laryngoscope) allows preservation of the airway and of ventilation before induction. A selection of tracheal tubes in various sizes should be available.

Upper Respiratory Infection (URI). This is a common preoperative problem, especially in children. Often anesthesia is delayed until the patient is asymptomatic for fear that a bacterial infection in the upper airway will be spread to the lower respiratory tract by the anesthetic and airway manipulation. Additionally, the profuse airway secretions associated with URI's can produce partial airway obstruction. This can be blocked by atropine, and the nasal mucosal edema can be treated with a topical vasoconstrictor, providing a more patent airway. These maneuvers may not always be successful, and the more direct action is to delay operation until the patient has recovered from the URI.

THE PATIENT WITH CENTRAL NERVOUS SYSTEM DISEASE

Acute CNS Disease. The patient with an acute head or spinal cord injury not infrequently requires anesthesia for diagnostic procedures or definitive operation. In the patient with cervical spine injury, great care must be taken to keep the head and neck stable and immobile, lest any injury to the spinal cord occur. This may require the effort of one person whose only assignment is to hold the head stable during induction and tracheal intubation. The latter can be difficult since the usual head extension position cannot be used. An awake blind nasotracheal intubation is sometimes used in these instances.

Increased intracranial pressure commonly accompanies acute head injury and intracranial bleeding. Though initially such bleeding and cerebral edema will have only modest effects in raising intracranial pressure (ICP), as the lesion enlarges a greater effect on the ICP will occur. Thus, it is most important to be aware of this possible problem, to measure ICP via a subarachnoid bolt or screw, and to take measures not to increase ICP further. For the anesthesiologist this includes the avoidance of drugs that increase cerebral blood flow, such as halothane or narcotics, which can increase $PaCO_2$ and thus cerebral blood flow. Maintenance of a patent airway is crucial. Airway obstruction or coughing, when the airway is instrumented, can raise ICP even further. Hyperventilation to lower $PaCO_2$ and cerebral blood flow and administration of osmotic diuretics, steroids, and barbiturates are measures that the anesthesiologist can use to lower ICP to tolerable levels.

The patient with an open eye injury poses problems similar to those of head-injured patients. Again, elevation in airway and intracranial pressures must be avoided if extrusion of ocular contents (vitreous) is to be prevented. Care during tracheal intubation to avoid patient coughing and straining, as well as use of nondepolarizing muscle relaxants rather than depolarizing agents, which raise intravascular pressure, are guidelines.

Psychotropic Drug Therapy. Despite widespread use of psychotropic drugs, they generally add no great hazards to anesthesia. An exception to this is the MAO inhibitors. They interact with narcotics, vasopressors, and perhaps general anesthetics to produce unpredictable changes in blood pressure and heart rate. If possible, they should be replaced with other antidepressant drugs two weeks before operation. If this is not possible, the anesthesiologist should be prepared to treat sudden hypertension or hypotension.

THE PATIENT WITH RENAL AND METABOLIC PROBLEMS

Chronic Renal Failure. These patients are often undergoing routine hemodialysis. Dialysis is best performed as close to operation as possible, thereby permitting the patient to enter the perioperative period with near normal fluid volume and electrolyte levels. Renally excreted drugs that might ordinarily be given by the anesthesiologist, such as phenobarbital, gallamine, and curare, are best avoided or given in smaller than usual doses. Care also must be used when placing intravenous catheters to minimize infection in individuals with a renal transplant and immunologic suppression.

Acute Renal Failure. Careful fluid and electrolyte management during anesthesia is crucial. Generally only enough fluid should be given to replace insensible and operative losses. With urine output no longer a valid indication of fluid volume requirements, other indices such as central venous or pulmonary artery pressure become even more important if fluid overload is to be avoided. The same drugs should be avoided as in chronic renal failure.

THE PATIENT WITH ENDOCRINE PROBLEMS

Adrenal Steroids. Usually patients who have received adrenal steroids in the 6 to 12 months preceding anesthesia are routinely given supplemental steroids in the preoperative period. This "overtreatment" is used since little harm occurs thereby and serious complications may be avoided. The alternative would be to assess the adrenal status of each patient at risk of developing addisonian crisis and then treat those showing adrenal insufficiency. The usual steroid dosage consists of hydrocortisone 300 mg on the operative day, which is then tapered over the next few days. Need for additional steroids would be indicated clinically by hypotension in the postoperative period unexplained by blood loss or drug overdose.

Diabetes Mellitus. Patients on diet therapy, oral hypoglycemic agents, or small doses of insulin (less than 25 U per day) can be managed preoperatively simply by withholding the preoperative insulin or oral drug on the day of operation. Juvenile and more severe adult diabetics can be managed by numerous regimens. Commonly a fraction (one-half or one-third) of the usual insulin dose is given in the morning and an intravenous infusion of dextrose is begun. Further management is dictated by blood or urine sugar levels, generally using small doses of regular insulin intravenously. It is preferable to err on the hyperglycemic rather than the hypoglycemic side. The latter state can quickly result in neurologic injury; the former will cause metabolic derangement much more slowly.

CHOICE OF ANESTHETIC — TECHNIQUE AND DRUGS

Anesthetic choice is often dictated more by avoidance of possible problems than by indications for a particular drug or technique, a testimony to the overall efficiency and safety of modern anesthetic drugs and techniques. Of course, there are well-publicized exceptions. Because methoxyflurane is metabolized to fluoride, a nephrotoxin, the use of this anesthetic in patients with renal disease is unwise. Some anesthesiologists avoid halothane in patients with liver or biliary tract disease, although evidence favoring avoidance of this combination is scanty at best.

Other factors are important too when considering choice of anesthesia. The patient's, surgeon's, and anesthetist's preferences must be considered. Some surgical procedures must be performed under general anesthesia, such as thoracotomy, which requires tracheal intubation and positive pressure ventilation. For other operations a variety of techniques are suitable. For example, inguinal hernia repair can be carried out successfully under general, spinal, epidural, or field block anesthesia. After a decision has been made to use a particular technique, a variety of agents can be chosen. General anesthesia can be given with a single drug such as halothane or a combination of several drugs such as a muscle relaxant, narcotic, barbiturate or tranquilizer, and nitrous oxide. Numerous drugs are available and suitable for local or regional anesthesia. The end result in all cases should be an anesthetic that is acceptable and safe for the patient and that provides good operative conditions for the surgeon. All modern drugs and techniques can be utilized successfully by a well-trained anesthesiologist, and in most cases it would be impossible to prove that one drug or technique is preferable to another either in efficacy or safety.

MANAGEMENT OF PROBLEMS ENCOUNTERED IN THE POSTANESTHESIA PERIOD

PAIN

Postoperative Pain. Techniques to relieve postoperative pain begin with the preoperative interview. A full explanation of how the patient will feel after surgery and a description of relaxation techniques used in the presence of pain will decrease to some extent the need for postoperative analgesics.

The most common type of drug used for pain relief is the narcotic analgesic. When it is given in small doses intravenously, a more sustained level of analgesia is achieved than when larger intramuscular doses are employed. Nerve blocks too are successful for pain relief. Examples include intercostal and continuous thoracic epidural block following thoracotomy and upper abdominal surgery and continuous lumbar epidural block for lower abdominal and lower extremity pain. Catheters to facilitate reinjection of local anesthetic can be left in place for several days without great fear of infection or bleeding. The newer long-acting local anesthetics bupivacaine and etidocaine provide analgesia for three to four hours.

Myalgia and Headache.   Myalgia is especially common in healthy patients after short diagnostic procedures when a depolarizing muscle relaxant has been given. This pain can often be prevented by preceding the depolarizing agent with a small dose of a nondepolarizing agent, thereby stopping the fasciculations that follow a depolarizing muscle relaxant, the presumed source of myalgia. Myalgia and headache are relieved by simple analgesics ordinarily. Headache after spinal anesthesia is secondary to leakage of cerebrospinal fluid through the hole made by the lumbar puncture needle in the arachnoid membrane. Though self-limited, it can be relieved by measures that raise cerebrospinal fluid pressure, such as recumbent posture, hydration, and an abdominal binder. On rare occasions, autologous blood is injected into the epidural space at the level of the previous lumbar puncture. The blood then clots and seals the hole, stopping leakage of cerebrospinal fluid.

Sore Throat.   Laryngoscopy and tracheal intubation are followed by a sore throat as one of their common, though minor, complications. This too is self-limited and can be treated with analgesics if needed.

NAUSEA AND VOMITING

To some extent this complication can be prevented by careful administration of anesthesia. Minimal use of drugs (such as morphine) that may cause nausea, especially in the sensitive individual, and avoidance of inflation of the stomach with air will help. Some anesthetic drugs commonly associated with nausea (such as ether and cyclopropane) are rarely used today, but surgical procedures in the abdomen are likely to produce nausea regardless of what other drugs or procedures are employed. When nausea and vomiting does occur it can be relieved in part with tranquilizers or benzquinamide, though these agents are not completely successful and may have unwanted side effects such as hypotension. Their use prophylactically before anesthesia is probably unjustified in view of their low success rate and potential side effects.

CARDIOVASCULAR COMPLICATIONS

Altered Blood Pressure.   Hypotension is a common blood pressure abnormality that occurs after anesthesia and operation. Likely causes include partly unreplaced or continued blood loss, continued cardiovascular depression from anesthetic drugs, or a cardiovascular catastrophe such as myocardial infarction or pulmonary embolus. After immediate treatment has been accomplished with oxygen, fluid administration, change in position, and vasopressors (if needed), a definitive diagnosis must be made. To rule out residual anesthetic effect, the reversal drugs naloxone (for narcotics) and physostigmine (for scopolamine and other sedatives) can be given. Over time, anesthetic effects will diminish as the drugs are metabolized or excreted. A test infusion of several hundred milliliters of fluid while noting arterial and central venous pressures yields some estimation of the patient's intravascular volume. An unchanged arterial and venous pressure suggests hypovolemia, while a marked rise in central venous pressure indicates normovolemia. A 12-lead electrocardiogram, when compared with the preoperative study, might indicate occurrence of myocardial infarction or pulmonary embolus.

Hypertension is a less frequent postanesthesia complication and one for which a cause cannot always be found. Some etiologic factors include pain, emergence excitement, distended urinary bladder, hypothermia and shivering, and hypercapnia or hypoxia. Many of the patients have a history of hypertension under poor control. These various causes are sought and treated. Usually postanesthesia hypertension is a self-limited complication, with onset shortly after the cessation of anesthesia and a return to preoperative levels within a few hours. Since complications such as pulmonary edema, heart failure, cardiac arrhythmia, and cardiovascular accident are more likely to occur with prolonged hypertension, drug treatment is best begun when it appears that the hypertension is serious and persistent. Nitroprusside or trimethaphan given by continuous infusion or hydralazine, diazoxide, or chlorpromazine are some of the drugs that can be useful.

Heart Failure.   With the cardiac depression and fluid shifts that occur during and after operation, congestive heart failure often results. Common symptoms and signs include dyspnea, venous distention, rales, wheezing, cyanosis, and tachycardia. Narcotics and diuretics are the therapeutic mainstays, though rotating tourniquets and digitalization are still frequently used. Treatment of arrhythmias and oxygen administration (after IPPB) are also necessary.

Arrhythmias.   A variety of cardiac arrhythmias have been noted in the postoperative period. Of most concern are those of ventricular origin. Ventricular tachycardia can be treated with lidocaine or, if necessary, direct current countershock. Ventricular fibrillation is treated in the same way. Ventricular extra beats will usually respond to lidocaine infusion, though a search for a precipitating cause, such as abnormal arterial CO_2, O_2, and pH, serum potassium level, or blood pressure, should be made. Atrial tachycardias usually respond to vagal stimulation or propranolol, as does atrial fibrillation.

PULMONARY COMPLICATIONS

Ventilatory failure is characterized by increased $PaCO_2$ and thus signs of sympathetic hyperactivity, that is, sweating, tachycardia, and hypertension. This rather common complication is suspected when one observes extremes in respiratory rate or shallow ventilation (measured with a ventilometer). The diagosis is usually confirmed by measurement of arterial blood gases with demonstration of increased $PaCO_2$.

Of the numerous causes for postoperative ventilatory failure, perhaps the most common are residual effects of anesthetic drugs and muscle relaxants. When residual anesthetics are the cause, the respiratory response to CO_2 is depressed. When residual relaxants are the cause, muscle strength is inadequate to maintain adequate alveolar ventilation, especially when an element of airway obstruction is present. Pain secondary to operation can inhibit deep breathing and expulsion of airway secretions. Aspiration of blood or stomach contents can occur during any course of anesthesia, general or regional, and this can lead to ventilatory failure. When any of these events occurs in a patient with preexisting lung disease, ventilatory failure is even more likely to occur.

The therapy for ventilatory failure consists primarily of an increase in the alveolar ventilation to decrease elevated CO_2 tension. If residual relaxant effect is present, it can be reversed pharmacologically with an anticholinesterase. Narcotics can be reversed by naloxone, and physostigmine may reverse the CNS depression of several different etiologies. When residual drug effects cannot be reversed, the patient is supported with mechanical ventilation via endotracheal tube until the drug effects have substantially disappeared. Ancillary modes of therapy are used as needed, such as antibiotics, steroids for aspiration pneumonia, and nerve block or narcotic drugs for pain relief.

Hypoxemia is a common occurrence after anesthesia and operation, often in the absence of ventilatory failure. In the presence of an unexpectedly low PaO_2 in relation to the inspired oxygen concentration, patients may exhibit cyanosis, tachypnea, and agitation. Causes for hypoxemia are numerous. Increased lung water resulting from aggressive fluid therapy or heart failure, aspiration, bronchospasm, and atelectasis are some of the more common precipitating conditions. In addition to a widened A-a gradient for oxygen, there may be auscultatory or roentgenographic signs to confirm the diagnosis. Often the hypoxemia responds favorably to diuresis as well as to oxygen therapy. The latter can be administered via a face mask or preferably via an endotracheal tube, which then allows the use of positive end-expiratory pressure

(PEEP) or functional residual capacity (FRC). Other standard measures include tracheal suction, chest physiotherapy, bronchodilator agents, and bronchoscopy.

Nervous System Complications

Occasionally patients fail to awaken promptly and completely at the end of anesthesia. The degree of difficulty ranges from complete unresponsiveness to simple slowness in answering questions. The most common cause is residual effect of anesthetic drugs. Some anesthetics can be reversed pharmacologically, such as with naloxone or physostigmine. However, inhalation anesthetics and barbiturates depend upon redistribution, metabolism, and excretion for cessation of their action. In these instances supportive care of the patient and maintenance of adequate pulmonary, cardiac, and renal function can allow time to diminish their action and effect.

Although relative overdose is the most common cause of postoperative stupor, other diagnoses should be considered. CNS catastrophes such as stroke or severe hypoxia might cause similar clinical symptoms and signs. A neurologic examination can help to determine the etiology. Metabolic imbalance, hyponatremia, hypoglycemia, severe hypercapnia, and nonketotic hyperosmolar coma can also cause postanesthesia somnolence. These conditions can be diagnosed by the appropriate laboratory tests. Finally hypothermia, deliberate or unintentional, can cause patients to awaken slowly.

Muscular weakness, like prolonged somnolence, is occasionally noted at the end of anesthesia. Again the most likely cause is overdose of muscle relaxant, although a deep anesthetic state will also cause muscle weakness. The latter can be differentiated by the use of a nerve stimulator because in this case the effect will not fade and post-tetanic facilitation will not occur. These phenomena, however, can be evident in the presence of a "curare" block. An attempt can be made to reverse the block with neostigmine or other anticholinesterase drugs. This is not always successful, and one may have to ventilate the patient mechanically until strength returns and he or she is able to sustain an adequate minute ventilation. Certain factors predispose patients to prolonged muscle paralysis. Renal failure is associated with prolonged block, as are latent (or overt) myasthenia gravis, certain antibiotics (aminoglycosides), and electrolyte imbalances. If any of those factors are present, their correction may hasten recovery from the effects of muscle relaxants.

Nerve palsy after anesthesia usually manifests itself within 24 to 48 hours as muscle weakness and anesthesia or paresthesia over the innervated area. Usually involved are the long, superficial nerves that pass near bony prominences. Hence, the brachial plexus and superficial peroneal nerve are most frequently affected. Such injuries can be prevented by care in positioning, insuring that the arm is not hyperextended and that nothing hard rests on the legs. These measures prevent pressure upon and stretching of nerves, which lead to either intraneural hematoma or ischemia with subsequent palsy. Prognosis is good with supportive care, though return of function may require three to six months.

RENAL COMPLICATIONS

Renal injury and subsequent oliguria may follow transfusion of mismatched blood or a prolonged period of hypotension during anesthesia. Another cause of oliguria is the antidiuresis that occurs after anesthesia, especially when narcotics have been used. The use of a rapidly acting diuretic like furosemide can be useful. Water loading is attempted but not continued if diuresis does not occur.

Certain anesthetics, especially methoxyflurane, yield fluoride ion as one of their metabolic products. When after prolonged exposure to methoxyflurane a high concentration of fluoride is present, renal damage can occur. In this case polyuria and dilute urine are the predominant findings. The prognosis for recovery from this condition is better than in the case of the oliguric renal failure that follows ischemia.

CONCLUSION

The principles of good preanesthesia and postanesthesia care have been outlined. Obviously the interests of the surgeon and anesthesiologist are similar: to prepare the patient as well as possible before operation and to minimize the incidence of postoperative problems. Following the principles herein suggested should achieve the desired results.

REFERENCES

Egbert, L. D., Battit, G. E., Turndorf, H., et al.: The value of preoperative visit by an anesthetist. J.A.M.A., 185:553, 1963.

Goldman, L., Caldera, D. L., Nassbaum, S. R., et al.: Multifactorial index of cardiac risk in noncardiac surgical procedures. N. Engl. J. Med., 297:845, 1977.

Marsh, M. L., Marshall, L. F., and Shapiro, H. M.: Neurosurgical intensive care. Anesthesiology, 47:149, 1977.

Prys-Roberts, C., Meloche, R., and Foéx, P.: Studies of anesthesia in relation to hypertension. Br. J. Anaesth., 43:122, 1971.

Riggs, J. R. A., and Jones, N. L.: Clinical assessment of respiratory function. Br. J. Anaesth., 50:3, 1978.

Stein, M., and Cassara, E. L.: Preoperative pulmonary evaluation and therapy for surgery patients. J.A.M.A., 211:787, 1970.

Symposium on the postoperative period. Br. J. Anaesth., 47:91, 1975.

Wollman, H., and Dripps, R. D.: Pre-anesthetic medication. In Goodman, L. S., and Gilman, A. (eds.): Pharmacologic Basis of Therapeutics. New York, MacMillan, 1970.

12

Respiratory and Circulatory Failure

LLOYD D. MACLEAN

The minimal requirement of preoperative, intraoperative, and post-operative management of any patient is the maintenance of normal blood flow to vital organs. This chapter is concerned with inadequacies of the circulation in patients and how to measure and treat them. We are also concerned with certain constituents and characteristics of the blood, such as oxygen content, hematocrit, pH, colloid osmotic pressure, lactate content, and distribution of the flow.

The goals of management are to detect respiratory and circulatory failure early, to correct the dysfunction, and to eliminate the underlying cause. Eight measurements (Table 12–1) are useful in assisting history and physical examination to establish a hemodynamic diagnosis and to monitor the adequacy of cardiovascular and pulmonary responses.

ARTERIAL BLOOD PRESSURE

Arterial blood pressure should be measured accurately with an intra-arterial catheter placed in patients with circulatory failure or in patients who fall into the high-risk categories, but this means of monitoring alone does not confirm or rule out circulatory failure. The blood pressure can be decreased with adequate flow, or flow may be markedly decreased accompanying an elevated peripheral arterial pressure due to vasoconstriction. A discharging pheochromocytoma produces many features of shock in afflicted patients with evidence of ischemia of the brain, heart, and kidney despite a high blood pressure. A low peripheral arterial pressure may not indicate as serious a circulatory problem as might be expected if on palpation of central vessels, carotid or femoral, good pulses are detected. The pulse pressure is more closely related to flow. It is preferable to have a blood pressure of 90/60 than 120/110. A

226

Table 12-1. Assessment of Hemodynamic Status

Primary measurements	Normal values	Secondary measurements	Normal values in adult humans
Arterial blood pressure (BP)	120/80 mm Hg	Pulse pressure	40 mm Hg
		Position change	0 mm Hg
Pulse rate	70/min	EKG	Sinus rhythm
Central venous pressure	5 ± 2 cm saline	Pulmonary capillary wedge pressure (PCWP)	5 ± 2 cm saline
Cardiac index (CI)	3.20 ± 20 l/min/m^2	Stroke index	46.0 ± 50 ml/m^2
		Systemic vascular resistance	2100 ± 200 dyne-sec/cm^5/m^2
		Left ventricular stroke work index (LVSWI)	56.0 ± 6.0 gm meters/m^2
		Starling performance curves	See text
Urine flow	50 ml/hour	Specific gravity	1.003–1.030
		Urine to plasma creatinine ratio	>20
		Urine sodium concentration	<20 mEq/l
Arterial blood Po$_2$	100 mm Hg	Arterial oxygen content	19.0 ± 1.0 ml/100 ml
Pco$_2$	40 mm Hg	Arteriovenous oxygen content difference	4.60 ± 0.40 ml/100 ml
		Oxygen consumption	140.0 ± 25.0 ml/min/m^2
		Alveolar-arterial oxygen content difference	100 mm Hg
Arterial blood lactate	1 mm/l		
Hematocrit	35–45%	P$_{50}$	27 ± 1.5 mm Hg

precipitous fall in blood pressure or pulse pressure on assuming the erect or sitting position indicates a contracted blood volume.

Despite these shortcomings and limitations, the monitoring of arterial blood pressure, especially when measured both serially and accurately, is extremely important in managing patients with circulatory failure.

PULSE RATE

A continuous (oscilloscopic) monitor of pulse rate and rhythm is essential in patients with acute circulatory failure and those undergoing general anesthesia. Treatable arrhythmias that precede asystole or ventricular fibrillation are frequently detected by this means alone. Cardiac output may also be reduced if the rate is either too slow (<60 beats per min) or too rapid (>150 beats per min). Both direct current countershock and drug therapy may be used to terminate tachyarrhythmias. Specific therapy depends on the arrhythmia, its cause, and the patient's clinical state.

CENTRAL VENOUS PRESSURE (CVP)

This measurement reflects the competence of the right ventricle to accept and propel the venous return. Therefore, it is an indirect measure of blood volume and capacity of the central veins. The central blood volume is large. The tip of a CVP catheter "sees" 50 per cent of the total blood volume. By comparison, the tip of a pulmonary artery catheter in the wedge position "sees" only 18 per cent of the blood volume (Fig. 12–1). The latter reflects more rapidly and sensitively the changes in blood volume, assuming there is no difference between right and left ventricular function.

Valid determination of CVP depends on several factors. The first is accurate localization of the catheter tip. This is done by using a radiopaque catheter, injecting a few milliliters of radiopaque material into the catheter, and obtaining a chest film or performing fluoroscopy; by noting respiratory fluctuations; or by noting an abrupt increase in pressure when the catheter enters the right ventricle and then withdrawing the catheter a few centimeters. The silicone rubber (Silastic) catheter is ideal for this purpose. This type of catheter may be introduced through a large-diameter, 15- or 16-gauge needle. The internal jugular and subclavian veins are currently favored as locations for catheter placement. The catheter should be secured firmly to the skin by placing several small tabs of adhesive tape circumferentially around the catheter and suturing the tape to the skin. A blunt needle with a hub is inserted into the Silastic catheter. This connection is reinforced with rigid material such as a tongue blade; otherwise, the needle will eventually

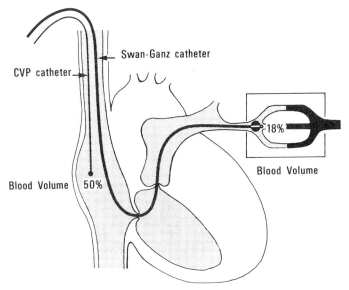

Figure 12–1. The central venous pressure catheter is in direct communication proximal to the venous valves with 50 per cent of the total blood volume. The left atrial (LA) catheter "sees" only 18 per cent of the blood volume. Therefore, smaller changes in volume will affect the left atrial wedge pressure sooner and greater than the central venous pressure.

perforate the tubing. Sterile dressing changes using povidone-iodine ointment are performed daily. Tunneling the catheter prior to its entrance into the vein decreases movement and infection rates.

The second factor is the zero point of the manometer. This is adequately fixed at one-half of the anteroposterior diameter of the chest and the fourth interspace with the patient in the supine position. Relative changes in the pressure with time related to treatment are much more important than the absolute value, which may reflect an erroneous zero point.

The third factor is interpretation of findings. A low CVP usually means hypovolemia. A prompt response to volume replacement indicates that the deficit has been corrected. If other indications of hypovolemia, such as hypotension and oliguria, still exist, then a pulmonary capillary wedge pressure (PCWP) measurement is necessary.

An elevated CVP (greater than 12 to 15 cm of water) suggests right heart failure. In patients with cardiorespiratory disease it is quite common to have a normal CVP with an elevated PCWP, which indicates left heart failure.

Remember that any cause of increased intrathoracic pressure can raise the CVP or PCWP, such as intermittent positive pressure ventilation (IPPV), pneumothorax, or abdominal distention. Cardiac tamponade will cause an elevated CVP even in the presence of hypovolemia.

The Swan-Ganz catheter, a soft, flexible, double lumen (sizes 5, 6, and 7) or triple lumen (size 7) catheter can be passed into the pulmonary artery at the bedside without fluoroscopy in most patients. Measurement of pulmonary capillary wedge pressure is indicated for patients in whom circulatory instability is associated with (1) coronary artery disease requiring a complicated intravenous fluid regimen; (2) high-risk cardiac surgery and severe trauma; (3) increased pulmonary resistance (chronic obstructive lung disease); (4) severe multisystem trauma, generalized peritonitis, decompensated cirrhosis, and severe pancreatitis; (5) massive transfusions, and (6) high CVP in the presence of underperfusion of peripheral tissues.

TECHNIQUE OF SWAN-GANZ CATHETERIZATION

The Swan-Ganz catheter can be easily positioned with the aid of a pressure monitor, electrocardiogram, and oscilloscope. Fluoroscopy may occasionally be necessary to ascertain proper position. The catheter can be inserted percutaneously into the antecubital, subclavian, internal jugular, or femoral veins through an introducer or by venotomy. The balloon should be inflated when the catheter tip is in the thorax. Air, never liquid, should be used for inflation because flotation is better; liquid may be impossible to withdraw, and it transmits high pressures to the containing wall, which can damage the pulmonary vasculature and parenchyma. Pressures are recorded as the catheter is advanced, and characteristic pressure contours for the right atrium, right ventricle, and pulmonary artery are noted. The catheter is advanced until the pressure approximates pulmonary artery diastolic levels — the pulmonary capillary wedge pressure (PCWP). In the absence of valvular heart disease the PCWP is a good estimate of left ventricle end-diastolic pressure. As the balloon is deflated, the phasic pulmonary artery pressure should reappear. An anteroposterior chest roentgenogram will confirm optimal position of the catheter tip. In time, the transcardiac loop of the catheter may shorten, resulting in migration of the tip into smaller branches or even into the wedged position. If at any time the pressure is dampened and a contour other than that characteristic of the pulmonary artery (PA) is observed and *gentle* flushing does not eliminate the distortion, the possibility of wedging should be considered and the catheter should be pulled back 1 to 2 cm.

Whenever the balloon is reinflated for recording wedge pressure, it is possible that the catheter tip is in a small pulmonary artery branch. Inflation to recommended volume in a small branch may cause lateral tension sufficient to rupture the pulmonary vessel and injure the parenchyma. Therefore, reinflate slowly and cautiously. Insert increments of 0.2 ml of air into the balloon while observing the pulmonary artery pressure contour until a change from PA to PCWP is observed. If at volumes substantially less than the recommended inflation, values consistent with PCWP are obtained, the catheter should also be withdrawn 1 to 2 cm.

Table 12–2. COMPLICATIONS OF CENTRAL
VENOUS AND PULMONARY ARTERY CATHETERS

BOTH	PULMONARY ARTERY
Infection	Pulmonary artery perforation
Loss of catheter	Ischemic lung lesion
Thromboembolism	Catheter kinking and heart murmurs
Perforation of right ventricle	Intracardiac knotting of the catheter
Low impedance pathway to the central circulation with risk of ventricular fibrillation	Cardiac arrhythmias

Catheters have been left in place for more than seven days, but 48 hours is considered the upper limit of safe usage (Table 12–2).

CARDIAC OUTPUT

The determination of cardiac output is valuable but not essential in the management of seriously ill or injured patients. The thermodilution technique has simplified this measurement. The Swan-Ganz catheter, by incorporating thermistors, permits measurement of the change in temperature of a bolus of cold saline injected into the right atrium or superior vena cava that is sampled in the pulmonary artery. Cardiac output is then proportional to the fall in temperature. The method has several advantages, which include (1) a physiologic indicator is used, (2) blood withdrawal is not required, and (3) no recirculation of the indicator occurs.

Total flow (cardiac output) is not the best indicator of perfusion in patients who are in shock. If cardiac output is quite low (less than 2 liters per min per m²), then inadequate perfusion almost certainly exists. It is possible during incidents of sepsis and in trauma to have a total flow greater than normal with failure of perfusion of one or more vital organs. Even within a single organ, total flow does not reflect the situation accurately, for some capillary beds may be wide open with many times the usual flow, while neighboring capillary beds, such as those in the renal cortex, are closed, and the cells supplied by these capillaries are ischemic and dying. The brain and kidney are sensitive indicators of perfusion adequacy, so much so that mental status and urine flow are probably as important for the vital sign sheet as blood pressure, pulse rate, respiratory rate, or body temperature. If the patient is alert, calm, and intellectually intact and if urine flow is of adequate volume and appropriate osmolarity, then shock is unlikely regardless of the blood pressure and cardiac output values recorded.

URINE OUTPUT

The incidence of primary acute oliguric renal failure has decreased owing to improved fluid resuscitation during and after operation and trauma. Less severe forms of renal failure with normal or increased urine output are now frequently recognized. Measured urine flow in patients under close scrutiny for a circulatory problem should be 50 ml per hour. The differentiation between prerenal and renal failure can be made by the measurement of urine electrolyte concentration, specific gravity, and the ratio between plasma and urine concentrations for creatinine. In prerenal failure, the sodium concentration is usually less than 20 mEq per liter in the urine, and specific gravity is greater than 1.018 and is not fixed. The urine-to-plasma ratio for creatinine is greater than 20. In renal failure, the sodium concentration is usually greater than 20 mEq per liter, the specific gravity is less than 1.018 and is fixed, and the urine-to-plasma ratio for creatinine is less than 20.

It is especially important to recognize nonoliguric renal failure, because a rapid progression of hyperkalemia after the administration of potassium salts with the threat of cardiac arrest can occur. In addition, mild azotemia may be converted to severe renal failure by the administration of drugs with a nephrotoxic potential. Similarly, drugs that normally do not produce toxicity may do so in the presence of reduced renal function. Especially dangerous are the aminoglycosides (streptomycin, kanamycin, and gentamicin), polymyxin, tetracycline, and vancomycin.

ARTERIAL BLOOD GASES AND pH

Monitoring pulmonary function can be conveniently divided into three general components: (1) evaluation of oxygenation; (2) ventilation; and (3) lung-thorax mechanics. Fortunately, the measurement of arterial blood gases and pH reflect all three of these. The partial pressure of oxygen in arterial blood PaO_2 is the most direct method to determine the adequacy of oxygenation. It must be interpreted concomitantly with the knowledge of the inspired oxygen concentration (FIO_2). The normal difference between PaO_2 and FIO_2 is between 350 and 500. A value below 250 is definitely abnormal.

The adequacy of ventilation is determined by the arterial partial pressure of carbon dioxide ($PaCO_2$). Tidal volume (VT), the amount of air breathed during one respiratory cycle, is another indication of the adequacy of ventilation. This can be readily measured with a modestly priced respirometer. The effective compliance may be quite valuable as an assessment of the ease of distensibility of the lung and thoracic cage and is obtained by dividing the VT by the peak airway pressure. Therefore, an adequate assessment of pulmonary function can be achieved by the serial measurement of arterial blood gases, VT, minute ventilation (tidal volume multiplied by the respiratory rate), and effective compliance.

HEMATOCRIT

In the microcirculation when capillary pressure falls, there is a net movement of extracellular fluid into the capillaries, restoring plasma volume and at the same time lowering the hematocrit. Normal transcapillary refilling does not produce hypoalbuminemia. With infusion of salt solution there is a simultaneous movement of salt and water out of the circulation and a net movement of albumin into the circulation. Serial measurements of hematocrit are a valuable indication of losses from the intravascular space. If blood is lost, the hematocrit will of course drop, but it will rise if large losses of plasma are occurring, as with pancreatitis.

ARTERIAL BLOOD LACTATE

Lactate elevation can be due to tissue hypoxia and oxygen debt, but in most instances of circulatory failure an elevation probably reflects a change in food substrate utilization. Animals with sepsis and other forms of circulatory failure show (1) an increased production as well as utilization of lactate even though both oxygen uptake and carbon dioxide production are within normal limits, (2) a decreased metabolic clearance of lactate, and (3) abnormal substrate utilization, that is, decrease in oxidation of fatty acids and increased metabolic breakdown and oxidation of liver and muscle glycogen and amino acids. The reason the lactate and pyruvate are elevated in this setting is that the substrates being utilized must pass through lactate and pyruvate to enter the Krebs cycle. Serial measurements of arterial blood lactate are useful for prognosis and might indicate a need for total parenteral nutrition.

THERAPY

The specific therapy of circulatory failure is the identification and treatment of the underlying cause. Immediate therapy is designed to maintain the patient long enough to discover the fundamental causes and to institute appropriate therapy.

INTRAVASCULAR VOLUME

The first consideration is to optimize intravascular volume. Hypovolemia causes vasoconstriction, hypotension, hypoperfusion, and ultimately vital organ failure. The absolute volume may be measured by radiolabeled albumin or inferred from changes in the hematocrit, but the absolute volume is not as important as the relationship of volume to capacitance. If the capacitance vessels (capillaries and veins) are widely dilated, a blood volume much greater than normal may be needed to maintain adequate venous return as reflected by heart filling pressures. If the capacitance vessels are tightly constricted, a normal blood volume may result in a high filling pressure.

FILLING PRESSURES

Central venous pressure and left ventricular end-diastolic pressures can both be measured. Of greatest importance is the left ventricular filling pressure, for it determines both the output from the left ventricle and the likelihood of pulmonary edema. The pulmonary artery wedge pressure is an accurate reflection of left ventricular end-diastolic pressure. Most patients, even after myocardial infarction, will increase cardiac output as pulmonary wedge pressures are increased to 14 or 18 mm Hg. A ventricular function curve can be constructed very simply by increasing wedge pressure, increasing fluids, or elevating the patient's legs and measuring directly the changes in cardiac output. The goal is to increase cardiac output to normal or one liter above normal without evoking pulmonary edema.

COLLOIDS VERSUS CRYSTALLOIDS

What determines pulmonary edema? We recognize two types of pulmonary edema: (1) that due to fluid overload, which is frequently only interstitial but may become florid air space pulmonary edema; and (2) the acute respiratory distress syndrome of the adult, which is almost always associated with sepsis. The normal capillary alveolar membrane is illustrated in Figure 12–2. Forces tending to cause movement of fluid out of the capillary are the hydrostatic pressure in the capillary and the colloid osmotic pressure (COP) of the interstitial tissues, a net force of 23 mm Hg in humans. Forces tending to move fluid back into the capillary are interstitial pressure and the colloid osmotic pressure of plasma (a force of 22 mm Hg). There is a continuous flow of lymph with a high protein content into the interstitial space that can be sampled via the right thoracic duct. The negative interstitial pressure protects the alveolus. Fluid in the alveolus passes normally into the interstitial space and into the circulation.

The protein content of the right thoracic duct or lung lymph has been measured in several animals and is normally between 3 and 4 gm per cent. This is a higher protein concentration than is found in systemic lymph, which suggests a greater permeability for protein molecules in

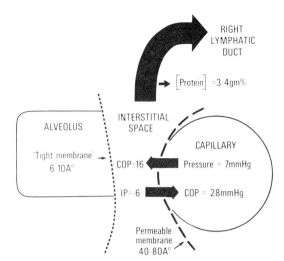

Capillary-Alveolar Membrane

Figure 12–2. Forces at and characteristics of the capillary-alveolar membrane (see text).

the pulmonary capillary. The albumin-globulin ratio is higher than in the plasma, suggesting that pore size limits passage of the larger molecules.

When increased hydrostatic pressure at the pulmonary capillary occurs owing to fluid overload or to elevated left atrial pressure, lymph flow increases and protein concentration decreases linearly with the elevation of hydrostatic pressure. Lung water content does not change until the microvascular hydrostatic pressure doubles. The increased lymphatic flow, together with washout of interstitial protein, protects the lung from edema. Thus, it follows that decreased colloid osmotic pressure of plasma is not an important cause of pulmonary edema.

When sepsis intervenes, lymph flow increases markedly without elevation of left atrial pressure. Protein concentration of the lymph remains the same as the baseline values, and alveolar edema is prompt and much more frequent. This suggests damage to both membranes with an increase in pore number and pore size, in contrast to fluid overload, which suggests an increase in pore number but not in pore size.

In summary, the lung has a built-in protection against edema initiated by increasing lymphatic flow and lowering interstitial protein content. Cardiovascular failure, as we see it clinically, alters the capillary membrane but does not permit passage of more protein. Sepsis alters both the capillary and alveolar membranes and permits passage of protein even when the lesion is reversible. Elevation of left atrial pressure will aggravate the lung lesion, especially in the presence of sepsis. How corticosteroids affect the membranes and transport mechanisms is not known at this time. It is not even clear whether albumin and plasma should be administered to a patient with a pulmonary alveolar membrane that is leaking protein.

The timing of specific therapy intervention remains a controversial subject. Our own policy for patients in circulatory failure is to provide crystalloid solutions first (Ringer's lactate or buffered saline solution) and to correct hematocrit and serum proteins later. The hematocrit should usually be corrected within 24 to 48 hours. The protein concentration of plasma might conveniently be altered and corrected over several days by administering total parenteral nutrition or by normal feedings but rarely by the use of albumin, never by plasma protein fraction (Plasmanate), and infrequently by plasma. There is no convincing evidence that lung lesions associated with circulatory failure are altered by the use of colloid preparations.

DRUGS

Ionotropic Drugs. If hypoperfusion persists after filling pressures have been corrected, the next approach is to augment contractility and thereby increase cardiac output. Many drugs are available, but only the directly acting catecholamines are appropriate. There are four reasonable possibilities: norepinephrine, epinephrine, dopamine, and isoproterenol. They all have equivalent effects on heart force but quite different effects on heart rate and systemic vascular resistance. Norepinephrine constricts most peripheral vessels, increasing afterload of the heart to the greatest extent. This may be appropriate during cardiopulmonary resuscitation, but for patients in shock this diminishes essential organ perfusion and may precipitate pulmonary edema.

Epinephrine dilates bronchi, and in the rare instance in which bronchodilatation is required, it will be important to use either epinephrine or isoproterenol for this purpose.

Isoproterenol causes tachycardia and tachyarrhythmias and dilates vessels in skeletal muscle. It is likely that the fraction of cardiac output reaching the kidneys diminishes when isoproterenol is given. It may well aggravate myocardial ischemia by the combined effects of tachycardia and diastolic hypertension, which minimize oxygen delivery and maximize oxygen utilization.

Dopamine has emerged as the most useful ionotropic drug. In doses of 200 to 500 μg per minute it dilates directly the renal, mesenteric, cerebral, and coronary vessels. It must be remembered that coronary perfusion is determined more by myocardial oxygen demands than vasomotor action. In doses of 500 to 2000 μg per minute given to adults, dopamine increases heart force to the same extent as the other catecholamines at comparable doses, an effect that might triple heart force and myocardial oxygen requirements. At doses above 2000 μg per minute, there is progressive alpha-adrenergic vasoconstriction resembling the action of norepinephrine. The patient with mild hypoperfusion will respond to small doses that largely redirect blood flow to essential organs yet increase heart force minimally. At higher doses, the ionotropic effects are predominant, but vasodilatation maintains appropriate perfusion distribution. If the patient is very refractory to therapy and a pressor response is required to maintain arterial pressures at viable levels, then the vasoconstriction that occurs with higher doses of dopamine will accomplish this action as well as any other alpha-adrenergic agonist.

Vasodilators. Vasodilators first became popular in treating cases of shock when it was common to give inadequate intravascular volume replacement, and tightly vasoconstricted patients given vasodilators were better perfused as an additional volume was obviously required. Now we see the reverse. The patient is given excessive intravascular volume, and as pulmonary edema supervenes, the patient is treated with vasodilators. Only a few patients with circulatory failure should receive vasodilators as primary therapy.

Some patients with myocardial infarction present with pulmonary congestion, high filling pressures, and profound vasoconstriction. Careful vasodilatation in such cases may improve perfusion, diminish myocardial oxygen requirements, and increase filling pressures, thereby relieving pulmonary congestion.

There are three vasodilators to consider: (1) phentolamine (Regitine) is an alpha-adrenergic antagonist with an active duration of action of about 30 minutes. It dilates both veins and arteries, and its effects are more prominent in patients with high levels of sympathetic tone or during administration of large doses of norepinephrine, epinephrine, or dopamine. Phentolamine is given by constant intravenous infusion at doses from 50 to 500 μg per minute, and it may be mixed with a catecholamine in the same infusion solution. (2) Nitroprusside (Nitride) directly dilates smooth muscle and blood vessels, possibly with greater action on arterial vessels. It is given as a constant intravenous infusion at doses of 20 to 1000 μg per minute. It has a short active duration (one or two minutes), but care must be taken that no bolus is given, such as during the flushing of an intravenous catheter. (3) Nitroglycerine when given intravenously may have a predominant action on capacitance vessels, and there is some evidence that it may improve collateral flow to ischemic myocardium to a greater extent than nitroprusside.

There are certain basic principles that must be followed in using vasodilators. Adequate filling pressures must be maintained, arterial pressures must be monitored carefully, the patient's position should never be changed suddenly, minimal doses of the vasodilator should be administered, and every effort should be made to stabilize arterial pressure at about 10 to 20 mm Hg less than normal values.

SPECIFIC TREATMENT FOR RESPIRATORY FAILURE

Respiratory failure in surgical patients is usually an acute problem secondary to (1) ventilation-perfusion inequality, as in atelectasis; (2)

increased dead space, as in hypotension; (3) increased work of breathing, as in pulmonary edema; or (4) decreased oxygen transport, as in decreased cardiac output. Many factors are known to predispose the patient to these abnormalities: (1) pain (consider epidural analgesia for postoperative pain), (2) abdominal distention, (3) restrictive binders, (4) narcotics, (5) sepsis, (6) chronic obstructive lung disease, (7) smoking, (8) severe obesity, and (9) neurologic diseases that affect thoracic excursion.

OXYGEN THERAPY

The PaO_2 is normally 80 to 100 mm Hg when ambient air is inspired at sea level and decreases normally to 70 mm Hg at age 70. Tolerance to hypoxia is variable, but it is generally wise to administer oxygen to hospitalized patients who have an acute decrease in PaO_2 to less than 55 to 60 mm Hg. If hematocrit and cardiac output are low, a higher PaO_2 than 55 to 60 mm Hg may be necessary.

How to Administer Oxygen

Nasal Cannulas and Catheters. This method is simple and efficient, and flow rates of 6 to 8 liters per min deliver 30 to 40 per cent inspired oxygen. Higher rates are uncomfortable for the patient. All oxygen should be humidified. Therapy is possible while the patient is eating.

Plastic Face Masks. Loose-fitting plastic face masks deliver 30 to 50 per cent of oxygen at a flow rate of 8 to 10 liters per min.

Venturi Masks. These plastic masks are designed to deliver variable and adjustable concentrations of oxygen of 24 per cent, 28 per cent, 34 per cent, and 40 per cent using a Venturi system. A constant proportion of air is entrained when oxygen flow exceeds 2 liters per min.

Rubber Face Masks. The Boothby, Lovelace, and Bulbulian (BLB) masks are more tightly fitting and can deliver up to 80 per cent oxygen but are too hot, heavy, and uncomfortable for the patient to use for longer than 15 to 20 minutes or during resuscitation.

Face hoods and oxygen tents are no longer recommended because of inconvenience, expense, and fire hazard potential.

T-Piece System. This system is often used to deliver oxygen and humidity to patients with endotracheal tubes or tracheostomies. It is a simple, safe method without valves. The oxygen delivered will depend upon the concentration and flow of oxygen. A flow rate of three times the minute volume is required to eliminate rebreathing. Rebreathing or air entry, both of which will dilute oxygen delivery, is also determined by the length of the expiratory limb of the T.

Mechanical Ventilation

Respiratory support is indicated if a patient who is receiving oxygen at 10 liters per minute by a face mask has a PaO_2 of 60 mm Hg or less or a $PaCO_2$ of 55 mm Hg or greater and there are signs that these values are deteriorating, or if a poorly oxygenated patient has rapid, shallow respiration and is tiring. Positive pressure ventilation by use of a tightly fitting face mask with bag is useful in emergency resuscitation only.

A cuffed endotracheal tube is passed through the mouth if the situation is urgent or through the nose if feasible; the latter procedure is more comfortable for most patients.

Elective tracheostomy is performed only if there is (1) an anatomic or traumatic abnormality that precludes intubation from above; (2) obvious long-term need, i.e., more than two weeks; and (3) an inability to cope with excessive secretions or bleeding without tracheostomy.

There are certain important requirements for patients on a ventilator. A competent attendant must always be present when an intubated patient is on mechanical ventilation. The patient should be well oxygenated prior to suctioning, and ventilation should be interrupted for not more than 15 seconds at any one time. In order to avoid drying of secretions in the airway, the respiratory gas mixtures should be humidified by passage through heated water and then should be diverted at 30° C. Mist should be visible but not dense. Laryngeal or tracheal ulceration and stenosis are common after prolonged intubation, but the incidence can be decreased by using low-pressure pliable cuffs on endotracheal and tracheostomy tubes. Inflation should be just sufficient to prevent air leakage. The cuff can be deflated for about five minutes every hour if the patient can tolerate being off mechanical ventilation for that period of time. Suctioning of the oropharynx prior to deflating the balloon may prevent aspiration.

Types of Ventilators

The types of ventilators in common use are those that are pressure-cycled (Bird) and volume-cycled (Bennett MA1, Emerson, and Engstrom). The pressure-cycled ventilators do not make alterations for changes in lung and chest wall compliance; hence, tidal volume must be monitored. With the volume-cycled ventilators, the inflation pressure must be monitored. The volume-cycled ventilators are more expensive than pressure-cycled machines, but they are easier to use.

Oxygenation

Oxygenation of the blood is maintained if possible at a minimum PaO_2 of 80 to 90 mm Hg, and this is accomplished by increasing the fraction of oxygen in the inspired air (FIO_2). It is conventional to begin with 40 per cent humidified oxygen. Clinical experience suggests that oxygen concentration of 50 per cent or higher is likely to produce serious pulmonary damage due to oxygen toxicity when used for prolonged periods (over 48 hours).

Patients on controlled ventilation at normal tidal volumes of 7 ml per kg often complain of dyspnea and inadequate chest expansion, even though blood gases are normal. Tidal volumes of 10 to 15 ml per kg are therefore recommended and usually well tolerated. Excessive hypocapnea can be corrected by the introduction of a mechanical dead space.

Positive End-Expiratory Pressure (PEEP)

Another alternative to changing FIO_2 and tidal volume is to reinflate collapsed or partially collapsed alveoli by increasing end-expiratory pressure. Volume ventilators have the capability of instituting PEEP without modifying the equipment. The usual beginning level is 5 cm of water. Cardiorespiratory monitoring is done after 15 minutes to assess the effects. If no beneficial effect is noted, further increases in PEEP are made in increments of 3 to 5 cm of water pressure. While some patients respond with an immediate increase in PaO_2, others may not show improvement for 30 to 60 minutes or longer. Benefits are rarely accrued with pressures greater than 10 cm of water.

Weaning from the Ventilator

Sustained spontaneous ventilation requires a minimum vital capacity of 15 to 20 ml per kg, or a volume twice the normal tidal volume. If the PaO_2 is maintained at 200 mm Hg or above on the ventilator with FIO_2 of 40 per cent, it is probable that the patient will tolerate a short trial period off the ventilator. Weaning can begin with 5 to 15 minutes per hour or half hour of spontaneous respiration off the ventilator but with a T connector to the tracheal tube delivering 60 per cent to 80 per cent humidified oxygen. The process of weaning must be gradual if the patient has had acute respiratory failure, a long period of mechanical ventilation, or an unstable chest wall. In addition to measured blood gases and pH, the electrocardiogram, the depth and rate of respirations, and alertness of the patient are valuable indicators of the ventilation adequacy.

SUMMARY

Successful treatment of cardiovascular and respiratory failure demands attention to many details, and the surgeon must evaluate other patient needs ranging from the nutritional to the psychological. All of these requirements are best met in a specialized unit staffed and equipped specifically for these patients, the surgical intensive care unit. The details of resuscitation after cardiac arrest are widely known and practiced. The question is frequently asked, "How many survive and leave the hospital?" In our own general hospital as measured over a recent 10-year period, 1204 patients were resuscitated with an overall survival rate to discharge of 20 per cent. Of the survivors who left the hospital, 75 per cent were alive one year postdischarge, 59 per cent at two years, and 51 per cent at three years. A random study of the survivors shows that their functional capacity before and after resuscitation was unchanged. The endeavor here to clarify treatment of cardiovascular and respiratory failure patients is in part supported by our own experience.

REFERENCES

Berk, J. L.: Monitoring the patient in shock: What, when and how. Surg. Clin. North Am., 55:713, 1975.
Blaisdell, F. W., and Lewis, F. R., Jr.: Respiratory Distress Syndrome of Shock and Trauma. Philadelphia, W. B. Saunders Co., 1977.
Carrico, C. J., and Horovitz, J. H.: Monitoring the critically ill surgical patient. Adv. Surg., 11:101, 1977.
Staub, N. C.: Pathogenesis of pulmonary edema. Am. Rev . Resp. Dis., 109:358, 1974.

13

Renal Function and Renal Failure

SAMUEL POWERS

Appropriate preoperative preparation and timely postoperative assessment of renal function usually insures normal clearance of nitrogenous wastes and virtually eliminates acute tubular necrosis as a postoperative complication. Prevention of acute tubular necrosis is important because postoperative acute renal failure continues to have a high mortality rate. The key to preventing postoperative disorders of renal function is to prepare the kidney preoperatively with an optimal internal environment. A priority of postoperative management is to recognize and correct any disturbance in the internal environment before established renal failure supervenes. If normal renal function is to be preserved and the renal parenchyma is to be protected from cellular damage, then accurate preoperative assessment followed by appropriate preoperative preparatory measures must be carried out. Preoperative assessment begins with identification of the "high risk" and clinical setting.

THE HIGH-RISK PATIENT

The highest risk for the development of postoperative acute renal failure exists for those patients who have been seriously injured prior to operation. The three classes of injuries that may have occurred are loss of body fluid, damage to body tissues, and sepsis.

Loss of body fluid, whether it be whole blood from active hemorrhage or extracellular fluid from vomiting or diarrhea, is rarely, if ever, associated with acute renal failure secondary to acute tubular necrosis. Patients who develop the clinical state of shock as a result of bleeding from a duodenal ulcer, for example, recover their renal function rapidly when the source of bleeding is controlled and the lost volume is replaced. Although hypotension appears to be a common factor in the development of tubular necrosis, it will not by itself lead to acute renal failure.

242

Crushed soft tissue, especially in association with a period of hypotension, frequently results in acute renal failure. The first clinical description of post-traumatic acute renal failure was reported as a complication of crushing injuries due to falling masonry during the civilian bombing of London in World War II. This association led to the term "crush kidney" as the name of a new syndrome. The first detailed studies of patients suffering from this disorder were carried out by the Army Surgical Research Team during the Korean conflict. The combination of damaged tissue, massive fluid loss, and circulating myoglobin was most frequently associated with the development of a uremic state. Blast injuries resulting from exploding land mines were the most frequent cause of post-traumatic renal failure. The mortality in this combat setting approached 90 per cent.

Systemic sepsis may be associated with impaired renal function, especially if it is associated with hypotension and fluid loss. If all these factors occur in conjunction with extensive soft tissue damage, a cascade of sequential organ failures may follow in which acute renal failure is an early and prominent event in the inexorable fatal course. Patients who experience a combination of hypotension, tissue damage, and systemic sepsis make up the highest-risk group. Little can be done for such patients unless the source of infection can be identified promptly and corrected surgically.

There are certain operative procedures that are associated with a significant increased incidence of postoperative acute renal failure. Foremost among these are surgical procedures for ruptured abdominal aortic aneurysms. Elective resection of abdominal aortic aneurysms may also carry an increased risk of renal damage, although modern anesthesia methods and surgical techniques have virtually eliminated this problem. Other operative procedures that may be associated with an increased incidence of renal dysfunction in the postoperative period include extended operations on the biliary tract and pancreas. Surgical treatment of acute pancreatitis with drainage of its associated intrapancreatic abscesses is a notable example.

Prevention of acute renal failure is best accomplished by correction of all preexisting abnormalities of the internal environment prior to the surgical procedure. This can usually be accomplished by accurate replacement of blood loss and sufficient fluid to provide an optimal environment for normal renal function. Inability to restore renal function by these means suggests that tubular necrosis may have developed preoperatively. Assessment of the adequacy of preoperative preparation requires an accurate assessment of the patient's renal function.

THE ASSESSMENT OF RENAL FUNCTION

The response of the kidney to the replacement of lost blood and the restoration of the extracellular fluid volume usually provide a reliable guide to the state of renal function. Single measurements of renal function under one set of conditions and at any specific time provide little reliable information concerning the status of the kidneys, whereas sequential observations following therapeutic intervention provide an accurate assessment of renal function. The urine volume may be abnormally high if the glomerular filtration rate is reduced to the point of renal failure, and the increased urine volume represents an additional failure of tubular function. Similarly, an abnormally low urine volume may occur in the presence of perfectly normal kidneys. Furthermore, a systolic blood pressure in the range of 90 mm Hg may be associated with relatively normal renal perfusion, whereas with the crush syndrome, a normal blood pressure may be associated with severe renal vasoconstriction and almost complete cessation of glomerular filtration. In each of these situations, however, the response to an administered fluid load is frequently diagnostic of the underlying disorder. The renal response to a fluid load may not be a reliable indication of renal function, and therefore, the response of the total patient should be evaluated. For example, severe volume depletion generally produces oliguria with a rapid heart rate and low central venous pressure. The administration of isotonic saline solution at a rate of 400 to 500 ml per hour usually demonstrates the adequacy of fluid repletion. If volume depletion is still present, the central venous pressure remains low in spite of the rapid rate of infusion, but the pulse rate usually slows, and urine output improves at least transiently. However, an increase in central venous pressure with the first 300 to 500 ml of infused fluid, especially if it is not accompanied by an increase in urine output, suggests that fluid volume is normal and the difficulty lies elsewhere. Frequent determinations of the serum sodium concentration are important because failure of the serum sodium concentration to increase following an infusion of isotonic saline suggests serious volume depletion. A salt load in a normally hydrated individual, on the other hand, will result in either an increase in sodium excretion in the urine or an increase in the serum sodium level. In either case, the test infusion provides valuable information concerning the patient's physiologic status.

The response of central venous pressure to a fluid load is frequently employed to estimate the adequacy of the volume replacement. There are several pitfalls in this measurement that may lead to an erroneous conclusion. The term "central venous pressure" means that the tip of the catheter must be either in the vena cava or the right atrium. Verification of this assumption can be obtained only by means of a chest roentgenogram. Measurements of the length of catheter inserted are totally unreliable because catheters introduced through the antecubital space may pass cephalad to the jugular bulb or downward into the abdomen, lodging in the hepatic or renal veins. It is essential to the technique of central venous pressure monitoring to include a chest roentgenogram to ascertain the position of the catheter. Pressure measurements should be carried out with the bed completely flat because changes in the position of a patient exert a variable gravitational effect on the manometer and may yield fallacious values. The bottom of the manometer should be placed at the level of the midaxillary line and, of more importance, should be repositioned at the same point each time the central venous pressure is measured. A useful maneuver is to place a short piece of adhesive tape marked with an "X" to indicate the proper point for serial measurements. If the central venous pressure is determined in this way, the pressure response to fluid therapy can be a useful clinical guide.

The accurate and continuous measurement of urine volume is essential in the management of any patient with suspected renal failure. The risk of an indwelling catheter must be accepted in order to obtain moment-to-moment information concerning urine output. The modern urine collecting apparatus provides a closed system between the catheter and the graduated measuring device, which can be emptied into the reservoir without disconnecting the catheter. In this way, the danger of gross contamination is minimized while the necessary monitoring information is still provided. Persistent oliguria below 25 ml per hour for more than two hours is an ominous sign and requires the most urgent and aggressive corrective therapy. Oliguria is an important part of the clinical setting in which renal cell necrosis may develop. Failure of the urine volume to increase with a fluid load, especially if associated with an increased central venous pressure, indicates that the normal renal control mechanisms may no longer be operative; the urine:plasma osmolar ratio will help to make this determination. Identical concentration of dissolved materials in both plasma and urine suggests that acute renal failure has already occurred. Remember that renal failure may occur in the presence of a diminished urine volume, in the face of complete anuria, or with a normal or excessive urine output. It is the quality rather than the quantity of urine that provides diagnostic information.

Variations of renal function in the preoperative or postoperative surgical patient can be divided into two groups. The first consists of variations that represent appropriate responses of the renal control mechanism and the renal parenchyma to an abnormal physiologic state; the second consists of failure of the renal system responses due to parenchymal damage or inappropriate control mechanism. The distinction between these two conditions may be clinically obscure because in each case, a low or high urine volume may result, and the urine may consist of dilute or concentrated fluid. This differentiation is important because in one case, a superbly functioning system is carrying out its appointed task, and in the other, there is a pathologic state that can lead to death. The distinction hinges on the urine:plasma ratio of concentrations of dissolved material and the deviation of this ratio from unity. Normal kidneys are invariably associated with some processing of the glomerular filtrate during its passage through the tubular system. This processing may yield a urine that is more or less concentrated than plasma but will never result in a urine whose composition is identical

Table 13–1. COMMON VALUES OBTAINED FROM
OLIGURIC PATIENTS WITH NORMAL KIDNEYS

	URINE	PLASMA	U:P	GFR (ML/MIN)
Creatinine (mg/ml)	100	1	100	
If urine volume	= 30 ml/hr	(0.5 ml/min)		50
Osmols (mOsm/l)	400	300	1.3	
Sodium (mEq/l)	20	140	0.14	

with that of plasma. Urine:plasma ratios seen in patients with a normal renal parenchyma are shown in Table 13–1.

A further estimate of renal function may be obtained from measurements of the glomerular filtration rate (GFR). This function is measured in milliliters per minute and is a quantitative statement of the amount of fluid that must have passed through the glomeruli in order to account for the quantity of a nonresorbable substance, such as creatinine, which appears in the urine. If the urine:plasma ratio of creatinine is 100 and the urine volume is 60 ml per hour, then 1 ml of urine was made per minute. Multiplying the urine:plasma ratio of 100 by the volume of urine per minute (1 ml) yields a glomerular filtration rate of 100 ml per minute, which is normal for the usual adult patient.

Studies in experimental animals and humans suggest that a fall in blood pressure to a mean value of about 80 mm Hg is not associated with a significant change in glomerular filtration rate, whereas a fall in blood pressure below this level produces a precipitous decline in GFR. Prompt restoration of blood pressure to normal will restore the GFR. If the quantity of a metabolic end product such as urea is produced faster than it is cleared through the glomerulus, then the blood level of this substance will rise, and renal failure has occurred. The urine:plasma ratios of sodium, creatinine, and osmolarity in patients with established acute renal failure are shown in Table 13–2.

Table 13–2. COMMON VALUES OBTAINED FROM
PATIENTS WITH ACUTE RENAL FAILURE

	URINE	PLASMA	U:P	GFR (ML/MIN)
Creatinine (mg/ml)	20	2	10	
If urine volume	= 10 ml/hr	(.16 ml/min)		1.6
Osmols (mOsm/l)	300	290	1.03	
Sodium (mEq/l)	110	130	0.9	

PREOPERATIVE ADJUSTMENT OF THE RENAL CONTROL MECHANISM TO ALLOW FOR POSTOPERATIVE EXCRETION OF SALT AND WATER

Sodium restriction, especially when accompanied by water restriction for even a few hours, may result in activation of aldosterone. This is an example of a normal control system that acts to enhance sodium resorption under conditions in which further loss of sodium from the body might represent a threat to survival. This is considered a disorder of renal function because a normally functioning kidney will excrete almost any administered sodium load. Inability to excrete excess sodium poses a potential threat during the postoperative period. The mechanism for activation of aldosterone appears to be associated with the release of renin from the kidney and its subsequent action on a plasma globulin to produce angiotensin. The control mechanism resides in the distal tubules in the cells of the macula densa, which detect alterations in sodium concentration and govern the release of renin granules from the juxtaglomerular apparatus. This mechanism is of considerable clinical importance because of its relatively long active duration of action. The release of aldosterone from the adrenal cortex requires several hours from the time of onset of the sodium depletion, and after this substance has appeared in the bloodstream, it will continue to circulate for a period of many hours or even days. During this time, the ability of the kidney to excrete sodium is markedly reduced. The clinical implications of aldosterone release are apparent when one considers that this release is associated with sodium depletion, but when the sodium is replaced by intravenous infusion, the kidney will be unable to excrete this substantially, and sodium overloading may occur. Patients with congestive heart failure and expanded extracellular volumes may well suffer from aldosterone release, especially if they are prepared for operation by a period of fasting with deprivation of salt and water. Attempts to restore sodium balance by the intravenous administration of sodium chloride solution can easily result in further overexpansion of the extracellular space or may interfere with the kidneys' inability to excrete the administered sodium load. This control mechanism has unquestioned survival value when sodium cannot be readily replaced. Unfortunately, the ability of the physician to administer sodium chloride intravenously is an unanticipated bit of human meddling that removes the necessity and even the survival value of this control system. Sodium retention as a result of activating production of aldosterone might be considered a failure by the physician to understand and correctly manipulate the internal environment to the advantage of the patient. Preoperative intravenous administration of salt and water prior to the release of aldosterone insures that the patient undergoes the stress of surgery with a sodium control mechanism set for free excretion of excess sodium ion.

POSTOPERATIVE RECOGNITION OF IMPENDING RENAL FAILURE

The earliest evidence of impending renal dysfunction is an inappropriate urine volume. A high urine volume (greater than 100 ml per hr) in a patient who appears volume-depleted is just as ominous as a low urine volume (less than 30 ml per hr) in a patient with apparently adequate fluid replacement. In either case, the kidney may be reacting normally to correct an abnormal fluid and electrolyte state, or renal damage may have already developed. The first requirement for accurate assessment of postoperative renal function is to have a precise knowledge of the functional state of the body fluid composition. The words "functional state" are used deliberately rather than the more usual term "fluid and electrolyte balance." The body fluid composition is optimal when cardiovascular, pulmonary, and central and autonomic nervous systems are functioning normally. This may involve positive or negative total fluid balance compared with the preoperative state. An extended operation that exposes the intestines to evaporative losses for several hours and results in a paralytic ileus with fluid sequestration in the gut can deplete the patient's functional fluid volume. The net fluid balance and even the patient's weight may suggest that the proper amount of fluid has been provided. However, a serious appropriate restriction of fluid and the use of diuretics may result in a large negative fluid balance, which has improved the function of the cardiopulmonary systems in patients with congestive heart failure. Therefore, the accuracy of fluid volume replacement in the postoperative period must be judged by the presence of adequate central venous pressure (or pulmonary capillary wedge pressure), a normal systolic blood pressure and pulse pressure, normal blood gases, the presence of a clear sensorium, and the absence of signs of sympathetic hyperactivity, such as pale, cool, clammy skin. Ordinarily, these clinical signs will provide a clear evaluation of the patient's fluid volume status.

In especially high-risk situations, such as occur with patients suffering from preexisting cardiovascular disease, it may be necessary to insert a thermal dilution pulmonary artery catheter to measure cardiac output. This device permits frequent repeated measurements of both the cardiac output and cardiac filling pressures. Adequate fluid therapy can then be assessed as that quantity that is required to maintain the cardiac index of 3.5 l per M^2 without raising the pulmonary capillary wedge pressure above 8 mm Hg. This technique is most reliable, but because of its invasive nature, its use should be restricted to those patients for whom the standard clinical evaluation has not achieved the desired therapeutic effect.

MANAGEMENT OF POSTOPERATIVE OLIGURIA

The measures for optimizing the patient's internal environment recommended before usually result in restitution of a normal urine volume of normal composition. If oliguria persists, there is often a strong temptation to administer a loop diuretic such as furosemide. Although this drug may produce an increase in urine volume, there is little evidence to suggest that any improvement in renal function occurs. If oliguria persists following apparently adequate fluid replacement, then glomerular filtration rate should be measured. A simple calculation will illustrate the problem. In a patient with acute tubular necrosis, the glomerular filtration rate may be reduced to 10 ml per min (normal value is approximately 100 ml per min). This reduced rate still produces 600 ml of filtrate per hour. If the effect of a high dose of furosemide was to block the absorption of one-half of the filtered sodium load, there would still be a urine volume of 300 ml per hour. The clearance of nitrogenous waste would not be improved by this maneuver; only the quantity of water and electrolytes excreted would be increased. This can easily be confirmed in any oliguric patient by repeated determinations of the glomerular filtration rate. The GFR will be unchanged after the use of furosemide under these conditions. Persistent oliguria following apparently adequate fluid resuscitation may be improved by the timely use of the osmotic diuretic mannitol.

There is a transition period between depression of renal function by normally acting control mechanisms and the initial breakdown of renal function that leads to functional renal failure. An opportunity to reverse the chain of events leading to renal cell death exists during this period. Unfortunately, the period of functional renal failure may last for only two or three hours; therefore, prompt and energetic action is required. Fifty gm of a 20 per cent solution of mannitol should be given intravenously over a period of approximately one hour. Since mannitol acts as a volume expander, it is imperative that cardiac filling pressure as determined from the pulmonary capillary wedge pressure be continuously monitored during this infusion. If the wedge pressure rises more than 5 mm Hg from its initial value, mannitol infusion should be promptly discontinued. Administration of mannitol may result in reversal of functional renal failure, as evidenced by an increase in the urine:plasma osmolar ratio. If tubular damage is already severe before therapy has begun, mannitol may still be useful, since it appears to provide an increased urine flow through the still functioning portions of the kidney. Under these circumstances, there will be chemical evidence of renal failure as evidenced by an increasing serum creatinine and blood urea nitrogen, but the continued urine volume will make the problems of water and electrolyte balance considerably easier to manage than they might have been in an anuric state.

Acute renal failure is, therefore, a generally preventable complication of surgical trauma. Prophylaxis can almost invariably be accomplished if aggressive therapy is carried out within a short time of the acute process. A high index of suspicion for the high-risk clinical setting in which acute renal failure may occur, combined with frequent measurements of the quantity and composition of the urine, provide early clues to impending difficulty. Measurements of the urine:plasma osmolar ratio are most helpful, but important additional information is also obtained from urinary sodium and creatinine determinations. A urine volume that is inappropriately low (less than 35 ml per hour) or high (greater than 80 ml per hour) deserves further investigation and immediate corrective action. Prevention of postoperative acute renal failure is usually accomplished by series of steps designed to raise the sodium concentration in the distal tubule. This increase can be accomplished in most cases by the simple administration of adequate quantities of isotonic electrolyte solution, but under special circumstances it may require the addition of an osmotic diuretic. Each of these maneuvers should be carried out rapidly, one after the other, until urine volume is restored to a level of approximately 60 ml per hour. Because of the ever-present danger of fluid overload, it is essential that such aggressive therapy be performed with a flow-directed pulmonary artery catheter in place so that the pulmonary capillary wedge pressure can be monitored at least every 15 minutes. Under these circumstances, successful prevention can be accomplished with minimal risks.

POSTOPERATIVE RECOGNITION OF RENAL DYSFUNCTION DUE TO APPROPRIATE SECRETION OF ADH

Conservation of water during volume depletion represents a normal biologic response. This control system also operates in the other direction by suppressing release of ADH when excretion of excess water from the body is desirable. These biologic principles apply to overexpansion of the extracellular fluid compartment, especially in association with hyponatremia. Serious abnormalities of the internal environment occur if the ADH control system is inoperative or ineffective during water depletion or, conversely, if the system is activated by the secretion of ADH when excessive water is present in association with hyponatremia. Both of these pathologic states may be seen in postoperative patients.

INAPPROPRIATE RELEASE OF ADH

This syndrome of ADH secretion consists of water retention in the face of an expanded extracellular space in conjunction with hyponatremia. It is further characterized by inability to increase the serum sodium concentration by intravenous administration of isotonic solutions. At a time when the internal environment calls for excretion of dilute urine, urine is processed that is more concentrated than is appropriate for a dilute plasma. Recognition of this disorder is important because treatment of the decreased serum sodium concentration by the usual program of intravenous sodium administered as an isotonic solution will worsen the situation. Water will be retained in preference to sodium, resulting in a further fall in serum sodium concentration. After the diagnosis has been established, the only effective therapy is rigid water restriction, which results in an increasing serum osmolarity as water is lost by evaporation. Fortunately, this disorder is self-limited, and if further overloading of the extracellular space can be avoided, no serious consequences ensue. The differential diagnosis of other causes of hyponatremia is easily made if urinary sodium concentration measurements are obtained. Other causes of hyponatremia may elicit low urinary sodium (less than 10 mEq per l), whereas patients with inappropriate release of ADH excrete an inappropriately high sodium urinary value (greater than 30 mEq per l).

NEPHROGENIC DIABETES INSIPIDUS

Complete failure of the ADH control system may occur following administration of certain fluorinated hydrocarbon anesthetic agents. Such failure is frequently associated with the anesthetic agent methoxyflurance (Penthrane). Complete absence of ADH, such as that seen in patients with diabetes insipidus, causes massive water loss via the urine and severe dehydration. The urine under these circumstances characteristically is maximally dilute, being much more dilute than plasma. The tubular mechanism is functioning normally, as is the glomerular filtration rate. Sodium resorption is maximal, as one would expect with adequate functioning of the aldosterone mechanism. The characteristic feature of Penthrane nephropathy, therefore, is the total absence of ADH activity. Patients become severely dehydrated owing to excessive water loss, and since sodium is not excreted along with the water, severe hypernatremia may ensue. This syndrome is differentiated from true diabetes insipidus in that administration of ADH fails to correct the abnormality. Because of the resistance to ADH administration, the condition is often referred to as nephrogenic diabetes insipidus. The marked dehydration that may occur if this condition is uncorrected will result in elevations of the blood urea nitrogen simulating the picture of high-output acute renal failure. The distinction, however, is of great importance. The glomerular filtration rate and tubular function in nephrogenic diabetes insipidus are within normal limits. In acute renal failure, tubular function is reduced, and an underlying renal abnormality is appreciated. The loss of large volumes of water in the urine requires supplementation of as much as 9 liters of water per day for the patient to maintain normal hydration. When normal hydration is achieved, the blood urea nitrogen will return to normal, and since this disorder is self-limited, restoration of normal urine volume and normal urine:plasma osmolar ratio will soon occur spontaneously.

MANAGEMENT OF ESTABLISHED RENAL FAILURE

A patient's failure to produce a urine flow of 40 ml per hour or better is tantamount to the diagnosis of acute renal failure. Complete absence of urinary output is most unusual, however, in the early stages of tubular necrosis. Indeed, the appearance of immediate anuria suggests that the difficulty lies in obstruction of urine outflow rather than in the production of urine. Obstruction of the lower urinary tract at the bladder neck is a common postoperative occurrence, although it is unfortunately not always diagnosed immediately. A less common form of immediate anuria occurs following intra-abdominal operations in which the ureters may have been inadvertently damaged. It is most unusual for a surgeon to believe that his or her operative procedure could possibly have resulted in damage to the upper urinary tract, but the clinical facts speak loudly that even in the hands of the most experienced surgeon, occasional obstruction to the ureters may occur as an inadvertent complication of intra-abdominal surgery. The appearance of immediate postoperative anuria is suggestive evidence of urinary tract obstruction until appropriate roèntgenographic contrast studies have been obtained to eliminate this diagnosis.

MANAGEMENT OF ESTABLISHED ACUTE TUBULAR NECROSIS

Acute tubular necrosis is established when the kidneys are no longer able to maintain the composition of the internal environment within normal limits. The exact point in time at which this diagnosis becomes manifest is impossible to identify, because a large fraction of the renal parenchyma can be destroyed before evidence of renal insufficiency is demonstrated. Pathologic studies indicate that tubular necrosis has a patchy appearance with microscopic areas of apparently normal renal tissue interspersed between areas of severe tubular damage. The cardinal principle of managing acute tubular necrosis is the maintenance of a normal internal environment; when the kidneys are unable to function adequately, supplemental measures must be applied.

Acute renal failure may occur in either an oliguric or a polyuric form, and the management of each condition is somewhat different. In either case, the management is best divided into considerations initially of the metabolic consequences of inadequate renal function and later of the complications that arise from the background of disordered metabolism. The clinical syndrome of oliguric renal failure is associated with retention of potassium, water, and sodium and nitrogen and anion accumulation. The most serious of these is the retention of potassium. Hyperkalemia can cause sudden death from cardiac arrest with little or no warning, whereas the other aspects of renal insufficiency proceed slowly with ample time for thoughtfully considered selection of the best method for correction. Potassium intoxication may be associated with a patient who is symptom-free one hour and dead from cardiac arrest the next. As soon as the diagnosis of acute tubular necrosis is made, an immediate serum potassium level should be obtained and an electrocardiogram tracing should be recorded. Cardiac arrhythmias due to hyperkalemia can be detected more rapidly than the electrolyte concentration can be determined by the clinical laboratory. For this reason, electrocardiographic monitoring assumes prime importance in the management of this disorder. The typical recorded electrocardiographic changes in hyperkalemia, as shown in Figure 13–1, should be recognizable by the entire staff, including those nurses who are engaged in the immediate care of the patient. The changes seen in Stage III indicate an emergency requiring the most aggressive measures for rapid decline of the serum potassium level toward normal. Early stages are indicative of impending disaster but can generally be managed by more conservative means. Management of hyperkalemia requires immediate cessation of potassium intake. It is surprising how often one finds patients in renal failure receiving oral fluids or intravenous solutions containing potassium. Fruit juices, coffee, tea, and broth are all sources of considerable potassium and should be rigidly eliminated from the diet. An oral regimen consisting of water and special diets composed only of fat and carbohydrates should be used. Ringer's lactate solution contains potassium and should be avoided.

Hyperkalemia in oliguric renal failure can usually be controlled by a combination of cessation of potassium intake and removal of potassium from the body by sodium polystyrene sulfonate. This material (Kayexalate) is administered in 30 ml of sorbitol to which sufficient water has been added to make the mixture ingestible. This combination is best given orally, but if the gastrointestinal tract is not functioning, it can also be administered rectally. Repeated instillations of Kayexalate will result in control of the level of serum potassium in the vast majority of patients, and indeed, hyperkalemia as an indication for dialysis should rarely occur.

The next most serious compound retained in oliguric renal failure is water. Most patients enter the phase of oliguric renal failure with an

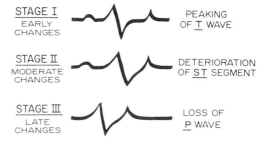

Figure 13–1. Stages of electrocardiographic evidence of hyperkalemia.

STAGE I
EARLY CHANGES
PEAKING OF T WAVE

STAGE II
MODERATE CHANGES
DETERIORATION OF ST SEGMENT

STAGE III
LATE CHANGES
LOSS OF P WAVE

expanded extracellular fluid compartment because vigorous attempts have been made to institute adequate urine flow. Careful avoidance of overhydration by repeated measurement of the central venous pressure will minimize the likelihood of overhydration, although its presence must be assumed in the majority of instances. The day-to-day water requirement of a patient in oliguric renal failure is much less than is generally appreciated. If there are no extrarenal losses of water, then the total loss consists of the basal insensible water loss from the skin and lungs and amounts to 12 ml per kg per day. The loss is partially offset by the production of water that results from the metabolism of glucose. In the postoperative period, this may yield 300 to 400 ml of water per day so that the average-sized adult patient's water deficit is as little as 500 to 600 ml. A useful guide to the state of hydration is the serum sodium concentration. If there are no extrarenal sodium losses, then accurate water replacement will result in a constant concentration of sodium in the extracellular fluid. When extrarenal sodium and water losses are present, such as those that occur from gastric drainage, enterotomies, and fistulas, then these losses must be accurately measured with regard to both volume and electrolyte composition, and they should be quantitatively replaced. A second useful guide to the degree of hydration is accurate daily weighing of the patient. If the patient is fasting, then a weight loss of approximately one pound per day should occur. Maintenance of a steady weight indicates a continuing degree of overhydration.

Modern dialytic therapy is aimed at maintaining the internal environment within normal limits. There is considerable evidence that the maintenance of the blood urea nitrogen in the normal range by frequent dialytic therapy will lessen the incidence of infection and wound disruption, which are so frequently the terminal complications of the patient with acute renal failure. It is our practice to prepare patients for dialysis with an arteriovenous shunt as soon as the diagnosis of tubular necrosis has been made. The frequency of dialysis is determined by the metabolic state of the patient, the degree of tissue damage, and the presence of infection. Clinical evidence of uremia should never be allowed to develop in these patients, and, indeed, with frequent and adequate dialysis, a near normal metabolic state can be maintained.

Peritoneal dialysis can be used in situations in which the necessary equipment for hemodialysis is not available. Unfortunately, peritoneal dialysis is frequently inapplicable to the surgical patient because of the presence of intraperitoneal drains and open retroperitoneal areas or other factors that destroy the fluid-containing properties of the parietal peritoneum. Peritoneal dialysis may have a place in the treatment of acute renal failure in association with open-heart or thoracic surgical procedures when the peritoneal cavity has not been disturbed. This is particularly true when the presence of suture lines in the heart or major blood vessels makes the use of heparin dangerous. Several recent studies have indicated that early aggressive peritoneal dialytic therapy is helpful in the management of postperfusion renal tubular necrosis.

After the patient has been successfully managed through the period of oliguric renal failure, a period of polyuric renal failure generally occurs prior to complete recovery. This period of polyuric failure is identical with the high urine output form of acute renal failure that occurs in patients who have been well hydrated prior to the development of the renal insult. It is imperative that an appreciation of the nature of the diuresis and the overall state of hydration of the patient be continuously assessed. In certain patients, the magnitude of the diuresis represents a restoration toward normal hydration by a recovering kidney in a patient who was previously suffering from fluid overload. In this circumstance, it is a serious therapeutic error to attempt to keep up with the diuresis. The replacement of the lost fluid will result in the development of further fluid overload and possible congestive heart failure. On the other hand, the excessive urine volume may result from failure of the tubular mechanism to produce a concentrated urine and, therefore, is a signal that glomerular filtrate is being lost quantitatively from the body. Measurements of urine:plasma osmolar ratio and the glomerular filtration rate are helpful. If renal function is improving, the diuresis will be associated with a rising GFR and urine:plasma osmolar ratio. If the renal function tests remain at their previous abnormal levels, then the diuresis must be quantitatively replaced since it represents uncontrollable losses. Sodium losses at this time may be very large owing to the high sodium content of urine in high output renal failure. The safest procedure is to obtain daily electrolyte determinations of both urine and plasma and then to quantitatively replace the measured losses. Certain patients in the recovery phase of oliguric acute tubular necrosis will demonstrate a continuing rise of the blood urea nitrogen in the diuretic recovery phase. If the urine:plasma ratio remains at unity, further dialysis may be required, just as in the management of high-output renal failure. Therapy should not be terminated until the internal metabolic environment has returned to normal.

14

Multiple Systems Failure

ARTHUR E. BAUE

As our knowledge and capabilities improve, the problems that we encounter change. Previous problems decrease in frequency and importance, and new problems appear. In recent years, improvement in the evaluation and care of patients before, during, and after operations and after injury has resulted in a new clinical syndrome of multiple organ or systems failure. The purpose of this chapter is to review the present problems of organ failure as they relate to preoperative and postoperative care and the relationships between organ systems that are now being studied. This syndrome also reminds us of our continuing limitations in the care of the injured patient. Formerly, failure of one system or organ, such as the circulation or the lungs, heart, or kidneys, would often be fatal. Now, prevention or treatment of these problems has allowed for survival of many of these patients. With severe injuries or complications, however, a number of organs may fail together or in sequence, resulting in what we have called multiple, progressive, or sequential system or organ failure (Baue, 1975; Baue and Chaudry, 1980; Eiseman et al., 1977; Tilney et al., 1973). Ways to prevent these problems are not yet well understood, and support of multiple organ failure is difficult; moreover, it is accompanied by excessive morbidity, a high mortality, and great emotional and financial cost to the patient, family, and society.

In previous chapters, the evaluation and methods of support of individual organ systems, including the cardiovascular system, lungs, and kidneys, have been reviewed. Chapters are included in this edition on other physiologic functions, each of which must be considered a system that can fail. These include the liver, the central nervous system, gastrointestinal system, musculoskeletal system, coagulation, host defenses, and metabolism.

EVOLUTION OF THE CONCEPT OF MULTIPLE SYSTEMS FAILURE

At any particular time in recent surgical history, there has been a single limiting organ system that was the primary factor resulting in morbidity and mortality after injury. At the beginning of World War II, the cardiovascular system and shock were the major problems. Hypovolemic shock and adequate volume replacement were not well understood. As these concepts and an understanding of the problems involved were developed, the treatment of shock greatly improved. The mystique of wound shock was eliminated by hemodynamic studies, and shock was no longer the single, most important limiting factor in survival. Throughout the Korean conflict, the kidney became the limiting organ system. The U. S. Army Surgical Research Unit used the phrase, "post-traumatic renal insufficiency," which occurred 20 to 30 times more commonly in Korea than in the Vietnam conflict. As an understanding of the factors producing renal insufficiency developed, this problem was more frequently prevented by rapid resuscitation of the patient and support of the kidney. Moreover, when renal failure did occur, it was treated more satisfactorily. Nothing was written about the lung by the Army research team during the Korean war. During the Vietnam war, however, the lung increasingly became a problem referred to as "post-traumatic pulmonary insufficiency." The lung then became the limiting organ system, both in civilian and military practice. This raised the question as to whether this happened because better resuscitation and support of the cardiovascular and renal systems exposed the lung as the next limiting organ, or whether aggressive and perhaps, on occasion, excessive fluid resuscitation jeopardized the lung. Probably both of these were contributing factors in this development. In the past 15 years, surgeons have identified and studied this problem, and respiratory failure is now being prevented more regularly. When it is not prevented, it can often be treated satisfactorily. Mortality from ventilatory failure as an isolated problem should now be fairly low.

In recent years mortality has not been secondary so much to failure of a single system but rather to the complex of multiple organ failure. Morbidity and death after operation or injury still occur from thromboembolism, acute vascular occlusions or infarction, shock, posttraumatic renal failure, post-traumatic pulmonary failure, sepsis and peritonitis, and other complications. However, each of these problems occurring by itself can be treated reasonably well. Renal failure associated with sepsis and respiratory or liver failure still has a grave prognosis, but renal failure in itself is no longer a critical event. The incidence of renal failure in the injured in Vietnam was only 0.2 per cent, but the mortality in those who developed it was 63 per cent, owing to associated injuries and sepsis rather than to renal failure itself. When these problems occur in combination or in sequence, we often reach the limiting edge of our present capabilities for providing support and promoting survival of such patients. Recognition of multiple or sequential systems failure as a current problem is now leading to study and description of how some of these sequences or simultaneous events occur and how they might be prevented.

DEFINITION OF MULTIPLE SYSTEMS FAILURE

When more than one system cannot support its activities spontaneously, then the problem of multiple systems failure is present. Failure of the cardiovascular system is defined as hypotension, low or marginal cardiac output, or in general terms as an inadequate circulation that requires pharmacologic and/or mechanical circulatory assistance. Ventilatory failure is defined as the requirement for assisted ventilation in order to maintain adequate gas exchange, including elimination of carbon dioxide and oxygenation. Renal failure is defined as the inability of the kidneys to regulate water volume and electrolytes and remove waste products. The definition of hepatic failure is inexact at present but includes an elevated bilirubin, markedly elevated hepatic enzyme levels, and an end stage that is manifested by hepatic coma. Gastrointestinal failure is the inability of the gut to function in maintaining nutrition by oral intake and/or gastrointestinal bleeding that becomes life-threatening. Failure of the metabolic or muscular system or both is a twofold problem: (1) failure to provide for anabolism and to prevent the central metabolic problems of catabolism and (2) the catabolism of skeletal muscle with loss of strength, producing problems with coughing, ventilation, inability to ambulate, development of decubitus ulcers, and other problems. Failure of the immune system is exemplified by the development of sepsis that is unexpected or difficult to control or cannot be eliminated. Failure of the coagulation system could present as diffuse intravascular coagulation on one hand or primary bleeding problems on the other. Failure of the central nervous system is defined as decreased or depressed sensorium or coma. When the central nervous system is injured, however, it often becomes the limiting system that prevents survival. Whether or not several organs fail progressively or sequentially or whether organ failure occurs all at once depends upon the severity of the insult and the preinjury or preoperative state of the individual.

There are numerous lethal combinations in which several organs failing together may produce a fatal result because of certain specific relationships. Renal failure and ventilatory failure occurring together are a potentially lethal combination because, as renal failure is diagnosed or as it occurs, there usually are efforts to prevent it or alter it by infusing large amounts of fluid. This overloads the lungs, and there may be no immediate way to excrete this excess fluid other than by dialysis. Another combination that produces a particular problem is that of ventilatory failure and metabolic failure. A patient who requires a ventilator and is catabolic with decreased muscular strength may not be able to be weaned from the ventilator because of an inability to breathe spontaneously. An example is the patient with end-stage valvular heart disease and cardiac cachexia. It may be possible to replace the valves, thereby restoring good cardiovascular function, but the patient still has such loss of muscle mass that spontaneous ventilation is impossible and secondary complications occur. A ruptured aneurysm with renal failure has been a particularly lethal combination owing to shock, problems of cross-clamping the aorta, atherosclerotic embolization, and vascular disease of the kidney. However, patients with this problem have survived when other problems did not develop. Cardiac failure and ventilatory failure occurring together are difficult because the treatment of ventilatory failure, including high levels of positive end expiratory pressure, may alter cardiac output and adversely influence cardiovascular function. Finally, the combination of peritonitis, ventilatory failure, and cardiovascular instability is a common one that is often lethal unless the primary problem of peritonitis can be controlled.

FACTORS CONTRIBUTING TO THE DEVELOPMENT OF MULTIPLE SYSTEMS FAILURE

By reviewing the clinical characteristics of patients who develop these overwhelming problems, recognizable patterns begin to emerge. From these patterns the beginning steps toward prevention can be derived. Although some patients before operation or injury may have altered organ function as a result of chronic and degenerative diseases such as atherosclerosis, many are otherwise healthy young individuals with no prior organ limitations. The common factors in patients who develop this syndrome include the following: (1) multiple systems injury or extensive soft tissue injury and/or a major extensive operation; (2) a period of shock accompanying injury or operation (successful resuscitation of the patient from the initial circulatory depression may have taken place); (3) requirement for multiple blood transfusions; (4) continued cardiovascular instability with a marginal cardiac output; (5) renal injury or an alteration in renal blood flow that may not be evident initially and not documentable until renal insufficiency becomes overt; (6) marginal ventilatory function with atelectasis, aspiration, fat embolism, and other problems; (7) hepatic dysfunction, which may only be evident later; (8) severe catabolism, which is often a contributing factor with a depressed immune response; (9) major bleeding, which may have occurred during the initial insult or later; and (10) invasive sepsis, particularly within the peritoneal or thoracic cavities, which is often the final insult or which may begin the process of organ failure. In recent reviews of this syndrome, invasive sepsis has been the most common and characteristic ingredient.

Thus, the setting for this problem exists most frequently in a patient (1) with a severe metabolic insult secondary to trauma, operation, or both; (2) in whom a clinical or technical error may have occurred; and (3) a patient who develops sepsis, particularly peritonitis. Multiple organ failure can occur of course without recognizable clinical or technical errors or sepsis.

A common sequence in the injured patient is to have an initial period of shock or circulatory instability and decreased renal function immediately after the injury, which seems to respond favorably to adequate resuscitation. The patient then is operated upon or treated for the injuries and subsequently develops pulmonary failure. This is associated with decreased cardiac function, particularly right ventricular failure, which is followed by hepatic failure. Following this, there may be failure of the kidneys, sepsis, metabolic failure, coagulation changes, and other problems (Border et al., 1976).

THE ORGAN ASSOCIATIVE OR SYSTEMS RELATIONSHIP PERIOD

We are now entering a period in which it is necessary to learn more about the relationship between various organs and how they influence one another. Although much has been known about this in the past, many critical relationships have not been understood. As relationships between systems and the occurrence of sequential events like a domino effect are studied, the hazards of post hoc ergo propter hoc reasoning must be recognized. Two events occurring simultaneously or sequentially may or may not have a cause-and-effect relationship.

An important area of study has been that of the frequency and possible causes of an organ failing in association with a disease process that is remote to that organ. Pancreatitis, for example, is frequently associated with ventilatory failure and pulmonary edema. There has been speculation that this may be due to pulmonary alveolar–capillary membrane damage produced by some factor liberated from the necrotic pancreas, such as pancreatic enzymes (phospholipase A), vasoactive substances, or circulating free fatty acids. Many other factors, however, may contribute to this problem in pancreatitis; the patient is catabolic and may have sepsis, the abdomen is distended, the hemidiaphragms are elevated, pleural effusions may be present, and the circulation is altered, all of which can contribute to the development of ventilatory failure. Patients with pancreatitis may also have myocardial depression. It is now recognized that the combination of peritonitis and intra-abdominal sepsis is commonly associated with pulmonary failure. There has been speculation and laboratory experimental evidence that the septic process produces a circulating factor that may cause capillary endothelial damage in the lung. The earliest evidence for an effect of sepsis on the lung may be a rise in pulmonary vascular resistance and an increase in pulmonary extravascular water. The mechanisms for this could be the effects on the pulmonary microcirculation and permeability of immune complexes, granulocyte aggregation, complement activation platelets, fibrin, the kallikrein-kinin system, or the prostaglandin system through arachidonic acid and lipoxygenases. There are also other features of sepsis that could be involved in the production of ventilatory failure. The same is true for sepsis and renal failure. Infection now seems to be a much more common cause of renal failure than other factors, such as shock. Gram-negative infection was recognized in the Vietnam war as the cause of acute renal failure in some surgical patients. There may be some specific factor produced by the septic process that alters renal function and sets the stage for organ failure. Septic patients with a hyperdynamic circulation will usually have increased renal blood flow and decreased renal vascular resistance. They also often initially have polyuria, which could be due to increased serum osmolality secondary to sepsis or an injury to the glomerulus or the juxtaglomerular tubules, causing decreased medullary hypertonicity and decreased reabsorption from the collecting tubules (Lucas, 1976). The final insult to the kidney that produces failure with sepsis is probably insufficient blood fiow and cortical ischemia. Polyuria in the septic patient suggests good renal function, satisfactory renal perfusion, and adequate hydration, which may delude the unwary.

The hepatorenal syndrome is an example of an organ associative problem that has been recognized for a long time but has not been well understood. Liver disease produces alterations in the metabolism of aldosterone, and through the renin angiotensin mechanism may produce changes in renal blood flow by a redistribution of the intrarenal circulation and decreased cortical flow. The deposition of false neurochemical transmitters producing intrarenal shunting has also been suggested, as has an effect on endotoxin. The decreased cortical flow may not be sufficient in itself to damage the kidney but does place the organ in jeopardy if any further, albeit minor, insult occurs. The addition of a minor circulatory change, such as a small hemorrhage or paracentesis with a fluid shift, which in itself may be innocuous, may produce renal failure. Thus, a kidney from a patient with the hepatorenal syndrome and renal failure may be transplanted and work satisfactorily in the recipient.

Another example of this organ associative phenomenon is the finding that recently recognized deficiency states can alter organ function. For example, hypophosphatemia, identified with increasing frequency as a cause of a number of systemic problems, has now been found to be a factor in ventilatory failure. Patients have been reported with ventilatory failure that responded completely to inorganic phosphate administration.

The nutritional state of an individual has now been found to be related to his or her ability to increase ventilation in response to hypoxia. Semistarvation for 10 days in otherwise normal individuals produces no change in their ability to increase ventilation in response to hypercapnia. However, the ability of the individual to respond to hypoxia is severely blunted so that reduction of the arterial PO_2 to approximately 45 mm Hg produces little change in minute volume of ventilation. The injured and semistarved individual is susceptible then to hypoxia and may be less able to compensate for it. Thus semistarvation, which occurs in many of our injured and operated patients, seems to blunt a physiologic response that should be protective for that individual.

The relationships of host resistance and immunologic defense mechanisms to injury, operation, and starvation are now being explored more thoroughly. Hemorrhagic shock, even when treated adequately, seems to predispose to infection by mechanisms such as vasoconstriction, decreased opsonization of bacteria and neutrophil phagocytosis, and depression of the reticuloendothelial system. A surgical procedure in itself may be associated with a number of temporary deficits in the immune system. An important recent development has been the documentation that patients with protein-calorie malnutrition or brief periods of starvation have altered immunocompetence and host resistance. Acquired failure of host defenses does occur. Anergy or relative anergy to the injection of skin antigens has been associated with decreased neutrophil chemotaxis, decreased lymphocyte rosette formation, and a high mortality rate from infection (MacLean et al., 1975). If such anergic or relatively anergic patients were given adequate nutrition and the infection was treated, their responsiveness to skin antigens increased and their mortality rate decreased. It has been documented that the thymus (T) and bone marrow (B) cell immune systems are impaired by protein-calorie malnutrition and that adequate nutrition will restore immunocompetence (Law et al., 1973). Other measures of altered host resistance have been the decrease in opsonic proteins, particularly the C3 component of complement in patients who did not have adequate nutritional support. Such patients also had an alteration in neutrophil function. A severe depression in the ability of a factor called fibronectin in the plasma to support Kupffer cell phagocytosis has been found in injured patients who did not survive. Another associated problem is the increase in risk infection and of coagulation problems in patients with renal failure. Renal insufficiency is associated with impaired wound healing, diminished cellular immunity, and decreased lymphocyte activity.

The association of sepsis, pulmonary failure, and right ventricular failure is recognized but not well understood. This is another example of an organ associative phenomenon of impaired cardiac output and increased pulmonary vascular resistance in patients with acute respiratory failure. In normal individuals, pulmonary vascular resistance is fairly independent of cardiac output. However, in patients with acute respiratory failure who have a low cardiac index, the pulmonary vascular resistance may be extremely high. Conversely, with a high cardiac index, pulmonary vascular resistance may be much lower in such patients. This is an enigma, but it could be the reason why patients with a decreased cardiac output and ventilatory failure develop right heart failure. The right ventricle may be jeopardized by having to work excessively against the high pressure of increased pulmonary vascular resistance. The reason for the increase in pulmonary vascular resistance, which occurs in some patients after injury or with sepsis, has not been established.

Intestinal ischemia occurring without mesenteric vascular occlusion is believed to be caused by severe vasoconstriction of the mesenteric arteries in response to a reduction in cardiac output. This can occur in patients with a variety of cardiovascular diseases and can progress to infarction. Underlying causes are many — hypovolemia, cardiogenic shock, digitalis toxicity, severe sepsis, and intracardiac operations. The mesenteric vasoconstriction and ischemia may be manifested clinically by abdominal pain and distention, fever, hemoconcentration, high hematocrit, and leukocytosis. Less severe ischemia may be masked by other problems. There may be deterioration of renal function as well. Confirmation of the diagnosis requires selective catheterization of the superior mesenteric artery to demonstrate narrow, thin vessels, indicating mesenteric vasoconstriction. Management consists of infusion of papaverine into the superior mesenteric artery at 30 to 60 mg per hr by a continuous infusion pump following or concomitant with appropriately indicated measures to improve cardiac output or restore it to normal. The course of the patient determines whether or not a laparotomy is necessary because of the possibility of infarcted gut. Intestinal ischemia due to decreased cardiac output may also result in inability of the gut to function adequately even though it does not progress to infarction.

The importance of the liver in this syndrome has recently been recognized, and the term "post-traumatic hepatic failure" is now being used. The factors that can contribute to postoperative or postinjury jaundice include (1) anesthetic agents, particularly halothane, (2) an increased pigment load from red cell breakdown following massive transfusions, (3) infection and septicemia, (4) hemolysis, (5) various drugs, (6) congestive heart failure, (7) extravasated blood, (8) underlying liver disease and unrecognized hepatitis, and (9) hepatic ischemia and/or hypoxia from circulatory depression or shock. After a severe injury many patients develop a small increase in serum bilirubin level. In most patients, particularly those who survive, this reaches a peak four to eight days after the injury and usually returns to normal by 10 to 12 days. The degree of jaundice in this early period does not seem to be related to the presence of sepsis, ventilatory support, operation, or anesthesia. The one factor common to many of these patients is a period of hypotension after the injury. Thus, hepatic dysfunction after trauma seems to occur often and is probably related to a period of hypotension and decreased hepatic blood flow with cellular hypoxia or anoxia. The primary alteration in function is an impairment of hepatic cellular excretory function resembling intrahepatic cholestasis. In patients who do not survive a severe injury, there may be a rapidly and progressively rising serum bilirubin level that does not peak and return toward normal, suggesting an unfavorable prognosis related to a more severe liver injury.

There seem to be three somewhat separate time courses of hepatic difficulty following an injury or an operation. The early mild elevation of serum bilirubin is probably secondary to transfusions, hematoma absorption, the anesthetic agent, and other such transient phenomena. If the hyperbilirubinemia becomes more marked and persists for a longer period of time, reaching its peak about 8 to 12 days after the insult, then the problem is probably hepatic dysfunction secondary to the injury, hypotension, decreased hepatic perfusion, and hypoxic injury to hepatocytes. In the third type, the rise in serum bilirubin is even more marked, peaks later, and seems clearly to be associated with sepsis. After a period of shock there is enzymatic and also morphologic evidence, both by light and electron microscopy, of cellular damage and intrahepatic cholestasis in the liver. In experimental shock studies, the liver has been found to be injured earlier and more severely than other organs. Right heart failure and elevated venous pressure can produce acute alterations in the liver just as they occur in cardiac cirrhosis. Changes in the hepatic reticuloendothelial system with injury may be very important in the development or perpetuation of infection, particularly from the peritoneal cavity. Thermally injured patients seem to have an alteration in liver function in which hepatic cell membrane transport is depressed. This seems to be related to a deficiency of glucose and can be corrected by provision of large amounts of glucose. Parenteral nutrition with intravenous amino acids and glucose frequently results in elevations of serum hepatic enzymes and bilirubin. Explanations for these findings have not been clearly documented but include the toxic effects of breakdown products of tyrosine or tryptophan, essential fatty acid deficiency, an excessively high calorie:nitrogen ratio, and other theoretical possibilities yet to be studied. These findings serve to emphasize the importance of the liver in the ability of a patient to respond to injury and support metabolism. Post-traumatic hepatic insufficiency is still incompletely defined but is an important and perhaps critical event in multiple organ failure.

There is now increased recognition of a combination of metabolic defects in injured and operated patients that could best be called energy problems. Certainly the reduction in lean body mass and loss of muscle strength with prolonged catabolism are energy problems that can threaten the viability of an individual. Now we have learned that there are other problems that occur with decreased energy or produce an energy crisis, either acute or chronic, in a patient with ischemia, hypoxia, and/or decreased blood flow. The requirements of the wound for energy, particularly for glucose, are now being documented. The wound and its constituents — cells for defense and repair — are high-glucose and high–energy-requiring cells. Altered host resistance occurs if energy needs are not met. Physiologic defenses are depressed with starvation as previously indicated. Decreased visceral proteins and now altered organ function can be documented if adequate glucose as an energy source is not provided. Reserves against ischemia are diminished, and cell function is altered with depletion of energy, substrates and the high-energy phosphate compounds (ATP and ADP) in the cell. These are all related to the problem of providing for cell and organ energetics and function.

Thus, nutrition has become a problem not merely of maintaining muscle strength and body weight but also a matter of maintaining the overall integrity of the entire organism.

Detailed studies of the metabolic effects of sepsis with multiple systems organ failure in patients have been described in a series of papers by Border and Cerra (McMenamy et al., 1981) and their group. They have defined a peripheral metabolic defect which reduces oxidative catabolism of conventional energetic fuels, glucose, fatty acids and triglycerides and enhances the catabolism of essential branched chain amino acids. Along with this there is reduced hepatic protein synthesis and increased albumin catabolism. This produces an "autocannibalism" of skeletal muscle, and they ascribe the ultimate death of such a patient to metabolic exhaustion.

CLINICAL APPROACH TO THE PROBLEMS OF MULTIPLE SYSTEMS FAILURE

Although better methods of support of failing organs will be developed, this syndrome should be preventable in many patients by not allowing the organs to fail, either singly or in multiples. This requires an understanding of the etiology of the problem and adequate evaluation and organ support during and after the injury and operation, including (1) preoperative evaluation of organ function, (2) preoperative improvement in organ function whenever possible by precise treatment or delay of urgent or elective procedures while support is being provided, (3) accurate and adequate support during the operation with monitoring of the various organs and their functions, (4) a concise operation without defects, and (5) postoperative care that anticipates the possibility of organ failure in various settings and studies interorgan relationships and dependencies.

PREOPERATIVE EVALUATION

The evaluation must go beyond determining whether the patient will tolerate an operation or not. In patients approaching an elective or urgent operation, evaluation of the limits or weak links in each of the various organ systems is necessary unless the function and reserve of an organ system is completely normal by history and physical examination. Obviously in an emergency the systems evaluation must be cursory during resuscitation and initial treatment. Proper timing of the operation is a critical decision. Postponing an elective operation for several days to improve pulmonary function by exercises, postural drainage, and medications may be lifesaving. In a patient with a large incisional hernia, preoperative decompression of the gastrointestinal tract may make repair easier and prevent ventilatory embarrassment and wound separation after the procedure. On the other hand, allowing intraperitoneal sepsis to continue without intervention for even a few hours may contribute to death in the postoperative period.

Ventilatory Reserve. Not every patient having a major operative procedure requires in-depth evaluation of pulmonary function. Adequacy of ventilation can be documented by a brief history and observation of the patient. If these are not totally normal, then measurement of arterial blood gas tensions with the patient breathing room air and simple exercises such as climbing stairs should be carried out. This should provide information as to whether more detailed studies are in order. If a patient is known to have limited pulmonary function, heavy smoking, asthma, emphysema, or other problems, then methods of improvement in lung function should be considered before the operation. A patient with chronic lung disease who has an intensive respiratory care program for a few days may be able to tolerate an operative procedure without ventilatory failure. Such patients, when recognized, can also be supported during and after the operation so that this organ system does not begin the cycle of progressive organ deterioration.

Cardiovascular Function. Estimation of capability and reserve of the cardiovascular system is essential. The patient with marginal cardiac function and borderline congestive heart failure may seem normal except for a gallop rhythm. Excess fluid may not be apparent. The possibility of arrhythmias must be considered. Intermittent or prolonged uncontrolled hypertension can be a problem. Again, these can be evaluated by history and physical examination. If this system seems to have marginal reserve, particularly in myocardial function, blood pressure control, or rhythm, then measures should be taken to insure optimal function before an elective procedure. If cardiovascular function is quite limited but an operation or repair of an injury is mandatory, then support measures may be required in the preoperative period. This may require vasoactive drugs such as inotropic agents to improve ventricular performance. Elective digitalization preoperatively may decrease myocardial stress when a higher cardiac output is required or may control heart rate if an arrhythmia occurs. Stabilization of blood pressure before operation may prevent fluctuations in blood pressure, which jeopardize organ perfusion. With severe circulatory depression, support mechanisms such as the intra-aortic balloon may be required.

Renal Function. Evaluation of renal function by measurement of creatinine and blood urea nitrogen gives some evidence that the kidneys can cope with the patient's present situation. It does not give much indication, however, as to renal reserve with stress, and, in certain individuals, this should be tested by appropriate studies. If renal function is impaired, then one is forewarned that renal blood flow and a diuresis must be maintained at all costs and that it may be necessary to use external support such as dialysis early after the operative procedure. Patients with permanent and complete renal failure can now undergo operations for a number of problems. If they are properly cared for with well-planned dialysis and fluid programs, they should have excellent possibilities for survival.

Liver Function. The recognition of decreased hepatic reserve or liver disease such as cirrhosis indicates the need for as much nutritional and metabolic support as is possible preoperatively and for early nutritional and metabolic support in the postoperative period while minimizing the insult to the liver.

Gastrointestinal Function. A history of prior gastrointestinal problems, particularly ulcer disease, prior bleeding episodes, and inflammatory diseases may alert the surgeon to careful postoperative care in support of this organ system.

Metabolic Function. Evaluation of the metabolic system of an individual presently consists of an estimation of weight loss and weakness. In the future the reserve of this system will be evaluated in more detail. The ability of the metabolic system to support host resistance against infection can be estimated now by various skin tests.

With injury, where preoperative evaluation must of necessity be limited, it is important to recognize the types of injury, the extent of shock, and other factors that will contribute to organ dysfunction. The recognition that hepatic dysfunction frequently occurs after injury when the patient has had a period of shock indicates that in the immediate postinjury phase, metabolic support of the liver becomes a critical matter. The recognition that after a period of shock the kidney may, for a period of time, have increased renal vascular resistance and decreased cortical blood flow alerts one to the necessity of protecting the kidney even after the period of shock seems to have been solved by fluid replacement.

SUPPORT DURING THE OPERATIVE PROCEDURE

This must be emphasized in four areas: (1) selection of an anesthetic technique that maximally supports organ function and does not introduce agents that may depress or jeopardize a particular organ such as the liver, the cardiovascular system, or the kidneys; (2) careful monitoring of organ performance, particularly the cardiovascular system, the lungs, and the kidneys, maintaining organ function at optimal levels; (3) an appropriate and carefully done operation. The possibility of technical error must be minimized to eliminate wound dehiscence, anastomotic breakdown, inadvertent occlusion of ducts and vessels, and other problems. (4) Potential complications that can be predicted in a particular patient must be considered during the operative procedure, and preventive measures must be taken.

Elderly patients having hip operations and others who have a high incidence of thromboembolic complications should have a preventive program such as minidose heparin instituted before and during the operative procedure. With peritoneal contamination and bowel injury, precautions must be taken to eliminate the possibility of continuing peritonitis and abscess formation. Exteriorization of bowel or proximal decompression is preferable to a marginal anastomosis that may leak. The prevention of dehiscence by an all-layer closure, the prevention of wound infection by delayed primary closure, and a decrease in intra-peritoneal abscess formation by thorough irrigation, appropriate drain-age, or insertion of lavage catheters can greatly reduce the insults that set the stage for multiple systems failure. The most important key then to prevention of this syndrome is to prevent complications after the injury and the operation.

POSTOPERATIVE CARE

Excellent postoperative care that maximally supports all organs should help to prevent multiple systems failure. A number of specific recommendations and guidelines can now be provided because of recent experiences with this syndrome.

1. Adequate monitoring of the various systems is critical in provid-ing early support to prevent organ failure rather than cope with it after it becomes an established problem. Cardiovascular monitoring must in-clude accurate measurement of arterial blood pressure and, in the severely injured patient, an estimate of both left and right atrial pres-sures to determine adequacy of circulating vascular volume and ventric-ular capability. Since in many of these patients a marginal cardiac output may be the key problem (in spite of an adequate blood pressure), measurement of cardiac output by the thermodilution technique should be available. This has become an increasingly important factor in preventing this syndrome (Chap. 40). Monitoring of renal function must include not only urine volume measurements but also intermittent assessment of the ability of the patient to concentrate and excrete waste products. Ventilatory functions must be monitored not only by ausculta-tion, observation of ventilation, and chest roentgenograms as necessary but also by periodic arterial blood gas tension measurements. Accurate assessment and monitoring of the metabolic system and of the liver do not as yet provide information that can be used prospectively, but this may be forthcoming.

2. The lungs are often the first system to fail. Therefore, ventilatory support should be continued after operation or injury whenever prob-lems are anticipated. This is particularly true in patients with peritonitis, pancreatitis, or severe multiple injuries. Cardiac surgeons have learned to relieve the patient of the extra burden of spontaneous ventilation during the first 12 to 24 hours after a cardiac operation. Ventilatory support during this critical period will preserve pulmonary function and

often prevent failure. Such patients should not be extubated in the recovery room but should have the endotracheal tube left in place. Ventilatory support should be provided until the patient can ventilate satisfactorily and the physician is satisfied that the patient will not deteriorate and develop ventilatory problems later. This may require a day or as long as a week of support, depending on the severity of the problem. In the critical period after an operation for peritonitis, there may be residual infection and continuing pulmonary damage. If such a patient is required to breathe spontaneously and to maintain his or her own alveolar inflation, it may set the stage for the development of multiple systems failure.

Ventilatory failure should be prevented by early support before the lungs fail. The technology of ventilatory support is such that it can be accomplished safely and with minimal risk. Intubation with an indwelling endotracheal tube by the oral or nasal route should be done as the patient begins to have difficulty and long before this becomes critical for immediate survival. It has been documented repeatedly that it is much easier to maintain alveolar inflation and ventilation than it is to try to get the lung reinflated after a period of extensive alveolar collapse. Early use of low levels of positive end expiratory pressure (PEEP) may help to prevent the adult respiratory distress syndrome. This effect is exerted by increasing functional residual capacity and balancing regional ventilation and perfusion.

3. An adequate circulation and cardiac output must be maintained by circulatory support, using vasoactive agents early to support the circulation before it fails and produces remote organ failure. There is no single agent that is best for this purpose. Patients requiring an inotropic agent to improve myocardial contractility may have a trial of isoproterenol, epinephrine, or dopamine, each of which may be appropriate in certain patients. There seems to be little doubt that a marginal or inadequate circulation lies at the root of most multiple systems failure problems. This is probably true with sepsis as well; some of the mysterious effects of sepsis thought presently to be due to toxins are very likely due to circulatory alterations and inadequate organ perfusion related to the demands of the septic process. Of particular importance is the recognition that the right ventricle may dilate or fail in itself and then seemingly have an adverse effect on the left ventricle if the pericardium is intact.

4. A clear understanding of the pharmacology of the vasoactive agents is necessary, particularly those that produce vasoconstriction as a primary event and those that have an inotropic effect. Ventilatory support, particularly high levels of PEEP, may decrease cardiac output and add to circulatory inadequacy. This potential problem must be recognized, measured, and the circulation supported appropriately, often by more fluid volume. Studies in patients with the adult respiratory distress syndrome suggest that cardiac output is higher with spontane-

ous ventilation using intermittent mandatory ventilation (IMV) in combination with continuous positive airway pressure (CPAP) than with
controlled mechanical ventilation and corresponding levels of PEEP.
CPAP was more effective than the same amount of PEEP in improving
arterial oxygenation by the lung without adversely affecting cardiac
output.

5. It must be recognized that for the patient in shock, adequate and
rapid resuscitation that supports the cardiovascular system and provides
excellent renal function and urine output may require more fluid than
the lungs can tolerate. This does not mean that excess fluid was given
during the resuscitative period. The amount of fluid that is appropriate
and required during the early resuscitation period may subsequently
prove to be excessive and jeopardize the lungs. This may be a dilemma
for the surgeon early after injury. An adequate circulation and reasonable renal function must be provided. If the ventilatory system is
overwhelmed with a falling arterial PO_2 and interstitial edema, then
ventilatory support must be instituted. The volume and rate of fluids
must be carefully monitored to maintain the circulation and renal
function and to begin to restore equilibrium in the lungs.

At this time, a urine output of 25 to 50 ml per hr is adequate in most
individuals, and a higher urine output usually indicates excess fluid
administration. As soon as circulatory stability and reasonable renal
function are present, then fluid support should be reduced to a maintenance level. In order to improve pulmonary function, it may then also be
appropriate to begin to induce excretion of some of the water previously
given. Fluid restriction and diuretics such as the loop diuretic furosemide may be necessary to improve lung function after resuscitation
has been completed. Careful assessment of the circulation is required
so that hypovolemia is neither produced nor perpetuated.

6. Caution must be exercised in the infusion of large volumes of
colloid after injury and during operation. Patients have been described
who, after an injury and resuscitation with sizable amounts of colloid,
have had a period of hypertension, elevated central venous pressure,
and what seems to be fluid overload. This is probably colloid overload
and suggests that the patient should have received less colloid and more
electrolyte solution. Albumin has been used for resuscitation but is
probably not necessary. If there is respiratory failure, then albumin must
be used cautiously, if at all. In post-traumatic pulmonary insufficiency
there may be an extensive pulmonary capillary endothelial leak. Albumin may then get out into the interstitial space and into alveoli,
producing diffusion problems rather than helping to prevent them. It
may thus produce a reverse oncotic effect and lung and renal tubular
dysfunction. However, some physicians have reported improvement in
pulmonary failure when albumin and a diuretic were used together.

7. The first 36 to 72 hours after injury is the sequestration period, or
time when the third space, the wound, is taking up and secluding

extracellular fluid. When oliguria occurs during this time, fluids must be given first to try to increase urine output. Only if one is sure that the patient is normovolemic and fluids have not produced a diuresis should the use of diuretics be contemplated. The hazards of diuretics and of fluid restriction must be recognized. The mortality with oliguric renal failure requiring dialysis after injury is still high. It is mandatory, therefore, not only to try to prevent oliguric renal failure but also, if renal failure seems to be developing, to try to convert this to nonoliguric renal failure. High-output or nonoliguric renal failure allows a better survival rate; recent series report a mortality of zero. Prevention of renal failure, then, during the initial resuscitative and postoperative period requires maintenance of renal blood flow, recognition that renal vascular resistance may remain elevated for some period of time after an insult such as shock, and maintenance of diuresis to handle excessive pigment or protein loads that may be presented to the kidneys. The best way to maintain renal function is to maintain an adequate cardiac and vascular volume so that renal blood flow is adequate. After doing this it may also be helpful, if oliguria tends to recur because of other factors, to use a loop diuretic to maintain urine output even though there has been renal damage. Mannitol may be helpful in improving the intrarenal distribution of blood flow. The fine line between trying to prevent oliguric renal failure and trying to convert it to high-output renal failure may be a difficult one. A transient period of polyuria has been described immediately after operation, particularly in injured patients who have previously been in shock. The exact mechanism of this phenomenon is not understood, but it usually lasts for only a few hours and then there is return to normal urine output.

8. Later in the recovery period, or initially if the patient's primary disease is sepsis or peritonitis, a different problem with the kidneys may be present and must be recognized. Many patients with sepsis have a hyperdynamic circulation initially, particularly if they have had adequate resuscitation and fluid therapy. Such a patient may have polyuria — increased urine output. This is inappropriate in the sense that it is not due to excess fluid administration. In fact, the polyuria associated with sepsis may occur even though the patient is becoming hypovolemic. Failure to recognize this may lead to withholding fluids in the septic patient and can result in the production of renal failure due to decreased renal perfusion. The reasons for the polyuria are not well understood. It may be due to a glomerular lesion and/or injury to the juxtaglomerular tubules. A seemingly good urine output of up to 50 ml per hr in a septic patient may not be adequate, and circulatory insufficiency may be developing in spite of this. Septic patients have been reported to have urine outputs of 200 ml per hr without fluid overload. Careful monitoring of intake and output of these patients, who will often have other tubes and drains as well, is necessary. In this situation, the presence of a low urine sodium level, below 20 mEq per l, indicates inadequate renal perfusion

and the need for more intravenous fluids. Periodic measurement of urine sodium concentration is important in septic patients. In the septic patient, this situation may again jeopardize the lungs. It may be necessary to support the lungs by mechanical means while this renal response is corrected and the sepsis is brought under control.

9. Excessive sodium and particularly sodium bicarbonate should be avoided. Patients with circulatory failure develop metabolic acidosis that can be corrected only by improvement in the circulation. Correction of a low pH by sodium bicarbonate administration will not be maintained unless the circulation is improved by blood volume expansion, use of inotropic agents, or other approaches. Giving large amounts of sodium bicarbonate empirically will not produce permanent improvement in the depressed circulation with coexisting metabolic acidosis.

10. Microembolization to the lungs by particles in transfused blood occurs, but its clinical significance has not been established. Certainly there are particles of leukocytes, platelet aggregates, red cell ghosts, fibrin debris, and other material that accumulate in stored blood. This material does embolize to the lungs of patients who receive transfusions. The measurement of screen filtration pressure indicates that these particles increase the resistance of blood going through such a screen. The significance of this problem in patients with multiple transfusions and postoperative or postinjury pulmonary complications, however, is not clear. Evidence has been provided recently to suggest that these particles probably do not make very much difference. They may be so small and so few or may be lysed so rapidly in the pulmonary circulation that they do not produce pulmonary problems. Some have recommended that all patients receiving more than two blood transfusions should have the blood filtered through one of the microfilters that removes particles as small as 20 to 40 microns. It seems likely, however, that these particles do not have pathophysiologic significance in most patients. They could be a factor, however, in the marginal, elderly, or otherwise jeopardized patient. The experience in Vietnam indicates that those patients who received multiple transfusions but did not have extensive soft tissue injury did not develop post-traumatic pulmonary insufficiency. Post-traumatic pulmonary insufficiency developed in patients with massive soft tissue injuries. Thus, the use of the microfilters may be a little safer in the patient with marginal status, but in most patients it probably makes little difference. In an extracorporeal system, such as the heart-lung machine, such filters are important to prevent microembolization in the arterial system.

11. Sighing and deep breathing should take place intermittently during the operation and in the immediate postoperative period in order to maintain alveolar inflation. This should continue during the resuscitation period and afterward. The stage is often set for pulmonary complications in the recovery room where the patient is quiet, ventilation is not stimulated, and the shallow, nonsighing ventilatory pattern of the

injured and postoperative patient contributes to the beginning of severe atelectasis.

12. Dopamine is now a commonly used vasoactive agent and certainly can be a very useful and helpful one. The limitations of the drug must be understood. Dopamine, if given in high doses, may in some patients produce pulmonary hypertension. This might place a patient with right-sided cardiac insufficiency in jeopardy. The patient with ventilatory failure may already have high pulmonary vascular resistance, producing an increased workload for the right ventricle. Dopamine, by further increasing pulmonary vascular resistance, may set the stage for progressive circulatory failure. This effect could be interpreted as cardiac failure rather than an effect of dopamine.

13. It should now be possible to prevent or totally eliminate problems of stress ulceration and gastrointestinal bleeding after injury and operation. It has been well documented in patients having cardiac operations that the use of a nasogastric tube to empty the stomach before the operation, keeping the stomach empty during and after the procedure, and the periodic instillation of antacids into the stomach can virtually eliminate stress bleeding and acute ulceration. The benefits of this approach have now been confirmed in burn patients and in ICU patients, in whom the problem can be practically eliminated by careful titration of the gastric pH up to 4.0–7 with antacid, with evacuation of the stomach in between antacid administrations. There is also some evidence that cimetidine may be helpful in prospectively eliminating this problem. In most studies, it has not been as effective as antacid titration. Once stress bleeding occurs, another organ has failed, further jeopardizing the patient.

14. Early nutritional support by enteral or parenteral means must be provided, particularly in any patient for whom one would predict that adequate oral intake and adequate nutrition would not be possible during the first five days after injury. The biggest hazard has been waiting one day after another, hoping that the next day the gut will begin to work again and that the patient will take sufficient food by mouth to insure adequate nutrition. Even the young, otherwise normal individual can have changes that will jeopardize his or her chances for survival after one week of marginal nutrition supplied only by 5 per cent glucose and water. The support and preservation of muscle mass for strength, the maintenance of the various host resistance factors, and other energy needs now mandate early nutritional support within the first few days after injury. Waiting for a week or two to see what happens is no longer justifiable. The risk of parenteral nutrition is low if a careful protocol is followed (Chap. 5). Placement of a small jejunostomy catheter if a laparotomy was done will allow use of the small bowel for nutrition in many patients.

15. The use of steroids in pharmacologic doses in patients, particularly those who develop sepsis and circulatory failure, is controversial.

Evidence has been developed for and against this common practice. Prospective randomized trials of the use of steroids in the treatment of septic shock in patients suggest that there may be improvement in survival rates when such patients have received steroids. The timing of the use of these massive pharmacologic doses of steroids is another matter. If they are given early in the process, they probably are not needed. All reasonable approaches to sepsis and septic shock should be carried out first, including administration of fluids and appropriate antibiotics, drainage, and the use of inotropic vasoactive agents. If this does not rapidly support the patient and produce improvement, then steroids can be given. There should be little objection to the use of steroids when other accepted approaches do not work. The critical factors, of course, in the treatment of sepsis and septic shock are selection of the appropriate antibiotic for the organisms producing the problem, early and adequate drainage, and elimination of continuing contamination. If this is carried out and the circulation is supported, then the patient will very likely survive, and steroids will usually not be necessary. There is also recent evidence that there are variations in the adrenocortical responsiveness of individuals during severe bacterial infection. It may be that in such situations some patients may have relative adrenal insufficiency or impairment of adrenal cortical function related to the septic process. More must be learned about this, but it is another bit of evidence supporting the utilization of pharmacologic doses of steroids after a patient does not respond rapidly to conventional treatment.

16. The fact that an injury and ischemia or shock produce tissue edema and cell swelling has certainly been recognized for a long time. The anterior compartment syndrome in the calf of the individual with an acute occlusion of the common femoral artery is well recognized, as is the brain edema that occurs following a central nervous system injury. There is abundant laboratory evidence in experimental animals that cell and organ swelling and their attendant problems may be important factors in limiting restoration of the circulation after shock and ischemia. Swelling in the kidneys could well be a factor in the persistence of increased renal vascular resistance after a period of shock, in addition to the effect of aldosterone through the renin-angiotensin system. Postischemic oliguric renal failure has responded to renal decapsulation so that renal swelling does not produce increased pressure within the kidney due to a taut capsule. Evidence is now accumulating that the prevention of cell swelling in such circumstances or compensation for it may allow better organ function after an ischemic period. Preservation of organ function by cooling the kidney, the liver, or the heart during a period of ischemia to decrease metabolic load is commonly done. Methods to decrease cell swelling after an ischemic or anoxic injury, such as by infusion of hypertonic solutions (mannitol), must now be considered.

17. Whether or not skin tests should be performed on patients who might have altered host resistance in order to document this, or whether

one should move on to support nutrition in all such patients, is presently a moot point. Certainly skin tests have provided the documentation of anergy or relative anergy in depleted patients, suggesting that all such patients should have early nutritional support. The use of skin tests may be most valuable in indicating a satisfactory response to nutritional support. The provision of fresh frozen plasma or whole blood periodically in such patients will provide the complement and properdin system factors needed for host resistance.

18. With tissue injury, antibiotics should be used during the critical period of bacterial invasion. Antibiotics given several hours after the insult or invasion are ineffective, do not decrease the ability of organisms to produce infection, and may allow infection due to resistant strains. There is abundant evidence that appropriate antibiotics given immediately after the insult in appropriate concentrations can be helpful in decreasing the possibility of a bacterial inoculum becoming established in a contaminated area.

19. Early drainage of septic foci and the elimination of continuing peritoneal contamination are the cornerstones of prevention or elimination of many problems of multiple or sequential systems failure. In fact, the failure of several systems, particularly the lungs and kidneys, some time after the injury or after the operation suggests the presence of sepsis and particularly intra-abdominal sepsis of occult origin. The development of systems failure is now strongly suggestive of the diagnosis of hidden or obscure foci of injection in many patients.

The possibility of intra-abdominal sepsis must now be considered in febrile or toxic patients who develop ventilatory failure postoperatively (Vito et al., 1974) or if ventilatory function worsens in a patient with stable ventilatory failure. Although the most common early postoperative problems are still pulmonary in origin, ventilatory failure alone should rarely be fatal. When it occurs with severe intraperitoneal sepsis, then there is a high mortality in part because of the difficulty of recognizing the septic process. The same is true of renal failure. Ventilatory failure, renal failure, or hepatic failure after abdominal injury or operation may be the first clues to occult abdominal sepsis. The core body temperature measurements, leukocyte count, left shift of the leukocyte count, and gallium scan may not be helpful until it is too late. Should an exploratory laparotomy be carried out empirically in all patients who develop these problems? Certainly this should be seriously considered (Polk and Shields, 1977). Recently it has been suggested that the presence of a blood culture positive for *Bacteroides* is another indication of an intra-abdominal septic process that requires operation and drainage. The gallbladder must be considered as a site for occult abdominal infection and necrosis. The search for intra-abdominal abscesses can be helped by gray-scale ultrasonography.

20. In patients who develop renal failure, dialysis should be carried out early. With renal failure the incidence of sepsis is increased, and

there are secondary coagulation problems. Early and repeated dialysis may help to decrease these complications and maintain the patient in a better overall condition until renal function returns to normal. The criteria for dialysis in the otherwise normal individual are quite different from those in the severely injured patient, in whom catabolism, altered host resistance, and other factors play a role. Dialysis may be necessary in the immediate postinjury and postoperative period if there has been excessive fluid given for resuscitation or renal failure prophylaxis. Excess water can best be removed by peritoneal dialysis if the peritoneal cavity is clean and not injured; otherwise, hemodialysis will be necessary. Although the mortality of renal failure after injury is still said to be high, renal failure per se does not seem to play the major role in the death of an individual. The complications and other systems failures that occur in association with renal failure prevent greater survival rates.

21. In patients with severe peritoneal contamination and perhaps pancreatitis, particularly if the kidneys are jeopardized, consideration should be given to leaving catheters in for lavage and dialysis in the immediate postoperative period. Peritoneal lavage with antibiotics may provide high local levels along with removing foreign particles, devitalized debris, and digestive enzymes. This is an aggressive approach that may be lifesaving when it is necessary not only to cleanse the peritoneal cavity but also to dialyze the patient simultaneously.

22. The problem of oxygen delivery to tissues must be considered. A deficiency in the organic phosphate compound 2,3-diphosphoglycerate (DPG) increases the affinity of hemoglobin for oxygen and therefore tends to decrease the release of oxygen from hemoglobin in the capillary circulation. Deficiencies of 2,3-DPG occur in injured and operative patients owing to hypophosphatemia, acidosis, and transfusion of DPG-deficient blood. Hypophosphatemia can be treated by hyperalimentation providing adequate phosphate supplementation. Transfusion of blood with CPD used as a preservative will maintain more normal 2,3-DPG levels. Again, however, there has been debate as to whether these alterations of DPG have biologic significance in most patients. Compensation for this problem can occur by a modest increase in cardiac output. In the elderly, stressed, or marginal patient, a deficiency of this factor may contribute to peripheral hypoxia if cardiac output cannot increase. Certainly, maintaining a normal oxyhemoglobin dissociation curve is in the best interest of the severely injured and jeopardized patient.

23. For the injured, stressed, or failing liver, adequate nutrition with glucose and amino acids providing for positive nitrogen balance is necessary. For hepatic failure, more specific therapy would include provision of branched-chain amino acids and sufficient calories without aromatic amino acids to try to shut off the muscle source of aromatic amino acids, which may adversely affect the brain. Others have treated liver failure with glucagon and insulin. In liver disease and perhaps with

sepsis as well, total renal blood flow may be adequate, but there is intrarenal shunting with relatively reduced cortical flow. Thus, with hepatic failure the advice is do not diurese the failing liver.

The studies of metabolic exhaustion in patients with multiple organ failure and sepsis (McMenamy et al., 1981) indicate that better support would be provided by giving branched-chain amino acids along with short-chain fatty acids.

CONCLUSIONS

The ultimate goal is to prevent organ failure and, in particular, the development of multiple organ and systems failure so that this syndrome will gradually decrease in frequency and severity. A number of methods were described that should decrease the occurrence of this problem. The next limitation in our capability to support and help injured and operated patients will then emerge. In the meantime, there are certain specific areas in which additional study and information are necessary.

1. We must learn to better support the circulation and the kidneys without jeopardizing the lungs.

2. The relationship of sepsis, pancreatitis, and other problems to pulmonary damage and renal failure must be further defined. The frequency of pulmonary problems, ventilatory failure, and renal failure with severe sepsis, pancreatitis, and other difficulties indicates some associations that are not well understood as yet and therefore are not preventable.

3. The host resistance–immune defense mechanisms and their relationship to protein-calorie malnutrition are now being elucidated. The time course and day-to-day relationships of these factors now require definition and, particularly, further information as to the timing for intervention with parenteral nutrition in order to maintain host resistance. The possibility of circulating immunosuppressive factors must be further defined and their importance evaluated:

4. More must be learned about potential biochemical support of cell function and, therefore, organ function. This area of activity is now in its infancy. There is little information that has gone further than the experimental laboratory. This should be a very fruitful area to study and bring into the intensive care unit for support of injured patients.

5. Further definition of the effects of impaired hepatic function must be provided. Certainly post-traumatic hepatic insufficiency is now a pivotal feature in multiple systems failure. Marginal hepatic activity may play a much greater role in the organism's overall economy than is presently recognized.

6. Other combinations of events must be studied to determine whether one insult in itself not sufficient to produce organ failure may

combine with another insult and together become a critical or organ failure–producing factor. An example of this is the combination of hypoxemia and underperfusion or ischemia. Each of these problems may not be severe enough to produce a catastrophe but together could produce renal failure. There may be other combined events that together produce a significant insult.

7. The critical role of sepsis and particularly peritonitis in producing multiple organ failure requires further definition. It is predicted that the major problem with sepsis is inadequate blood flow to the various organs. Therefore, cell and organ failure probably develop on the basis of hypoxemia and ischemia. This requires further definition and better support for the circulation during septic processes.

8. Finally, methods to increase an individual's resistance to invasive infection would eliminate many of these problems.

The injured or operated patient who has experienced a severe metabolic insult has the potential for multiple systems or organ failure. Careful evaluation, a well-planned operative procedure, and excellent supportive postoperative care with elimination of clinical or technical errors and prevention of sepsis should result in survival of most such patients.

REFERENCES

Baue, A. E.: Multiple, progressive, or sequential systems failure. A syndrome of the 1970s. Arch. Surg., *110*:779, 1975.

Baue, A. E., and Chaudry, I. H.: Prevention of multiple systems failure. Surg. Clin. North Am., *60*:1167, 1980.

Border, J. R., Chenier, R., McMenamy, R. H., La Duca, J., Seibel, R., Birkhahn, R., and Yu, L.: Multiple systems organ failure: Muscle fuel deficit with visceral protein malnutrition. Surg. Clin. North Am., *56*:1147, 1976.

Clowes, G. H. A., Vucinic, M., and Weidner, M. G.: Circulatory and metabolic alterations associated with survival or death in peritonitis: Clinical analysis of 25 cases. Ann. Surg., *163*:866, 1966.

Eiseman, B., Beart, R., and Norton, L.: Multiple organ failure. Surg. Gynecol. Obstet., *144*:323, 1977.

Law, D. K., Dudrick, S. J., and Abdou, N. I.: Immunocompetence of patients with protein-calorie malnutrition. The effects of nutritional repletion. Ann. Intern. Med., *79*:545, 1973.

Lucas, C. E.: The renal response to acute injury and sepsis. Surg. Clin. North Am., *56*:953, 1976.

MacLean, L. D., Meakins, J. L., Taguchi, K., Duignan, J. P., Dhillon, K. S., and Gordon, J.: Host resistance in sepsis and trauma. Ann. Surg., *182*:207, 1975.

McMenamy, R. H., Birkhahn, R., Oswald, G., Reed, R., Rumph, C., Vaidyanath, N., Yu, L., Cerra, F. B., Sorkness, R., and Border, J. R.: Multiple systems organ failure. I. The basal state. J. Trauma, *21*:99, 1981.

Polk, H. C., Jr., and Shields, C. L.: Remote organ failure: A valid sign of occult intra-abdominal infection. Surgery, *81*:310, 1977.

Tilney, N. L., Bailey, G. L., and Morgan, A. P.: Sequential system failure after rupture of abdominal aortic aneurysms: An unsolved problem in postoperative care. Ann. Surg., *178*:117, 1973.

Vito, L., Dennis, R. C., Weisel, R. D., and Hechtman, H. B.: Sepsis presenting as acute respiratory insufficiency. Surg. Gynecol. Obstet., *138*:896, 1974.

II

The Pediatric
Surgery Patient

15

General Principles

MARC I. ROWE
MICHAEL B. MARCHILDON

Infants and children have unique morphologic and physiologic characteristics that profoundly alter their preoperative and postoperative management. These are related to the infant's adaptation to the extrauterine environment, differences in physiologic maturity of individual newborn infants, demands created by rapid growth and development, and the relatively small physical size of the pediatric patient. This chapter presents some of the problems created by these unique factors and outlines practical methods of recognizing and dealing with them effectively.

THE LOW-BIRTH-WEIGHT (LBW) BABY

A normal full-term infant has a gestational age of over 38 weeks and a body weight of greater than 2500 gm. The majority of babies who weigh under 2500 gm are prematurely born, but at least one-third are more than 38 weeks gestational age. However, because of intrauterine problems they are small for their gestational age (SGA). The surgeon must be aware of several important physiologic differences between the preterm and SGA baby.

THE PRETERM INFANT

Infants born before 38 weeks of gestation, regardless of recorded birth weight, are premature. This diagnosis is established if the gestational age is accurately known. Without an accurate gestational history, the diagnosis must be made by physical examination. Small infants with head circumferences below the 50th percentile are usually premature, since small-for-gestational-age infants have a relatively normal-sized head. The skin of the preterm infant is thin and semitransparent, and there is absence of plantar creases. The ears are soft and malleable, and the cartilage is poorly developed. Breast tissue is not palpable, and the areolae are not visible. The testicles are usually undescended, and the scrota are undeveloped, whereas in females the labia minora appear enlarged while the labia majora are relatively small.

Physiologic Characteristics

Small preterm infants can develop serious nutritional problems in the postoperative period because of inability to consume an adequate diet. The suck reflex is often weak and ineffective, gastrointestinal absorption may be inadequate, and the gastric volume may be small. Jaundice may rapidly develop after operation because of the preterm infant's impaired ability to conjugate bilirubin; this may be dangerous because of the increased susceptibility to the neurotoxic effects of unconjugated bilirubin. The lungs and the retinas of the preterm infant have increased susceptibility to high oxygen levels. Even relatively brief exposures may result in permanent blindness. There is a high incidence of hyaline membrane disease in premature infants, and this serious illness may complicate postoperative recovery. It is most frequent (35 per cent incidence) in the moderately premature infant at 31 to 36 weeks gestational age. Apnea episodes are common and may develop any time during the preoperative and postoperative period. These episodes may be brief or of prolonged duration, accompanied by cyanosis, bradycardia, and finally cardiac arrest. They may occur spontaneously, particularly in the very premature infant, or may be nonspecific signs of problems such as sepsis of hypothermia.

An increased incidence of hypoglycemia, hypocalcemia, anemia, and intraventricular hemorrhage occurs in preterm infants. The most common circulatory problem is associated with the transitional circulation and the high incidence of patent ductus arteriosus. Persistence of the patent ductus arteriosus may lead to bidirectional shunting and serious congestive heart failure, particularly if large volumes of fluid and electrolyte solutions are delivered to the postoperative infant.

Practical Considerations

Preoperative and postoperative chest roentgenograms of the preterm infant who has respiratory difficulties are essential in detecting hyaline membrane disease and can be helpful in recognizing congestive heart failure. All premature babies should have electrocardiographic pulse monitoring with the warning alarm set for a pulse rate below 110 beats per minute. Besides being a helpful guide to the cardiovascular status of the baby, this is the most efficient method of identifying serious apneic episodes. When respiration stops, the pulse rate is maintained briefly and then gradually falls until bradycardia and cardiac arrest develop. A pulse rate below 110 beats per minute suggests significant hypoxia and demands immediate action by the nursing and medical staff. The majority of these episodes are interrupted readily by stimulating the infant. Recurrent or prolonged attacks may require endotracheal intubation and artificial ventilation. Whenever apneic episodes develop or their frequency increases, a careful search should be made for an initiating cause, such as infection.

Preterm infants who receive oxygen therapy require arterial blood PO_2 monitoring to detect levels that might result in retinal and lung injury. Because the transitional circulation allows right-to-left shunting across the ductus arteriosus, it may be necessary to monitor blood gases from the upper extremities or the temporal artery. These samples represent blood above the ductus that perfuses the eyes and brain rather than blood from below the ductus that perfuses the abdominal viscera. Blood sugar, serum bilirubin and calcium, hemoglobin, and hematocrit levels should be monitored on a regular basis in the postoperative period. Following operation, it is often necessary to maintain the weak, premature infant on total intravenous nutrition or gastrostomy feedings with special formulas because of the poor suck reflex and sluggishly functioning gastrointestinal tract.

Small-for-Gestational-Age Infants

Babies born after 38 weeks of gestation that weigh less than 2500 gm are thought to suffer from intrauterine growth retardation and are labeled small-for-gestational-age (SGA) infants. Factors that lead to growth retardation may reside in the fetus or may result from placental or maternal abnormalities. The SGA infant can usually be recognized by his or her physical characteristics. Although body weight is low, body length is often normal, and head size usually approaches that of a normal full-term infant. The plantar creases are well developed, and the testicles are descended into a well-formed scrotum. The ears and ear cartilages are well developed, and breast tissue is palpable. In the female, the labia majora cover the labia minora.

Although SGA babies may be the same body weight as premature infants, they face different physiologic problems because of their longer gestational period and resultant well-developed organ systems. Their metabolic rate is much higher in proportion to their body weight, and, therefore, fluid and caloric needs are increased. Because of their larger body surface area, lack of body fat, and high metabolic demands, they frequently present problems in thermal regulation. Hypoglycemia is common as a result of inadequate liver glycogen stores. Even without placental transfusions, SGA infants are usually born with marked polycythemia, which may lead to high blood viscosities and circulatory problems. Hyaline membrane disease is uncommon, but there is an increased incidence of meconium aspiration syndrome.

Practical Considerations

The surgeon must be aware of the high metabolic activity of the SGA infant and must provide a relatively large maintenance fluid volume and caloric intake. Rapid hypoglycemia can develop soon after birth or operation, and close monitoring of the blood sugar is essential. Because of the frequent occurrence of polycythemia, hematocrit levels should be monitored in the first few weeks of life. If the preoperative hematocrit levels are extremely high, bleeding may occur, and replacement with plasma or electrolyte solutions may be required.

TEMPERATURE CONTROL

Unless protective measures are taken, all pediatric patients must expend energy above basal levels to maintain body temperature in a cold environment. If the cold challenge persists for an unprotected individual, there is eventual exhaustion of energy supplies, a significant energy debt, a marked fall in body temperature, and in the newborn infant, an increased mortality. The infant is thermodynamically at a disadvantage in comparison with the older child. Small infants have a relatively large heat-losing surface area in relation to body weight. All newborns, but particularly preterm and SGA babies, lack adequate insulation because of a low ratio of body fat to body weight. The infant also has a high thermal neutral zone. At an environmental temperature below thermal neutrality, metabolic activity must increase above basal metabolic levels for the individual to maintain normal body temperature. The baby also cannot generate heat by shivering and must rely on nonshivering thermogenesis utilizing brown fat. Finally, aside from the physiologic differences between the older individual and the infant, mature patients challenged by cold can manipulate their environment — add more clothing and blankets, complain, turn up a thermostat, or leave the area — options that are not available to the infant.

Practical Considerations

Once environmental temperature drops below the infant's thermal neutral zone, metabolic work increases, calories are burned to maintain body temperature, and energy is then unavailable for other essential metabolic functions and responses to surgical stress. For this reason, environmental temperature must be kept at close to the thermal neutral zone for each individual surgical infant. Thermal neutrality is about 34 to

35°C for the low-birth-weight (LBW) infant up to 12 days of age and 31 to 32°C at six weeks of age. Larger babies (2000 to 3000 gm body weight) have a thermal neutrality zone of about 31 to 34°C on the first day of life and 29 to 31°C at 12 days. These environmental temperatures can be effectively maintained by setting the temperature control of an incubator and then monitoring the ambient temperature.

An alternative method for maintaining temperature close to thermal neutrality is to control an incubator or radiant heater with a servocontrol system. A temperature probe is placed on the skin of the right upper quadrant of the abdomen, and the servosystem is set at a skin temperature that reflects the basal metabolic activity for the individual baby. The heat output of the incubator or radiant warmer increases if the skin temperature is below the set point, and it shuts off if the set point is exceeded. The skin temperature, which represents basal metabolic activity, is approximately 36.2°C for the full-term infant and 36.5°C for the LBW infant.

When an infant must be placed in a cool environment, heat loss can be reduced by covering much of the body surface. This can be accomplished by wrapping the extremities in sheet wadding and placing a stockinette cap on the baby's head. Plastic sheets and aluminum foil serve a similar purpose.

Measuring the gradient between the skin and rectal temperature is an effective method of determining if an infant has increased its metabolic output in order to maintain a normal core temperature. A fall in skin temperature in the face of a constant rectal temperature suggests that there is increased metabolic activity. The optimal gradient between rectal and skin temperature is 1.5°C.

GLUCOSE AND CALCIUM METABOLISM IN THE PEDIATRIC SURGICAL PATIENT

Fetal blood levels of glucose and calcium are maintained by transplacental passage of these substances, but at birth, a critical period of adjustment begins during which the newborn infant's own metabolic processes take over this homeostatic regulation. Several factors, some hereditary, some iatrogenic, can upset this balance and cause critical derangements in serum chemistry. In addition, surgical stress in infants and even in older children can surpass limitations in their abilities to meet such challenges.

GLUCOSE HOMEOSTASIS

The fetus receives glucose by facilitated diffusion across the placenta, maintaining its blood glucose at 70 to 80 per cent of maternal levels. It builds up glycogen stores in liver, skeletal, and cardiac muscle, which are proportionately higher than in the adult, but almost never synthesizes glucose de novo (gluconeogenesis).

Following delivery, the newborn infant rapidly catabolizes its hepatic glycogen stores, depleting them almost completely in two to three hours. Muscle glycogen is less available, but these levels also fall greatly in the first few days of life. Within a few hours, the neonate becomes almost totally dependent on gluconeogenesis to maintain its blood glucose levels. Though fat catabolism occurs, as evidenced by a rise in free fatty acids, the availability of substrates for synthesizing glucose, particularly amino acids, is severely limited, and serum glucose progressively falls. The nadir is usually reached at four to six hours of age. How rapidly and how low serum glucose levels fall depend both on the adequacy of substrate stores related to the gestational age and on the energy demands of the infant. Babies at very high risk for the development of hypoglycemia are SGA infants, the smaller of twins, and "distressed" infants, particularly those of toxemic mothers. Also at risk are neonates with hyperinsulinemia, i.e., those with diabetic mothers and babies with erythroblastosis fetalis (Rh incompatibility). The institution of oral feedings decreases the risk of hypoglycemia, but this feeding method is frequently not possible in the pediatric surgical patient.

Symptoms of hypoglycemia are nonspecific and include a weak or high-pitched cry, cyanosis, apnea, "jitteriness" (coarse trembling), apathy, and seizures. The differential diagnosis must always include sepsis and other metabolic disturbances. It is essential to note that many babies may exhibit no symptoms whatever in spite of very low blood sugar levels.

Neonatal hypoglycemia is generally defined by a serum glucose level less than 30 mg per 100 ml in a full-term infant and less than 20 mg per 100 ml in a LBW infant. This is not a clinically useful definition, since brain damage has been reported at or above these levels. Prevention of symptomatic hypoglycemia in the pediatric surgical patient is essential because over 50 per cent of those with symptoms are later found to have significant neurologic damage. Monitoring of high-risk babies, especially LBW babies undergoing surgery, should consist of Dextrostix screening determinations every one to two hours, confirmation of low levels by serum glucose values, and prompt therapy of developing hypoglycemia. Nursery personnel must be able to perform these tests competently and also must be able to recognize the clinical signs of hypoglycemia.

Although the newborn infant is at highest risk for developing hypoglycemia, the older infant and child are not immune. Because of proportionately less muscle and fat reserves, children do not tolerate prolonged fasting well. Hence, hypoglycemia must be anticipated and avoided in older pediatric surgical patients.

Practical Considerations

All pediatric surgical patients, particularly neonates, should be considered at risk for developing hypoglycemia. Fasting plus surgical stress can be a dangerous combination for any infant. LBW infants, particularly SGA babies and infants of diabetic or toxemic mothers, are very susceptible to hypoglycemia. Frequent Dextrostix (every one to two hours) and serum glucose determinations are mandatory. When non–dextrose-containing solutions are being administered to a pediatric surgical patient, such as during blood transfusion, blood glucose can fall precipitously, and close monitoring and prompt therapy are essential. Most authors recommend vigorous therapy when blood glucose falls below 40 mg per 100 ml. If the infant is symptomatic, he or she should receive 50 per cent dextrose, 1 to 2 ml per kg intravenously immediately. The infant can then be maintained on intravenous 10 to 15 per cent dextrose at 80 to 100 ml per kg per 24 hrs.

CALCIUM METABOLISM

Calcium is supplied to the fetus by active transport across the placenta, 75 per cent of the total amount being transferred after week 28 of gestation. Fetal serum calcium levels are maintained at higher than maternal levels throughout the pregnancy.

At birth the neonate has a natural tendency toward hypocalcemia. The causes appear multiple and include (1) decreased calcium stores, especially in LBW babies; (2) renal immaturity with decreased phosphate excretion; and (3) relative hypoparathyroidism, possibly secondary to suppression by high fetal serum calcium.

Between 24 and 48 hours of age, serum calcium levels are lowest. Hypocalcemia during this period is defined as values less than 7 mg per 100 ml. Over 80 per cent of babies experiencing neonatal hypocalcemia fall into three categories: (1) LBW, especially preterm; (2) complicated pregnancy or delivery (toxemia, maternal diabetes, or low Apgar scores); and (3) those receiving bicarbonate infusions.

Symptoms of hypocalcemia may include "jitteriness," high-pitched crying, cyanosis, vomiting, twitching, or seizures. Chvostek or Trousseau signs are not reliable indicators of calcium levels in the neonate, and serum calcium levels must be determined. In most cases, depression of serum calcium is transient, and values return to normal by the time the infant is three to four days of age. If serum calcium is extremely low or if signs of tetany appear, therapy is indicated. In most cases, calcium supplementation is necessary only for a few days. Although symptomatic hypocalcemia should be treated promptly, the prognosis for this is much better than for significant hypoglycemia. Even when tetanic seizures occur, neurologic sequelae are very rare.

Magnesium and calcium metabolism are interrelated. SGA babies and infants with diabetic or toxemic mothers are also at risk for hypomagnesemia. If an infant has hypocalcemia-associated seizures that do not respond to calcium therapy, magnesium deficiency should be suspected and confirmed by obtaining a serum magnesium level. Appropriate treatment for magnesium deficiency is administration of 50 per cent magnesium sulfate, 0.2 ml per kg intramuscularly every four hours, followed by oral magnesium sulfate, 30 mEq per day.

Practical Considerations

A "jittery" baby should have an immediate Dextrostix determination as well as serum glucose and calcium measurements. Therapy should be prompt, especially when hypoglycemia is suspected. Although most seizures occurring in the newborn period are not secondary to hypoglycemia or hypocalcemia, these etiologies must be strongly suspected in high-risk infants — LBW babies and "stressed" infants, particularly those of toxemic or diabetic mothers. Therapeutic manipulations that alter the ionized fraction of calcium can result in clinical hypocalcemia without great reduction of serum calcium levels. Pediatric surgical babies receiving sodium bicarbonate or undergoing exchange transfusion are susceptible to iatrogenic calcium depression. Calcium therapy is appropriate if the clinical situation suggests hypocalcemia. Intravenous calcium therapy should always be considered potentially dangerous and should be administered with great caution only to infants who are severely symptomatic or in whom oral calcium cannot be given. When indicated, intravenous 10 per cent calcium gluconate should be given slowly with constant monitoring of an electrocardiogram. Dosage may range from 10 ml for a full-term infant to 6 ml for a LBW infant, at a rate not exceeding 1 ml per min. Calcium gluconate may also be given as maintenance therapy, 1 to 2 gm per 24 hrs intravenously or 2 gm per day orally.

BLOOD VOLUME

It is only in the first few months of life that there are significant differences between the blood volume values of the pediatric and the adult patient. Total blood, plasma, and red blood cell volumes are all at their highest point at delivery. After six hours, plasma shifts out of the circulation, and the total blood volume continues to remain high, owing primarily to an elevated red blood cell volume. The red blood cell volume then gradually falls with growth and by the fiftieth day reaches adult levels. At about three months, total blood volume in all infants is nearly equal to adult levels.

During the newborn period, the proportion of total blood volume made up by the red blood cell mass and the plasma varies according to three factors: (1) the maturation of the infant; (2) its size in relation to maturation; and (3) the presence or absence of placental transfusion. Plasma volume is larger than red blood cell volume in preterm and full-term infants who have not received a placental transfusion. Infants who have had a placental transfusion and all SGA babies have a red blood cell volume that is higher than the plasma volume.

Practical Considerations

In evaluating the blood volume of an infant, it is important to consider whether the baby has had a placental transfusion. A significant placental transfusion can increase total blood volume by as much as 25 per cent. The hematocrit has value as a rough guide to the presence or absence of placental transfusion and the volume of placental transfusion. Hematocrit values over 50 per cent suggest that some degree of placental transfusion has taken place. High hematocrits over 65 per cent suggest a significant placental transfusion.

The red blood cell volume of the newborn infant can be estimated by the formula: RBC volume (ml per kg) = hematocrit -11. The total blood volume can be calculated by the following formula: Total blood volume (ml per kg) = $0.46 \times$ hematocrit $+ 63$. It is easier to refer to one of the published tables to estimate the blood volume. It is generally safe to use adult values for total blood volumes (75 to 80 ml per kg) after one or two months of age.

THE JAUNDICED INFANT

At birth the newborn infant is abruptly separated from its mother's sophisticated metabolic apparatus, and the baby must perform several vital functions on his or her own for the first time. The liver must maintain glucose homeostasis, conjugate and excrete bilirubin, detoxify drugs, and inactivate endotoxins and bacteria absorbed through the intestinal tract. This section deals with bilirubin metabolism, while drug detoxification and glucose homeostasis are discussed elsewhere.

The spleen and liver catabolize heme pigments, mostly hemoglobin, to produce bilirubin. Bilirubin is a lipid-soluble substance and, in the fetus, can be transported across the placental membranes for clearance. After birth, bilirubin becomes bound to albumin, is transported into the hepatocyte, and then is conjugated with glucuronic acid. This water-soluble product enters the bile through the canalicular system and is excreted into the intestinal tract. The overall result is transformation of a lipid-soluble substance (unconjugated or indirect bilirubin) into a water-soluble substance (conjugated or direct bilirubin) for elimination through the gut. This mechanism also converts a potentially toxic product, which can cross the blood-brain barrier and produce central nervous system damage, into a polar, nontoxic form.

The neonate has several problems in handling this metabolic load. During the fetal period, it was disadvantageous to solubilize bilirubin, since this would prevent its passage across the placenta. Hence, most of these steps are minimally active in utero, and enzyme activities must rise significantly after birth. In addition, the fetal intestine contains an enzyme, beta glucuronidase, that can hydrolyze conjugated bilirubin and return it to the circulation for placental clearance. The presence of this enzyme persists after birth and increases the bilirubin load of the newborn via this enterohepatic route. The bilirubin load is already proportionately greater than in the adult because of a shorter red blood cell lifespan. Hence, a full-term infant's liver has a metabolic and excretory capacity for bilirubin about equal to its load, whereas a normal adult has a sevenfold reserve capacity. During this period of adjustment, even healthy full-term babies show a rise in unconjugated bilirubin, so-called physiologic jaundice, peaking about the fourth day of life and returning to normal levels by the sixth. Rarely does the total bilirubin rise much above 10 mg per 100 ml in these babies. A level over 12 mg per 100 ml in a full-term infant warrants investigation. SGA babies peak later and higher, while preterm babies show the latest and highest bilirubin levels of the three groups.

Excessive levels of unconjugated bilirubin in the neonate can result in severe and permanent brain damage (kernicterus). The toxic product appears to be the unconjugated bilirubin, which is not bound to albumin; hence, kernicterus can occur at relatively low bilirubin levels when factors are present that upset this dynamic binding equilibrium. These factors include hypoalbuminemia, acidosis, cold stress, hypoglycemia, caloric deprivation, hypoxia, and competitive binding substances such as drugs or free fatty acids.

In sick LBW babies, normal or accelerated bilirubin production can exceed the infant's metabolic capabilities and reach toxic levels. Hemolysis secondary to ABO or Rh incompatibility can also result in dangerous bilirubin elevations in any infant. Traditionally, high-risk infants have undergone exchange transfusion to decrease bilirubin when it becomes clinically apparent that toxic levels will be reached. Recently, preloading of the infant circulation with albumin has been performed to increase the amount of bilirubin removed. Exchange transfusion remains effective and the treatment of choice in many instances, but it carries a mortality rate of about 1 per cent in most series.

Within the last 10 years, increasing numbers of high-risk infants have been treated prophylactically with phototherapy to decrease circulating bilirubin. The mechanism of action appears to be through photodegradation of bilirubin in peripheral tissues (skin) to water-soluble products. Although most investigations have suggested that these products are not toxic to the developing organism, many clinicians have reservations about phototherapy. The photodegradation process is a nonspecific one and could theoretically produce alterations in albumin or lead to hormonal imbalances in the newborn infant. Nevertheless, most major institutions utilize phototherapy early for their high-risk infants, especially preterm babies, as the risk seems less than that of exchange transfusion.

Elevated levels of bilirubin may signal an underlying pathologic condition that warrants investigation. An early, rapid rise (greater than 8 mg per 100 ml in less than 48 hrs) suggests hemolysis, either secondary to inherited enzyme defects or to maternal-newborn blood group incompatibilities (ABO or Rh). Prolonged bilirubinemia is often the conjugated type and may herald biliary obstruction or hepatocellular dysfunction. Breast milk jaundice very commonly appears between one to eight weeks of age. Intestinal obstruction can intensify jaundice by increasing the enterohepatic circulation of bilirubin. Jaundice is often one of the earlier signs of sepsis, which can appear at any time in the newborn period.

Practical Considerations

Clinically apparent jaundice in the newborn occurs only at bilirubin levels of 7 to 8 mg per 100 ml. Hence, clinical assessment of the course of jaundice, particularly in patients receiving phototherapy, is notoriously inaccurate, and serial serum bilirubin levels must be obtained. Jaundice that is too early, too late, too much, or too conjugated may be secondary to a significant pathologic condition and should be investigated. If hemolysis is suspected, serial hematocrits, reticulocyte counts, peripheral blood smears, and Coombs' test are appropriate. Sepsis should always be considered a possible cause of unexplained jaundice. Evaluation for neonatal sepsis, consisting of complete blood count (CBC), platelet count, chest roentgenogram, and cultures of blood, urine, and cerebrospinal fluid (CSF), should be seriously considered in any case of undiagnosed jaundice. Phototherapy on the first day of life in LBW babies with rising bilirubin may be useful. Phototherapy should be continued in any patient until bilirubin is less than 10 mg per 100 ml and is falling. Exchange transfusion should be performed in any baby with indirect bilirubin greater than 20 mg per 100 ml or greater than 15 mg per 100 ml in the first 48 hours of life. Exchange transfusions should be utilized even earlier when hemolysis is the underlying etiology or in infants with very low birth weights. Many factors increase the risk of kernicterus. Several of these factors are particularly pertinent to surgical patients: small size, poor nutrition, acidosis, and intestinal obstruction. Often the treatment of the contributing factors is as important as the therapy for jaundice. Several pharmacologic agents can compete with bilirubin for albumin-binding sites and increase the risk of kernicterus. Synthetic penicillins and free fatty acids are two such agents. Therapy with these antibiotics or with parenteral lipid emulsions must be carefully considered in babies at risk for kernicterus.

CALORIC REQUIREMENTS

The pediatric patient requires a relatively large caloric intake because he or she has a high basal metabolic rate, must often expend considerable energy to maintain body heat, consumes calories for growth and development, and frequently has low or reduced energy reserves.

At birth, the full-term infant has a basal metabolic rate of 32 cal per kg per 24 hrs. This rises to a peak of 48 cal per kg per 24 hrs by two weeks of age. It then remains stable until the early teens, when there is a fall to the adult level of 23 cal per kg per 24 hrs. SGA infants tend to be hypermetabolic and increase their metabolic rates more rapidly than full-term infants. The premature infant reaches his or her highest metabolic rate of 58 cal per kg per 24 hrs at about six weeks of age.

The greatest caloric expenditures for growth and development occur in infancy (33 cal per kg per 24 hrs) and then fall to 18 cal per kg per 24 hrs by three months of age and 12 cal per kg per 24 hrs by six months of age. The number of calories utilized for growth then remains stable until the adolescent growth spurt at age 12 to 13 years.

Other caloric needs are dependent on the patient's age and condition. The young patient must expend large quantities of calories to maintain body temperature when he or she must deal with a cold environment. Surgical operations increase caloric demands in all patients as much as 10 to 25 per cent; infection increases needs more than 50 per cent and burns 150 per cent.

The newborn infant has meager energy stores in comparison with the older child and the teenager. Although liver glycogen is rapidly consumed in the first three hours of life in all babies, preterm, SGA, and stressed infants have even less than usual stores of glycogen at birth. Fat stores, a significant source of energy reserve, are deficient in the small baby and represent as little as 1 per cent of the body weight.

Practical Considerations

In order to decide whether the patient can tolerate a period of relative starvation or if he or she requires intensive nutritional therapy such as total parenteral nutrition or special formulas, the following questions must be considered: (1) What are the basal energy needs of the patient? (2) Is the patient subject to cold stress that will result in increased heat production? (3) What are the caloric requirements for growth and development? (4) Are there adequate energy reserves? (5) Are there existing energy deficits? (6) Are factors such as infection or trauma present? After these questions have been answered, the total requirement for the individual can be estimated. It is possible to determine the caloric requirements in various age groups utilizing Table 15–1, which takes into account the basal metabolic needs and the calories required for growth and development. To these values must be

Table 15–1. Caloric Requirements of Various Age Groups

Age	Growth Calories Cal/Kg/24 Hrs.
Birth	33
3 months	18
6 months	12
1 year	12
Teen	18
Basal Metabolism **Full-Term Infant**	
Birth	32
2 weeks	48
1 year	40
Teen	23
Total Calories Maintenance + Growth ++	
Newborn term (0–4 days)	110–120
Low birth weight	120–130
3–4 months	100–106
5–12 months	100
1–7 years	90–75
7–12 years	75–60
12–18 years	60–30

added calories for special factors such as cold stress, surgical trauma, and infection.

FEEDING THE PEDIATRIC SURGICAL PATIENT

In the adult surgical patient, the process of initiating postoperative feedings is generally straightforward. When nasogastric drainage is acceptably low, bowel sounds are present, and flatus or stools are passed, the nasogastric tube is removed, clear liquids are begun, then advanced to full liquids, and then the patient may begin a regular diet. In the pediatric surgical patient, the indications for beginning a postoperative diet are frequently the same. When the decision is made to begin feeding, the next decisions involve what feeding to order, how much, and how often. The surgeon must also be aware of signs of dietary intolerance in the small patient and must know how to monitor the infant's nutritional progress and make appropriate adjustments in management.

Neonatal Pancreatic Function

Although measured levels of amylase, trypsin, and lipase are proportionately lower in infants than in adults, it is only in rare cases that pancreatic insufficiency is primarily responsible for malabsorption in the pediatric surgical patient. An exception is the patient with cystic fibrosis.

Carbohydrate Absorption

The limiting step in carbohydrate absorption in infants is the cleavage of disaccharides into monosaccharides in preparation for transport into the mucosal cells. The disaccharidase enzymes responsible for this function are found in the microvilli of the intestinal cells, the so-called brush border. The enzymes for hydrolysis of sucrose and maltose are present in full titers several weeks before birth. Lactase appears only in the second half of gestation and increases to the time of delivery. Hence, preterm infants often demonstrate lactase deficiency. Because of their superficial location in the microvilli, disaccharidases are particularly vulnerable to any disease damaging the small bowel epithelium. Following inflammatory bowel disease, for example, lactose digestion is often abnormal and may remain so for weeks. In severe cases, other disaccharidases may be diminished, and even monosaccharide absorption may be affected, possibly by damage to transport mechanisms.

In patients with carbohydrate malabsorption, sugars retained in the bowel lumen can produce a secondary osmotic diarrhea. In the colon, the sugars are metabolized to lactic acid, further increasing the osmotic load and resulting in watery, acidic stools.

In the pediatric surgical patient, one can test for carbohydrate malabsorption in three ways: (1) fecal pH (Combistix or pH paper) — care must be taken to avoid contamination of the stool specimen with urine. A pH less than 6 is abnormal and strongly suggests carbohydrate intolerance. (2) Fecal reducing substances or fecal glucose (Clinitest tablets or Combistix) — reducing substances greater than 0.25 per cent or glucose greater than 1+ is abnormal. (3) Disaccharide tolerance tests — the disaccharide to be tested (for example, lactose) is given orally at 2 gm per kg diluted in a 1 to 5 ratio. Serial serum glucose levels are measured. A rise of serum glucose greater than 20 mg per 100 ml within two hours is considered normal.

Protein Absorption

Protein digestive mechanisms are well developed even in the LBW baby. With a single exception, peptidases are found in epithelial cell cytoplasm rather than in the brush border. Hence, their deficiency, even in pathologic states, is virtually unknown. Tests for protein malabsorption are not available and, fortunately, are almost never indicated.

Sensitivity to cow's milk protein may appear during the first six months of life. Manifestations of this disorder vary but may include diarrhea, vomiting, rhinitis, skin rashes, and failure to thrive. The presumptive diagnosis is confirmed by a favorable clinical response to withdrawal of cow's milk protein from the diet.

Fat Absorption

Absorption of lipids in infants is relatively poor, especially in LBW babies. Of particular importance is a measured bile salt pool, which is only 50 per cent of that of adults. This represents borderline levels for formation of micelles and a precarious balance for fat digestion. Ileal resections may result in decreased bile salt absorption. This can produce steatorrhea by depleting the bile salt pool or "bile salt diarrhea" by the irritant effect of these substances on the colon.

Fat absorption is further complicated by the nature of individual lipids. Human milk lipid is absorbed best, but even in healthy full-term babies, 10 to 15 per cent is lost in the stools. Cow's milk lipid (butterfat) is most poorly absorbed (60 to 70 per cent), while corn, coconut, and soy lipid absorption is comparable to that of human milk. Medium-chain triglycerides (MCT), composed of fatty acids of 8 to 10 carbon atoms, are absorbed directly into the portal circulation and require neither lipase nor bile salts for digestion. They are useful adjuncts for difficult patients and are included in some special infant formulas (Table 15–2).

Steatorrhea in the pediatric surgical patient can be documented by two methods. Grossly, fecal fat can be detected by microscopic examination after staining with Sudan III. Complete fecal collection over three to six days for quantitative chemical determination is tedious and difficult but is the only accurate method of assessment.

General Comments

The full-term infant has 8 to 10 feet of small bowel, about one-third that of the adult. The musculature and elastic fiber of the bowel are not well developed at term, but the digestive and absorptive surfaces are. The stomach empties more slowly in the newborn period than at any other time. Air swallowing begins almost immediately after birth. Air reaches the jejunum in 15 minutes and the cecum by two hours. The quickness and consistency of intestinal air transit is an important aid to diagnosing GI malformations in the newborn infant.

Lactose is the principal sugar in breast milk and in regular infant formulas. Though it is the most difficult sugar to absorb, it is well tolerated by most infants who do not have serious intestinal problems. It has the added advantages of increasing calcium absorption and of promoting a fermentative, less putrefactive intestinal flora.

Ideal oral protein intake for neonates, including LBW infants, is between 2.25 and 5.0 gm per kg per day. Adequate weight gain occurs in infants who breast-feed, although protein intake may be less than the

Table 15-2. INFANT FORMULAS

	CARBOHYDRATE	PROTEIN (CONC.°/SOURCE)	FAT (CONC./SOURCE)	OSMOLALITY mOsm/l	CLINICAL USAGE	COMMENTS
Human breast milk	Lactose	1.1%/Human (mostly whey)	4.5%/Human	273	Preferred when feasible and no contraindications to lactose or fat	Much higher in cholesterol than commercial formulas
Similac Enfamil	Lactose	1.5%/Cow (mostly casein)	3.6%/Coconut and soy	262	Standard formulas; indications as for breast milk	
SMA	Lactose	1.5%/Casein + whey	3.6%/Butterfat, coconut, soy, safflower (SMA)	271	As for standard formulas	"Humanized" protein composition, which may have theoretical value
Similac-PM60/40			3.8%/Coconut, corn (PM60/40)	239	Low renal solute load; useful in babies with congestive heart failure	PM60/40 has low phosphate content
Isomil Neomullsoy Prosobee	Sucrose ±corn syrup solids	1.9–2.5%/Soy	3.6%/Soy ±coconut	228–245	Primarily for patients with cow's milk protein sensitivity	May be useful in patients unable to tolerate lactose
Portagen†	Sucrose Starch	2.3%/Casein	3.4%/MCT (85%) Corn oil (12%)	203	Lactose intolerance Steatorrhea Cystic fibrosis Short gut syndrome	Low osmolality a plus

	Carbohydrate	Protein	Fat	Osmolality	Indications	Comments
Pregestimil‡	Glucose Starch	2.2%/Casein hydrolysate	2.8%/MCT (86%) Corn oil (13%)	539	General disaccharide intolerance Steatorrhea Cystic fibrosis	High osmolality warrants close monitoring The most predigested formula aside from elemental formulas Possible metabolic acidosis (see Nutramigen)
Nutramigen†	Sucrose Starch	2.2%/Casein hydrolysate	2.6%/Corn oil	416	Protein sensitivity Lactose intolerance	Also hyperosmolar Metabolic acidosis sometimes occurs secondary to casein hydrolysate
Vivonex‡ standard (unflavored)	Glucose Glucose Oligo-saccharides	2.0% (est)/Amino acids	0.15%/Safflower	333‡	Severe intestinal disturbances Short-gut syndrome	Flavored or High Nitrogen Vivonex have significantly higher osmolality Some infants may refuse oral feedings with unflavored Vivonex Patients must be observed for essential fatty acid or protein deficiency

°Concentrations reported as wt/vol, e.g., gm/100 ml
†Powder—requires mixing at home
‡Osmolalities reported for formula concentrations of 20 cal/oz

suggested figure. This appears secondary to the high quality of the protein in breast milk. Dietary protein greater than 5 gm per kg per day is not generally desirable and may produce a number of metabolic disturbances.

The total caloric requirement of growing infants is about 100 cal per kg per day; LBW infant requirements vary between 110 and 150 cal per kg per day. Most infant formulas contain 20 cal per oz.

Practical Considerations

LBW infants and babies with conditions associated with mucosal epithelial damage, such as necrotizing enterocolitis, gastroschisis, or malnutrition, have the highest risk for developing carbohydrate intolerance. The stool pH and sugar content should be monitored. Formula change is often indicated (Table 15–2). The same conditions also predispose the infant to steatorrhea. If diarrhea without sugar spillage or low fecal pH occurs, steatorrhea should be suspected. An MCT formula may be of clinical benefit (Portagen, Pregestimil). Following ileal resection, either steatorrhea or bile salt diarrhea may result. If fat absorption seems adequate, addition of cholestyramine to feedings will bind bile acids and diminish bile salt diarrhea. If diarrhea increases after giving cholestyramine, steatorrhea should be suspected, and the patient should be reevaluated. Steatorrhea is associated with increased fecal losses of calcium, magnesium, and the fat-soluble vitamins A, D, E, and K. Deficiencies of any of these nutrients may occur.

Osmotic diarrhea can result secondary to carbohydrate malabsorption or to hyperosmolar formulas. (Bile salt diarrhea is also a form of osmotic diarrhea.) The osmolarity of the formula being administered (Table 15–2) should be confirmed by laboratory studies if there is any question. This is of particular importance when elemental formulas, such as Vivonex, are used. True short-gut syndrome can result after massive bowel resections, especially those including the ileocecal valve. Conditions with extensive mucosal damage, such as necrotizing enterocolitis, can produce a functional short-gut syndrome, though adequate anatomic bowel length is present.

When feasible, breast milk feeding has many advantages — low osmolarity, high-quality protein, easily absorbed fat, and many immunologically active substances. Table 15–3 outlines an approach to the feeding of babies, but obviously feedings must be individualized. Most LBW infants will require intravenous supplementation of their oral intake for several days. Babies less than 34 weeks of gestational age have uncoordinated sucking and swallowing mechanisms and generally require gavage or gastrostomy feedings. If enthusiasm for oral feedings declines unexplainably, sepsis should be suspected.

Table 15-3. Guidelines for Feeding Babies

Infant Weight	Frequency of Feeding	Method of Feeding	Formula	Volume of Feeding
<1500 gm	q2h	Gavage or gastrostomy tube	Sterile distilled water (SDW) × 2 feedings Half strength standard formula (HSSF) (10 cal/oz) or 13 cal/oz formula × 48–72 hrs; full strength standard formula (FSSF).	4 ml/kg initially Increase 1–2 ml/feeding each day to total 15–20 ml/kg/feeding by days 8–14
1500–2500 gm	q3h	Gavage and/or nipple	SDW × 2 feedings HSSF or 13 cal/oz formula × 24 hrs; FSSF	4 ml/kg initially Increase up to 10 ml/feeding each day in larger babies to 20–25 ml/kg/feeding by days 5–10
>2500 gm	q4h	Nipple	SDW × 2 feedings HSSF or 13 cal/oz formula × 2 feedings; FSSF	4 ml/kg initially Increase 10–15 ml/feeding each day to 25–30 ml/kg/feeding by days 4–8

FLUID AND ELECTROLYTE MANAGEMENT

Effective fluid and electrolyte management, regardless of age, level of maturation, or size of the patient, involves seven steps: (1) Calculate the quantity of water and electrolytes necessary to maintain metabolic functions; (2) estimate fluid and electrolyte deficits; (3) measure and estimate ongoing losses; (4) construct a tentative fluid and electrolyte program, taking into consideration the maintenance needs, the losses, and the deficits; (5) write specific fluid orders for a finite period of time; (6) serially monitor the patient's responses to the program; and (7) adjust the program according to the analysis of the patient's responses.

CALCULATING MAINTENANCE NEEDS

Maintenance needs are met if losses from the skin, lungs, and kidneys are replaced. Unfortunately, it is possible to estimate these needs only roughly by applying one of the formulas or rules described in most textbooks. All fluid programs must be constantly modified by the feedback from the patient's responses. Attention to responses is particularly important in the pediatric patient because of the great variability in insensible and renal water losses resulting from differences in body surface area, skin characteristics, respiratory rate, renal function, basal metabolic rate, pathologic lesions, environmental conditions, and surgical trauma.

Although fluid and electrolyte maintenance needs can be safely estimated utilizing body weight as a guide in the adult, it is obvious that a close relationship between weight and fluid and electrolyte needs for all ages does not exist. Nevertheless, fluid calculations based on weight may be helpful occasionally as a guide to maintenance requirements in a specific narrow weight and age group, particularly the LBW newborn infant group.

The physiologic approach to calculating maintenance requirements for all ages is based on the fact that fluid and electrolyte needs are fundamentally related to energy expenditure — the amount of calories necessary for the body to perform its vital functions. Since there are no simple measuring devices available that accurately reflect the metabolic activity, formulas must be used to calculate metabolic activity. Metabolic activity can be estimated by relating surface area to metabolic rate, assuming that metabolic rate is equal to about 1000 cal per m^2 per 24 hrs over a wide range of body sizes. Utilizing this relationship, maintenance fluid requirements are thus equal to 1200 to 1500 ml per m^2 per 24 hrs. Sodium and potassium maintenance needs are 30 to 40 mEq per m^2 per 24 hrs. However, as more information has become available, multiple deviations from the general rule of relationship of surface area to metabolic rate have modified the use of this method.

The caloric method has largely replaced the surface area method in

Table 15–4. FORMULAS FOR DETERMINING CALORIC EXPENDITURE

WEIGHT	CALORIC EXPENDITURES
3–10 kg	100 cal/kg
11–20 kg	1000 cal + 50 (wt [kg] −10)
>20 kg	1500 cal + 20 (wt [kg] −20)

calculating maintenance fluid and electrolytes of pediatric patients. The total caloric expenditures of an individual patient are determined from a graph that plots body weight against calories expended in 24 hrs. A relatively simple formula to determine caloric expenditure is described in Table 15–4. Total water maintenance is generally calculated as 100 ml per 100 cal metabolized per 24 hrs. Sodium and potassium requirements are estimated at 1 to 3 mEq per 100 cal per 24 hrs.

The simplest way to calculate maintenance needs for the older infant and child is to utilize either the square meter or calorie method. For newborn infants, particularly LBW babies, it is probably easiest to estimate fluid requirements by body weight. All three systems are safe if it is recognized that they allow only a rough estimate of true maintenance needs, and the quality of fluids and electrolytes must be constantly readjusted according to the patient's responses to the initial therapy.

CALCULATING FLUID AND ELECTROLYTE LOSSES AND DEFICITS

Body fluid losses can usually be collected and measured but may be immeasurable if they accumulate in body cavities or tissues. The volume of gastric, small bowel, biliary, pancreatic, and diarrheal fluids can be measured directly, and the electrolyte concentrations can be estimated by referring to published tables. These steps are sufficient if losses are brief and only moderate in quantity. Minor electrolyte adjustments are usually made by the kidney. However, when losses are large or prolonged or when renal function is compromised, the electrolyte content of the lost fluid must be analyzed frequently, and replacement must be made on a milliliter for milliliter and milliequivalent for milliequivalent basis. The characteristics and the volume of immeasurable losses and existing deficits can be estimated by clinical and laboratory assessments.

MONITORING THE FLUID AND ELECTROLYTE PROGRAM

Clinical Observations

Severe isotonic and hypotonic dehydration are usually accompanied by signs of impending or frank shock. The skin is cool and mottled, and the turgor is reduced. There is poor capillary filling, and the peripheral veins are collapsed. The mucous membranes are dry, and the anterior fontanel is severely sunken. The presence of these findings indicates that there is a 9 per cent reduction of body fluid in a child and 14 per cent in an infant. Less severe dehydration without cardiovascular signs usually suggests 6 per cent dehydration in a child and 10 per cent in an infant. Hypertonic dehydration is more difficult to diagnose clinically. In spite of as much as 20 per cent reduction in body weight, there may be only a 7 per cent reduction in blood volume. For this reason, signs of shock occur late, and central nervous system signs predominate early. Initially, the patient may be lethargic or stuporous, but seizures can occur frequently, particularly when there is a rapid correction of hypertonicity.

Urine Flow Rate

Monitoring urinary output is an extremely valuable guide to the fluid balance of the young patient. At any age, the individual produces significant urine when well hydrated and scant urine when underhydrated. All patients must maintain a urine flow rate that will allow the excretion of the solute load at a reasonable concentration. The full-term newborn infant usually has a urine flow of about 25 ml per kg per 24 hrs, the LBW infant 50 to 100 ml per kg per 24 hrs, and the child 600 to 700 ml per m^2 per 24 hrs, or about 55 ml of urine per 100 calories metabolized. In the severely dehydrated pediatric patient, it is helpful to insert an indwelling bladder catheter in order to measure hourly urine output.

Urine Osmolality and Specific Gravity

Serial measurements of urine osmolality or specific gravity together with urine flow rates serve as valuable checks as to whether sufficient volumes of fluid have been delivered. The maximal concentrating ability of the kidney varies with the age and maturity of the patient. The newborn infant can concentrate to 450 mOsm per kg, the older infant and child to 700 mOsm per kg, and the teenager and adult to 1200 to 1400 mOsm per kg. The trend of serial measurements in response to fluid therapy is more important than individual values. Generally, urine specific gravity parallels urine osmolality and can be estimated on a very small volume of urine by using the refractometer.

Body Weight

Serial measurements of body weight are an excellent guide to total body water in the infant. Fluctuations over a 24-hour period are primarily related to loss or gain of body fluids. Roughly 1 gm of weight loss or gain can be equated to the loss or gain of one ml of water.

Hematocrit and Refractometer Total Protein

Serial hematocrit and refractometer total protein measurements are simple, rapid techniques for estimating plasma water changes with dehydration and rehydration. Serial changes in hematocrit over a 24-hour period in the absence of hemolysis or bleeding suggest a loss or gain of plasma water. Changes in the total protein, as measured by refractometer in the absence of massive protein loss, are usually directly related to changes in serum water and can confirm the changes of the hematocrit.

Serum Electrolytes, Blood Urea Nitrogen, and Sugar and Osmolality

The hematocrit and refractometer measurements principally serve as a guide to the adequacy of the volume of fluid administered to the patient. Measurements of serum electrolytes, blood urea nitrogen, osmolality and blood sugar, and calculation of serum osmolality are helpful in planning the program that will replace ongoing losses and deficits of electrolytes. Once a tentative program has been initiated and the fluid orders have been written, the responses of the patient can then be simply monitored by measuring serum osmolality frequently.

An increase in osmolality suggests that too little water or too great a quantity of electrolytes, usually sodium, has been given. A fall in osmolality suggests that sodium replacement is inadequate or that too great a quantity of water is being administered. An unexpected change in osmolality, particularly an increase, requires immediate determination of serum electrolytes, blood urea nitrogen, and sugar values and a calculation of the osmolality. Serum osmolality can be calculated by the following formula:

$$\text{Osmolality} = \text{Sodium} \times 1.86 + \frac{\text{Blood Urea Nitrogen}}{2.8} + \frac{\text{Glucose}}{18} + 5$$

It is then possible to determine whether the rise in osmolality is due to an increase in serum sodium, the development of hyperglycemia, or a high blood urea nitrogen. Occasionally, the measured serum osmolality is higher than calculated osmolality. This suggests that the increase in serum osmolality is due to some unidentified osmolar active substance such as a metabolic byproduct resulting from sepsis or shock or radiopaque contrast material.

DRUG METABOLISM IN THE INFANT SURGICAL PATIENT

It has been estimated that the average 1500 gm premature infant is exposed to 20 prescribed drugs between the time of conception and discharge from the nursery. How well the infant copes with these multiple pharmacologic challenges depends on the infant's gestational and postnatal age, as well as the characteristics of the drug itself — its absorption, distribution, metabolism, and excretion. Adding to the clinician's dilemma is the fact that few studies on drug effects and metabolism in neonates and infants have been reported. Hence, information regarding pharmacology in the pediatric surgical patient is often conjectural and theoretical rather than well established.

Like bilirubin, most drugs are bound to plasma proteins while circulating in the blood. The unbound fraction is responsible for the pharmacologic activity. This fraction is often larger in infants than in adults, so the neonate may show a much greater drug effect at similar serum concentrations. Whether this difference is attributable to lower serum albumin concentrations, qualitative protein differences, or increased binding competition from endogenous substances is not clear.

Drug metabolism involves oxidation or conjugation or both. Oxidation appears to be the more important pathway and involves a cascade of enzyme steps in the microsomal fraction of hepatocytes, similar to conversion of heme to bilirubin. Conjugation mechanisms are important in detoxification of steroids, salicylates, and chloramphenicol. During gestation, the placenta is the major excretory organ for waste products and transports lipid-soluble substances specifically. As with bilirubin, mechanisms leading to water solubilization such as oxidation or conjugation are to the fetus' disadvantage and are not well developed at birth. In the newborn infant, both oxidative metabolism and conjugation enzymes are decreased. These deficiencies result in a prolonged half-life of many drugs and may be extremely dangerous if not appreciated, for example, the "gray syndrome" following chloramphenicol administration.

Renal excretion of drugs is dependent on glomerular filtration rate (GFR) and renal blood flow (RBF), which are both low in the newborn infant. These deficits are roughly proportional to the gestational age of the infant and are especially significant in the first week of life. Hence, administered dosages of drugs (such as gentamicin) can be very different during this period. Nephrotoxicity of drugs is related to the concentrating ability of the kidney for the particular agent. It has been suggested that newborn infants have a decreased susceptibility to nephrotoxicity effects because of their diminished renal concentrating ability. When correct dosages are used, it does not appear that any drug has a distinct kidney-damaging effect in the newborn period.

Maturation of oxidative and conjugative hepatic function as well as renal mechanisms begins at birth, but the newborn period represents a complicated and critical period of transition, which may be even more prolonged in LBW infants. In summary, newborn infants have very different absorption and volume distribution of drugs, decreased protein binding, and a greatly diminished ability to metabolize and excrete drugs. By two to three years of age, drug absorption and elimination become very efficient, even exceeding adult levels.

Practical Considerations

Digoxin. (1) Serum digoxin half-life in preterm infants averages 1.5 times that of full-term babies. Digoxin should be administered cautiously, particularly to the more immature newborns. (2) Therapeutic digoxin serum levels are 1 to 2.5 ng per ml in normokalemic patients. Conduction disturbances can occur when levels exceed 3.0 ng per ml (3.5 ng per ml in infants). One must always look for signs of toxicity: vomiting, anorexia, and arrhythmias. If the pulse rate of a newborn infant receiving digoxin falls below 100, consideration should be given to holding the next digitalis dose. A serum digoxin level should also be obtained. (3) Digoxin should not be given by intramuscular injection to either neonates or infants because of the slow and unpredictable rate of absorption and because of the possibility of local tissue necrosis. Digoxin is well absorbed by the intestinal tract, so dosage should be administered either orally or by careful intravenous infusion.

Furosemide (Lasix). Pharmacokinetic studies have demonstrated that furosemide is cleared much more slowly in newborn infants than in adults. The mechanism, as with digoxin, is probably secondary to immature renal function. Prolonged diuretic and saluretic effects of furosemide in the neonate are common and must be kept in mind.

Gentamicin. Recommended dosages: Infant less than one week of age, 2.5 mg per kg intramuscularly or intravenously every 12 hours; older neonates, 2.5 mg per kg intramuscularly or intravenously every eight hours; infants and children with septicemia, 2 mg per kg intramuscularly or intravenously every eight hours; infants and children with urinary tract infections, 1 mg per kg intramuscularly or intravenously every eight hours. (2) Therapeutic serum gentamicin levels are 4 to 5 gm per ml; toxic levels are 12 to 15 gm per ml. Ototoxicity and nephrotoxicity are manifested as progressive damage, which is usually reversible if detected early. Serum creatinine determinations should be performed once or twice a week. (3) Gentamicin penetrates poorly into the CSF, even when meninges are inflamed. It also reaches only low concentrations in the bile, about one-fourth to one-half of normal serum levels. These characteristics make aminoglycosides less desirable antibiotics to utilize in patients with meningitis or biliary infections. Gentamicin is well concentrated in renal lymph, making it a satisfactory agent for treating urinary tract infections. Unless bloodstream infection is present, however, other agents are usually preferable.

Chloramphenicol. Chloramphenicol is an appropriate antibiotic for pediatric patients in selected situations, such as meningitis and some enteric infections, but its use in peritonitis is controversial. Because neonates may develop a form of cardiovascular collapse, the "gray syndrome," secondary to diminished conjugation of chloramphenicol, the drug is not recommended for usage in young infants if serum levels cannot be accurately determined.

Clindamycin. The incidence of clindamycin-associated colitis appears much less common in children than in adults, particularly when the parenteral form is used. Though this agent should not be used indiscriminately, it should be considered when infection may be secondary to *Bacteroides fragilis*. *Bacteroides* is also usually sensitive to chloramphenicol and, reportedly, to some of the newer cephalosporins.

Summary

Although variable serum protein binding of drugs can occasionally yield misleading serum drug levels, these levels are still the most objective indices to follow in very ill patients. It is important to measure serum drug levels, not only to detect toxic concentrations but also to ascertain that the administered dosage is appropriate to obtain the desired therapeutic levels.

REFERENCES

Klaus, M. H., and Fanaroff, A. A. (eds.): Care of the High Risk Neonate. Philadelphia, W. B. Saunders Co., 1973.

Smith, C. A., and Nelson, N. M. (eds.): The Physiology of the Newborn Infant, 4th ed. Springfield, IL, Charles C Thomas, 1976.

Winters, R. W. (ed.): The Body Fluids in Pediatrics. Boston, Little, Brown & Co., 1973.

16

The Newborn and Young Infant

ROBERT M. FILLER

The most common symptoms and signs indicative of a surgical problem in the neonate are respiratory distress, vomiting, abdominal distention, failure to pass meconium, diarrhea, defects of the abdominal wall, abdominal masses, and sepsis. The abnormalities most often responsible for these clinical findings include diaphragmatic hernia, esophageal atresia, pyloric stenosis, intestinal obstruction due to atresia, malrotation, or meconium ileus, Hirschsprung's disease, anorectal malformations, necrotizing enterocolitis, omphalocele, and gastroschisis.

GENERAL CONSIDERATIONS

DIAGNOSTIC STUDIES

Almost any test can be hazardous for the infant because of his or her small size and the fragility of the mechanisms that maintain homeostasis. The surgeon should consider each test carefully to be certain that it is necessary to establish a diagnosis or to manage an altered or malfunctioning physiologic state.

Those individuals caring for neonates should realize that even a series of blood tests that require as little as 5 ml of blood per test can soon produce hypovolemia or anemia in a patient whose normal blood volume ranges from 80 to 300 ml. In fact, blood transfusion is often necessary for those acutely ill infants for whom serial determinations of electrolytes or blood gases are indicated. The use of micro methods in the clinical laboratory can significantly reduce the volume of blood necessary for a test. However, not all laboratories have this capability.

Similarly, roentgenographic examinations or other special diagnostic studies must be carefully planned to minimize the neonate's exposure to an unfavorable environment. The procedure room, the equipment, and all personnel must be in readiness before an infant is removed from the protection of an incubator. If the child is to be exposed to an external environment for more than a few minutes, a method for maintaining body temperature, such as an infrared heating lamp, must be available. Special care is necessary to avoid disruption of any intravenous lines and drainage tubes. Intravenous infusions must be maintained, especially when hypertonic radiopaque media such as meglumine diatrizoate (Gastrografin) are introduced into the intestinal tract because their osmotic effect can cause sequestration of fluid in the gut and lead to hypovolemia and shock in the infant. The diagnostic study room must have facilities for suctioning, oxygen administration, and cardiorespiratory resuscitation. For maximal safety and efficiency, the attending surgeon should accompany the infant and remain with him or her until the study is completed.

Fortunately, the diagnostic tests needed for the most commonly occurring surgical conditions in infants need not be complicated or time-consuming. For example, a standard anteroposterior roentgenogram of the baby, which includes the chest and abdominal area, usually suffices for an infant suspected to have a diaphragmatic hernia or omphalocele. Even a more complicated study, such as a barium enema, can be completed within five minutes if preparations have been adequate.

INTRAVENOUS FLUIDS BEFORE AND DURING SURGERY

Preexisting acid-base fluid and electrolyte abnormalities should be corrected preoperatively whenever possible. However, in certain conditions it is unwise to delay operation. For example, in infants with diaphragmatic hernia, the correction of respiratory acidosis and hypoxia may not be possible until the intestinal contents are removed from the thorax. Similarly, a delay in operation to treat metabolic acidosis in an infant with suspected midgut volvulus may be dangerous because intestinal injury may become irreversible during an attempt to reverse metabolic acidosis.

Because of the infant's small vascular and extravascular spaces, accurate assessment of blood and fluid requirements is necessary. Intraoperatively, fluid should be administered at a rate calculated to meet the infant's maintenance requirements (4 ml per kg per hr) and/or to correct preexisting deficits. Since a deficit is rarely more than 10 per cent of body weight (100 ml per kg) and since gradual rather than rapid correction is desirable, an additional 4 ml per kg per hr suffices for most depleted patients. Although it has been shown that dissection and manipulation during operation may increase fluid requirements by inducing losses into a third space, the magnitude of the surgical procedures performed in neonates is such that fluid loss during operation need not be considered a major factor in postoperative fluid assessment.

During operation, the need for blood transfusion is determined by the infant's pulse, blood pressure, hematocrit, and losses measured in suction bottles and in sponges that are carefully weighed before and after use. As a rule, a rapid transfusion of 20 ml per kg will be tolerated in infants without heart disease even if the actual volume of blood loss is significantly less.

ANTIBIOTICS

Prophylactic antibiotic therapy is advisable for all neonates who require major chest, abdominal, or genitourinary surgery. The neonate is especially prone to sepsis from certain organisms because of the state of the immune system. Of primary importance is that the infant's serum has only trace quantities of IgM; hence, humoral protection against E. coli and other gram-negative organisms is decreased. IgM is not synthesized by the fetus, and unlike some immunoglobulins, IgM does not pass the placental barrier. Concentrations of components of serum complement also are reduced, and normal antibody-antigen reactions and phagocytosis may be affected. In addition, the infant's local inflammatory response to noxious stimuli is slower and less intense than that of an older patient. Staphylococcal infection is also a special hazard for the neonate because of colonization with virulent staphylococci at the time of delivery or in the nursery. A combination of gentamicin (5 to 7.5 mg per kg per day in three divided IV doses) and ampicillin (100 to 200 mg per kg per day in four divided IV doses) will provide protection against those organisms that are most likely to produce infections in newborns. Other antibiotic combinations also have been successful in minimizing the incidence of sepsis. Ideally, antibiotics should be started before operation, so that they are present in the blood and tissues at the time of the incision. Antibiotics are discontinued after three days in the absence of septic complications. At some centers, 0.5 ml gamma globulin is given intramuscularly before operation for additional protection. However, there is little evidence that this decreases the incidence of septic complications.

VITAMIN K

Although clotting factors VII', IX', and X are present in normal quantities in umbilical cord blood, serum levels fall rapidly in the first three days of life. In some babies levels fall so low that bleeding (hemorrhagic disease of the newborn) occurs. To prevent this complication, most hospitals administer vitamin K routinely shortly after delivery. Before any operation in a neonate, the surgeon must confirm the fact that vitamin K has been administered. If not, 1 mg vitamin K should be given intramuscularly or intravenously.

PREMEDICATION

For the newborn, narcotics are never used as preoperative medication, nor are they needed postoperatively for control of pain. Neonates are especially sensitive to the respiratory depressant effects of opiates and barbiturates, and the use of these agents is unwise since their psychological effects are not necessary, and pain and restlessness are not a problem for this age group. Atropine is necessary to block the effects of vagal stimulation during surgery; to insure its optimal effect, atropine should be given after the patient arrives in the operating room and before anesthesia is induced. An intramuscular dose of 0.1 mg is satisfactory for most infants.

GASTROINTESTINAL DECOMPRESSION AND GASTROSTOMY

The importance of adequate gastrointestinal decompression before and after operation for almost all neonatal surgical problems cannot be overemphasized. For example, infants with untreated intestinal obstruction usually die from aspiration pneumonia, not dehydration or starvation. In those with diaphragmatic hernia, respiratory function deteriorates rapidly as air and fluid fill the herniated intestines. In infants with gastroschisis, omphalocele, and diaphragmatic hernia, the ability to replace the intestine into the abdominal cavity is markedly impaired by intestinal distention.

A variety of nasogastric tubes can be used to accomplish decompression. For most infants, a tube with a diameter of 10 French is satisfactory. When a straight, single lumen tube is used, a suction apparatus (approximately 10 mm Hg intermittent suction) used for the older patient is suitable for the infant. When a double lumen sump tube is used, continuous suction is necessary, and negative pressure of 40 to 60 mm Hg should be maintained. Whichever tube is used, it should be carefully taped in place and should be fixed in such a position that the tube does not rest against the cartilage of the ala nasae; otherwise, necrosis of the nose will occur.

Stamm gastrostomy is preferable to nasogastric intubation when it is anticipated that decompression may be necessary for more than one week. In addition, gastrostomy is needed for decompression and feeding in infants with esophageal abnormalities that preclude the passage of a nasogastric tube. Ordinarily, a 16 French mushroom-type catheter is ideal for infant gastrostomy. A Foley catheter, commonly used in the older patient, should be avoided in the infant because the distal catheter tip, which protrudes beyond the balloon, can cause perforation of the posterior gastric wall. Gastrostomy tubes drain best by gravity, and suction may be harmful to gastric mucosa. Even when gastrostomy tubes are sutured to the skin and fixed with tape, dislodgment may occur. To minimize the possibility of passing a tube into the peritoneal cavity when it is replaced, the stomach should always be sutured to the anterior abdominal wall at the tube exit site when the gastrostomy is established. As an additional precaution, the position of a replaced tube should be determined radiographically by injecting radiocontrast material through it.

Gastrostomy is helpful when feedings are started postoperatively. Prior to each feeding, the gastrostomy tube is aspirated, and the volume of gastric residue is measured by the nurse. Gastric residuals of less then 10 ml imply the absence of significant intestinal obstruction. Repeated low gastric aspirations indicate that the volume of feedings can be increased safely. If a large gastric residual is encountered (greater than 25 ml after a two-hour fast), the next feeding should be decreased or not given. When the volume of feeding is adjusted to the gastric residual, vomiting can be avoided and the chance of aspiration decreased.

TEMPERATURE CONTROL DURING OPERATION

Without appropriate preparation, all infants will become hypothermic during surgery. Although many devices have been manufactured to avoid this problem, most are so cumbersome that they interfere with the surgeon's maneuverability and visibility. However, the best method of maintaining or restoring normothermia is available to most surgeons. First, the ambient temperature of the operating room is raised to 80°F before the infant enters the room. The arms and legs are wrapped with bandages to reduce heat loss. A portable infrared heating light is focused on the baby during the preparation for operation and the induction of anesthesia. Solutions used for preparation of the skin are warmed. A heating blanket is placed under the child for use intraoperatively. Although maintenance of the 80°F temperature in the operating room may be uncomfortable for the operating team, it is the most important step to be taken. Fortunately most operations in neonates can be completed within an hour or two, and the discomfort is tolerable and insures an optimal environment for the infant.

POSTOPERATIVE NURSING CARE

Newborns who have undergone operation should be nursed in a section of the hospital that is specially equipped and staffed, preferably a neonatal intensive care unit. The infant should be kept in the isolated, controlled environment of an incubator whenever possible. Special incubators outfitted with appropriate ports for multiple intravenous and intra-arterial lines and gastrostomy or nasogastric drainage are necessary. Better access to the critically ill child can be obtained by nursing him or her in an infant warmer, but the ability to isolate the infant from a hostile microbial environment is thereby lost. Despite all recent advances in electronic monitoring, there is no substitute for the surgical nurse experienced in the special care of infants.

TRANSPORT

Since management of abnormalities in neonates often requires special expertise, the possibility to transfer to a center specially equipped to handle neonatal problems is often considered. Factors that will influence this decision include the need for a more accurate diagnosis, the capabilities of the anesthesia team, the experience and training of the surgeon, the sophistication of the institutional support services, and the urgency of the clinical problem.

If a decision is made to transfer the patient to a neonatal center, proper arrangements must be made to insure a safe trip. Details should be coordinated with specialists at the referral center before transfer. Often the center can dispatch a specially equipped transfer vehicle. The child always must be accompanied by a properly trained professional who can monitor important physiologic indices and provide the care that might be necessary during transport.

The most common complication encountered during transport is hypothermia, often because of faulty or inadequate equipment available in the transport vehicle or because the infant's attendants failed to take steps to avoid this problem.

In addition to the need to maintain normothermia during transport, nasogastric suction is required for almost every neonate who is to undergo a surgical procedure. Ventilatory support may be needed for those with respiratory difficulties. Except in rare cases, fluid therapy is usually not critical during the relatively short transfer time. Standards for neonatal transfer have been well established in manuals published by the American Academy of Pediatrics and the American College of Surgeons.

SPECIAL CONSIDERATIONS FOR SPECIFIC PROBLEMS

DIAPHRAGMATIC HERNIA

Although some children with this abnormality have relatively few symptoms, many have severe respiratory distress, hypoxemia, and hypercapnia from birth. Fetal lung growth is impaired because the abdominal contents have been in the chest since the first trimester of pregnancy. Although hypoplasia of the lung usually is more severe on the side of the hernia, hypoplasia of the contralateral lung can be significant when mediastinal shift to that side occurs early in pregnancy.

As soon as the diagnosis of diaphragmatic hernia is made, a nasogastric tube should be inserted to prevent further accumulation of air and fluid in the intestine. If transport is necessary, the infant should be propped up and turned toward the affected side. Rarely, insertion of an endotracheal tube is necessary to assist ventilation while preparations for operation are made. For the desperately ill infant, some physicians have advised decompression of the chest on an open ward, but this is seldom advisable.

Preoperatively, attempts should be made to achieve at least partial correction of hypercapnia and hypoxemia. However, in those with severe respiratory insufficiency, complete correction will not be possible until the abdominal viscera are removed from the thorax, and then only if total lung volume is sufficient.

Postoperative support depends on the infant's status. In all infants, a chest tube can be of critical importance. Application of too much suction to the affected chest can move the mediastinum to a position that will decrease venous return and overdistend the contralateral lung. Application of too little suction will fail to relieve mediastinal compression and pressure on the contralateral lung. These problems usually can be avoided by attaching the chest tube to water seal drainage without additional negative pressure. When there is doubt about the optimal position of the mediastinum, air can be withdrawn or added to the affected thorax while the infant's vital signs and blood gases are monitored carefully. In infants who will require respiratory support following operation, it is our opinion that a chest tube should be placed in the uninvolved thorax prophylactically because pneumothorax is likely in many infants. Without a tube for decompression, contralateral pneumothorax can be fatal in a child whose pulmonary function is barely adequate.

Other resuscitative measures also must be considered for those with persistent severe respiratory insufficiency. Recently, it has been shown that increased pulmonary vascular resistance increases hypoxemia because it causes blood to shunt from right to left through a patent ductus arteriosus for a foramen ovale. In some infants, the injection of tolazoline (1 to 2 mg per kg) into a pulmonary artery catheter has produced pulmonary vasodilation and reduced shunting and hypoxemia. When low cardiac output and poor urine output compound the clinical problem, an intravenous infusion of dopamine may be helpful. Unfortunately, despite the use of these agents, many infants still do not have sufficient lung function to survive.

ESOPHAGEAL ATRESIA AND TRACHEOESOPHAGEAL FISTULA

The definitive diagnosis of this condition depends on the demonstration of complete esophageal obstruction. A nasal catheter that does not pass into the stomach is strong suggestive evidence of this anomoly, but radiographic confirmation is necessary. In some cases, the presence of a dilated, air-filled, upper esophagus on a lateral chest roentgenogram is diagnostic, but in other cases the obstructed esophagus is best seen radiographically by filling it with radiopaque medium. To avoid aspiration during this study, the contrast medium should be injected into the esophagus through the catheter during continuous flouroscopic observation. The catheter should have only a single opening at its distal end, and less than 1 ml of medium should be injected. A contrast medium used for bronchography is preferred in case aspiration occurs.

During preparation for operation or for transport to a neonatal center, the obstructed esophagus must be kept empty to prevent aspiration of saliva. This can be accomplished by frequent intermittent suction applied to a small (8 to 10 French) nasoesophageal catheter or by continuous suction applied to a small sump tube especially designed for this purpose.* In addition, an infant who also has a tracheoesophageal fistula should be kept in an upright position to minimize the reflux of gastric juice into the tracheobronchial tree. When repair of the esophagus is to be delayed for more than six hours, decompression of the stomach by gastrostomy provides more reliable protection against the possibility of gastric reflux.

As already noted, antibiotic therapy is appropriate for all neonates requiring major operations. In those with esophageal atresia, antibiotic usage is therapeutic and not prophylactic because some aspiration has occurred in all infants, and pneumonia complicates the postoperative course for many. Gentamicin and ampicillin offer appropriate protection at least until the specific bacteria are identified.

One of the most common complications of repair is a leak at the esophageal anastomosis. Therefore, following operation, oral feedings are withheld for five to seven days, and feedings are given by gastrostomy or nasogastric tube beginning 48 hours after operation. The chest tube placed at the time of operation is not removed for 10 days because an anastomotic leak is not always apparent immediately postoperatively. Usually the leak is small, and it drains well through the chest tube. Feedings are given by gastrostomy, and spontaneous closure generally occurs in a week or two. However, when the esophageal opening is large, the leak persists longer, and adequate nutrition cannot be maintained with gastrostomy feedings if significant gastroesophageal reflux is present. In these cases, insertion of a feeding tube beyond the pylorus or intravenous hyperalimentation is necessary until the opening in the esophagus closes.

Stricture at the site of anastomosis may become apparent when oral feedings are begun. Since esophagoscopy and esophageal dilatation may disrupt a recently constructed anastomosis, treatment of a stricture

---

*Argyle Replogle Catheter, Sherwood Medical Industries, Inc., St. Louis.

should be delayed until three weeks postoperatively. Decompression of the esophagus with a sump tube is necessary if aspiration of saliva occurs during this interval.

PYLORIC STENOSIS

Hypertrophic pyloric stenosis is the most common gastrointestinal problem in infants requiring operation in the first two months of life. Dehydration and hypokalemic alkalosis are the greatest threats to life, and these abnormalities should be corrected preoperatively. In those patients with severe prolonged vomiting, serum chloride may be as low as 60 mEq per l and serum bicarbonate as high as 60 mEq per l. In most cases, more moderate abnormal values are noted. Ordinarily, acid-base balance and fluid and electrolyte balance can be restored in 12 to 24 hours by the intravenous infusion of 0.45 per cent NaCl in 5 per cent dextrose with 4 mEq KCl per 100 ml at a rate of 6 ml per kg per hr. However, for the markedly depleted and malnourished infant, several days of fluid therapy may be required, in addition to blood transfusion and albumin administration.

Potassium chloride is an essential component of the replacement solution. Even though serum potassium measurements may be within normal limits, total body potassium is depleted as a result of the potassium concentration in gastric juice and the potassium losses that occur as the kidney tries to conserve hydrogen ion. In addition to its cardiac effects, potassium depletion interferes with the ability of the kidney to excrete an alkaline urine and, therefore, further aggravates alkalosis. Persistent alkalosis can be responsible for serious respiratory depression in the recovery room.

During the period of preoperative fluid and electrolyte therapy, oral feedings should be stopped. Nasogastric suction is not necessary except for the severely depleted, critically ill infant or one with gastritis, as indicated by blood in the vomitus. However, in all infants the stomach should be intubated and emptied just before operation to avoid the possibility of aspiration during induction or emergence from anesthesia.

Usually, small feedings (15 to 30 ml) of 5 per cent dextrose and water every two hours are started four hours postoperatively. If tolerated, 30 ml of milk formula is begun 12 hours later. The volume of each feeding is increased so that the infant is taking 60 to 90 ml every three or four hours by the third postoperative day. In some, the progression of postoperative feeding must be slowed because of vomiting, which may persist for several days even though pyloromyotomy has been adequate. In infants with gastritis or in those in whom the duodenum was entered at operation, resumption of feeding should be delayed, and nasogastric decompression should be maintained for 24 hours postoperatively.

INTESTINAL OBSTRUCTION

In infants suspected of having intestinal obstruction, a nasogastric tube should be inserted and diagnostic studies obtained. Ordinarily, supine and upright roentgenograms of the abdomen are sufficient to indicate the presence of obstruction. However, a barium enema is always desirable to aid in determining the site and cause of obstruction and to rule out the possibility of an associated colonic atresia in those with atresia at higher levels.

For infants whose obstruction might be due to midgut volvulus, immediate operation is necessary to avoid irreversible ischemic damage to a large portion of the intestine. In other patients, such as those with duodenal atresia, a reasonable delay is acceptable to correct fluid and electrolyte imbalance or to determine the presence of Down's syndrome. In infants with meconium ileus and no evidence of intestinal perforation, operation should be delayed until attempts at relief of obstruction by Gastrografin enema have proved unsuccessful.

The major problem encountered following surgical correction of intestinal obstruction in infancy is prolonged abnormal gastrointestinal function. In some cases this is the result of persistent mechanical obstruction due to edema at the site of an anastomosis or early postoperative adhesions. In others, intestinal motility is inadequate, especially when a dilated loop of proximal intestine has been left in the abdomen. Diarrhea and malabsorption often develop as the result of residual short intestinal length, absence of the ileocecal valve, partial intestinal obstruction, or bacterial overgrowth in a blind or dilated loop of intestine. If adequate nutrition can be maintained, experience has shown that most of the causes of inadequate intestinal function will resolve spontaneously.

In some cases, nutrition can be maintained by the enteral route. For example, in a child with a malfunctioning duodenojejunostomy, feedings can be given through a tube that traverses the anastomosis. In the infant with mild absorptive abnormalities, elemental diets may be tolerated. However, in many situations, intravenous hyperalimentation is necessary until at least partial resolution of the underlying abnormality occurs. For those with postoperative intestinal obstruction, total parenteral nutrition may be necessary for as long as six or eight weeks. When mechanical obstruction persists longer, it is likely that surgical correction will be necessary. For those with malabsorption after operation, total parenteral nutrition may be necessary for even longer periods.

The following measures have been helpful in the management of postoperative malabsorption: special diets, cholestyramine to bind bile salts, oral antibiotics to alter intestinal bacterial flora, and drugs to decrease intestinal motility.

ANORECTAL ABNORMALITIES

In all infants with an imperforate anus, a nasogastric tube should be passed for decompression and to rule out the possibility of esophageal atresia, which is present in about 10 per cent of cases. Because of the high incidence of urinary anomalies, the urinary tract also should be evaluated by an intravenous pyelogram sometime during the initial hospitalization.

Before deciding on an appropriate operative procedure for the infant with imperforate anus, it is necessary to determine if the distal end of the rectum is below the puborectalis muscle (low imperforate anus) or above it (high imperforate anus). A perineal or visible rectovaginal fistula is indicative of a low lesion. In infants with no visible fistula, the determination of the site of the distal end of the intestine can be aided by lateral roentgenograms of the pelvis taken when the patient is 12 to 24 hours of age, after swallowed air has passed into the colon. Vomiting and overdistention of the bowel can be prevented during this period by continuous nasogastric suction. Often the distal bowel can be visualized by retrograde urethrogram in boys and vaginogram in girls when radiocontrast material enters the colon through a fistula.

For low imperforate anus, definitive repair can be performed safely by a perineal operation at an early age. If repair is delayed for any reason, such as the baby's size, the presence of other congenital anomalies, or the surgeon's preference, adequate decompression of the colon can be maintained by dilatation of the fistula every week or two. For those with high imperforate anus, definitive repair should be delayed for 6 to 12 months, when the anatomy of the puborectalis is better defined and the chance of achieving continence is increased. In these infants temporary colostomy is necessary.

A loop colostomy in the transverse or sigmoid colon is used in pediatric surgery for imperforate anus and Hirschsprung's disease. When the colostomy is established, the peritoneum and rectus sheath should be sutured to the entire circumference of the stoma to prevent herniation of the small intestine. The loop should be supported by a glass or plastic rod, which should remain in place for 10 days to prevent retraction of the colon into the peritoneal cavity. The stoma can be covered with a diaper, but a small appliance is preferred by most families. When colostomy is performed for Hirschsprung's disease, the stoma should be biopsied to be certain that it contains ganglion cells. Prolapse of the distal colostomy limb may occur a month or more postoperatively. This complication has been noted when the skin opening has been too large and, paradoxically, when it has been too small. Diarrhea may be troublesome early after colostomy if the stoma is placed in the ascending colon. With supplemental intravenous feedings and proper skin care, this problem is self-limited. However, in the child with diarrhea, the possibility exists that the material discharged at the stoma is urine that has entered the colon through a rectourethral fistula. These infants develop hyperkalemic, hyperchloremic acidosis that requires not only appropriate fluid therapy but also urgent division of the fistula.

NECROTIZING ENTEROCOLITIS

Premature infants with respiratory distress and those who have had exchange transfusion or who have required catheters in the umbilical artery or vein are especially prone to develop necrotizing enterocolitis. This condition is first suspected in the neonate who develops abdominal distention, bloody diarrhea, or both. The diagnosis is usually confirmed radiographically by findings that can include nonspecific bowel dilatation, pneumatosis intestinalis, air in the portal vein, and pneumoperitoneum. In untreated cases, intestinal necrosis leads to perforation, peritonitis, and death.

Initial management of the infant without intestinal perforation includes continuous nasogastric suction, systemic broad-spectrum antibiotic therapy, oral antibiotic therapy, intravenous hyperalimentation for nutrition, and the removal of umbilical catheters if present. Thrombocytopenia is noted in infants who are septic. Abdominal roentgenograms are obtained every eight hours to follow the progression of the disease. Nonoperative treatment must be continued for at least 48 hours after all symptoms and signs of illness have disappeared. Currently, surgical intervention is indicated for those with evidence of intestinal perforation.

When operation is performed, the extent and location of necrosis varies, although the terminal ileum and right colon are most frequently involved. Exteriorization of necrotic bowel is preferable to resection and anastomosis. Following operation, gastrointestinal decompression, total parenteral nutrition, and antibiotic therapy are maintained. Intestinal stomas are closed when sepsis is no longer evident and the infant's general condition is satisfactory.

In many infants whose acute illness is successfully managed by nonoperative means, operation may be required one to three months later for intestinal stricture that develops at a site of prior injury.

DEFECTS OF THE ABDOMINAL WALL

Nasogastric suction is an important initial step in the management of infants with omphalocele and gastroschisis to prevent intestinal distention and minimize the difficulty of replacing the herniated viscera in the abdominal cavity. In addition, during preparation for operation and/or transport, an extra effort must be made to prevent evaporative and radiant heat loss, which is a major hazard for these infants because of the exposed moist viscera. To minimize heat loss, it is helpful to cover the omphalocele membrane or exposed intestinal tract with moist gauze and then wrap the baby in a plastic sheet or place him or her in a plastic bag from the neck to the toes.

Surgical repair is indicated as soon as possible. Problems encountered during operation or afterward are related to the size of the abdominal wall defect, the volume of the herniated mass, and whether or not the peritoneal membrane is intact.

If the abdominal cavity is too small to accept the viscera, repair of the defect may cause respiratory embarrassment secondary to elevation of the diaphragm or hypotension and low cardiac output secondary to compression of the inferior vena cava. Since these problems can be resolved by reopening the abdominal wound, the infant should be kept in the operating room for 20 to 30 minutes following operation to be certain that cardiorespiratory function is satisfactory. When the size of the abdominal cavity is inadequate, techniques have been developed so that the exposed viscera can be covered temporarily by an envelope of synthetic material that is sewn to the edges of the abdominal wall defect. The envelope tends to pull the defect up over the viscera and aids in enlarging the abdominal cavity. Since the peritoneal cavity expands rapidly, tucks can be taken in the envelope every two or three days until the edges of the defect come together. Eventually all the synthetic material is removed. During this staged closure, intestinal decompression by gastrostomy or nasogastric tube is necessary. Since decompression may be needed for two or three weeks, intravenous nutrition must be provided until final closure is completed and intestinal function is satisfactory. Because sepsis is a definite complication of this method, all dressings and manipulations of the envelope must be done aseptically. If sepsis occurs, all synthetic material must be removed.

In infants with gastroschisis and ruptured omphalocele, some degree of mechanical intestinal obstruction exists because of adhesions that have developed between intestinal loops that were bathed in amnionic fluid in utero. Fortunately, in most cases obstruction will resolve after the intestinal tract is put at rest in the abdominal cavity. Occasionally intestinal atresia is responsible for persistent intestinal obstruction. Operative exploration is necessary when intestinal obstruction persists beyond six weeks after initial repair.

SUMMARY

Although the basic principles of preoperative and postoperative care are similar for all patients, certain modifications and considerations are necessary for the newborn because of size, immaturity of organ systems, and susceptibility to environmental hazards, especially cold and infectious agents. However, in many ways the neonate is able to tolerate operation better than the older patient because of a vigorous, responsive cardiovascular system, unusual tolerance to hypovolemia and hypoxia, and a remarkable capability to heal wounds, to regenerate certain organs, and to adapt to many anatomic deficiencies.

17

The Child and Adolescent

JAMES A. O'NEILL, Jr.

The primary aims of preoperative and postoperative care are maintenance of normal physiologic function and avoidance of complications that may delay operative procedures or convalescence. In the childhood age group, additional attention must be given to psychological considerations, which are important for postoperative cooperation as well as for the child's long-term well-being. Rooming in the hospital by one of the parents of young children is to be encouraged. Also, whenever possible, a child or adolescent should be prepared for an operation with a thorough explanation of procedures and expectations in an honest and straightforward fashion appropriate to the child's age and degree of maturity. If the patient will be admitted to an intensive care unit postoperatively, a preoperative visit to the unit, introduction to the nurses, and familiarization with equipment is helpful. In many institutions, the nursing service assists physicians with preoperative programs designed to acquaint the child with procedures such as blood drawing, intravenous fluid therapy, nasogastric drainage, endotracheal suctioning, dressing changes, and similar measures. Such programs are augmented by the use of dolls and photographs as well as visits to special care units where pleasant nurses may minimize childhood fears. These introductory steps appear to be helpful to all young individuals beyond the infant age group.

In this chapter, consideration is given to a variety of common conditions seen in toddlers and older children and to the special care often necessary for this group. The reader is encouraged to assume that general aspects of care given in other chapters should apply as well as the special considerations listed here. As is true for all patients, a thorough physical examination and an accurate diagnosis are essential to the management of surgical disorders.

HEAD AND NECK SURGERY

Common conditions involving the head and neck regions in children and adolescents include thyroglossal duct and branchial cleft cysts and sinuses; enlarged cervical lymph nodes due to infectious conditions, inflammatory disorders, and neoplasms, tumors and inflammation of the parotid and submaxillary glands; abscesses of the neck; and enlargements of the thyroid due to inflammation or neoplasms. If an extensive operative procedure is anticipated (such as corrective measures for patients with vascular malformations of the head and neck), appropriate amounts of blood should be typed and cross-matched preoperatively, and a large intravenous access should be established. Treatment of the vast majority of the above abnormalities requires the use of a general anesthetic. Children undergoing elective surgical procedures of this or any other type should not receive general anesthesia if they have any evidence of an upper respiratory tract infection, particularly if an endotracheal tube is to be utilized. This is an extremely important consideration if postoperative pneumonia and croup are to be avoided; it is far better to delay operation than to place the child in jeopardy from a potentially life-threatening airway complication. Secure control of the airway with an endotracheal tube is mandatory to insure the safety of the procedure. Loose teeth should be noted. Elective operations involving the head and neck are similar to other elective procedures in terms of the duration of time that food and fluids need to be withheld preoperatively. It is probably best for young children to fast for six hours, and for adolescents undergoing elective surgical procedures such as these, it is probably safer to withhold fluids for up to eight hours.

Preoperative antibiotics are appropriate therapy for those patients with obvious infectious conditions of the neck that require either excision or drainage. In these instances, streptococcal and staphylococcal infections are the most common offenders; therefore, unless another organism has been demonstrated, antibiotics effective against these organisms are indicated. Of course, it should be determined first whether the patient is penicillin-sensitive. Preoperative antibiotics are particularly important for children who have extensive abscesses of the neck, since operative manipulation may be associated with sepsis. Abscesses due to an infected branchial cleft usually contain bacteria that commonly inhabit the mouth; thus, penicillin in addition to a broad-spectrum antibiotic may be helpful in these instances. However, preoperative antibiotics are not indicated in the vast majority of noninflammatory and noninfectious conditions of the head and neck, which comprise the bulk of disorders in this region.

Special preoperative consideration should be given to adolescents with hyperthyroidism. These patients should be under adequate control and in the euthyroid state, confirmed by appropriate tests of thyroid function, if possible. We prefer to administer iodine preoperatively in order to diminish the size and congestion of the enlarged gland and to minimize intraoperative complications. Blood should be available for infusion during operation if needed for patients with large congested glands. Specific postoperative considerations are limited for most patients who have undergone surgical procedures in the head and neck since the majority of individuals recover rapidly and uneventfully. The first and most important postoperative aspect of care involves careful timing for the removal of the endotracheal tube. It is preferable to ascertain that the patient is fully awake before the tube is removed in order to avoid respiratory obstruction, a particular danger for those patients who have undergone removal of lesions associated with the airway or in the immediate vicinity. In this situation, it may be extremely difficult to reintubate these patients after they have developed respiratory obstruction.

A second major consideration concerns potential postoperative bleeding within the neck tissues. If the surgeon feels that the operative field is likely to have postoperative oozing, it is best to use either a soft rubber or suction drain to prevent accumulation of blood, which may potentiate airway obstruction as well as late infection. Dressings on the neck should be applied loosely enough to avoid undue pressure, which might accentuate respiratory obstruction or venous congestion. Elevation of the head of the bed may be helpful. If extensive procedures such as radical neck dissection have been performed, excessive edema may occur in the cervical region, and under these circumstances, constant observation and frequent nasotracheal suctioning are essential to optimal care. Most of these patients are able to resume oral feedings rapidly, but it may be best to withhold feedings for approximately 24 hours if there is edema or intraoral suture lines. Postoperative antibiotics should be continued as indicated for infectious conditions or when suture lines extend into the nose, mouth, or pharynx.

ABDOMINAL CONDITIONS

For most surgical patients with abdominal conditions, preoperative and postoperative care is related to the magnitude of the procedure and whether the operation is elective or an emergency. The greater the physiologic derangement, the more intense the attention to supportive care should be. Although specific examples are given below, they are meant to serve as general guidelines to be observed for a variety of similar surgical procedures.

ANOMALIES OF THE INGUINAL CANAL

Elective surgical procedures for umbilical and inguinal hernias, hydroceles, and undescended testes may usually be performed during a one- to two-day hospitalization and in some cases may be done on an outpatient basis. Patients should fast in the normal manner preoperatively. Most anesthesiologists prefer that the child's hematocrit be in the range of 30 volumes per cent to insure adequate oxygen-carrying capacity during the period of general anesthesia. If a child is anemic, it is necessary for the surgeon and the anesthesiologist to decide whether it is safe to wait until the child's hematocrit improves with iron therapy or whether transfusions should be administered. If transfusion is the procedure of choice, packed red cells should ordinarily be administered in the range of 5 ml per kg of body weight. A diagnostic sickle cell preparation should routinely be performed as a screening measure in Negro children in order to avoid anesthetic complications. This type of screening is particularly important for those black children who are anemic or who have a family history of sickle cell disease. In the case of a young child in diapers, it is important for the surgeon to instruct the mother that operation must be delayed if an extensive ammonia rash due to urine is present, since a rash of this nature may harbor *Staphylococcus* or *Candida*. If a rash is present, it is best to instruct the mother to leave the diaper off for 12 to 24 hours, as a dry environment ordinarily results in a rapid resolution.

Adequate preoperative sedation and atropine should be ordered by the anesthesiologist or surgeon. For patients over six months of age, secobarbital, 1 mg per kg of body weight, meperidine, 1 mg per kg, and atropine, 0.005 mg per kg, administered approximately one to 1½ hours prior to anesthesia are helpful. Infants under six months of age require no sedation, but atropine is still helpful. Other preanesthetic drug regimens are also available and useful. As children approach adulthood, dosages should be modified upward toward adult dose levels. Whatever method is used, it is desirable to have most patients undergoing these elective procedures asleep when they enter the operating room.

Intraoperative management of patients involves anesthesia administered either by mask or endotracheal tube. Again, it should be stressed that patients should be free of upper respiratory tract infection at the time of operation in order to avoid respiratory complications. For the same reason, an intravenous route should be established so that drugs may be administered by the anesthesiologist as required for problems such as improper endotracheal tube placement, laryngospasm, and vomiting. A 0.25 normal saline solution in 5 per cent dextrose administered at a rate of 4 to 6 ml per kg of body weight per hour is ordinarily sufficient.

Postoperatively, most children who have undergone elective operation upon the inguinal canal are able to resume oral feedings within four hours, provided they have sufficiently recovered from anesthesia. One exception to this may be the patient with an undescended testis that has required extensive retroperitoneal dissection and mobilization during repair. In this circumstance, intestinal ileus may persist until the morning following operation. As soon as patients who have had inguinal operations are able to retain oral feedings and to void, the intravenous infusion may be discontinued. Patients who have inguinal incisions should not be diapered tightly in order to keep these areas dry, and they should not be permitted to lie prone in bed. Swelling in the operative area is usually minimal, but this may be further reduced by limiting mobility and ambulation for the first 12 hours. The majority of these patients are ready for discharge the morning following operation with the exception of patients who have undergone extensive orchiopexy and may require further observation.

Complications of inguinal hernias occasionally require emergency management. Approximately 10 to 15 per cent of children with inguinal hernias suffer incarceration. This problem is preponderant in younger children. Only about 5 per cent of incarcerated inguinal hernias become strangulated. Occasionally, incarceration that is particularly tight results in testicular infarction from engorgement of the testis. Most incarcerated hernias can be safely reduced by simply sedating the child while he is positioned in a head-down position. If spontaneous reduction of the hernia does not occur within 15 minutes, gentle manual reduction may be attempted. Incarcerated hernias in children typically traverse the inguinal canal, and after exiting from the external inguinal ring, they may tend not only to advance downward toward the scrotum but also to curve upward above the external ring. For this reason, reduction is usually most readily performed in a sedated child by first gently pushing the incarcerated mass downward toward the scrotum and then gently upward, applying slow, steady pressure. If reduction is successful, it is best to wait 48 hours before performing surgical repair in order to allow edema within the inguinal canal to subside. When reduction cannot be performed or when there are signs of strangulation, such as local redness, signs of intestinal obstruction, fever, leukocytosis, or vascular instability, urgent surgical exploration is warranted. Since these patients tend to have intestinal ileus, it is worthwhile to utilize a nasogastric tube to evacuate the stomach prior to operation. Intravenous fluids should be given appropriately, depending upon the severity of the clinical situation, in order to correct any electrolyte imbalance and to insure adequate vascular volume and urinary output. Such preoperative preparation rarely requires more than one or two hours. Intravenous antibiotics should be given in anticipation of the possibility of gangrenous bowel.

Following operation for incarcerated and strangulated inguinal hernias, intravenous fluids are continued until intestinal function has returned and the child has passed stool. Subsequently, nasogastric suction may be discontinued and light feedings begun with rapid progression thereafter. Most young children have very little pain following repair of inguinal hernias, but older children may require narcotics for a day or two postoperatively. Early ambulation is also helpful in diminishing postoperative discomfort.

Patients with torsion of the testis should be treated preoperatively in much the same fashion as patients with incarcerated or strangulated inguinal hernias. Under most circumstances, unless the testis is obviously completely necrotic, the gonad is left in place after decompressing it by incising the tunica albuginea. These particular patients may have a great deal of early swelling and pain associated with fever, which may require bedrest for three to five days. Antibiotics are continued until the patient is afebrile and comfortable. Patients with torsion of the appendix testis may be treated as if they had elective inguinal hernia repairs.

APPENDICITIS

The most common acute abdominal problem in childhood that requires operation is appendicitis. Although the disease has the same characteristics in both the child and the adult, complications can be quite different for these two age groups. In general, older children respond more like adults, and younger children tend to have a more complicated course related to frequent perforation. For example, in the very young age group, the criteria for diagnosis are different, and the untreated disease runs a much more rapid course. Older children, usually in the 10- to 14-year age group, present with typical adult complaints or abdominal pain gradually localizing in the right lower quadrant, and pain is associated with mild vomiting. These children are rarely dehydrated and ordinarily do not have any electrolyte imbalance. They may, however, develop an intestinal ileus with gastric retention so that passage of a nasogastric tube preoperatively is usually the safest procedure before anesthesia is induced. Indeed, we feel that it is safest to pass a nasogastric tube preoperatively in all young patients undergoing an abdominal operation. Mild sedation frequently eases insertion, since children sometimes object to passage of the tube. If patients with early appendicitis have no signs or laboratory findings suggestive of gangrene or perforation, minimal amounts of preoperative intravenous fluids are required, and antibiotics are probably not needed.

Postoperatively, patients with simple acute appendicitis without gangrene or rupture ordinarily may have nasogastric drainage discontinued the following morning, and clear, noncarbonated oral fluids may be begun. Intravenous fluids are discontinued as soon as adequate oral intake has been established. Early ambulation is helpful as well. Most of these patients are able to go home by the third postoperative day.

Unfortunately, some patients progress from simple appendicitis to transmural disease, resulting in thrombosis of the blood supply of the appendix, gangrene, and rupture. In older individuals, the process may be localized by adjacent mesenteric surfaces and by the omentum. In infants and young children, this mechanism is deficient since the omentum is undeveloped and mesenteries are devoid of fat. This is presumably the reason that appendicitis progresses to rupture more rapidly in very young children than in older ones, and it also explains why generalized peritonitis is the rule in children under the age of four (although sometimes this may be associated with localized abscesses in the pelvis, between intestinal loops, or in other parts of the abdomen). In patients with ruptures, there may be severe inflammation of all peritoneal surfaces with outpouring of fluid into the peritoneal cavity and within bowel loops. Under these circumstances, vomiting may be severe, and occasionally diarrhea occurs simultaneously.

As a result of massive fluid loss, these patients may first present with marked abdominal distention, tachypnea, oliguria, vascular instability, high fever, and extreme acidosis. Generally, a rapid infusion of Ringer's lactate solution (supplemented with 5 per cent albumin in extreme instances) given rapidly at the rate of 5 ml per kg of body weight followed by an infusion at the rate of approximately 3000 ml per square meter of body surface will be sufficient to produce resumption of urine output, stabilization of vital signs, and reduction of acidosis. Nasogastric suction will alleviate vomiting and to some extent abdominal distention. Fever may be controlled with tepid water sponging, rectal antipyretics, and small doses of intravenous morphine. Ice packs should not be used since they frequently cause shivering and further increase body temperature.

The choice of antibiotics is usually indicative of the surgeon's individual experience. However, in our experience, various gram-negative organisms, such as *Enterococcus, Staphylococcus*, and *Bacteroides*, can be isolated. Thus, we use a combination of intravenous penicillin and ampicillin, with the addition of clindamycin when anaerobic organisms are thought to be present. If particularly foul-smelling, thin, purulent fluid is obtained at operation, *Bacteroides* is often isolated. Various other antibiotic regimens are available and effective. Patients who have tachycardia should not be given atropine preoperatively since it may accentuate hyperpyrexia and tachycardia. Also, operation should not proceed until urine output, vital signs, and body temperature are brought to near-normal levels. Operative management is dictated individually, but, if at all possible, the appendix should be removed and drains utilized whenever there are localized abscesses. Thorough saline irrigation of the abdomen is also helpful.

Postoperatively, children with severe forms of advanced appendicitis should be maintained in an intensive care unit. The patients should be elevated in semi-Fowler's position. Intravenous fluids should be administered at a sufficient rate to keep urinary output adequate, with a sodium and potassium content sufficient to maintain normal electrolyte levels. Gastric suction losses may be replaced with one-half normal saline solution in 5 per cent dextrose with 30 mEq of potassium chloride per liter. If tachycardia continues, it may be worthwhile to administer additional amounts of 5 per cent albumin in a volume of 5 ml per kg of body weight daily for one to three days. Most patients do not require blood. Nasogastric suction should be continued until patients pass flatus and stool and until abdominal distention is relieved. This is important because segmental intestinal ileus continues in the presence of resolving peritonitis, and return of total intestinal function may take a little longer than the first appearance of stool.

We prefer to continue sedation with intravenous morphine in small doses for 48 hours postoperatively and then to use narcotics only as indicated. Antibiotics are continued until the patient no longer has a fever, and then they are gradually withdrawn. If drains have been used, it is preferable to begin to withdraw them by the second postoperative day so that they are removed by the fifth or sixth postoperative day, unless profuse drainage occurs. If so, the drains may be left in a day or two longer. Patients are not ready for discharge until their wounds are healing properly, rectal examination is normal, temperature is normal for at least 24 hours, and white blood cell count and differential count are normal. For the young patient with ruptured appendicitis, it may be three to seven days before nasogastric drainage and intravenous fluids may be discontinued. Although some patients occasionally develop postoperative obstruction from recurrent abscess or adhesions, the majority recover uneventfully. It should be mentioned that other related inflammatory abdominal conditions, such as Meckel's diverticulitis, severe enterocolitis, and primary peritonitis, are ordinarily managed in the same fashion as described for appendicitis.

Intussusception

Typically, intussusception involves invagination of the terminal ileum into the cecum and colon for varying distances and occurs in children between the ages of three months and two years. The signs and symptoms of intussusception are well described, and it is known that approximately 70 per cent of such patients with this condition may be relieved by hydrostatic barium emena reduction if the diagnosis is made prior to the appearance of symptoms suggesting bowel compromise. It is wise to prepare patients for whom barium enema reduction will be attempted as if they will require operation, in an effort to avoid sudden clinical deterioration that may occur during radiologic manipulation if the subject has a marginal vascular status. Those patients who have any suggestion of bowel necrosis, early perforation, or long-standing mechanical intestinal obstruction should not be candidates for barium enema reduction. Children in whom intussusception is recognized in its early stages may behave almost as if they were completely healthy, while those for whom diagnosis has been late may have extensive bowel gangrene, complete intestinal obstruction, shock, and sepsis.

The principles of care for intussusception may be applied to a wide variety of other emergent abdominal disorders in childhood as well. Depending upon the severity of the condition, children with intussusception are treated in a fairly standard fashion. A nasogastric tube is passed in order to evacuate the stomach and to prevent further intestinal distention. A secure intravenous route is established, and intravenous fluids are begun. We prefer to start Ringer's lactate solution in 5 per cent dextrose while awaiting laboratory determinations of serum electrolytes, urea nitrogen, glucose, osmolality, and complete blood cell count. The intravenous fluid regimen may be altered in response to these results. When the child has attained satisfactory circulatory condition, he or she is taken to the radiology suite if hydrostatic reduction is to be attempted; otherwise the child is taken to the operating room. The technique of barium enema reduction has been well described and will not be repeated here. If criteria for complete reduction have been satisfactorily accomplished, the aforementioned regimen is followed until intestinal function returns.

When barium enema reduction is unsuccessful or when it is not attempted because bowel compromise is suspected, the child is brought to the operating room as soon as his or her clinical condition is stable. This is an exceedingly important procedure to follow because manipulation of gangrenous bowel at the time of attempted reduction in the operating room may result in sudden and unexpected shock unless there has been preoperative preparation. We prefer to begin the administration of intravenous penicillin and ampicillin preoperatively. When the surgeon encounters a very sick child, it is wise preoperatively to place a central venous catheter in the superior vena cava via the subclavian or jugular vein for monitoring purposes. In such patients, there may be limited time for the blood bank to cross-match blood when there is a significant length of gangrenous intestine present. Under these circumstances, it may be necessary to administer 5 per cent albumin solution and Ringer's lactate solution intraoperatively. After a few hours, it is usually possible to perform the cross-match, and packed red blood cells may be administered if necessary. Careful monitoring of arterial blood and central venous pressures is helpful in making decisions concerning infused fluids. Of course, during procedures involving infants and young children, body temperature should be carefully monitored during operation, and efforts should be made to insure that it remains close to normal.

Once the operative procedure has been completed, the seriously ill patient should be managed in an intensive care unit so that central venous pressure, arterial blood pressure, hourly urine output, and general clinical status can be monitored. Serum electrolytes, blood urea nitrogen, hematocrit, and osmolality values should be determined as indicated. Patients who develop hyperosmolality should have this condition corrected gradually over a period of at least 24 hours rather than attempting rapid correction, which might result in central nervous system damage.

Total serum protein concentration may fall following resection for gangrenous intussusception, as in any other extensive surgical condition, because of third space losses of protein-rich fluid. Total proteins may be measured either directly or indirectly using the Goldberg refractometer. The latter determination, along with measurement of hematocrit and venous pressure, may be quite helpful in terms of indicating whether the patient requires additional crystalloid, albumin, or blood. Daily measurement of body weight is a good indication of the status of hydration. In the early postoperative period, the seriously ill patient with intussusception may have derangements of acid-base balance either as a result of the pathologic condition itself or as a result of infusion of large amounts of stored blood. While restoration of adequate circulatory volume usually corrects acidosis, administration of sodium bicarbonate may be indicated as well.

Mechanical ventilatory support may be necessary for the first 12 to 24 hours following operation in infants and children who have been severely acidotic or very lethargic either preoperatively or in the early postoperative period. The extreme work of breathing may be an intolerable burden from a metabolic point of view, and under these circumstances, it is best to err on the side of being overly aggressive in utilizing a ventilator to diminish the work of breathing. Antibiotics should be continued as long as indicated by the patient's clinical condition. Also, nasogastric suction should be continued until abdominal distention has regressed and intestinal function is well established. As with virtually all other abdominal conditions involving intestinal obstruction or severe ileus, the first type of bowel movement to be expected is green, watery, or sometimes bloody diarrhea. After a few days, the stool will be of a more normal character. Finally, severely ill patients should be moved from side to side in bed and encouraged to sit in a bedside chair and ambulate as soon as their condition permits. This minimizes pulmonary complications and also promotes the resumption of gastrointestinal function.

It is thought that most children do not experience as severe postoperative pain as adults do; however, significant pain does occur and needs to be treated. The surgeon must balance the child's comfort against possible postoperative respiratory complications that may result if depression is too profound or too prolonged. This is particularly an important consideration for infants under the age of six months. Over that age, meperidine 1 mg per kg of body weight or morphine 0.1 mg per kg of body weight intramuscularly every four to six hours (or lesser doses given intravenously) is effective in relieving pain.

TRAUMA AND MAJOR ELECTIVE SURGICAL PROCEDURES

Since extensive elective surgical procedures may involve considerable hemorrhage and third space loss, the preoperative, intraoperative, and postoperative management of these patients is similar in many ways to the management of young children who have sustained extensive trauma. The most obvious differences may be in the magnitude of injury or in the fact that extreme physiologic derangement in the case of elective procedures may be anticipated and perhaps prevented. Elective operations in this category would include anorectal pull-through procedures for Hirschsprung's disease or imperforate anus; extensive intestinal resections or gastrectomy for inflammatory bowel disease, ulcerative colitis, or gastrointestinal bleeding disorders; operations for portal hypertension; extensive resections of retroperitoneal tumors and hepatic lesions; lengthy operations on the pancreaticobiliary tree involving intestinal bypass; and a wide variety of other procedures of similar magnitude. Complicated genitourinary procedures for urinary diversion and obstructive uropathies also fall into this category.

The most common form of childhood trauma encountered is that of a blunt nature involving multiple organ systems, including head trauma, thoracic crush, and blunt abdominal injuries with or without associated extremity fractures. The abdominal organs injured listed in the order of frequency include the spleen, kidney, liver, pancreas, intestine, and bladder. The pathophysiologic considerations are those of extensive, continuing hemorrhage, peritoneal soilage, and urinary leaks. Evaluation of the severity of intra-abdominal injury may be impeded because of the presence of injuries to other parts of the body. The first priority is to establish an adequate airway and maintain normal respiratory function. The second priority (which should be attended to almost simultaneously) is placement of a large-bore secure intravenous catheter inserted either percutaneously or via cutdown. In most instances, it is preferable to place a catheter in a central vein above the diaphragm for central venous pressure monitoring. In children under the age of four years, we prefer to perform a cutdown on a neck vein. In children over the age of four, it is usually possible to position the central venous catheter percutaneously via the subclavicular route. Traumatized young patients may move about wildly, so the latter technique tends to have a higher incidence of complications, particularly if the patient is under four years of age. Complications may reflect the operator's prior experience and familiarity with the procedure. Only one subclavian vein catheterization should be attempted at a time in order to avoid bilateral complications occurring simultaneously.

If the child is in shock following a severe injury, this ordinarily indicates a loss of at least one-fourth of the blood volume. It is usually best to administer Ringer's lactate solution, 5 ml per kg of body weight, until blood is available. Five per cent albumin solution may be used alternatively until blood is available. Only under unusual circumstances is it necessary to administer untyped or un–cross-matched blood immediately. However, as soon as cross-matched blood is available, it should be administered in increments of 5 ml per kg of body weight (this is the equivalent of one unit transfusion in an adult) until the patient's cardiovacular status stabilizes. Normal vital signs and values are listed in Table 17–1. Nasogastric suction should be initiated immediately in order to prevent vomiting and pulmonary aspiration, an ominous danger, particularly for the depressed patient. A monitored adequate urinary output is a good indication of satisfactory cardiac output (Table 17–1). It is usually best to pass a urinary catheter into the bladder. A Foley catheter is useful in all females and in males over the age of 10 years. A straight catheter or small feeding tube of appropriate size is preferable in males under the age of 10 in order to avoid the complication of membranous urethral stricture that occurs occasionally with a Foley catheter. We also prefer to avoid long-term use of a urinary catheter in patients who have undergone severe trauma or nephrectomy in order to protect the remaining kidney from infection.

Most severely traumatized patients are in satisfactory electrolyte balance preoperatively, but acid-base balance may be deranged. While ventilatory support with adequate amounts of oxygen is certainly helpful for patients in shock, adequate blood replacement and administration of sodium bicarbonate, one mEq per kg of body weight, is usually necessary. Appropriate serial pH and blood gas determinations indicate any need for additional sodium bicarbonate. We feel that it is best to administer antibiotics preoperatively to all patients who have sustained severe trauma and require operation and to all those who are to undergo extensive elective abdominal surgical procedures. The antibiotics selected should be appropriate to the situation involved, including such considerations as intestinal spillage, extensive skin loss, or involvement of the respiratory tree.

An additional consideration that should be mentioned with regard to major elective procedures involving the colon concerns preoperative preparation of the bowel. Cathartics are usually not required in infants and young children, and they should be specifically avoided in the presence of severe inflammatory bowel disease. Solid food is withheld, including milk, and only clear liquids are permitted. While adults may do well on this regimen, infants and young children tend to become ketotic. For this reason, we prefer to provide such small patients with adequate amounts of an elemental liquid diet that maintains positive nitrogen balance, prevents ketosis, and simultaneously does not provide

Table 17–1. NORMAL VITAL SIGNS FOR AGE

	RESPIRATIONS	HEART	BLOOD PRESSURE	URINE OUTPUT
First year	40/min	120/min	80/40	10 ml/hr
Age 1 to 5	30	100	110/60	20
Age 6 to 12	20	80	120/80	30

Another criterion of adequate urine output is 1 ml/kg/hr.

any stool bulk. Cleansing saline enemas rather than soap suds or other preparations are helpful. We use a 48-hour antibiotic oral bowel prep in addition to these measures and prefer to use neomycin, 40 mg per kg of body weight per day in four divided doses, in conjunction with erythromycin, 50 mg per kg of body weight per day in four divided doses. Appropriate doses of kanamycin or tetracycline may be substituted for these drugs.

Postoperative care is directed at further improving the patient's physiologic state and maintaining functions at a normal level until the child's condition stabilizes. The services of an intensive care unit especially designed for children are desirable. Respiratory support is continued as long as necessary to insure adequate oxygenation without labored breathing or as long as secretions are so profuse that the patient is too weak to cope with them. Sterile precautions must be followed. Blood should be administered until central venous pressure and arterial blood pressure stabilize and the child's hematocrit levels off between 35 and 40 volumes per cent. The nature and volume of intravenous fluids are determined by serial measurements of serum electrolytes, osmolality, serum proteins, hourly urine flow, and specific gravity. Body weight should be determined daily. Salt and water retention, a particular problem in infants and younger children, is usually indicated by excessive weight gain or pulmonary congestion as evidenced by radiography. Administration of diuretics may be helpful for those patients who have associated pulmonary injuries. Serum and blood sugar levels should be carefully monitored in patients with liver damage with or without hepatic resection, and overhydration must be avoided in patients with head injuries. Antibiotics should be continued as long as necessary; monitoring catheters should be removed as soon as it is practical in order to minimize the risks of infection. This is particularly important for severely injured children who may also have depressed host resistance to infection.

NUTRITION

An important consideration for the management of nearly all serious surgical conditions is nutrition. The more severe the physiologic insult, whether it results from trauma or an elective surgical procedure, the greater the degree and the longer the duration of hypermetabolism and negative nitrogen balance. The pathophysiologic implications of an inadequate nutritional status involve delayed wound healing, an increased incidence of infectious complications, and prolonged convalescence. Patients who require prolonged intravenous support because of delayed gastrointestinal function, such as those with intestinal, hepatic, or pancreatic injuries, benefit from intravenous hyperalimentation. Peripheral administration of dextrose and amino acids in conjunction with intravenous fat emulsion is indicated for those patients with modest degrees of trauma who will require intravenous support only for a week or so. Those patients who require support for longer periods of time are best treated with central venous administration of maximum amounts of dextrose and amino acids as well as fat emulsion in order to provide optimal nutritional support and to reverse negative nitrogen balance quickly. Temporary glucose intolerance may be managed by manipulation of the quantity of glucose provided or by the administration of small amounts of insulin.

Children who have suffered severe abdominal trauma may have characteristic signs of deliberate abuse. Invariably, the history offered to explain the injury is meant to be evasive and is clearly inadequate. In these cases, the physician should search carefully for the telltale signs of abuse. Most abused children have multiple soft tissue injuries in various stages of healing, and roentgenograms of the long bones may show fractures in various stages of healing. There is often a history of multiple hospital or emergency room admissions, often to several hospitals. Burn injuries are a frequent form of child abuse. Alertness to child abuse is the most effective weapon to prevent potentially lethal injuries.

THORACIC CONDITIONS

Thoracic surgical procedures include operations for trauma, pulmonary resection, vascular malformations of the aortic arch, resection of cysts and tumors of the mediastinum and thorax, and repair of chest wall deformities. Special considerations related to cardiac surgical procedures are discussed in Chapter 20. When possible, infants and children undergoing thoracic surgical procedures should be nutritionally evaluated and replenished if necessary to obtain an optimal preoperative condition. Patients must be free of upper respiratory tract infection; pulmonary infections and atelectasis should be treated with appropriate postural drainage, endotracheal suctioning, specific antibiotics, and sometimes bronchoscopy. Bronchoscopy may be extremely important prior to thoracotomy for bronchiectasis, lung abscess, and other conditions in which there is danger of endobronchial contamination during the time of thoracotomy. Blood and red cell volume should be evaluated and restored to normal levels preoperatively. In patients with anemia, it is preferable to infuse packed red blood cells at least 24 hours preoperatively in order that redistribution of plasma volume may be achieved. Thorough evaluation of all preoperative data and roentgenograms is necessary in order to determine whether a chest tube will be needed preoperatively to treat an unsuspected pneumothorax, whether a specific type of endotracheal tube will be required, and whether special precautions will need to be taken with intraoperative ventilatory techniques. A large-bore secure intravenous catheter is necessary, and when indicated, a central venous pressure catheter should be placed if blood loss is expected to be extensive, such as in patients with suppurative lung disease or large mediastinal tumors. Placement of a radial artery catheter may be helpful for monitoring changes in systemic pressure and blood gases.

Since pulmonary toilet and physiotherapy are such important aspects of postoperative care, children should be told explicitly preoperatively what will be expected of them postoperatively. The best individuals to orient children are the nurses and other personnel who will be working with them in the intensive care unit.

Regardless of the condition treated by thoracotomy, it is our preference routinely to use an intercostal tube appropriately positioned to drain the thoracic space of blood, fluid, and air. The amount of suction necessary on the drainage set should be adjusted to suit the needs of each individual patient. More suction is needed in the presence of large air leaks than when only fluid drainage is required. It is important to evacuate even a limited pneumothorax in order to allow for maximal pulmonary expansion and ventilation and for obliteration of dead space. The latter may be an extremely difficult goal to accomplish in those patients who have sustained severe thoracic trauma with pulmonary contusion, requiring assisted ventilation with high levels of positive end expiratory pressure. Once the chest tube is no longer needed, it should be removed as soon as possible, since the pain associated with the mere presence of the tube impedes breathing efforts and voluntary coughing.

Dressings on infants and small children should be as small in size as possible in order to minimize limitation of thoracic excursion. Patients should be encouraged to cough and deep-breathe voluntarily as frequently as possible; adequate analgesia should be given. Additionally, postural drainage, frequent changes in position, and endotracheal suctioning performed by both nursing and physician staffs are keys to preventing the accumulation of secretions in the tracheobronchial tree, which is necessary to prevent small airway closure, gross atelectasis, and pulmonary infection. The patient should be adequately hydrated, and external humidity should be provided if secretions are thick. Nasotracheal intubation may be helpful for a day or two if significant secretions are anticipated. The most common indication for a nasotracheal tube is the provision of assisted ventilation.

A variety of techniques for mechanical ventilation are now available. All are designed to provide adequate oxygenation and removal of carbon dioxide. If ventilatory assistance is anticipated to be needed for only 12 to 24 hours, placement of an endotracheal tube is probably adequate. However, nasotracheal intubation is far more comfortable for the patient, and it is a preferred choice to avoid laryngeal trauma when a tube is needed for over 24 hours. In general, if a nasotracheal tube is expected to be required in a child for longer than five days, tracheostomy is probably indicated at that time since the patient may be in jeopardy from subglottic stenosis, an extremely serious complication. The newborn infant is an exception because neonates can tolerate nasotracheal intubation for a longer period of time. The essentials of ventilator management are beyond the scope of this chapter, but important considerations include proper adjustment of oxygen delivery, adequate humidification without overhydration, occasional use of aerosols such as racemic epinephrine, selection of the appropriate ventilatory technique, and frequent pH and blood gas monitoring. Ventilatory assistance has probably reduced postoperative morbidity and mortality in the pediatric age group more than any other adjunct to care.

A frequent early complication following thoracotomy in the childhood group is gastric dilatation, which may result in vomiting and aspiration or impaired respirations due to diaphragmatic elevation. Intermittent passage of a nasogastric tube during the first 12 hours is ordinarily all that is required. In most instances, children are able to take oral fluids on the first postoperative morning, unless they are being artificially ventilated, which may prolong the postoperative ileus for 24 to 48 hours.

The risk of postoperative infection can be minimized if pulmonary atelectasis is prevented. Additionally, adequate pleural drainage prevents fluid accumulation, which may lead to empyema. Optimally, all patients who undergo surgical procedures involving entry into the tracheobronchial tube should receive appropriate preoperative and postoperative antibotics as indicated by frequent cultures of pulmonary or other secretions.

18

Mechanical Support and Monitoring Procedures

ARNOLD G. CORAN

Since the techniques of monitoring and mechanical support of children and adolescents are quite similar to those used for adults, this chapter will be devoted to the management of neonates and infants, for whom the procedures are often different.

Skillful preoperative and postoperative care of an infant undergoing operation is essential to a successful outcome. These patients are more difficult to manage than are older children primarily because of the technical problems created by their small size and their unique metabolic needs. Observations on which critical decisions are made must be quantified whenever possible. The bedside assessment of skin color, temperature, vigor of sucking, character of respiration, and other physical signs is very important, but it must be supplemented by additional, more precise information that can now be obtained via sophisticated modern techniques of patient monitoring. The more ill the patient, the more often precise observations are required, and, for some ill patients, continuous monitoring is necessary. The type of flow sheet we have found very helpful in organizing the data essential to caring for critically ill infants is illustrated in Figure 18–1.

Since infants require proportionately higher doses of most medication than do older patients, it is suggested that age-adjusted dosage schedules be consulted. A warm, well-fed infant rarely requires sedation, and when restlessness occurs, hypoxia or low cardiac output should be suspected. Small doses of morphine, 0.1 mg per kg, and chloral hydrate, 14 mg per kg by mouth or by suppository, are generally the only sedatives needed.

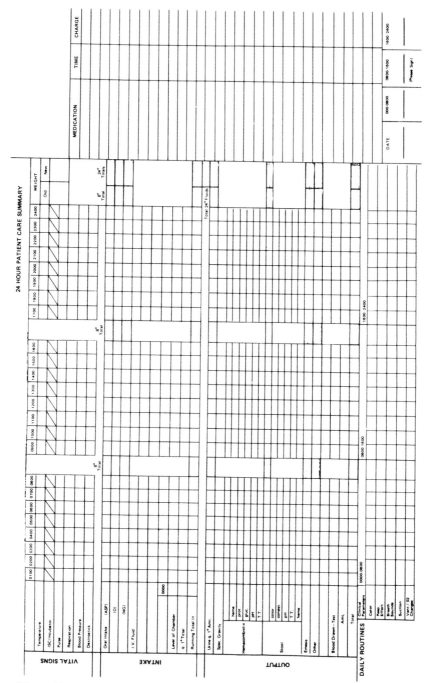

Figure 18–1. Example of a flow sheet used in an infant intensive care unit. This sheet maintains an accurate record of hemodynamic variables, intake and output, and blood chemistries.

DISTURBANCES IN THE CHEMICAL CONSTITUENTS OF THE BLOOD

Fluid and electrolyte management for infants is discussed in Chapter 15. However, there are additional chemical aberrations that occur in the infant that require careful monitoring.

All newborn infants have poorly developed mechanisms for regulating glucose and calcium levels in the blood. The small hepatic glycogen stores are rapidly depleted, and, particularly in newborn infants subjected to operation, significant hypoglycemia (below 30 mg per 100 ml in full-term infants; below 20 mg per 100 ml in premature infants) is likely to occur and can lead to convulsions. Fortunately, the blood glucose level can be monitored easily on an hourly basis with the clinical use of Dextrostix to supplement the more accurate blood glucose determinations obtained periodically from the laboratory.

Hypoglycemia is treated initially by cautious administration of 1 to 2 ml per kg of 50 per cent dextrose in water via central venous cannula, then increasing the dextrose concentration of the maintenance intravenous fluids to 10 to 15 per cent. Occasionally, even this treatment does not suffice, and corticosteroids must be administered (hydrocortisone 5 mg per kg every 12 hours). Resumption of oral or gavage feedings usually eliminates the problem, but in the transition, intravenous dextrose supplementation must be tapered slowly. Occasionally, the neonate suffering from hemorrhage or septic shock develops significant hyperglycemia. If the blood glucose remains below 250 mg per 100 ml, no treatment is necessary. Glucose levels above this value, however, require insulin therapy.

Hypocalcemia (that is, a serum calcium concentration less than 7 mg per 100 ml) also tends to occur in newborn infants undergoing operative procedures. Several factors may predispose such infants to this problem: (1) prematurity, with inadequate calcium stores and immature parathyroid glands; (2) stress leading to endogenous steroid production; (3) administration of sodium bicarbonate; and (4) administration of CPD anticoagulant during blood transfusion. Hypocalcemia may be manifested by twitching, irritability, and convulsions. It should be treated by prompt but slow administration of a 10 per cent calcium gluconate solution into a central venous line to a total dose of 10 ml for a full-term infant (6 ml for a premature infant); 1 to 2 gm are subsequently added to the 24-hour maintenance intravenous fluids for a day or two. Resumption of oral feeding also is frequently accompanied by resolution of this problem. Most laboratories measure total serum calcium content instead of the ionized portion that is physiologically important. Thus, when convulsions occur under conditions suggesting hypocalcemia, a therapeutic infusion of calcium gluconate may be indicated even when the total serum calcium level is reported as normal.

Hypomagnesemia occasionally coexists with hypocalcemia. Serum magnesium levels less than 1.4 mEq per liter are abnormal in the neonate. Tetany unresponsive to calcium therapy may be treated with 0.2 ml of 50 per cent magnesium sulfate solution administered intramuscularly every four hours.

Infants occasionally become jaundiced, and this tendency is more marked when bilirubin production is excessive, such as following massive transfusion. The serum bilirubin level should be measured daily postoperatively in the newborn infant. Levels greater than 10 mg per 100 ml require further investigation and prompt therapy to prevent kernicterus.

Hyperosmolarity

Sudden increases in an infant's serum osmolarity can result in brain damage and even intracranial hemorrhage secondary to sudden changes in cerebrospinal fluid pressure. A rise in serum osmolarity greater than 25 mOsm during any four-hour period is considered unsafe. Therefore, under these conditions, hypertonic agents should be administered slowly and sparingly. Sodium bicarbonate infused at a dosage of 3 mEq per kg of body weight will ordinarily raise the serum osmolarity by 7.5 mOsm per kg. No more than three doses of this magnitude should be given during a four-hour period. Ten ml of a 50 per cent dextrose solution exert 25.2 mOsm of pressure.

Coagulation Abnormalities

Older infants rarely have serious coagulation abnormalities unless they are severely polycythemic. However, newborn infants are normally deficient in vitamin K and should receive 1 mg intramuscularly before operation. Diffuse intravascular coagulation may be initiated by sepsis or severe hypoxia and should be suspected when troublesome bleeding persists postoperatively.

RESPIRATORY CARE

The provision of proper respiratory support is often the crux of postoperative care for infants who have undergone abdominal or thoracic surgery just as it is for adults. At the completion of the operation, a decision must be made regarding extubation. Vigorous infants who have had noncardiac procedures or one of the simpler cardiac operations may be extubated if they were not severely acidotic preoperatively. Most infants who have undergone major cardiac procedures should be ventilated postoperatively until they are fully awake, hemodynamically stable, and free of pulmonary edema; this can be carried out satisfactorily through either a nasotracheal tube or an oral endotracheal tube for as long as seven days. The nasotracheal tube is somewhat easier to place in position and is less likely to be dislodged by the infant. However, with proper technique, an oral endotracheal tube can be fixed in place securely (Fig. 18–2). The tube must be uncuffed and made of nonreactive plastic and, if gas-sterilized, must be thoroughly aired prior to insertion. To minimize tracheal trauma, it should fit the trachea loosely and not be allowed to slide in and out as the infant moves. The position of the tube must be confirmed with a chest roentgenogram in order to insure that it has not been inserted too deeply. This most commonly results in atelectasis of the upper lobe of the right lung, because the tube tends to enter the right main bronchus and thereby occludes the upper lobe bronchus.

The nurse caring for the patient should periodically auscultate the chest to be sure that both sides are aerating well and equally. If the infant requires mechanical ventilation for a prolonged period (greater than three to four weeks), tracheostomy should be performed in order to prevent permanent damage to the vocal cords. This should be done in the operating room via a transverse incision just above the sternal notch. A vertical incision is made in the second or third tracheal cartilage, and a

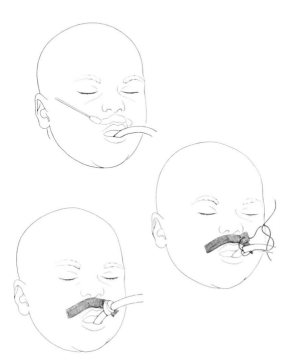

Figure 18–2. Method of fixing an oral endotracheal tube securely in an infant. Skin overlying maxilla is first painted with benzoin. Then a strip of Elastoplast is applied with the fold in the center. A heavy silk ligature is tightly tied around the tube, indenting the wall slightly; then the tube is sutured through folded Elastoplast. Finally, $\frac{1}{2}$ inch tape is applied over the suture to provide additional stabilization. By this method, the tube is secured to the maxilla, which moves relatively little, and saliva will not loosen its fixation.

nonreactive uncuffed tracheostomy tube is inserted. It is absolutely essential that no portion of the trachea be excised (as is sometimes done in adults) because this will result in a severe tracheal stricture.

The inspired gas must be fully humidified, either through the ventilator (if the patient is being ventilated mechanically) or by some other means such as a tent if the patient is breathing spontaneously through a tube. The day and night services of skilled chest physiotherapists are important. The airway of an infant is so small that retained secretions may quickly lead to pulmonary collapse if these precautions are not taken. A blocked tube is de facto indictment of inadequate nursing and physical therapy. When there is any suspicion that a tube is becoming compromised or occluded, it should be changed immediately.

Perhaps no other indices are as useful as the blood pH and arterial gas concentrations in monitoring an infant's respiratory status. These allow accurate repeated assessment of the adequacy of oxygenation, alveolar ventilation, and acid-base status. A significantly elevated PCO_2 indicates the need for intubation and mechanical ventilation. A diminished PO_2 may be caused by a ventilation-perfusion imbalance secondary to atelectasis, pneumonia, congestive heart failure, or by an obligatory right-to-left cardiac shunt. With atelectasis, the PO_2 can often be improved by augmenting the inspired oxygen tension (FIO_2) using a tent or incubator. With congestive heart failure, an operation is usually required to improve oxygenation significantly. The base deficit can be determined from the pH and PCO_2 measurements, and the amount of sodium bicarbonate necessary to correct metabolic acidosis can be calculated (Fig. 18–3). With practice, repeated arterial punctures can be performed safely in small infants. As in adults, it is preferred that the radial artery be punctured with a short 22-gauge needle attached to a heparinized 2 ml syringe. If precise measurement of PO_2 is not required and if peripheral circulation is good, a capillary sample taken from the infant's (previously warmed) heel will allow a reasonably accurate estimate of the arterial pH and PCO_2. When frequent arterial blood gas determinations are likely to be made or when a continuous recording of arterial pressure is needed, an arterial catheter is inserted into a radial artery (Fig. 18–4).

Oxygen toxicity occurs in infants for two reasons. First, retrolental fibroplasia is a hazard in premature infants who are given high concentrations of oxygen. Permanent eye damage has occurred when arterial PO_2 has exceeded 110 mm Hg for longer than one or two hours. Second, bronchopulmonary dysplasia occurs when ventilation with an oxygen concentration of more than 70 per cent is maintained for longer than four or five days. Therefore, arterial blood gas concentrations must be monitored closely and the inspired oxygen concentration reduced as much as possible in infants, especially if they are premature.

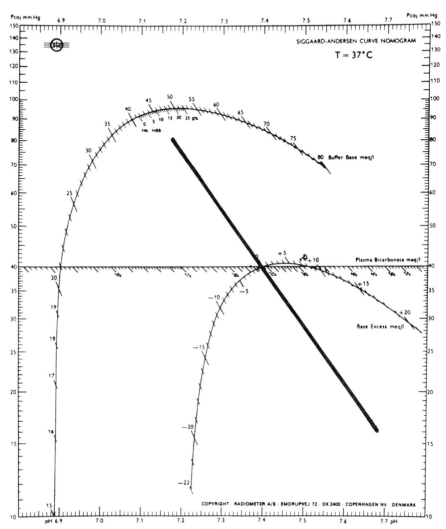

Figure 18–3. *See legend on opposite page.*

Figure 18–3. The Siggaard-Andersen curve nomogram.

1. To calculate base deficit, measure pH and P_{CO_2}. Plot these values on the nomogram and find the point at which these values intersect. Then with a straight edge draw a line through that point and parallel to the heavy black line. The point at which this line intersects the base excess curve defines the base excess. Then, to calculate the mEq of $NaHCO_3$ required to correct a metabolic acidosis:

$$mEq\ HCO_3 = \frac{\text{Base excess} \times \text{body wt (kg)}}{3}$$

For example, a pH of 7.27 with a P_{CO_2} of 23 gives a base excess of -15. Then for a 70 kg patient:

$$mEq\ HCO_3 = \frac{15 \times 70}{3} = 350\ mEq$$

It is generally a good practice to give half the calculated amount, then repeat the blood gas measurements before giving additional bicarbonate.

2. Common patterns of acid-base derangement:
   a. Respiratory acidosis—P_{CO_2} elevated, base excess 0. Treatment—increase minute ventilation if on ventilator or intubate and ventilate if breathing spontaneously (see text).
   b. Metabolic acidosis—P_{CO_2} normal, base excess negative. Treatment—determine and treat etiologic problems (e.g., poor perfusion), give sodium bicarbonate as per above formulas.
   c. Respiratory alkalosis—P_{CO_2} reduced, base excess 0. Treatment—reduce minute ventilation if on ventilator. (In general, slight respiratory alkalosis is helpful in reducing respiratory drive of a patient on a ventilator.)
   d. Metabolic alkalosis—P_{CO_2} normal, base excess positive. Treatment—none unless pH elevated significantly (above 7.60). Then give potassium chloride, which will correct the hypokalemia that is usually associated. In severe cases ammonium chloride can be used.
3. Combinations of the above are often encountered. Except in acute situations, it is unusual for pure patterns to persist, because normal compensatory mechanisms will intervene to correct the pH. Treatment consists of an appropriate combination of measures (as in 2a–2d).

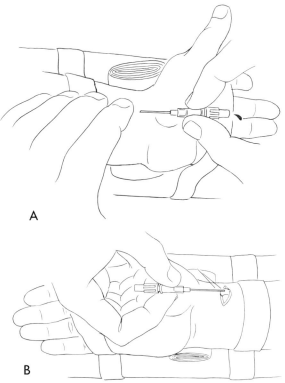

A

B

Figure 18–4. Methods of inserting radial artery pressure monitoring catheters. The wrist is extended and fixed to a padded board. A, To insert the catheter percutaneously, first puncture the skin with a No. 11 scalpel blade, then guide an Abbocath-T or similar needle with stylet into the artery by palpation. Once the artery has been entered, be sure to advance the needle into it 1 cm. before withdrawing the stylet. Rotating the needle 360 degrees as it is advanced helps to guide it up the lumen. B, To insert the catheter under direct vision, dissect the artery from its bed on the radial side of the flexor pollicis longus tendon, encircle it with a ligature for countertraction, insert the catheter, remove the ligature, and suture the incision. The catheter must then be secured by sutures and tape in such a way that it cannot be dislodged.

POSITIVE END-EXPIRATORY PRESSURE

Recently it has become evident that patients receiving respiratory assistance tend to accumulate interstitial water in the lungs, leading to decreased compliance and poor oxygenation. Possible causes include increased water permeability of damaged capillaries, decreased surfactant, diminished plasma oncotic pressure, increased antidiuretic hormone secretion, poorly understood effects of homologous blood transfusion, and left atrial hypertension. Increased interstitial water in the lungs may be reflected as an increased alveolar-arterial oxygen gradient (a-ADO_2) and decreased compliance. Vigorous diuresis often results in dramatic improvement in the PO_2 value and is one of the mainstays of postoperative respiratory care. With brisk diuresis, the blood volume may decrease, and infusion of salt-poor albumin, plasma, or packed cells may be required to maintain adequate intravascular volume as extravascular volume becomes contracted.

Another useful adjunct in the treatment of hypoxia is the application of positive end-expiratory pressure (PEEP), which reverses the progressive alveolar collapse resulting from constant volume ventilation and also inhibits the accumulation of interstitial water in the lungs. Positive end-expiratory pressure can be easily applied by connecting one end of a tube to the expiratory port of the respirator and submerging the open end of the tube the desired distance into a container of water, usually starting at a depth of 5 to 10 cm. Most respirators now have a built-in capability to deliver the desired PEEP simply by manipulating appropriate controls. Rarely, the cardiac output decreases because of the increase in pulmonary vascular resistance and the decrease in venous return caused by PEEP, thus limiting its usefulness. Usually, however, application of PEEP results in prompt improvement in arterial Po_2 followed by clearing of pulmonary edema when this is evident radiographically.

CONTINUOUS POSITIVE AIRWAY PRESSURE (Fig. 18–5)

Positive end-expiratory pressure can also be applied to patients breathing spontaneously. This technique was originally described as a way to improve the mortality rate of infants with hyaline membrane disease and was called continuous positive airway pressure

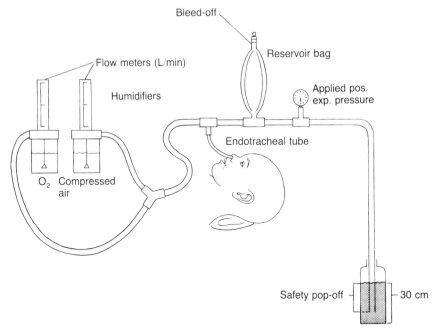

Figure 18–5. A continuous positive airway pressure (CPAP) can be administered to a spontaneously ventilating patient by a system such as this. Humidified oxygen and air are mixed to give desired FIo_2. Total flow rate of gases must be at least 2.5 times the patient's minute volume to prevent rebreathing of exhaled CO_2. Bleed-off from the reservoir bag is adjusted (Hofmann clamp) to result in the desired reading on the manometer dial (usually 3 to 10 mm Hg), which is the level of CPAP applied to the patient. A water trap provides a safety pop-off should airway pressure suddenly rise (for example, if the bleed-off valve should be inadvertently occluded).

(CPAP) breathing. We and others have used it principally in infants following cardiac surgery as a compromise between extubation and mechanical ventilation. It is sometimes difficult to ventilate small infants with a volume ventilator because they may breathe out of phase with the respirator or require heavy sedation. Furthermore, pulmonary dysfunction may be worsened by the combination of mechanical ventilation and oxygen toxicity. CPAP obviates these disadvantages, increases the arterial PO_2 so that FIO_2 can be reduced, prevents microatelectasis, and counteracts pulmonary edema. Of course, the patients must be sufficiently alert and strong to breathe spontaneously. Although we have applied CPAP postoperatively by means of an indwelling endotracheal tube, it may also be applied with specially designed nasal prongs. This method takes advantage of the fact that infants breathe exclusively through the nose.

One major hazard of both PEEP and CPAP applied at high levels of pressure is their tendency to produce tension pneumothorax. This complication must be ruled out immediately when the clinical condition of these patients deteriorates. We usually do not remove the chest tubes inserted intraoperatively until PEEP has been discontinued. If a baby develops a pneumothorax following the institution of PEEP and if no chest tube is already in place, then one must be inserted immediately. A No. 12 or 14 French rubber catheter is used. The safest technique is to make a small incision in the second or third intercostal space in the midaxillary line and then to spread the chest wall muscles with a hemostat until the pleural cavity is entered. This is by far preferable to the blind insertion of a trocar as is sometimes done in adults. The catheter is then inserted through the opening and is secured in place with a suture and adhesive tape. The chest tube is connected to an underwater seal with a negative pressure no greater than 5 cm of water; greater negative pressure will result in significant mediastinal shift in a neonate.

INTERMITTENT MANDATORY VENTILATION

An extremely useful variation of CPAP in infants has become possible by the recent introduction of a new type of ventilator, the "Baby Bird." In this system, the patient can breathe humidified gas spontaneously, which the respirator will augment with periodic "mandatory" breaths at any desired rate (Fig. 18–6). This is called intermittent mandatory ventilation (IMV). Since it is unnecessary to phase the patient's breathing with the machine, he or she need not be heavily sedated. The machine's rate can initially be set high, so that the patient's ventilation is effectively taken over. During weaning, the rate can be progressively reduced until the machine provides only a few breaths a minute. Use of this system allows the transition between total ventila-

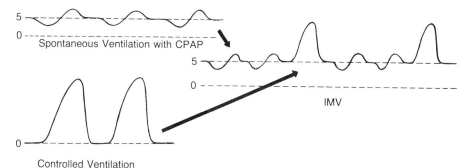

Figure 18–6. Intermittent mandatory ventilation (IMV). CPAP system is modified so that a ventilator can inflate a patient's lungs through a one-way valve periodically, thereby augmenting the patient's spontaneous breathing. This provides a useful compromise between spontaneous ventilation with CPAP (top left) and conventional, controlled mechanical ventilation (bottom left). It is unnecessary to sedate the patient so that he may be "controlled," since he is free to breathe independently of the machine. Weaning is smoothly accomplished by progressively reducing the backup rate of the ventilator until it is not needed.

tory support and spontaneous breathing to be made more smoothly and easily than with the older system of switching from the ventilator to a T-piece periodically. Furthermore, PEEP can easily be employed with this system by adjusting a dial on the respirator.

FEEDING (ENTERAL AND PARENTERAL)

It is generally agreed (without experimental support) that sucking is a severe exercise tolerance test for an infant. Certainly, one of the initial signs of congestive heart failure is poor feeding, and as the infant's cardiac condition improves, so does oral intake.

When the acute hemodynamic problems have subsided and the abdomen is soft (usually two to three days postoperatively), feeding orally through a gastrostomy or through a nasogastric tube is initiated. Starting with 5 ml hourly of 5 per cent dextrose in water, then advancing to half-strength and subsequently full-strength formula, the intravenous feedings are decreased as the enteral feedings are sequentially increased. It is easiest to specify the 24-hour fluid limit and to allow the nurses to increase the enteral feedings gradually and to decrease the intravenous feedings by equal amounts to maintain balance. If progress is satisfactory, the abdomen should remain soft, and spontaneous bowel movements should begin.

Not infrequently, diarrhea develops with resumption of enteral alimentation. Usually it is sufficient to switch to oral administration of 5 per cent dextrose in water until the diarrhea subsides. Then half-strength feedings and full-strength feedings are sequentially resumed as tolerated.

The infant may need a pacifier to satisfy the urge to suck. Once the patient is on full enteral feedings and is sucking well (usually after just a few days), completely oral feeding is begun with the feeding tube in place. Supplements are given through the tube until the infant is able to ingest all required food by mouth.

If the postoperative infant is unable to feed via the alimentary tract within five days after surgery, then intravenous nutrition should be initiated. The nutrient solution can be administered through a central venous catheter or into peripheral veins. Our preference is to utilize the peripheral route employing a fat emulsion; if this proves unsuccessful, which is rare, we then start central venous hyperalimentation.

PARENTERAL NUTRITION

Composition of Solution

Central Venous Hyperalimentation. The composition of the solution for central venous hyperalimentation is noted in Table 18–1. Half-strength solutions (basic formula diluted in half with 5 per cent dextrose in water) are also prepared by the pharmacy and are used primarily during the first day or two of therapy. During this period, the child adapts gradually to the very high dextrose load, and the high concentration of dextrose may produce an osmotic diuresis that will lead to hypertonic dehydration. As the patient's tolerance develops, as judged by diminishing glycosuria, full-strength solutions may be used. The administration of insulin is not necessary for nondiabetic children. Iron requirements are met either by weekly intramuscular injections of iron dextran or by blood transfusion. Trace metals are not routinely added to

Table 18–1. CONTENTS OF CENTRAL INFUSATE

CONSTITUENT	CONTENT PER LITER
Amino acids	4.25%
Dextrose (hydrous)	196.6 gm
Sodium†	15.0 mEq
Potassium†	16.0 mEq
Calcium	27.0 mEq
Phosphorus	19.0 mEq
Magnesium	7.6 mEq
Chloride*	10.8 mEq
Folic acid	0.5 mg
Multivitamin infusion†	5.0 ml
Vitamin K_1	0.2 mg
Vitamin B_{12}	6.6 μg

*Further adjusted at bedside
†U.S. Vitamin and Pharmaceutical Corp. Each liter provides 4.8 gm nitrogen and 800 cal.

Table 18–2. PERIPHERAL HYPERALIMENTATION WITH FAT
IN INFANTS

CONSTITUENT	AMOUNT PER KG PER 24 HR
Volume	160 to 200 ml
Intralipid	40 ml
Water	120 to 160 ml
Protein	2.4 to 3.2 gm
Glucose	14 to 19 gm
Fat	4 gm
Calories	111 to 134
Heparin	100 IU°
Sodium	2 to 4 mEq
Potassium	2 to 3 mEq
Chloride	2 to 4 mEq
Magnesium	0.6 mEq
Calcium	1.0 mEq
Phosphate	3.5 mm

°International Units

the basic mixture but are required if long-term total parenteral nutrition becomes necessary.

Peripheral Intravenous Feeding With Fat. The infusion consists of two separate bottles; one contains only the fat emulsion, Intralipid, and the other bottle contains the amino acids, dextrose, electrolytes, and vitamins. Table 18–2 lists the suggested contents of the infusion for infants. The total number of calories administered can be increased by infusion of more fat (up to 5 gm per kg per day) and/or more 10 per cent dextrose. The bottle containing the amino acids is prepared aseptically under a laminar flow hood in the hospital pharmacy. Essential fatty acids are present in Intralipid in large quantities.

Peripheral Intravenous Feeding Without Fat. A stock solution of 10 per cent protein hydrolysate is diluted with dextrose to make a 2 per cent protein hydrolysate in 12 per cent dextrose solution. The mixing is also carried out in the hospital pharmacy under a laminar flow hood, and the final solution contains 0.56 cal per ml. Electrolytes are added to the infusion to provide the recommended daily requirements plus additional needs based on the patient's clinical condition (Table 18–3). The electrolyte and vitamin concentrations are essentially the same as those recommended for central venous feeding and peripheral venous feeding with fat. Heparin (0.5 units per ml) is added to the solution to reduce the incidence of phlebitis. There is some evidence that a portion of the essential fatty acid requirement can be supplied through the application of sunflower seed oil to the skin of the infant's chest daily. For both peripheral venous methods of feeding, the administration of iron is the same as that described for central venous feeding. Trace metals are given as necessary.

Table 18–3. PERIPHERAL HYPERALIMENTATION WITHOUT FAT

Water	200 to 250 ml
Protein	4 to 5 gm
Glucose	24 to 30 gm
Calories	112 to 140
Heparin	100 IU°
Sodium	2 to 4 mEq
Potassium	2 to 3 mEq
Chloride	2 to 4 mEq
Magnesium	0.6 mEq
Calcium	1.0 mEq
Phosphate	3.5 mM

°International Units

Methods

Central Venous Feeding. Hypertonic infusions must be delivered through a central venous catheter to avoid peripheral venous inflammation and thrombosis. For this purpose, a silicone rubber catheter is passed through the internal or external jugular vein to the superior vena cava. This procedure is best carried out in an operating room or cardiac catheterization laboratory where adequate exposure is possible, proper instruments are available, and strict aseptic conditions are maintained. To minimize blood stream contamination, the venous catheter is tunneled from the vein entry point to a skin exit site 2 to 4 inches away. In the infant, it is brought out on the scalp, whereas in the older child, the exit site may be the neck or upper chest. Central venous intubation by percutaneous subclavian vein puncture has also been performed. The silicone rubber venous line may be left in place until the completion of therapy unless it becomes accidentally dislodged or septic complications develop.

The central venous catheter can be inserted with the use of local or general anesthesia. The head is turned to the contralateral side and the scalp is carefully shaved. A transverse incision 1 to 2 cm long is made over the sternocleidomastoid muscle at the junction of the middle and lower third of the neck. The external jugular vein is ordinarily the preferred choice, and it can usually be successfully cannulated even in the premature infant. However, if either external jugular vein is unavailable because of previous use or the vein's exceptionally small caliber, or if advancement of the catheter from the external jugular vein into the vena cava is not possible, the internal jugular vein can be used for cannulation. A long hollow needle with an obturator in place is passed beneath the skin of the neck from the incision to the scalp (Fig. 18–7). If the internal jugular vein is being used, the needle also pierces the belly of the sternocleidomastoid muscle. After the obturator is removed, the silicone rubber catheter (for an infant, the internal diameter is 0.025 in and the outside diameter is 0.047 in) is passed through the needle. As the

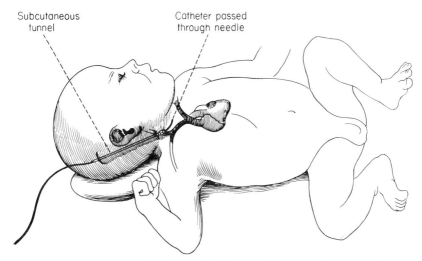

Figure 18–7. Insertion and fixation of a silicone rubber central venous catheter in an infant. The catheter is passed through a hollow needle that has created a subcutaneous tunnel from the venous cutdown site in the neck to the appropriate skin exit site behind the ear.

needle is withdrawn, the catheter is left to reside in its tract. Prior to cannulation, the vein is ligated distally and an incision is made between this point and a proximal controlling ligature. If the internal jugular vein has been selected, ligature of the vein can sometimes be avoided by passing the cannula into the vein through an incision made in the center of a purse string suture. The jugular vein is then cannulated and the tubing is advanced to the region of the right atrium (at the level of the second intercostal space at the sternum). Occasionally, some manipulation is necessary to obtain entry into the superior vena cava from the external jugular vein. The exact location of the catheter is confirmed radiographically via a single roentgenogram while the catheter is filled with radiopaque contrast material. This technique of central venous catheter insertion is also used when such a catheter is required for central venous pressure monitoring or for fluid infusion into a central vein; however, the tunneling under the scalp is usually not employed unless long-term placement is anticipated.

Antibiotics are administered only when indicated by the child's primary illness but not specifically to prevent sepsis that might result from the presence of a central venous line. An antimicrobial ointment and sterile dressing are applied to the skin exit site, and to avoid accidental displacement, a coil of catheter is included in the dressing. Every two days, the dressing and ointment are reapplied. Povidone-iodine ointment is now routinely used because of its effectiveness against both bacteria and fungi. Before the infusion is started, a Millipore filter (0.22 μ) is placed in-line to remove particulate matter and microorganisms that may have contaminated the solution. A calibrated buret is placed in the line next to the fluid reservoir to monitor the volume delivered accurately.

The infusion must be delivered at a slow uniform rate to insure proper utilization of the dextrose and amino acids. In the infant or child this is most readily accomplished by use of a constant infusion pump. The entire system, referred to as the "lifeline," is shown in Figure 18–8.

Peripheral Intravenous Feeding with Fat. The technique of infusion is depicted in Figure 18–9. In infants, a 21- to 23-gauge scalp vein needle (sometimes a 25-gauge needle) is inserted into a peripheral vein, usually in the scalp, and the intravenous tubing from the bottle containing the amino acids is connected to this needle. This technique of IV insertion is also used for the routine placement of an intravenous line into an infant. The tubing from the Intralipid bottle is then inserted into the rubber nipple at the end of the tubing from the first bottle ("piggy-

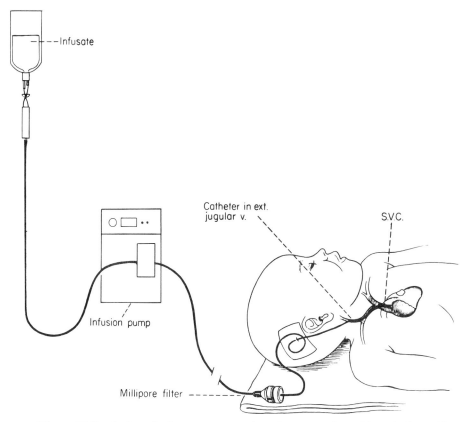

Figure 18–8. System for long-term central total parenteral nutrition. Amino acid-dextrose infusate flows through a calibrated buret. An infusion pump insures a uniform hourly flow rate. The Millipore filter in the circuit will remove any microorganisms that may have contaminated the system. The venous catheter enters the scalp behind the ear. The appropriate position of the catheter in the superior vena cava is confirmed radiographically.

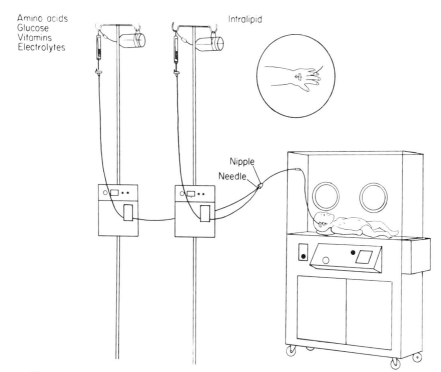

Amino acids
Glucose
Vitamins
Electrolytes

Intralipid

Nipple
Needle

Figure 18–9. Technique of intravenous feeding with Intralipid. In infants, a needle is inserted into the scalp; in older children, the veins on the dorsum of the hand are generally used. See text for details.

backed") and is secured to this tubing with tape. A calibrated buret is placed in each intravenous line, and both bottles are infused over a 24-hour period using two separate constant infusion pumps. The 24-hour infusion with two separate pumps is employed to insure proper utilization of the administered fat, dextrose, and amino acids. No filters are used since they would block the infusion of the fat. The needle usually requires changing every three to four days because of infiltration. Occasionally a peripheral venous cutdown is required when IV sites are scarce. The greater saphenous vein at the ankle is the easiest one to use initially. This vein is readily isolated by making a 1 cm transverse incision slightly anterior and superior to the medial malleolus. The vein lies anterior to the periosteum and is the only significant structure in this area. A small silicone rubber cannula is inserted into the vein using standard cutdown techniques.

Peripheral Intravenous Feeding Without Fat. The techniques involved here are no different from those used for routine intravenous infusions. The entire solution is contained in one bottle and is infused into a small needle placed into a peripheral vein in the scalp or extremity. A Millipore filter (0.22 μ) is placed in-line and the infusion is maintained for 24 hours for the various reasons already discussed. The intravenous sites remain viable for 24 to 48 hours and are changed promptly if signs of infiltration or phlebitis are noted. Warm soaks placed over the infiltrated skin reduce the swelling rather quickly. Rarely, a small skin slough results, which heals fairly rapidly with local care.

METABOLIC OBSERVATIONS

Clinical measurements that are essential include daily body weight, accurate volume of urine, and other body fluid losses. The urine sugar content is monitored at each voiding. The important blood tests and the frequency of study in the usual patient are given in Table 18–4. More frequent monitoring of some variables may be necessary in patients with specific metabolic abnormalities, such as those that occur with renal or hepatic disease.

Precise control of fluid and electrolyte administration is mandatory. Infusion pumps are useful if they work reliably. A skilled nurse can maintain patency of several intravenous lines with a fluid limit of 5 ml per hr. The volume of fluid used in flushing the monitoring lines must be included as input.

COUNSELING OF PARENTS

The parents of an infant undergoing major surgery are subjected to great emotional stress, especially if the child does not survive. Inevitably they experience guilt and may blame themselves or someone else for the loss. This attitude should be discussed with them, and they should be reassured that congenital anomalies are random events out of

Table 18–4. BLOOD VALUES MONITORED ROUTINELY DURING TOTAL PARENTERAL NUTRITION

FREQUENCY OF MONITORING		
At start of therapy and weekly	*At start of therapy and every two weeks*	*As indicated*
Na,K,Cl	SGOT, LDH, alkaline phosphatase	Copper
Urea	Bilirubin	Zinc
Glucose	Creatinine	Iron
Magnesium		Ammonia
Calcium, phosphorus		Osmolarity
Total protein		pH
Hgb, Hct, WBC		
Blood culture		
Candida precipitins		
Platelets		

their control. It is not helpful to suggest that earlier action on their part or earlier referral by the family physician might have altered the outcome.

Most parents are also concerned about the possibility that subsequent children might be born with defects. It is true that after one affected child is born in a family, the odds that another child will be affected increase somewhat compared with the incidence in the general population. However, the risk is still sufficiently low not to influence the parents' planning unduly, and we usually encourage parents to have more children if that is their wish.

REFERENCES

Behrendt, D. M., and Austen, W. G.: Patient Care in Cardiac Surgery. Boston, Little, Brown and Co., 1972.

Filler, R. M., and Coran, A. G.: Total parenteral nutrition in infants and children: Central and peripheral approaches. Surg. Clin. North Am., 56:395, 1976.

Mustard, W. T., Ravitch, M. M., Snyder, W. H., Jr., Welch, K. J., and Benson, C. D.: Pediatric Surgery. Chicago, Year Book Medical Pub., Inc., 1969.

III

The Organ Systems

19

The Lungs, Mediastinum, and Esophagus

LESTER R. BRYANT

Surgical treatment of pulmonary, mediastinal, and esophageal disorders constitutes the bulk of general thoracic surgery. Any operation that disrupts the integrity of the thorax must first be considered in terms of its potential effect on cardiopulmonary function. The preoperative care of a patient who is a potential candidate for a thoracic operation begins with the first encounter, whether an office consultation or an in-hospital bedside discussion with the referring physician. A deliberate effort must be made to resist a prematurely formulated management plan based on nothing more than chest roentgenograms or barium contrast studies. For example, a middle-aged cigarette smoker whose chest roentgenogram shows a left hilar mass is easily presumed to have bronchogenic carcinoma. This patient's mass, however, may be an unexpected thoracic aortic aneurysm. To perform mediastinoscopy, mediastinotomy, or exploratory thoracotomy would be inappropriate and dangerous. This does not imply that all possible diagnostic procedures are appropriate for every patient, but it does mean that the surgeon must exercise careful individual judgment.

Patients with esophageal, pulmonary, or mediastinal diseases that are ordinarily treated by surgical means may be placed in one of three categories on the basis of the surgeon's initial assessment. Those in the first category have a clearly defined lesion that is accessible to operative approach, and their general health is completely satisfactory. A third group of patients has advanced disease that has extended beyond surgical control or serious associated disorders that contraindicate major operative procedures. In between these two groups are the patients who require the greatest attention from the surgeon, because it is not immediately apparent whether or not their diseases are amenable to surgical treatment. Specific laboratory and diagnostic procedures must be done prior to making a definitive decision, and simultaneously, a more precise evaluation may be made of the patient's suitability for a major thoracic operation.

The history and physical examination, done with the consideration of a possible thoracotomy, constitute the basis of the evaluation of each patient. If the patient is younger than middle-aged, obviously in good health, and has normal values on the hospital admission blood tests and urinalysis, little additional evaluation is necessary. However, a standard electrocardiogram should be obtained because intraoperative and post-operative cardiac arrhythmias are common in thoracic surgical patients regardless of their ages. It is also important to have the preoperative electrocardiogram for comparison with subsequent tracings. When there is a history of cardiac symptoms, evidence of a previous myocardial infarction, or clinical findings of extensive cardiovascular disease (ar-teriosclerosis), a more detailed cardiologic evaluation is indicated. The risk of any thoracic operation is increased for a patient who has had a previous myocardial infarction, and the shorter the interval between the infarction and a major surgical procedure, the greater the risk of reinfarction. Every effort should be made to delay an operation for three to six months after a documented myocardial infarction.

Ordinarily, severe angina pectoris or uncontrolled congestive heart failure are contraindications to noncardiac thoracic operations. If these conditions can be corrected or significantly improved, it is then appropriate to reevaluate the patient for operative treatment. In addition, occasionally a patient has a mediastinal or pulmonary lesion that can be resected during the same operation that is done primarily for the cardiac disease.

EVALUATION OF PULMONARY FUNCTION

From a consideration of the symptoms and physical findings in conjunction with the chest roentgenograms, it is generally possible to estimate a patient's clinical pulmonary function. It is often possible to obviate the performance of formal pulmonary function tests in young or middle-aged patients who are scheduled for nonpulmonary operations. Elderly patients, however, are more likely to have disease that is undetected by history or physical examination. By obtaining pulmonary function tests in older patients, the surgeon is alerted to potential needs for specific additional preoperative preparation or consultation.

A decision to forego pulmonary function tests is based on the assumption that the patient has no respiratory symptoms or no evidence of lung disease, as demonstrated by either physical examination or by chest roentgenograms. Omission of the function tests is acceptable, for example, in patients who require operation for mediastinal tumors or cysts, in patients with benign esophageal disease, and in patients requiring simple chest wall procedures such as excision of a benign rib tumor. An important exception to this general approach, however, is the patient with myasthenia gravis who requires thymectomy or exploration for thymoma. In this situation, preoperative pulmonary function measurements are critical as baselines for comparison in evaluating the patient's postoperative progress.

There are some circumstances in which elective lung operations may be done without prior pulmonary function tests. Young patients with recurrent spontaneous pneumothorax are properly included in this category if clinical evaluation indicates good pulmonary function and the chest roentgenograms show no specific pulmonary lesions. These patients usually have small apical subpleural blebs that can be resected or obliterated with minimal loss of functional pulmonary tissue.

More frequently, the adult patient who is under consideration for a thoracic operation is an individual with a pulmonary or esophageal neoplasm or a cigarette smoker with symptoms of chronic bronchitis who is probably middle-aged. Any major operative procedure required will almost certainly interfere with cardiopulmonary function. If one side of the thorax is being operated upon, the ipsilateral lung is retracted or displaced in such a way that it can contribute little to respiratory gas exchange. If a pulmonary resection is necessary, the unilateral loss of function is even more significant. Therefore, the surgeon should evaluate overall pulmonary function and determine the functional status of the contralateral lung.

Despite the common use of estimates of pulmonary function, such as the patient's ability to walk rapidly up two flights of stairs, it is wiser to measure pulmonary function by reproducible objective techniques. The recent development of accurate electronic spirometers for office use makes it possible to perform satisfactory screening tests very conveniently. For the patient with compromised pulmonary function, a plan of management should be instituted before hospitalization. The patient should stop smoking cigarettes; if the patient cannot achieve complete withdrawal, a possible compromise is consumption of a few cigarettes a day of the recently marketed "low tar" brands, if they do not interfere with the patient's vigorous program of postural drainage, chest physiotherapy, and breathing exercises. For those patients who have borderline pulmonary function, as evidenced either by clinical evaluation or formal testing, it is entirely proper to delay a final decision about the operation for several weeks or more, even if they have a neoplasm.

No single test is available that provides an adequate overall evaluation of lung function in surgical patients. The specific measurements of greatest value include lung volumes, mechanics of breathing, and arterial blood gases. Carefully performed spirometry forms the basis of the pulmonary function data that are most often used for primary evaluation of patients with thoracic lesions. Recent developments in automated testing equipment, however, have extended the scope of function measurements that can be done on a routine basis. The thoracic surgeon should develop a strong relationship with the pulmonary laboratory in the hospital to facilitate maximal cooperation from that unit for repeat testing or for specialized tests that may be critically important in making decisions.

The studies that are most helpful for initial evaluation of pulmonary function include vital capacity (VC), inspiratory capacity (IC), forced expiratory volume at one second (FEV_1) and at three seconds (FEV_3), maximal voluntary ventilation (MVV), and the partial pressures of oxygen (PaO_2) and carbon dioxide ($PaCO_2$) in arterial blood. The FEV_1 is the most common flow measurement, and it provides a great deal of information when considered concomitantly with other data. In practice, the FEV_1 is usually reported as a percentage of the VC (FEV_1/VC) as well as an actual volume. If the measured VC is considerably less than the predicted value, the ratio FEV_1/VC may appear to be satisfactory while the actual volume exhaled is markedly abnormal. The FEV_3 has value in its ability to suggest small airway disease that is not generally detected at the high lung volume flows measured by the FEV_1. Recent interest has developed in utilizing flow-volume loops as an early indication of dysfunction of the small airways. The same measurement, however, often shows a more striking deviation from the normal curve with developing obstructive lesions in the trachea. Thus far, the flow-volume loop has not provided sufficient additional information to warrant its routine use in the evaluation of thoracic surgical patients.

Measurement of the MVV should give good correlation with the FEV_1, and the expected relationships are approximately $FEV_1 \times 34$ for males and $FEV_1 \times 40$ for females. If the actual measured value fails to correlate with the calculated value, first consideration should be given to an inadequate effort by the patient (it requires 15 seconds of sustained maximal breathing). This may be a result of the patient's illness, anxiety, or a failure to understand the instructions. In most laboratories, the patient is given an aerosol bronchodilator, and the spirometry is repeated. Failure of decreased function values to improve does not mean that the patient has irreversible pulmonary disease; aggressive therapy with well-motivated cooperation from the patient can often improve pulmonary function to the extent that a thoracic operation becomes feasible.

Measurements of PaO_2, $PaCO_2$, and pH should be routine in the preoperative evaluation of the candidate for thoracic surgery. While it would be inappropriate to depend on arterial blood gas measurements alone, occasionally a patient may exhibit hypoxemia or CO_2 retention that was not suspected at the time of clinical examination or spirometry. The $PaCO_2$ gives an immediate indication of the patient's alveolar ventilation, and any value above 46 torr defines hypoventilation. The ability of the lungs to excrete CO_2 is such that any persistent elevation of $PaCO_2$ suggests serious abnormalities in distribution of ventilation and perfusion. Most operations aggravate a ventilation-perfusion abnormality during the early recovery period. A mild elevation of the $PaCO_2$ in a patient with chronic lung disease may be treated aggressively so that the individual may become a better thoracic surgical candidate. If pulmonary resection is contemplated in such an individual, the risk of postoperative respiratory failure is high, and the final decision to operate may depend on whether *functioning* pulmonary tissue would be removed in the process.

The reported resting PaO_2 value should be interpreted with the knowledge that errors in blood collection or measurement can easily occur. At sea level the normal PaO_2 is above 85 torr, and the value decreases with elevation (i.e., the normal PaO_2 is approximately 70 torr at 5200 ft). However, it is impressive how frequently potential thoracic surgical patients 40 years of age and older have a PaO_2 below the normal range. If the patient who is being evaluated for either pulmonary or nonpulmonary surgery has a PaO_2 above 65 torr (sea level basis), we consider this status compatible with a reasonable operative risk. Of course, if other evidence of compromised function is present, it may be necessary to improve function before recommending operation. The etiology of the decreased PaO_2 should be considered, and more sophisticated function tests should be requested if the patient's respiratory abnormality requires further definition.

In considering the standard pulmonary function tests, surgeons have learned to place the greatest reliance on expiratory flow rates and MVV as the critical determinants of operability for the patient with respiratory disease, chronic illness, or advanced age. Several studies have shown a marked increase in postoperative cardiopulmonary mortality among patients who undergo thoracotomy with measured values of MVV that are less than 50 per cent of predicted values. This problem is more important for the patients who require pulmonary operations, but any major thoracic operation requires careful thought in this circumstance. If functioning pulmonary tissue is to be removed, it may be helpful in making a decision to operate to estimate the postoperative lung function by combined radioisotope and conventional spirometry. A split function test to predict the postpneumonectomy FEV_1 can provide the definitive data needed for a decision to operate on a patient with compromised pulmonary function. In studies on high-risk patients undergoing pneumonectomy, Boysen and associates (1977) showed that operative mortality did not exceed 15 per cent if the predicted postoperative FEV_1 was greater than 800 ml.

NUTRITIONAL EVALUATION

An assessment of the patient's nutritional status is a fundamental consideration in the preoperative evaluation since major thoracic operations may result in severe surgical stress. This is especially true in patients who require prolonged postoperative ventilatory support. Although the relationship between nutritional status and infection is not yet definitively established, many physicians feel strongly that a catabolic state increases susceptibility to infection. For young or middle-aged patients with no history of weight loss or recent dieting, the physical examination may be all that is required to determine that preoperative nutrition is adequate. If the patient is thought to have a benign lesion, and resumption of adequate oral food intake will be possible within a few days postoperatively, a return to good nutritional status may be expected without special nutrient therapy. The majority of patients with benign mediastinal lesions and most of those with congenital lung disorders not associated with infection are managed in this fashion.

Older patients should be considered more carefully. It is frequently more difficult to obtain an accurate dietary history, and weight loss may have occurred insidiously. Physical examination can be helpful diagnostically in a positive way for the muscular, active patient, but it may fail to provide an accurate assessment of nutrition in the obese individual who has lost protein mass and whose tissues have lost firmness. Therefore, total serum protein and albumin levels should be determined routinely, and any evidence of anemia should be investigated. In addition, the patient's weight may be compared with the ideal weight for his or her height and habitus from standard tables, and the dietetic service may be asked to determine actual daily caloric intake by the patient.

The goal of nutritional assessment is to estimate whether the patient is a good candidate for a major operation and its postoperative recovery requirements. If the patient has lost weight, has a serum albumin level below 3.2 gm per dl, or has a total lymphocyte count below 1500 per mm^3, it is wise to delay operation for several weeks if necessary to allow protein-caloric restitution. The need for nutritional therapy is infrequent in patients with benign mediastinal lesions, more frequent than is usually acknowledged in patients with malignant pulmonary neoplasms, and quite common in patients with esophageal lesions. It is preferable to use the enteral route for nutritional support, and if the patient's gastrointestinal tract is functional, an effort should be made to provide 40 to 50 kcal per kg per day. Again, the dietetic service should be requested to arrange the most attractive diet and provide nourishing supplements for the patient who can swallow satisfactorily. If swallowing is limited, either a tube feeding diet or a defined formula diet can be given. When the patient's serum albumin level is below 3.2 gm per dl, it is helpful to supplement the oral diet with daily peripheral vein infusions of amino acid solutions in the amount of approximately 1 gm per kg body weight per day. With the availability of the defined formula diets and crystalline amino acid solutions, it is seldom necessary to use a central venous catheter for total parenteral nutrition in the preoperative management of a thoracic surgical patient with the notable exception of a patient with esophageal cancer.

The optimal time to operate on a patient who is receiving nutritional support must often be determined by an improvement in general appearance, stabilization of body weight, normal skin test reactivity, and increased serum transferrin and albumin concentrations. If improvement does not occur despite maximal feeding efforts, it is possible that systemic spread of disease has occurred in those patients with malignant lesions, and the plan for operative treatment should be reconsidered.

ANTIBIOTICS

In some instances, patients have already been receiving therapeutic antibiotics for established infection when a decision for operative treatment is made. It is appropriate to continue the drugs during the operation and the postoperative period, with repeated cultures and sensitivity testing at intervals of 48 to 72 hours. The fact that an operation is done, however, is not an indication to change the antibiotic regimen or add additional drugs if the organisms remain sensitive to the antibiotics in use.

Prophylactic antibiotics have a clear-cut use for patients whose operations include expected contamination of the operative field. Therefore, prophylactic systemic antibiotics are indicated for those patients who undergo major pulmonary resection, tracheobronchial reconstruction, pulmonary decortication for empyema (if therapeutic antibiotics have been previously discontinued), esophageal resection, or esophagotomy for bypass procedures, ligation of varices, etc. During the endoscopic evaluation of patients with pulmonary or esophageal lesions, aspirates or washings should be taken for bacterial culture and sensitivity determinations. A resident flora can often be identified, especially in the presence of ulcerated neoplasms. If so, the appropriate prophylactic antibiotics should be administered. Additional contamination of the trachea and esophagus can be expected when the patient is anesthetized and intubated for operation.

Administration of cephalosporins has yielded good results in reduction of postoperative infection for patients who undergo either major gastrointestinal or pulmonary operations. When given prophylactically, a satisfactory regimen has been the intravenous infusion of 1 gm of cephalothin sodium up to one hour before the start of the operation and subsequent doses of 1 gm every six hours until the following morning. For patients who have an esophageal operation, the antibiotics may be continued by intravenous or intramuscular administration for three to five days. A similar regimen may be followed for patients who have a major bronchopulmonary operation, but it is often possible for the patient to begin consumption of restricted liquids by mouth on the day after operation. If so, cephalothin is replaced with 500 mg of cephalexin by mouth every six hours for three days.

When thoracotomy is performed for a solitary pulmonary nodule and only a small wedge of tissue is resected, there is usually no need to continue systemic antibiosis during the postoperative period. Irrigation of the thoracotomy incision margins and the pleural cavity with two antibiotic solutions is routinely done in those patients who undergo a major pulmonary resection in the presence of acute or chronic bronchopulmonary infection (with or without a pulmonary tumor) and in patients with esophageal operations for lesions with partial obstruction. The antibiotic solutions consist of 1 gm of cephalothin and 1 gm of kanomycin in separate liters of isotonic saline. Each solution is used for irrigation of the incision and operative field just before division of the bronchus or just prior to esophagotomy. The same solutions are then used for irrigation at several intervals before the chest is closed.

BRONCHOPULMONARY OPERATIONS

An attempt to establish the precise etiology and anatomic diagnosis before thoracotomy is worthwhile. In some instances, the extra effort allows confirmation of a suspected diagnosis, such as tuberculosis or a fungal infection, with the result that thoracotomy may not be necessary. Therefore, skin tests for tuberculosis and histoplasmosis should be done routinely in patients with undiagnosed pulmonary lesions and for coccidioidomycosis in the known endemic regions. These procedures are equally important as careful review of the patient's previous chest roentgenograms to determine if a newly found lesion really is a recent development. Bronchial brushing and flexible bronchoscopy have added significantly to the capacity for obtaining diagnostic material, and these techniques should be maximally employed.

It is important to establish, insofar as it is possible, the anatomic extent of disease prior to operation. For patients with congenital lesions such as pulmonary cysts, arteriovenous fistulas, or lung sequestration, the performance of bronchoscopy, pulmonary arteriography, and occasionally aortography allows an accurate classification of the disorder. With this information the surgeon can plan the operative treatment precisely, decide on the need for staged procedures, and consider the anomaly with the proper perspective. Bronchography is critical to decisions about operative treatment of bronchiectasis, but the decreasing frequency of this disease appears to parallel a decreasing availability of interest and skill in performance of bronchograms. Nevertheless, a complete mapping of the bronchial tree should be done preoperatively. Similarly, patients with empyema who have a history that suggests bronchiectasis should have bronchography prior to final consideration for decortication.

In the past, the increased ability to diagnose the extent of bronchial neoplasms has been a significant advance, allowing better selection of patients for curative operation. The procedures of mediastinal tomography, mediastinotomy, and mediastinoscopy must be considered for each patient suspected or proved to have bronchogenic carcinoma without obvious contraindications for curative resection. Each of these techniques has shortcomings, but if judiciously employed, they may markedly reduce the frequency of fruitless thoracotomy. In general, mediastinal tomography and mediastinotomy are indicated in all patients with central pulmonary neoplasms. Occasionally it is essential to enter the pleural cavity in order to adequately evaluate the extent of neoplasia or to obtain a lung biopsy. Mediastinoscopy is indicated in patients with lesions that are located more peripherally, particularly those greater than 3.0 cm in diameter and in patients with superior sulcus tumors.

Computerized tomography (CT) may become a valuable technique for demonstrating growth or spread of bronchogenic carcinoma into the posterior mediastinum, and the technique should be utilized when this is suspected. The CT scans are particularly useful for estimating the presence of multiple lesions in patients who are candidates for operative removal of pulmonary metastases.

The guidelines for the use of antibiotics have been described; however, specific comments should be made about the relationship of chemotherapy to the surgical treatment of tuberculosis. Presently, it is doubtful if more than 5 per cent of patients who develop tuberculosis will become candidates for pulmonary resection. For those patients, chemotherapy of 6 to 12 months' duration and conversion to a negative sputum should be considered an ideal preoperative status. Some surgeons feel that it is appropriate to add an additional drug to the patient's regimen at the time of operation and for three to six months postoperatively. When surgical treatment is required in patients infected with atypical mycobacteria or when drug-resistant organisms are present, operation may be necessary at an earlier time than that initially anticipated.

In all patients with bronchopulmonary infection, the preoperative preparation should include an aggressive approach to control of infection and reduction of tracheobronchial secretions. Chest physical therapy and postural drainage may be just as important for the patient with a bronchogenic carcinoma as they are for the patient with a lung abscess or bronchiectasis. Intermittent positive pressure breathing and incentive spirometry exercises can be helpful in acquainting the patient with respiratory therapy equipment and with the techniques of deep breathing. In addition, a program of orienting the patient to the surgical intensive care unit can be helpful for selected patients who have overt anxiety about their hospitalization and operation.

Preoperative digitalization is not recommended for prophylactic treatment of operative or postoperative cardiac arrhythmias. Patients requiring consideration for drug therapy for hypertension should be managed in cooperation with a physician who is skilled in this area. Preoperative radiation therapy is indicated for patients with superior sulcus tumors and for patients thought to have localized chest wall involvement. In the latter instance, the presumption is that the patient has a localized neoplasm and is otherwise an excellent candidate for curative resection. The course of radiation therapy should be short in duration, and operative treatment may be undertaken within a few days or a week after completion of radiation therapy.

ESOPHAGEAL OPERATIONS

The general considerations of pulmonary function and nutrition remain important items in the preoperative management of patients who require esophageal operations. A large segment of the patients who undergo operations on the esophagus consists of individuals with hiatus hernia, gastroesophageal reflux, and esophagitis. Their preoperative evaluation requires careful esophagograms, esophagoscopy, and manometry combined with objective tests for esophageal reflux. Because occasionally a patient has a primary motor disorder rather than true reflux esophagitis as the etiology of the symptoms, it is pertinent to review the contrast studies meticulously with the radiologist. Any evidence of thickening of the esophageal wall or barium retention in the lower esophagus is justification for reexamination with cinefluorography. Manometric studies allow a demonstration of differentiation of esophageal motility disturbances and provide objective data for preoperative and postoperative comparison. The pH reflux test should be done if there is any question of the occurrence of reflux.

Esophagoscopy is an appropriate examination early in the work-up of patients who have virtually any type of esophageal disorder. For patients undergoing attempted medical management of reflux esophagitis, repeat endoscopy may expedite determining whether progress is being made and whether any stricture formation will yield to dilatation. In patients with achalasia or with obstruction due to stricture, it may be necessary to restrict their diet to liquids for several days before attempting endoscopy so that visualization will not be impaired by retained foodstuffs. Because the selection of treatment for esophageal carcinoma may depend on the proximal extent of the neoplasm, it is crucial for the endoscopist to make this determination accurately.

Operations for esophageal bypass or replacement utilize either the stomach, small bowel, or colon as the substitute conduit. An important step in preoperative management is the roentgenographic study of the selected structure to confirm its suitability for use as an esophageal replacement. An adequate barium study of the stomach or small bowel may not be possible, however, in the patient who has near total esophageal obstruction from either stricture or carcinoma. If obstruction is present, the colon must be prepared for use as an alternate esophageal replacement in case the stomach or jejunum is found unsuitable for use at the time of operation.

Because esophageal obstruction is often associated with bacterial overgrowth in the lumen, either kanamycin or neomycin should be given by mouth for 36 to 48 hours before esophageal resection or bypass in conjunction with a liquid diet. If a colonic bypass is planned, mechanical cleansing of the colon is also done. The occasional patient who has a large esophageal diverticulum with retention should be prepared for operation with a liquid diet and with oral antibiotics in the same manner.

At present, there are sufficient data to suggest that there are benefits to be obtained from preoperative radiation in patients with esophageal carcinoma. For patients with carcinoma of the middle or lower third of the esophagus, the preferred treatment is 2500 rads administered during a period of 10 days to two weeks before operation.

MEDIASTINAL OPERATIONS

The principal activities in the preoperative management of patients with mediastinal lesions are concerned with differential diagnosis and general evaluation. Most operations involve removal of a mediastinal tumor or cyst, and it is often necessary to perform angiocardiography, tomography, and other contrast studies to estimate the extent of dissection needed. The operative approach may be through a lateral thoracotomy or via median sternotomy. The latter incision is tolerated better by patients with marginal pulmonary function. Occasionally, all evidence points to an extent of disease that precludes complete resection. Should this situation prevail, it is appropriate to obtain tissue for biopsy or to confirm the extent of disease by mediastinotomy or mediastinoscopy prior to making any other decisions regarding subsequent management.

Performance of thymectomy in patients with myasthenia gravis should be approached as a team effort with a neurologist and an anesthesiologist. Careful psychological preparation of the patient, including an introduction to the ICU staff and reassurance about postoperative respiratory support, cannot be overemphasized.

POSTOPERATIVE CARE

Patients who have undergone a major thoracotomy should be cared for in a surgical intensive care unit until their cardiopulmonary function has recovered from the unstable state that characterizes the first few postoperative days. This generally means that the patient is breathing and coughing well independently and cardiac output is satisfactory without evidence of significant arrhythmia. Younger patients who have had a simple thoracic procedure such as pulmonary wedge biopsy, excision of a benign mediastinal tumor, or an esophageal myotomy can often be discharged from the ICU the day after operation. However, the surgeon need not apologize for his or her reluctance to release a patient from the ICU if there is any question about the patient's adequate recovery.

The principal determinants of the nature of postoperative care are the patient's preoperative condition, the placement of central venous, arterial, nasogastric, and urinary catheters, and the operation performed.

For purposes of discussion, it is helpful to list postoperative considerations that are common to all thoracic surgical patients:

Pain relief	Fluids and nutrition
Monitoring	Urinary output
Thoracic drainage	Respiratory care
Chest roentgenograms	Wound care
Gastric decompression	Mobilization

This list is not intended to cover every facet of postoperative care, and it
is suggested that standard textbooks should be consulted for special
items that are unique to individual diseases or operations. Furthermore,
it is expected that those who are responsible for the patient's postoperative care will assess the status of recovery at regular intervals and decide
how strictly to follow a plan of management.

Pain Relief

Lateral thoracotomy incisions, supplemented by the tethering effect
of intercostal catheters, produce exquisite pain in the majority of
patients. Fortunately, there is adequate latitude between satisfactory
pain relief and respiratory depression to allow administration of effective doses of analgesics to all but a few patients. Inadequate doses of
analgesics, however, or inadequate frequency of administration force the
patient to use the primary mechanism of decreasing discomfort — immobilization of the hemithorax. This increases the likelihood of retained
secretions with subsequent atelectasis and may be followed by a
progressive ventilation-perfusion abnormality, hypoxemia, and a series
of related complications.

Either meperidine or morphine are satisfactory for pain relief in the
majority of patients, but small doses of intravenous morphine (3 to 5 mg)
at intervals of one to three hours are preferable for those patients who
require assisted ventilation for up to 24 to 48 hours postoperatively.
Intramuscular meperidine, in doses of 50 to 75 mg every two or three
hours, may be used as the initial postoperative medication for most
adults. The surgeon should change the dose or the schedule depending
on the patient's early responses. During the first 24 to 48 hours it is often
necessary to allow the patient to receive 100 mg meperidine or up to 15
mg of morphine as often as every three hours. For elderly patients and
for those with chronic lung disease, a similar dosage schedule must be
given only with great caution and with careful monitoring of respiration.
While there seems to be less pain associated with a median sternotomy
incision, the amount of narcotic analgesia required must be determined
by regular observation of the patient.

Occasionally, a patient is especially apprehensive during the first
few days after operation, and small doses of chlorpromazine (12.5 to 25
mg) may be used to supplement the primary analgesic. However, this is

recommended only if the function of the cardiovascular system seems stable and there is no evidence of a tendency toward hypotension. Obviously, it is critical first to exclude hypoxia or other threatening physical or chemical problems as the cause of the patient's anxiety.

Intercostal nerve blocks with 2 per cent lidocaine can be used for the occasionally encountered patient whose respiration is critically depressed by even small doses of narcotics. The injections must be repeated at intervals of no more than 12 hours, but several techniques have been described for placing small catheters adjacent to the intercostal nerves on each side of the incision during operation. Following operation, lidocaine can be injected through the catheters at whatever interval is necessary for adequate pain relief.

The nurses can help relieve the patient's discomfort by insuring that he or she is appropriately positioned in the bed and by insuring that the chest tubes do not pull on the chest wall. Removal of the tubes is usually accompanied by reduction of pain and greater freedom of movement.

MONITORING

Especially for older patients or for those with compromised cardiopulmonary function, a subclavian central venous catheter and an arterial catheter (radial or femoral) should be placed in the patient at the beginning of the operation. These catheters allow close monitoring of the patient's cardiopulmonary function in the postoperative period, and they should be maintained during at least the first 24 hours. Arterial samples should be drawn for blood gas analysis at the end of the operative procedure and again after one hour. If the patient's early ventilation is satisfactory, then arterial samples can be analyzed at 6- to 12-hour intervals until the catheter is removed, preferably at 24 hours postoperatively if there is no problem with respiration. If there is evidence of respiratory malfunction, samples of arterial blood may be analyzed as frequently as necessary to facilitate identification and correction of the problem, and the arterial catheter may be retained as needed beyond 24 hours.

It is recognized that central venous pressure (CVP) is inferior to pulmonary capillary wedge pressure for monitoring cardiac function, but the CVP is nonetheless a helpful guide for fluid therapy or transfusion in the postoperative period. The central venous catheter can be replaced with a Swan-Ganz catheter if there is a question of left ventricular function.

The patient's cardiac electrical activity and pulse rate should be monitored continuously during the first 24 hours after operation. Monitoring of cardiac activity should continue for longer periods for elderly patients, for those with any evidence of cardiac arrhythmia, and for those who have undergone pneumonectomy. If an arterial catheter was placed during operation, it should be used for continuous monitoring of blood pressure. In the absence of an arterial catheter, blood pressure should be checked every few minutes after the patient arrives in the recovery room and then at intervals of 15 minutes to one hour as the patient recovers from anesthesia.

THORACIC DRAINAGE

The pleural cavity is drained routinely after all types of operations that involve entering the pleural space. Effective drainage removes air and fluid in order to minimize dead space and to allow the lung the best opportunity to reexpand fully at the conclusion of the operative procedure. Continued drainage is crucial to maintain pulmonary expansion and prevent complications such as tension pneumothorax, hemothorax, massive atelectasis, and empyema. Drainage of the mediastinum should be provided after operations done through a median sternotomy, but the placement of the catheters depends upon whether or not the pleural space was entered. If the pleura has remained intact, satisfactory drainage can be provided by a single catheter drawn into the anterior mediastinum through a stab wound on either side of the xyphoid. After the sternotomy is closed, the catheter should lie in a retrosternal position and extend toward the superior mediastinum. If the pleura has been opened to an extent greater than a small fenestration, then the pleural cavity should be drained with an intercostal catheter placed in a low and somewhat posterior position. This may be adequate in simple cases in which there is no expectation of significant drainage. As an alternative, and especially if a wide dissection has been performed, a mediastinal drainage catheter should be used along with the intercostal catheter.

For some operative procedures done through a lateral thoracotomy, the pleural space can be drained by a single intercostal catheter. Examples of procedures that often require only a single catheter are resections of benign mediastinal tumors or cysts, transthoracic vagotomy, and pneumonectomy. Many surgeons do not use catheter drainage after pneumonectomy, but it is useful for obtaining accurate information concerning the amount of early postoperative blood loss. In addition, postpneumonectomy thoracic drainage prevents a shift of the mediastinum to the unoperated side and allows the initial postoperative fluid with its contained tissue debris and potentially contaminating bacteria to drain from the chest. In all cases, the intercostal catheter should be removed the day following pneumonectomy.

For the majority of thoracic procedures, drainage is better provided through two intercostal catheters. Following decortication for empyema, it is occasionally appropriate to use three or more catheters. Clear plastic catheters with multiple holes in sizes 28F to 36F should be used for adults, and similar catheters of 16F to 24F are recommended for children. The catheters should be connected to separate graduated water-seal bottles of one or two liter capacity by clear plastic tubing approximately six feet in length (⅜ or ½ in. diameter for adults, ¼ in. diameter for small children). It is appropriate to use either a single water-seal collecting bottle or the more elaborate disposable plastic collecting systems that incorporate a manometer and separate collecting chambers. The latter units tend to be expensive, and the majority of surgeons are not convinced of their superiority to the former method.

For all patients except those who have had a pneumonectomy, suction drainage is preferred over simple gravity drainage. Regardless of the source of suction, a high-volume system is needed, allowing 15 to 20 cm H_2O negative pressure to be applied to the catheters. When there is a large air leak from the lung surface, a reduction in pulmonary compliance, or anticipated difficulty in expansion of the pulmonary tissue to fill the hemithorax, a negative pressure of -30 to -50 cm H_2O may be needed. The volume of fluid or blood drainage should be noted hourly for the first six hours after operation and then at less frequent intervals if the hourly drainage falls as low as 25 ml. Beginning with the first postoperative morning, it is usually satisfactory to measure the drainage at the start or finish of each nursing shift.

Following operation, a continued hourly drainage of blood in an amount of 100 ml or more makes it mandatory to consider the possibility that the thorax may have to be reopened. This is necessary infrequently, but blood loss of more than 100 ml per hour signals the need to estimate or actually measure the hematocrit of the bloody drainage, to be certain the tubes are functioning well, and to determine by chest roentgenography that a hemothorax is not developing. The information suggested by the quantity and character of the drainage through the chest tube is correlated with any clinical evidence of inadequate circulating blood volume, and adequate blood transfusion or fluid replacement should be accomplished.

Whenever the early postoperative drainage contains a significant amount of blood, careful attention should be paid to the occurrence of clots in the intercostal catheters. The catheters and connecting tubing should be stripped at hourly intervals to discourage clot or fibrin adherence to the tube walls. With either postoperative bleeding or drainage of fibrinopurulent material, the intrapleural portion of the chest tubes may become blocked. It is possible to reestablish drainage by saline irrigation of the tubes, but this requires careful aseptic technique and the help of an assistant.

Assurance that the chest tubes and suction system are keeping the pleural cavity evacuated of air is critical for patients who have an air leak after a pulmonary operation. The necessity of mobilizing the lung in the presence of extensive pleural adhesions can result in postoperative air leaks after esophageal or mediastinal operations, and a daily portable chest roentgenogram is needed to evaluate lung expansion. Nursing personnel must be properly instructed about the danger of clamping the chest tubes in a patient who has an air leak. As a preliminary step to removing a chest tube after the air leak presumably has been sealed, some surgeons clamp the tube and obtain a portable chest roentgeno-gram an hour or more later. This practice is potentially hazardous because accumulating air could collapse the lung and conceivably produce a tension pneumothorax. It is safer simply to observe the drainage bottle for escaping air at frequent intervals and then to discontinue the suction for several hours or overnight after the last manifestation of an air leak. If a portable chest roentgenogram confirms lung expansion without pneumothorax, the chest tube can be re-moved.

When an air leak seems to be continuing longer than anticipated, several possibilities must be considered. The remaining pulmonary tissue may not be able to form a seal with the parietal pleura because of incomplete expansion of the lung. Another possibility is that one of the chest tubes may be situated exactly opposite a source of a leak from several small bronchioles, and the suction is keeping the leak from closing by streaming the air through the openings at high velocity. Occasionally, a chest tube becomes partly dislodged, and one or more of the holes in the tube may lie in the subcutaneous tissue outside the rib cage. When this happens, the negative pressure may draw outside air into the soft tissues around the tube and then into the tube drainage system. The result is an apparent continuing air leak that can continue indefinitely unless recognized. Therefore, each of these possibilities must be investigated and appropriate action taken.

A patient who has undergone lobectomy or segmental resection occasionally may continue to leak air for three to five days with no sign of a decrease, even though the chest roentgenogram suggests satisfactory expansion of the remaining pulmonary tissue. In this situation, an induced pneumoperitoneum can be especially helpful. By introducing 1000 to 1500 ml of air into the peritoneal cavity for several consecutive days, the hemidiaphragms can be elevated to help adjust the volume of the hemithorax on the operated side. The air can be introduced by needle paracentesis, but it is simpler to insert a small catheter into the peritoneal cavity and thus avoid the need for repeated punctures.

Chest tubes are generally left in place for a minimum period of 24 hours. Beyond this time they should be removed as soon as their need no longer exists. Thus, if two intercostal catheters were used to drain the pleural cavity after a surgical procedure that did not result in a continu-ing air leak, and a portable chest roentgenogram indicates adequate expansion of the lung on the morning following operation, the anterior tube can be removed. The posterior tube can be removed the same day if the fluid drainage following operation does not exceed a few hundred milliliters and if there has been no drainage for the previous 8 to 12 hours. Generally, however, it is wise to leave the posterior tube in place until the following morning (48 hours postoperatively), because the mobilization of the patient on the first day often results in drainage of 100 ml or more of fluid as the patient changes position. The tube should be removed when the drainage for the preceding 24 hours is 50 ml or less in an adult and 25 ml or less in a child. Under special circumstances, primarily those related to esophageal operations, it is appropriate to leave the posterior chest tube in place for a longer time.

Unfortunately, the need to leave a chest tube in place beyond five days seems to increase the likelihood of infection developing in the pleural space. Therefore, bacterial cultures should be taken from the pleural drainage at that time and a decision made about starting the patient on systemic antibiotics (if they are not already being used).

The technique of removing a chest tube includes synchrony of its swift, smooth withdrawal with prompt application of a Vaseline gauze over its exit site while the patient simultaneously holds his breath. A chest roentgenogram should be obtained shortly thereafter if there is any question that air may have entered the pleural cavity during tube removal.

POSTOPERATIVE CHEST ROENTGENOGRAMS

Following a thoracic operation, upright chest roentgenograms should be obtained at regular intervals to assess the completeness of pulmonary expansion and to detect any accumulation of fluid or blood. The films should supplement physical examination of the patient's chest rather than reduce the need for personal assessment. A portable roentgenogram is obtained soon after the patient arrives in the recovery room, and the film should be examined immediately by the surgeon. It may be appropriate to obtain another chest roentgenogram on the first evening postoperatively, depending on the volume of chest drainage and the patient's ability to cooperate. The frequency of subsequent chest roentgenograms depends on factors such as the patient's clinical course and the planned removal of chest tubes. While it can be expected that a daily chest roentgenogram may be appropriate for the first several days after operation, there should be a distinct justification for repeat chest roentgenography beyond that time.

Interpretation of chest roentgenograms after a thoracotomy can be difficult, and the radiologist should seek consultation with the surgeon in order to obtain the most accurate clinical correlation of information. It is especially helpful to establish a routine time of the day when the individual(s) responsible for the patient's care can review the roentgenograms with the radiologist. The variable quality of portable chest roentgenograms can make it difficult to be certain that the lung has expanded completely on the operated side, to distinguish postoperative atelectasis, or to detect unusual patterns of edema from pneumonitis. Clearly, the interpretation of the roentgenograms must be based on a correlation with the patient's clinical course and data such as temperature, respiratory rate, evidence of right-to-left pulmonary shunting, and peripheral blood counts.

GASTRIC DECOMPRESSION

For patients who have thoracic operations not involving the gastrointestinal tract, it is not routinely necessary to provide continuous postoperative gastric decompression. Instead, either before the patient leaves the operating room or just after arrival in the recovery room, a nasogastric tube should be passed into the stomach for aspiration of accumulated air and gastric secretions. If a large amount of secretions are removed, the tube can be placed on intermittent suction for a few hours or left in place overnight. When the patient requires assisted ventilation after operation, it is wise to insert either a plastic nasogastric tube or a sump-suction catheter and to use intermittent suction drainage at least until the following day.

Acute gastric dilatation can develop even a day or two after operation, and this potential complication must be kept in mind. The upright portable chest roentgenogram should be studied carefully for evidence of gastric distention, and the patient's abdomen should be examined each time the thorax is examined during the first few postoperative days.

FLUIDS AND NUTRITION

Most individuals who have undergone pulmonary or mediastinal operations are able to resume limited oral intake on the day after operation. Therefore, the postoperative fluid therapy need not include emphasis on intravenous calories or protein intake unless complications delay resumption of oral nutrition. A major consideration, however, is the risk of interstitial pulmonary edema due to excessive intravenous fluid administration during operation and in the early postoperative hours. The retraction and manipulation of the lung on the side of operation can accentuate the development of edema and result in decreased lung compliance with progressive increase in right-to-left shunting. For patients with borderline pulmonary function, this sequence is likely to mandate a period of assisted ventilation following operation. When the operative procedure has been prolonged and more than 2 liters of intravenous fluids have been administered, 20 mg of furosemide infused intravenously may help mobilize fluid from the lung. If there is palpable evidence of pulmonary edema before closure of the thoracic incision, an additional dose of 20 to 40 mg of furosemide should be given two hours after operation. A patient's elevated CVP may be helpful in suggesting the need for a diuretic, but edema is so often associated with a normal or low CVP that this decision should be based on other indices.

With the emphasis on restricted intravenous fluids in deference to the risk of pulmonary edema, the postoperative fluid and electrolyte management of patients who have had pulmonary or mediastinal operations differs in no major way from patients who have undergone intra-abdominal operations. Serum sodium potassium, chloride, blood urea nitrogen, and arterial blood gas measurements should be obtained immediately postoperatively. The initial orders for fluids should be based on the patient's estimated balance at the end of operation, including intraoperative urinary output. For the first 24 hours it is wise to limit the baseline fluids to 40 ml per kg given as 5 per cent dextrose in water. Up to 1 mEq per kg of sodium may be given as 0.25 per cent NaCl in 5 per cent dextrose in water, and 40 to 60 mEq of potassium should be included with the fluids if urinary output is satisfactory. Beginning with the first postoperative day, oral liquids may be started cautiously. If tolerated, intravenous fluids can often be discontinued by the morning of the second postoperative day.

For patients who undergo intrathoracic esophageal operations, the same caution about intraoperative and early postoperative pulmonary edema is applicable. Therefore, intravenous fluid administration for the first 24 hours should follow the same guidelines described for patients who undergo pulmonary or mediastinal operations. Oral nutrition should be withheld for 6 to 10 days for those patients who have had an esophageal anastomosis or major esophagotomy. Intravenous hyperalimentation can be started (or resumed) on the first postoperative day, using the subclavian venous catheter inserted at the time of operation. Daily measurements of serum electrolytes should be supplemented by a determination of the serum albumin concentration every third or fourth day. The patient should be weighed daily or at least every other day, and an esophagogram should be obtained on the sixth to eighth postoperative day. If there is no evidence of an esophageal leak, the patient can then start taking liquids orally, using an elemental diet initially to provide at least 2000 calories per day.

URINARY OUTPUT

It is appropriate to insert an indwelling urinary catheter at the time of operation for most patients who undergo major pulmonary or esophageal operations. This facilitates intraoperative and postoperative fluid administration by allowing continuous monitoring of urinary output. From the patient's standpoint, the mild discomfort of the catheter is easily outweighed by the convenience of not having to strain or be placed on a bedpan during the first 24 to 48 hours after thoractomy.

An output of 30 to 40 ml per hour for adults and 10 to 20 ml per hour for children is adequate on the day of operation and the first postoperative day. Especially if there are other fluid losses occurring, such as thoracic drainage or nasogastric drainage, urinary outputs in excess of these values suggest that excessive intravenous fluids are being given. The need to give furosemide to facilitate removal of intrapulmonary water alters the interpretation of urinary output as a guide to fluid therapy, but the diuretic effects are generally dissipated after two or three hours. It is preferable to remove the indwelling urinary catheter by the second postoperative day except for those patients who require prolonged assisted ventilation.

Respiratory Care

The two principal components of postoperative respiratory care for thoracic surgical patients are (1) periodic assessment of ventilation with supplemental oxygen or ventilatory support when necessary and (2) prevention and management of respiratory complications. These are closely related activities, and potential problems in either area can often be anticipated by careful consideration of the patient's preoperative respiratory status. In the discussions on pain relief and thoracic drainage, the potential complications of retained bronchial secretions, atelectasis, and pneumothorax were outlined. Even in patients without a long history of smoking or chronic airway disease, there is a risk of pulmonary atelectasis that can lead to inadequate respiratory exchange, pleural effusion, pneumonia, and empyema. The operative procedure and the placement of the endotracheal tube result in increased tracheobronchial secretions in many patients. Without an aggressive program to help the patient remove these secretions, the sequence of complications described above is likely to occur more often than is justifiable.

As soon as the patient has recovered from anesthesia, a routine schedule of hourly coughing and deep breathing exercises should be started. By holding a folded bath towel or a small sheet as a buttress over the area of the lateral thoracotomy incision, the nurse or physician can encourage the patient to cough less painfully. If some element of bronchospasm is present, and it often is in patients with chronic bronchitis, it is helpful to administer a topical bronchodilator by intermittent positive pressure breathing (IPPB) at four- to six-hour intervals. Similarly, saline and acetylcysteine may be administered by IPPB when the patient has dry, thick secretions that are difficult to expel. Unfortunately, IPPB has been disappointing when used alone as a technique for the prophylaxis of pulmonary complications. When used for the specific purpose of delivering medications to patients with established problems, however, it can be an important component of the total care program.

Humidified air can be provided for the patient with thick secretions by either an ultrasonic nebulizer or a heated aerosol unit. On the day following operation, chest physiotherapy may be started with postural drainage and "blow bottles" or an incentive spirometer. For those patients who refuse to cough or cannot do so, nasotracheal suctioning should be done at intervals of every one to three hours for the first few days after operation. This must be done carefully to minimize trauma to

Table 19–1. CRITERIA FOR ASSISTED VENTILATION

FUNCTION	NORMAL VALUES	VENTILATE
Pulmonary mechanics		
Respiratory rate, per minute	12–20	>35
Maximum inspiratory force, cm H_2O (minus values)	75–100	<25–35
Vital capacity, ml/kg	65–75	<15
Oxygen exchange		
PaO_2, torr	76–100 (air)	<65–70 (supplemental oxygen)
Alveolar-arterial oxygen difference, torr (100% oxygen)	30–70	>350
Carbon dioxide exchange		
$PaCO_2$, torr	35–45	>50
Dead space: tidal volume ratio	0.25–0.40	>0.6

the nose, larynx, and trachea and to prevent hypoxemia secondary to prolonged suctioning (i.e., not longer than 10 seconds).

The development of the flexible fiberscope has greatly facilitated the use of bronchoscopy for removal of secretions in patients with major atelectasis. When the techniques of induced coughing, postural drainage, and chest physiotherapy fail to result in reexpansion of a collapsed lobe, bronchoscopy should be done without hesitation.

A need for postoperative assisted ventilation can often be anticipated in the patient with chronic pulmonary disease. The endotracheal tube should be left in place so that the patient can receive assisted ventilation until he or she is fully awake. Then, based on the measured arterial blood gases and the patient's spontaneous ventilatory effort, a decision can be made either to continue assisted ventilation or to remove the endotracheal tube and give supplemental oxygen by mask or nasal catheter. An important aspect of supporting oxygen transport is the recognition that red cell transfusion is just as important as supplemental oxygen when the patient is anemic and the PaO_2 is 60 torr or higher.

Table 19–1 lists the general criteria that are most helpful for determining whether mechanical ventilation should be initiated or whether ventilatory support should be continued postoperatively. If assisted ventilation is required beyond the morning following operation, it adds entirely different dimensions to the patient's care, which are discussed in Chapter 40.

WOUND CARE

The postoperative care of thoracic incisions requires special attention. Because patients spend most of the time in the supine or semisupine position, the posterior aspect of a posterolateral thoracotomy incision may show effects of pressure by the third or fourth postoperative day. This is manifested as swelling and redness, which can be mistaken for wound infection by the inexperienced observer. Wound swelling and redness can be managed by the use of plastic foam strips or folded gauze sponges placed along either side of the incision to redistribute the pressure over a greater surface area away from the wound. In addition, the patient should be instructed to use a pillow under the shoulders in order to avoid lying flat against the mattress.

An arbitrary habit of removing the skin sutures or clips on a specific postoperative day (i.e., the seventh day) must be avoided. In general, it is advisable to leave the sutures of a posterolateral thoracotomy incision in place for several days longer than those of a simple abdominal incision (10 days to 2 weeks).

Dehiscence of a median sternotomy incision is a serious complication, but it can usually be avoided by the early detection of increasing movement ("rocking") of the sternal halves. The wound should be checked every day by applying gentle pressure on each side of the incision, particularly over the manubrium. If the two halves are obviously distracted, the sternotomy wound usually must be reopened. If infection is present, adequate débridement must be done, and the sternal halves must be reunited with new wire sutures. Catheters for topical antibiotic irrigation and drainage should then be placed before the wound is closed.

MOBILIZATION

From a practical standpoint, early mobilization of a patient with indwelling chest tubes is limited. Movement that is transmitted to the chest tubes causes pain, and once the patient has been hurt by accidental jerking or traction on the tubes, he or she will be less cooperative in continuing to initiate movement. In addition, vigorous efforts at ambulation before the patient has gained sufficient strength to help himself or herself can result in mishaps with the suction drainage system. Therefore, early mobilization should be encouraged on the first postoperative day but should be limited to movements such as sitting, coughing, deep breathing, and extremity exercises in bed. Depending on the patient's strength, it is generally possible to sit in a bedside chair and to take a few steps by the second postoperative day. As soon as the chest tubes are removed, the patient's mobilization should progress to full ambulation. Patients who have had a posterolateral thoracotomy must be encouraged to start active and passive movements of the upper extremity on the side of the incision to achieve satisfactory abduction and elevation by the time of hospital discharge. This is an important aspect of their convalescence, rehabilitation, and return to normal function and activity following major thoracic procedures.

REFERENCES

Boysen, P. G., Black, A. J., Olsen, G. N., Moulder, P. V., Harris, J. O., and Rawitscher, R. E.: Prospective evaluation for pneumonectomy using the ^{99}Tc quantitative perfusion lung scan. Chest, 72:422, 1977.

Cordell, A. R., and Ellison, R. G. (eds.): Complications of Intrathoracic Surgery. Boston, Little, Brown, and Co., 1979.

Deitel, M. (ed.): Nutrition in Clinical Surgery. Baltimore, Williams and Wilkins, 1980.

Postlethwait, R. W.: Surgery of the Esophagus. New York, Appleton-Century-Crofts, 1979, pp. 341–414.

Tisi, G. M.: Preoperative evaluation of pulmonary function. Am. Rev. Resp. Dis., 119:293, 1979.

20

Cardiac Surgery

L. HENRY EDMUNDS, JR.

In cardiac surgery, the principal objectives of preoperative care are to inventory the patient's pathologic processes and to assess the function of vital organ systems. These objectives are met by obtaining a careful history and physical examination, selected screening laboratory tests, and comprehensive review of the data collected from special cardiac studies. Proper preoperative care readies the patient for cardiac surgery and also prepares the operative team to deal with multiple diseases and compromised functions of organ systems. Such knowledge helps to anticipate and prevent complications.

Cardiac surgical patients require conscientious postoperative care, but since the heart's capacity to heal is great, attention to detail is usually rewarded with an uncomplicated convalescence. Clinical surveillance is greatly enhanced by continuous and intermittent quantitative measurements of circulatory and respiratory function. No other type of surgery requires vigilance on a beat-to-beat basis, and yet no other type of surgery permits as ready access to quantitative physiologic information.

PREOPERATIVE CARE

All patients should have a complete history and physical examination. Although all symptoms and signs referrable to the cardiac disease or disorder should be recorded, particular attention must be paid to latent or overt diseases of other organ systems. The history should audit drug intake, drug allergies, smoking, unusual anxiety, easy bleeding or bruising, recent trauma or infection, and any other noncardiac abnormality or disease. After the physical examination, a complete problem list should be developed; this list and the results of routine screening tests will determine subsequent preoperative investigations of diseased organ systems.

382

SCREENING LABORATORY TESTS

The following tests are recommended for all cardiac surgical patients preoperatively: hemoglobin, white blood cell count and differential count, anteroposterior and lateral chest roentgenograms, screening pulmonary function tests (if the patient is over 40 years of age), urinalysis, electrocardiogram, serum electrolytes, total serum protein, fasting blood sugar, blood urea nitrogen (BUN) and creatinine, prothrombin time, partial thromboplastin time, fibrinogen and platelet count, blood type, and crossmatch for 2 to 10 units, depending upon the proposed operation.

ADMISSION ORDERS

Admission orders will, of course, vary for individual patients. The orders should be specific for diet (low salt, diabetic, etc.), activity, amount of daily fluid intake, and medications. Nurses should record daily weights, fluid intake and output, and vital signs (temperature, heart rate, blood pressure, and respiratory rate). Laxative and sleeping medication orders help to insure patient comfort.

HEART

Digoxin and other digitalis preparations are routinely stopped 36 hours before the scheduled operation unless the drug is required to control heart rate, such as in patients with atrial fibrillation. Because of wide variation in serum potassium concentration during and immediately after cardiopulmonary bypass and because of variable washout of myocardial digoxin during bypass, low serum concentrations of digoxin during and after bypass avoid the potentially serious problems of digitalis toxicity. Coumadin is stopped at the time of hospital admission, and intravenous heparin (4000 to 6000 units for adults) is given every four to six hours to maintain anticoagulation until six to eight hours before operation. The dose of heparin can be monitored by obtaining partial thromboplastin times four hours after the heparin dose is given (twice normal indicates adequate heparin dosage). Diuretics are usually continued until the evening before operation; however, serum potassium must be monitored to avoid potassium depletion. Propranolol is generally continued at full dosage in the hospital until the day before operation. If the patient is comfortable, the drug dose is reduced by one-half and stopped completely six to eight hours before operation. If necessary to control cardiac ischemic pain, propranolol can be continued until the induction of anesthesia; the drug causes competitive blockade of beta receptors, and its effects can be overcome by isoproterenol.

In patients with ischemic heart disease or abnormal electrocardiograms, serum enzymes (HBD, LDH, CPK, SGOT) and myocardial-specific enzymes CPK-MB should be measured to rule out recent myocardial infarction. It is wise to postpone elective surgery for patients with a recent myocardial infarction; however, not infrequently operation must be carried out in the presence of an infarction because of unstable angina pectoris or life-threatening complications of the infarction. These patients require an indwelling arterial cannula and a Swan-Ganz catheter to measure pulmonary arterial blood pressure, central venous pressure, pulmonary arterial wedge pressure (a measure of left atrial pressure), cardiac output, and arterial blood gases preoperatively. Drugs to increase blood flow, increase cardiac contractility, and reduce left ventricular wall tension are often required, and some patients also benefit from insertion of an intra-aortic balloon.

Cardiac performance should be optimal prior to operation. Cardiac arrhythmias, particularly atrial flutter, atrial fibrillation, and premature ventricular contractions (more than six per minute), should be brought under control with appropriate drugs. Second- and third-degree heart block may require insertion of a temporary or permanent pacemaker before operation to regulate heart rate and to control heart failure.

Heart failure should be controlled as much as possible by salt restriction, diuretics, rest, digoxin, and if necessary, other measures. Patients in heart failure may develop hypokalemia and/or a metabolic alkalosis from diuretics; therefore, daily weights and measurement of serum electrolytes are required while the patient in chronic heart failure is prepared for operation.

LUNGS

Pulmonary function tests to assess lung volumes and respiratory mechanics should be performed in all patients over 40 years and in younger patients with historical, roentgenographic, or clinical evidence of lung disease. If lung disease is present, additional studies, including measurement of arterial blood gases, ventilation-perfusion ratios, diffusing capacity, and nitrogen washout, may be indicated. Cardiac function may affect pulmonary function; therefore, it is important preoperatively to improve lung function maximally and to determine the functional severity of any associated chronic lung disease.

Before elective cardiac surgery, atelectatic areas and pulmonary infiltrates visible on chest roentgenograms should be cleared. Large pleural effusions should be tapped to permit full expansion of the lungs. Smokers should abstain from smoking for one to two weeks if possible or drastically reduce their smoking if total abstinence is not possible. Sputum for culture and antibiotic sensitivity should be obtained in patients with chronic bronchitis. Patients with chronic bronchitis and those with moderately severe obstructive airway disease may benefit from daily chest physiotherapy, breathing exercises, antibiotics, bronchodilators, and abstinence from smoking for one to two weeks before operation. All patients should have preoperative instruction in breathing exercises, chest physiotherapy, and coughing.

BLOOD

Cardiopulmonary bypass reduces the platelet count and impairs platelet function so that bleeding times are usually prolonged postoperatively. Patients should avoid platelet inhibiting drugs such as aspirin, aspirin-containing compounds, other nonsteroidal anti-inflammatory compounds, and thiazides for at least 10 days prior to operation. A history of easy bruising or bleeding indicates the need for a full hematologic work-up. Abnormal measurement of four coagulation factors — prothrombin time, partial thromboplastin time, fibrinogen, and platelet count — indicates abnormalities of the intrinsic, extrinsic, and common coagulation pathways. Unexplained abnormalities of any of these screening tests indicate a need for hematologic investigation. Under special circumstances open heart operations can be performed in individuals who are deficient in one or more coagulation factors if platelet concentrates, fresh frozen plasma, and other specific coagulation factors are available for infusion.

During cardiopulmonary bypass, hematocrit is usually reduced to 20 to 30 per cent (depending upon the size and weight of the patient and to a lesser extent on the magnitude of the procedure) in an effort to reduce the need for transfused blood. Blood sequestered in the extracorporeal circuit after bypass stops is returned to the patient during the remainder of the operation or in the early postoperative period. Many patients do not require blood transfusions; however, for all patients some blood must be crossmatched in order to have a supply available for transfusion. The amount varies with the size of the patient and the procedure and ranges from 2 to 10 units.

Plasma coagulation proteins may be deficient owing to the small plasma volume in severely polycythemic patients. Preoperative bleeding is no longer necessary in these patients, as the hematocrit can be more easily reduced by dilution of the patient's blood with the priming fluid within the heart-lung machine. Administration of fresh frozen plasma after bypass stops will restore necessary coagulation factors.

KIDNEY

Compromised renal function does not preclude successful open heart surgery, even in anephric patients. The degree of impairment of renal function should be carefully determined preoperatively in patients with moderate or severe renal disease. A full renal work-up with clearance studies, measurements of renal blood flow, and measurements of urine and serum electrolytes and solutes may be necessary. Hemodialysis, if cardiac output is adequate, or peritoneal dialysis, if cardiac output is low, may be needed occasionally to supplement impaired renal function preoperatively. Patients with normal BUN, sodium creatinine, and urinalysis values do not need additional renal studies preoperatively.

The combination of low cardiac output, fluid restriction, and powerful diuretics may elevate the BUN without causing an increase in serum creatinine. Chronic furosemide diuretic therapy can cause an associated hypokalemic metabolic alkalosis. Usually this prerenal azotemia can be alleviated preoperatively by maintaining optimal cardiac output, adjusting fluid intake, reducing diuretics, and adjusting electrolyte replacement in the hospital. Improved cardiac output and renal blood flow postoperatively will allow healthy kidneys to correct the azotemia.

Patients with chronic urinary infections should have current cultures and sensitivity studies and should receive appropriate antibiotics just before, during, and after operation.

INFECTION

Ideally, patients should be free of infection before cardiac surgery. Occasionally patients with active endocarditis require operation before the bloodstream can be sterilized. Multiple blood cultures should be obtained before antibiotics are started. The choice of antibiotics is dictated by knowledge of the infecting organism, clinical and historical information, and the urgency of the operation. If the organism is unknown, blood cultures taken before broad-spectrum antibiotics are started may be important in controlling septicemia or recurrent endocarditis postoperatively.

In patients with active endocarditis, operation is preferably delayed until the bloodstream is sterilized by antibiotics effective against the cultured organism. When this is achieved, operation becomes feasible any time afterward, depending upon hemodynamic or clinical (e.g., emboli) considerations. A six-week waiting period before operation is not mandatory; however, effective antibiotics must be used before, during, and for two to six weeks after operation.

Prophylaxis is the best means of preventing infection in patients who have elective cardiac surgery. Potential sources of infection such as carious teeth, infected urine, severe acne, boils, or contaminated wounds are best eradicated before open heart surgery. This may require postponement of operation in order to remove infected teeth or clear infected urine. Patients with productive coughs or chronic bronchitis should have sputum cultures preoperatively.

Patients who have open heart surgery should receive broad-spectrum antibiotics effective against gram-positive and gram-negative organisms preoperatively. Before, during, and after open heart surgery, the exposure of the bloodstream to direct contamination via the heart-lung machine and vascular catheters is enormous. Prophylactic antibiotics reduce the risk that bloodstream contamination will result in bloodstream infection. Unfortunately, if infection occurs, the causative organism is likely to be resistant to the antibiotics used; however, other effective antibiotics are usually available if the infection is detected early by daily blood cultures as long as central venous and arterial catheters remain in place. Prophylactic antibiotics should be started 4 to 12 hours before operation in order to have an effective blood level during operation without causing a change in the patient's normal flora and subsequent selective growth of resistant organisms.

LIVER

Some patients with chronic right heart failure due to long-standing mitral and tricuspid valvular disease may develop hepatosplenomegaly and cardiac cirrhosis of the liver. Ultimately, portal hypertension with ascites, pleural effusions, hypoproteinemia, deficiency of coagulation proteins, and secondary thrombocytopenia may develop. Preoperatively, these patients should be closely managed to reduce the degree of heart failure and produce an effective diuresis. An attempt should be made to improve the patient's nutritional status; however, this is often difficult when fluids must be severely restricted. Although the cardiac operation may dramatically reduce central venous pressure postoperatively, liver function does not improve as fast. Poor clotting and fluid retention are common postoperative problems in these patients.

CENTRAL NERVOUS SYSTEM

Most patients are appropriately anxious before open cardiac surgery, and their anxiety is often intensified by the informed consent procedure. Basically, the relationship between the patient and surgeon should be one of mutual respect and trust. The operating surgeon who is responsible to the patient should discuss the operation with the patient, pointing out the indications, proposed plans, and benefits to be expected. Benefits should not be assured or exaggerated. In a general way, risks of complications and mortality should be covered, but unless specifically requested, a detailed list of potential complications and numerical risks of mortality are contraindicated in the patient's best interests. The surgeon's manner is extremely important, and answers to questions should be specific and truthful. Any questions the patient raises about the operative permit should be answered. Much of the patient's anxiety can be alleviated by the calm optimism and specific, truthful answers of the operating surgeon.

The patient's knowledge and attitude toward the operation can be favorably enhanced by a preoperative educational booklet or slide presentation. The booklet or presentation describes cardiac catheterization, the heart-lung machine, various common operations, the intensive care unit, convalescence, and rehabilitation. Illustrations should be cheerful and clear; the text must be understood by lay people and provide information they seek. The knowledge gained helps to alleviate anxiety.

The anesthesiologist should visit the patient preoperatively to explain the proposed anesthetic procedures and what the patient will experience before induction. Nurses can relieve anxiety by explaining procedures, answering questions, listening to the patient's fears and concerns, and offering reassurance and encouragement. Family members also can be very supportive. It is rarely necessary to consult a psychiatrist to help control a patient's emotions before heart surgery.

EMERGENCIES

During emergencies, diagnosis and treatment must proceed simultaneously, and the thoroughness of preoperative care is dictated by the urgency of the patient's condition. As a first priority, ventilation and circulation must be restored and maintained by whatever means available. If open cardiac surgery is necessary, the operating room staff and anesthesia and pump team must be called immediately to make preparations for operation. The diagnosis and anatomic location of the lesion or lesions must be known. In all except the most precipitous and desperate emergencies, results of history and physical examination are correlated with the electrocardiogram, chest roentgenogram, and other bedside diagnostic tests such as echocardiography and Swan-Ganz catheter measurements to determine the circulatory pathology. Often cardiac catheterization and angiography are necessary to localize lesions, particularly obstructive lesions of the coronary arteries. Blood should be sent for hemoglobin, electrolytes, BUN, creatinine, sugar, coagulation studies, and crossmatching; however, often the results are not available until during or after operation. The delayed results are still valuable for intraoperative and postoperative management. Preoperative preparation includes insertion of central venous, arterial, and bladder catheters, shaving proposed operative sites, crossmatching blood, and administration of antibiotics. A nasogastric tube may be needed to empty the stomach. Occasionally, patients must be intubated and ventilated prior to induction of anesthesia.

PREOPERATIVE ORDERS

The patient should have nothing by mouth six to eight hours before operation. All potential operative sites should be shaved widely. This often requires shaving from chin to toes circumferentially. The groin and axillae should be shaved for all cardiac operations.

The anesthesiologist will generally prescribe "on-call" sedatives and anticholinergic drugs for administration about one hour preoperatively. Prophylactic antibiotics should be given with the "on-call" medication. An operative permit should be signed before the patient receives preoperative medication.

Digoxin is usually stopped 36 hours before operation, and other drugs are tapered or stopped the evening before surgery. Orders for essential drugs (for example, antiarrhythmic agents such as propranolol) or replacement hormones (such as insulin and steroids) should be specified in the preoperative orders. If needed just before operation, these drugs should be administered parenterally at adjusted dosages rather than orally.

OPERATIVE CARE

After the patient reaches the operating table, electrocardiographic limb leads are connected and the electrocardiogram is continuously displayed on an oscilloscope. A monitoring stethoscope is placed over the patient's heart. A peripheral intravenous line is started. Depending upon the patient's condition and anxiety, arterial and central venous monitoring catheters are inserted before or after induction of anesthesia. The radial artery is usually cannulated percutaneously or via a cutdown. Alternatively the brachial, femoral, axillary, temporal, and umbilical (newborn infants only) arteries can be used for arterial cannulation. Arterial pressure is monitored continuously; arterial Po_2, Pco_2, and pH are measured intermittently. A standard blood pressure cuff with a Doppler probe over the brachial artery is used as an auxiliary to the intra-arterial pressure catheter. Occasionally peak systolic pressure in the radial artery is 10 to 20 mm Hg higher than aortic or cuff pressures (systolic wave overshoot); more often the catheter pressure tracing becomes dampened so that falsely low systolic blood pressures are recorded.

Frequently a Swan-Ganz thermistor quadruple lumen catheter can be introduced percutaneously over a wire into the right internal jugular vein (alternatively, either subclavian vein). When so introduced, a Swan-Ganz catheter is threaded relatively easily into the main pulmonary artery without the aid of fluoroscopy. When properly positioned, the Swan-Ganz catheter permits measurement of pulmonary arterial systolic, diastolic, and mean wedge pressure (distal port) and central venous pressure (proximal port). Thermodilution cardiac output measurements can be made by injecting cold or room temperature saline through the proximal port and recording the resulting temperature dilution curve from the catheter tip thermistor. Introduction of a Swan-Ganz catheter from the femoral vein is more difficult, and often the catheter must be placed directly into the pulmonary artery during cardiopulmonary bypass; otherwise, fluoroscopy must be utilized. Central venous pressure and/or pulmonary diastolic pressure are usually continuously displayed.

A Foley catheter is introduced into the bladder for intermittent measurements of urine volume. After intubation, an esophageal stethoscope is inserted to monitor heart rate and rhythm. Temperature is measured by a nasopharyngeal thermistor. This temperature most closely approximates the temperature of the brain and is preferable to an esophageal temperature probe, which is influenced by the blood temperature of the adjacent aorta and heart. When moderate or deep hypothermia is used, a rectal temperature probe is helpful and generally reflects the temperature of organs with small blood flow:mass ratios. During the operation, arterial blood gases, hematocrit, and serum potassium and ionized calcium levels are measured intermittently.

A variety of agents are used to anesthetize cardiac patients. Nitrous oxide, halothane, fentanyl, and morphine with pancuronium bromide (Pavulon) are commonly employed, but other agents that do not severely depress myocardial function can be used. All anesthetic agents depress myocardial function to some degree, but the depression can be minimized by skillful selection and administration of the various agents and relaxants available.

Before the aorta or femoral artery is cannulated, heparin (approximately 3 mgm per kg or enough to increase the activated coagulation time to 350 to 400 seconds) is given. One or two venous cannulae are used to cannulate the great veins through the right atrium. During cardiopulmonary bypass, flow rate is monitored by an electromagnetic flow probe, which is checked for accuracy by noting the pump revolutions per minute (a calibration chart correlates rpms and blood flow rate). Pump flow is maintained at 2.4 l/m² body surface area per minute. Blood pressure in the arterial perfusion line is monitored to detect kinking of the line or obstruction of the arterial catheter. Central venous pressure is also monitored to detect obstruction of venous cannulae. Body temperature is usually decreased during all except very brief periods of bypass to decrease body metabolism and to provide longer, safe periods of ischemia should problems of perfusion occur.

The cardiopulmonary bypass system requires a venous reservoir, heat exchanger, and membrane or bubble oxygenator. An arterial line filter is recommended. The cardiotomy sucker system is used to retrieve shed blood and must include a blood filter. The system is primed with blood, albumin, and/or electrolyte solutions in order that the hematocrit when mixed with the patient's blood will be between 22 and 30, depending upon the size of the patient and other factors. Mannitol can be added to the pump prime to increase urine output during bypass. Often furosemide is also given. Body (nasopharyngeal) temperature ranges between 18 and 38°C; however, blood is never warmed above 43°C. Flow rates may be reduced at lower body temperatures for varying periods of time to facilitate the operation.

Many operations require interruption of coronary blood flow and thus render the heart ischemic. Although exposed coronary ostia may be perfused through special cannulae, the use of cold cardioplegia has gained favor in recent years. The cardioplegic solution is chilled to 4 to 10°C and contains 25 to 30 mEq of potassium chloride per liter. A variety of other additives, including blood, bicarbonate, steroids, dextrose, insulin, and procaine amide, are sometimes included. The potassium arrests the heart in diastole, and the cold reduces cardiac temperature and the metabolic rate of cardiac muscle. The cold, arrested heart shows no electrical activity. During cold cardioplegia, it is helpful to monitor myocardial temperature (via a left ventricular thermistor) and the cardiogram and to reperfuse the coronary arteries with cardioplegic solution if electrical activity returns or if myocardial temperature increases above 22 to 24°C. Prolonged periods of ventricular fibrillation, even if the heart is not ischemic, are detrimental to subsequent cardiac performance.

The performance of the heart must be carefully monitored as bypass is discontinued. Distention should be assiduously avoided. Partial bypass, atrial or ventricular pacing, or the use of calcium, lidocaine, catecholamines, and/or vasodilators may be necessary to reestablish an adequate cardiac output and satisfactory cardiac rhythm. During this critical period, all of the hemodynamic pressure monitors must be operational, and blood samples must be frequently analyzed for arterial blood gases, pH, and calcium.

Occasionally the intra-aortic balloon is necessary intraoperatively to provide additional cardiac support. A 20 to 60 mm balloon can be inserted through a 10 mm woven dacron graft and sutured end-to-side to a patent femoral artery or to the ascending aorta. When properly timed with an electrocardiogram, the intra-aortic balloon reduces myocardial afterload and augments central aortic disastolic pressure and coronary blood flow.

Before closing the chest, the surgeon inserts two temporary atrial pacing wires and one or two temporary ventricular pacing wires. The pericardium may or may not be closed; if closed, a large-bore chest tube is left within the pericardium to prevent cardiac tamponade. Generally a second large-bore tube is left to drain the mediastinum. These tubes are connected to water seal drainage at 10 to 20 cm H_2O negative pressure.

The patient is transported to the intensive care unit using a battery-operated monitor to display the electrocardiogram and arterial pressure. All vascular catheters are left in place for use during the early postoperative period. Additionally a small polyethylene or Teflon catheter may be inserted directly into the left atrium or pulmonary artery (via the right ventricle) at operation if direct measurement and sampling of these chambers are desired. In infants who are too small for a Swan-Ganz catheter, a No. 2 French thermistor catheter inserted directly into the pulmonary artery via the right ventricle permits measurement of cardiac output by thermodilution.

POSTOPERATIVE CARE

Postoperative care of patients after cardiac surgery is most easily and safely delivered by a "systems" approach wherein the function of each major organ system is regularly assessed separately. Using available quantitative measurements, safe ranges of each measured index can be defined. Attention is thereby focused on deviations from the safe ranges or "limits." Therapeutic interventions can be made before serious problems or crises occur. The "systems" approach determines the functional adequacy of each organ system and correlates this information with the needs of the entire patient.

Immediate care of postoperative cardiac patients, who have potentially unstable circulatory and respiratory systems, takes place in an intensive care unit. Nurses and doctors are specially trained to make the required measurements and to deliver concentrated care. Ideally one nurse should care for only one to two patients simultaneously. Facilities for continuous electronic monitoring of important physiologic measurements, respiratory support, pharmacologic support of the circulation, and resuscitation must be available within the unit.

Some centers have also found computer-aided monitoring systems helpful in the care of postoperative cardiac patients. These systems record, display, store, calculate, and recall certain important physiologic measurements, automatically make some measurements such as urine output and chest drainage, and sound alarms when measurements deviate from "safe ranges." Newer systems are programmed to automatically infuse fluids, colloids, and even drugs under certain circumstances and can analyze cardiac arrhythmias.

MONITORED MEASUREMENTS

The electrocardiogram, arterial blood pressure, central venous pressure, pulmonary arterial pressure, and/or left atrial pressure are continuously measured and displayed in digital and analog forms on a bedside oscilloscope. In addition, temperature, urine volume, and the volume of chest drainage is measured at least every hour. Intermittently, arterial blood is analyzed for PO_2, PCO_2, and pH. Blood is also monitored for serum electrolytes, particularly potassium and ionized calcium concentrations, sugar, total protein, BUN, creatinine, osmolarity, hemoglobin concentration and platelet count, prothrombin time, and partial thromboplastin time. In some patients, myocardial enzymes, CPK-MB, HBD, CPK, LDH, and SGOT or measurements of liver function are also made.

Urine is intermittently analyzed (for specific gravity, protein, sugar, and cells), and occasionally urine electrolytes and osmolarity are measured. A 12-lead electrocardiogram and portable anteroposterior chest roentgenogram are obtained shortly after the patient arrives in the intensive care unit. Fluid balance is carefully measured and recorded. Cardiac output via dye or thermal dilution is measured periodically at the bedside. The frequency of each intermittent laboratory measurement depends upon the performance of individual organ systems and the patient's overall clinical condition.

ROUTINE POSTOPERATIVE CARE

Immediately after arriving in the intensive care unit, the patient is connected to the bedside monitor of the electrocardiogram and various vascular pressure. Heart rate, respiratory rate, and systemic arterial, central venous, and left atrial pressures are recorded on the bedside record every 15 minutes. Safe ranges or "limits" for these measurements and temperature, hourly urine volume, and hourly chest drainage are designated. Fluid intake and output are recorded hourly. The patient is nursed supine or, if reasonably alert and extubated, in the semi-Fowler position. A 12-lead electrocardiogram and an anteroposterior chest roentgenogram are obtained. Chest tubes are attached to water seal suction and are frequently stripped to prevent obstruction by clotted blood. Blood is sent for measurement of arterial gases and pH, hemoglobin, electrolytes, sugar, total protein, and screening coagulation tests.

Crystalloid fluids are usually limited to 500 ml per m² body surface area daily and given as dextrose and water. Potassium chloride and calcium chloride or gluconate are added to the crystalloid infusion (via a catheter in a central vein, since infusion of calcium in a peripheral vein may cause skin necrosis) as dictated by serum electrolyte measurements. Potassium is frequently required, sometimes in large amounts during the first 12 to 18 hours after open heart surgery. Colloids are infused as determined by drainage in the chest tubes and left-sided cardiac filling pressures (left atrial, pulmonary wedge, or pulmonary arterial diastolic pressure). The amount of infused colloids should be correlated with cardiac performance (see below). The type of colloid (whole blood, packed erythrocytes, 5 or 25 per cent albumin, plasma, and plasma derivatives) is determined by the hemoglobin and total protein concentrations.

Pulmonary care is designed to support respiratory function and to prevent pulmonary complications. Patients usually arrive in the intensive care unit with the endotracheal tube in place. Mechanical ventilation is required until the effects of anesthetic agents and relaxants disappear or are reversed. Intubated patients require careful regulation of the oxygen concentration, temperature, and humidification of inspired gases, tidal volume, respiratory rate, and peak inspiratory and end-expiratory pressures. The cuffed endotracheal tube should be securely fixed in place with the tip above the tracheal carina (position should be checked on the chest roentgenogram). Fixation of the nasoendotracheal tube is more easily secured than all other tracheal tubes. The cuff should be of safe design and inflated only enough just to occlude the airway during inspiration. Connections to the ventilator should be secure. If the stomach is distended, a nasogastric tube should be inserted to aspirate all air and fluid.

The adequacy of ventilation should be checked 10 to 15 minutes after each change in ventilatory control settings by measurement of arterial blood gases. Arterial P_{CO_2} between 30 and 42 torr ensures adequate alveolar ventilation; an arterial P_{O_2} between 80 and 120 torr is desirable. Postoperatively, arterial oxygen tension usually varies with changes in inspired oxygen tension (below 50 per cent prevents oxygen toxicity); positive end-expiratory airway pressure; extravascular lung water, which in turn is affected by left atrial pressure, plasma colloid osmotic pressure, and diuretics; compression of the lung by air or fluid; and the presence of atelectasis or pneumonia.

Intubated and recently extubated patients require vigorous measures to prevent atelectasis and pneumonia. The endotracheal tube should be aspirated at least hourly to remove secretions. Often 1 to 5 ml of saline or dilute sodium bicarbonate is instilled into the endotracheal tube to loosen secretions. The patient should be turned side to side every two hours. The lungs should be hyperinflated manually after aspiration with or without saline instillation. Chest physiotherapy should be administered frequently (as often as hourly) to loosen secretions and expand alveoli. Thick, purulent sputum should be gram stained and cultured.

The airway is extubated after the patient awakens from anesthesia and the effects of all relaxants have been reversed. The patient must have a stable and adequate circulation, must be free of serious arrhythmias and not likely to require reoperation for bleeding, and must demonstrate adequate alveolar ventilation. Usually the patient's endotracheal tube is connected to a T-piece, which provides oxygen-enriched, humidified air at no end-expiratory airway pressure while the patient breathes spontaneously. If arterial blood gases remain within the normal range, the patient is extubated and fitted with a face mask. The extubated patient should breathe high humidity gases and be encouraged to hyperventilate and cough deeply every hour. Changes in position and chest physiotherapy are continued. Most patients are extubated the afternoon or evening of operation.

Antibiotics are given parenterally (usually IV) for three to five days. Pain is alleviated by intravenous injections of 0.1 to 0.2 mg per kg (up to 20 kg) to 4 mg of morphine every two to four hours. Occasionally diazepam (Valium) or haloperidol (Haldol) are necessary for satisfactory sedation. Diabetics receive intravenous regular insulin in response to blood and urine sugar measurements. Other drugs that replace essential body chemicals are also prescribed as dictated by the patient's requirements. Chest tubes are removed when the drainage becomes mostly serous and less than 20 ml per hour is produced. Removal usually occurs the first postoperative morning.

A patient can be considered ready for discharge from the intensive care unit if all vital organ systems are performing well and have some margin of functional reserve. The patient should be alert, oriented, and relatively comfortable. Heart rate and rhythm must be stable; cardiac output must be adequate and stable and must not require continuous pharmacologic support. Measured values of cardiac output should be at least 2.4 l per m² per min, and the patient's peripheral pulses should be present. The extubated patient should have adequate respiratory function as evidenced by arterial blood gases, measurement of tidal volume, the chest roentgenogram, and the ability to cough and clear secretions. Preferably, chest tubes and the Foley catheter are removed. Urine volume should be adequate (0.5 ml to 1.0 ml per kg per hour). The fluid balance sheet should not indicate any major dislocations of crystalloids or colloids. Metabolic acidosis or significant electrolyte abnormalities should not be present. Doubtful or borderline patients should remain in the intensive care unit, but others may have systemic arterial and Swan-Ganz catheters removed and may be transferred to an intermediate facility or the equivalent. Usually one central venous catheter remains in place to facilitate administration of antibiotics, drugs, packed red blood cells, and other colloids and intravenous crystalloids.

Oral medications are usually resumed the day after operation. Pain often is controlled with acetaminophen (Tylenol) or codeine. Some or all of the patient's preoperative noncardiac medications are resumed. Many patients are restarted on digoxin and/or furosemide, depending upon their clinical conditions. Supplemental iron is given with or without a stool softener. The patient is encouraged to get out of bed briefly if able. Supplemental humidified oxygen delivered by nasal prongs or mask is helpful for some patients. All require continued breathing exercises, chest physiotherapy, and coughing. Some patients may require a medication for sleep. Routinely, total crystalloid fluids are restricted to 750 ml per m² per day, and the patient is carefully weighed daily. Heart rate, blood pressure, respiratory rate, and temperature are measured and recorded every four hours. Appetite usually does not return until the second to fourth postoperative day; however, some food is offered at each mealtime beginning the day after operation. Each day the patient is encouraged to increase his or her physical activity by walking or sitting out of bed. Elastic stockings are helpful in reducing leg edema.

For inpatients who require coumadin anticoagulation, the drug is started the evening that the chest tubes are removed. Daily prothrombin times are obtained until the coumadin dosage required to keep the prothrombin time in the therapeutic range (1.5 to 2 times control) is found. Many surgeons routinely prescribe subcutaneous heparin (1500 to 2500 units every six hours) to decrease the incidence of pulmonary embolism. Additionally, some surgeons prescribe platelet inhibitory drugs, aspirin, dipyridamole (Persantine), or sulfinpyrazone to reduce further the likelihood of early closure of aortocoronary grafts or of thrombus formation within the heart.

An electrocardiogram is obtained daily or every two days to monitor cardiac rhythm and to detect myocardial ischemic changes. A chest roentgenogram is also obtained every few days to monitor heart size, atelectasis, and pleural fluid accumulation. Hemoglobin, white blood cell count, urinalysis, serum electrolytes, and BUN measurements are obtained every two days, and abnormalities are corrected by administering appropriate therapy.

The patient is usually discharged 7 to 10 days after operation. It is important that each patient know and understand each oral medication that has been prescribed. It is helpful to prepare a card with each different pill or capsule taped to the card next to the name of the drug. The card should include instructions for taking the medication and a simple explanation of the medical reason. Additionally, the patient should receive explicit instructions regarding activities, diet, and any symptoms or signs that should be reported to the doctor. Preferably these instructions should be given in both verbal and written form. Finally, appointments should be made for the patient to return to the physician who will follow his or her out-of-hospital course.

MANAGEMENT OF COMMON PROBLEMS

Low Cardiac Output

Cardiac output is inadequate when the circulation cannot supply all body tissues with sufficient oxygen to maintain aerobic metabolism. Normally, oxygen consumption is approximately 155 ml per m^2 per min (newborn and other infants have higher oxygen consumption), and the normal arterial-venous oxygen difference is five volumes per cent. When hemoglobin and arterial oxygen saturation are constant, the requirement for cardiac output is directly proportional to oxygen consumption. Fever, muscular activity (such as shivering or labored breathing), and anxiety increase oxygen consumption and hence demand increased cardiac output.

Cardiac output may be low in the absence of suggestive clinical signs. Clinical signs of low cardiac output include pale, anxious, dry appearance, absent or weak peripheral pulses, tachycardia > 120 per min, systemic arterial hypotension (mean < 60 mm Hg), urine output < 0.5 ml per kg per hr, metabolic acidosis, and pulmonary arterial oxygen tension < 30 torr. The most reliable means to diagnose low cardiac output is to measure it in duplicate by dye or thermal dilution. The normal resting cardiac output is 3.5 l per m^2 per min; a cardiac output of

2.0 l per m² per min is barely adequate to meet postoperative metabolic needs, and an output < 1.8 l per m² per min requires urgent treatment.

Cardiac output is a product of heart rate and stroke volume. Preload, afterload, and myocardial contractility are the determinants of stroke volume. Preload is the term used to indicate ventricular end diastolic volume, which is directly proportional to resting myocardial sarcomere length. The Frank-Starling relationship describes the interaction between resting sarcomere length and ventricular stroke work (grammeters per min). Ventricular stroke work equals force times velocity per unit time. For cardiac and all muscle, velocity of shortening is inversely proportional to the load resisting shortening (force). Thus, force times velocity is a measure of myocardial contractility. The Frank-Starling property of cardiac muscle states that within limits an increase in ventricular end diastolic volume (resting sarcomere length) results in an increase in myocardial contractility, primarily as an increase in the force of contraction rather than velocity.

Afterload is defined as ventricular wall tension and is proportional to ventricular systolic pressure times the radius of the ventricular cavity (LaPlace's law). An increase in ventricular pressure or ventricular volume increases afterload. Stroke work is the sum of stroke volume (the amount of blood ejected with each beat) plus afterload (ventricular wall tension). Thus, for a given stroke work (myocardial contractility per unit time), an increase in afterload decreases stroke volume.

Proper management of low cardiac output requires optimizing cardiac rate, preload, myocardial contractility, and afterload. Sinus rhythm at 90 to 110 beats per minute is usually optimal for most postoperative adult cardiac patients. Optimal preload is more difficult to determine, and, of course, an increase in preload also increases afterload. To determine optimal preload, a measure of end diastolic volume of the weakest ventricle, usually the left in adults, must be obtained. Since ventricular compliance is generally linear, ventricular end diastolic *pressure* can be used as an index of end diastolic *volume*. In the absence of mitral valvular disease, mean left atrial pressure approximates left ventricular end diastolic pressure, and pulmonary wedge pressure, when properly measured, equals mean left atrial pressure. In a pinch, pulmonary arterial diastolic pressure can also be assumed to approximate left atrial pressure. Pulmonary wedge and diastolic pressures can be measured via a Swan-Ganz catheter inserted either at operation or afterward. Thus, changes in left ventricular preload are reflected as changes in left atrial or pulmonary wedge pressures.

Postoperatively, optimal preload depends in part on the left ventricular end diastolic pressure preoperatively. In patients with long-standing left ventricular dysfunction, left ventricular pressure is chronically elevated and left atrial pressures between 14 and 22 mm Hg may be necessary to obtain the maximal myocardial contractility available through the Frank-Starling relationship. In patients with normal left ventricular end diastolic pressures preoperatively, such elevated pressures may produce acute pulmonary edema; lower pressures, between 6 and 14 mm Hg, will generally load the left ventricle optimally. Additionally, ventricular function is improved when the atrial contraction precedes ventricular systole, as occurs in sinus rhythm or during atrial or atrioventricular sequential pacing. The improvement in cardiac output from properly timed atrial contractions may be as much as 25 per cent.

Many factors affect myocardial contractility. Digitalis preparations, catecholamines, and ionized calcium all increase both the force and velocity of sarcomere shortening. Hypoxia, acidosis, hypercapnea, elevated serum potassium (> 6.5 mg), barbiturates, anesthetic agents, propranolol, procaine amide, quinidine, lidocaine, and certain other drugs reduce myocardial contractility. In addition, a ventriculotomy, ventricular distention, a period of ventricular fibrillation during cardiopulmonary bypass, and insufficient coronary blood flow also reduce myocardial contractility. Obviously, drugs or conditions that reduce myocardial contractility in patients with low cardiac output should be avoided; however, antiarrhythmic drugs may be required because the myocardial depressant effect on contractility is less serious than the effect of the arrhythmia.

Coronary blood flow largely occurs during diastole. The most vulnerable area to ischemia is the subendocardium of the left ventricle. Subendocardial ischemia adversely affects myocardial contractility. Several factors that may be present in postoperative patients with low cardiac output may affect subendocardial blood flow. Subendocardial blood flow is reduced if diastole is shortened, if diastolic ventricular pressure (i.e., left atrial pressure) increases, or if aortic diastolic pressure decreases. Furthermore, when regional or total myocardial flow is marginal, factors such as temperature and catecholamines increase myocardial oxygen consumption and may produce myocardial ischemia if coronary blood flow cannot increase to meet the increased demand for metabolic substrates.

Afterload of the left ventricle is increased by an increase in systemic vascular resistance (vasoconstriction), aortic stenosis, increased systemic blood pressure, and increased ventricular volume (preload).

Management of low cardiac output after open heart surgery is based upon intelligent manipulation of the multiple factors that affect oxygen consumption and the determinants of cardiac output. Hematocrit above 30 aids oxygen transport, and oxygen consumption can be reduced by controlling fever, preventing shivering, sedation, and mechanical ventilation with or without pharmacologic skeletal muscle paralysis. Removal of the work of breathing may reduce oxygen consumption as much as 15 to 25 per cent.

Cardiac rate is preferably sinus at 90 to 110 beats per minute. Ventricular loading by properly timed atrial contractions (sinus rhythm, atrial pacing, or atrioventricular sequential pacing) is preferable to junctional rhythm and ventricular pacing (see Arrhythmias).

Optimal preload for the weakest ventricle (usually the left) is determined by trial and error. Serial measurements of cardiac output are very helpful. Left ventricular preload is manipulated by increasing or decreasing blood volume using left atrial, pulmonary wedge, or, less satisfactorily, pulmonary diastolic pressures as a guide. Blood volume is increased by colloid infusions or vasoconstrictor drugs; blood volume is decreased by diuresis, vasodilatation, or phlebotomy.

Conditions that decrease myocardial contractility should be corrected. Hypoxia and hypercapnia require manipulation of ventilatory support systems; acidosis should be corrected by $NaHCO_3$. Deficiencies in measured ionized calcium and hyperkalemia are corrected (see Renal Problems). Unnecessary myocardial depressant drugs are stopped. Within the confines of the clinical situation, measures to increase aortic diastolic pressure, reduce aortic systolic pressure, reduce heart rate (duration of diastole increases more than systole), and reduce left atrial pressure will increase subendocardial blood flow. Digoxin is given, and one or more catecholamines are infused continuously via a mechanical infusion pump to increase myocardial contractility.

The choice of catecholamine is determined by the properties of each drug and by the patient's clinical condition. All five drugs (Table 20–1) have a beta-adrenergic effect and result in increased myocardial contractility, an increase in heart rate, and mild dilatation of the systemic arterial vasculature. Norepinephrine, epinephrine, and dopamine also have alpha-adrenergic effects that cause systemic vasoconstriction. These drugs must be given through central venous catheters to avoid skin necrosis.

Norepinephrine is used sparingly because of its strong vasoconstrictor effect. Dobutamine is a new drug similar to isoproterenol but with less tendency to cause tachycardia. Isoproterenol, like dobutamine, is a pure beta-adrenergic agent that increases cardiac contractility. High doses of the drug increase cardiac rate and irritability and also increase

Table 20–1. CLINICAL DOSE RANGES FOR INTRAVENOUS CATECHOLAMINES

	STARTING DOSE	"USUAL" DOSE ±	"HIGH USUAL" DOSE ±	HIGH DOSE
		($\mu g/kg/min$)		
Isoproterenol	0.01	.025	.05	.2
Epinephrine	0.05	.1	.2	.4
Norepinephrine	0.05	.1	.2	.4
Dopamine	2–4	6–10	15	25
Dobutamine	2–4	6–10	15	25

myocardial oxygen consumption more than cardiac contractility. This may cause myocardial ischemia if coronary blood flow is limited.

Dopamine and epinephrine are used most often to increase myocardial contractility. Epinephrine is less likely to cause tachycardia than dopamine and causes more systemic vasoconstriction; dopamine, however, increases renal blood flow and urine output in therapeutic doses. Both drugs can be used in combination with vasodilators. Dose ranges for each catecholamine are given in Table 20–1.

Afterload can be reduced by infusion of vasodilators or insertion of the intra-aortic balloon. Nitroprusside (0.05 to 0.2 μg per kg per min) and trimethaphan (2 to 20 μg per kg per min) are most commonly used. Tachyphylaxis may occur with trimethaphan in 18 to 24 hours and occurs with nitroprusside in three to five days. Either drug is infused at a rate sufficient to reduce mean systemic arterial pressure to 65 to 75 mm Hg. Nitroglycerin (1.0 to 5.0 μg per kg per min) is a potent coronary and systemic arterial dilator and is used particularly in patients with electrocardiographic evidence of coronary ischemia. Serial measurements of systemic vascular resistance, calculated in dynes-sec-cm^{-5} from the difference between mean arterial pressure and pulmonary wedge pressure (mm Hg) divided by the cardiac output (L/min) and multiplied by 80 are helpful in administering vasodilator drugs.

Postoperatively, the intra-aortic balloon is inserted through a prosthetic graft and anastomosed end-to-side to the common femoral artery. The balloon (20 to 60 ml capacity) is positioned in the thoracic aorta with the balloon tip just distal to the left subclavian artery. When properly timed, the balloon reduces peripheral vascular resistance during ventricular systole and increases central aortic diastolic pressure. The effect of the balloon is to reduce left ventricular afterload, end diastolic volume, and left atrial pressure and to increase coronary blood flow, particularly to the subendocardium.

Clinical application of partial cardiopulmonary bypass systems or left ventricular assist devices to supplement inadequate cardiac output is still experimental.

ARRHYTHMIAS

Abnormalities in cardiac rate and rhythm are exceedingly common after open heart surgery. Factors that favor the development of postoperative arrhythmias include electrolyte imbalance (particularly low serum potassium), acidosis, hypoxia, high serum concentration of digoxin, intraoperative cardioplegia, cardiac injury, and preexisting rheumatic or ischemic heart disease. Because arrhythmias are so common, temporary insulated wires should be placed in pairs (1 cm apart) on the right atrium and on a ventricle at operation. These wires can be used for diagnosis or treatment of any postoperative arrhythmia.

Unipolar atrial electrocardiograms are easily recorded by connecting one atrial wire to each arm lead of the electrocardiographic machine. Then either lead 2 or 3 records a unipolar atrial electrocardiogram, which characteristically records a small spike for the atrial contraction and a large QRS complex. When the selector switch is turned to lead I, a bipolar atrial electrocardiogram is recorded. This characteristically shows a large atrial spike and a small QRS complex. For atrial pacing one lead is connected to the negative pole and the other to the positive pole of the external pacemaker. When the positive pole is connected to the ventricular lead, atrial pacing should occur, but in practice ventricular pacing often supervenes. Ventricular pacing is best achieved by connecting the negative pole of the pacemaker to the ventricular pacing wire. Atrioventricular sequential pacing requires two atrial and two ventricular pacing wires.

Recognition of cardiac arrhythmias is usually made by observation of the bedside monitor; however, accurate diagnosis requires a standard 12-lead electrocardiogram. Additionally, unipolar or bipolar atrial electrocardiograms are helpful in differentiating nodal and atrial arrhythmias.

Supraventricular Arrhythmias

Sinus tachycardia is usually associated with fever or is a transient phenomenon. Reduction in temperature reduces cardiac rate approximately 15 beats per minute per degree centrigrade. Excessive sinus tachycardia (> 150 beats per min) may be due to hypovolemia, pericardial tamponade, or hypoxia but also may occur for unexplained reasons. Therapy is directed toward correcting the underlying cause. If the etiology remains unexplained, neostigmine (Prostigmin) (0.5 to 1.0 mg) may slow the sinus node. Digoxin can also be tried, but the drug has relatively little effect on the sinus node. Sinus bradycardia may be treated by intravenous atropine (0.2 to 1.0 mgvIV), isoproterenol, or atrial pacing.

Paroxysmal atrial tachycardia, wherein an ectopic atrial focus originates the heart beat, can be slowed or stopped by increasing vagal tone by carotid massage, Prostigmin, or edrophonium chloride (Tensilon, 10 mg IV). Elevation of systemic arterial pressure by a vasoconstrictor or overdrive atrial pacing (at a rate faster than the tachycardia) may also interrupt the arrhythmia.

Atrial flutter at an atrial rate of 280 to 340 beats per minute may cause rapid ventricular contractions and hypotension if every other beat causes ventricular contraction (2:1 block). Sometimes the block is 4:1, causing a slower than desired ventricular rate. If circulatory hemodynamics are stable and serum potassium is normal, digoxin (0.125 to 0.5 mg IV) can be given to increase the duration of atrioventricular conduction and thus reduce the ventricular rate. Overdrive atrial pacing (at a rate higher than the atrial rate) usually converts the rhythm to atrial fibrillation. Atrial fibrillation is relatively easily controlled by digoxin. Electrical countershock can also be used to stop the arrhythmia. Propranolol (0.1 to 3.0 mg IV) may be needed if digoxin fails to control recurrences of the arrhythmia.

Atrial fibrillation is a common postoperative rhythm. The ventricular rate can generally be held between 80 and 120 beats per minute with increments of intravenous digoxin. If hemodynamics are unstable, electrical countershock may restore sinus rhythm, but generally digoxin, quinidine, or procaine amide are necessary to prevent recurrence of atrial fibrillation. Unfortunately, recurrence is the rule. Atrial pacing is ineffective. Fortunately, atrial fibrillation at controlled rates is well tolerated by most postoperative cardiac patients.

Junctional arrhythmias originate in the atrioventricular node or bundle of His and may be fast or slow. Digoxin and drugs that slow atrioventricular conduction are contraindicated in patients with junctional tachycardia; lidocaine (50 to 250 mg per minute bolus IV or an infusion at 1 to 2 mg per minute) may be helpful. Rapid junctional tachycardias may be extremely difficult to control. Paired ventricular pacing (two ventricular pacing wires are needed) or propranolol occasionally may be effective. Junctional rhythms at 80 to 120 beats per minute are usually well tolerated; if not, overdrive sequential atrioventricular pacing can be tried. Junctional bradycardia is best treated by atrial pacing.

VENTRICULAR ARRHYTHMIAS

Ventricular ectopic beats are not usually treated unless more than six occur each minute or if couplets and triplets develop. Intravenous lidocaine (50 to 250 mg), procaine amide (up to 750 mg over a 15-minute period), or propranolol will usually control frequent ventricular ectopic beats. Electrical countershock is used to stop ventricular tachycardia, which usually results in hypotension and low cardiac output. Lidocaine and/or procaine amide, propranolol, diphenylhydantoin, or bretylium are used to prevent recurrences.

Ventricular fibrillation requires immediate electrical defibrillation (100 to 300 watt-seconds) and external cardiac massage during the interim. If defibrillation is not successful, ventilation with oxygen and external cardiac massage must be continued until adequate cardiac contractions are restored. Resuscitative drugs that may be useful include sodium bicarbonate, lidocaine to suppress ventricular irritability, and calcium or epinephrine to make the fibrillatory pattern more coarse and hence more susceptible to electrical countershock.

Postoperatively, second- and third-degree heart block require ventricular or atrioventricular sequential pacing. If persistent, a permanent pacemaker is required.

PERICARDIAL TAMPONADE

Pericardial tamponade may occur after open heart surgery even if the pericardium is not closed and even if one or more chest tubes are draining satisfactorily. The diagnosis should be considered in every patient with low cardiac output. The diagnosis is suggested by a progressive rise in central venous pressure with steady or falling left atrial (pulmonary wedge) pressure, cessation or abrupt slowing of chest tube drainage, muffled heart sounds, variation of systemic arterial pressure with respiration (paradoxical pulse), a widened mediastinum on chest roentgenography, and a decreasing cardiac output. Chest drainage may actually increase if new bleeding is the cause of the tamponade.

If the patient is not hypotensive and has an adequate cardiac output, obstructed chest tubes may be aseptically irrigated with sterile saline or dilute Betadine solution. If cardiac output is decreased, the patient should be immediately returned to the operating room for exploration of the chest wound, control of bleeding, and evacuation of clot. If the diagnosis is made late and serious systemic hypotension occurs, the chest should be opened in the intensive care unit. Evacuation of clot with replacement of shed blood will usually restore cardiac output to pretamponade levels.

PERIOPERATIVE MYOCARDIAL INFARCTION

Myocardial infarction is reported after operations to bypass obstructed arteries in 5 to 10 per cent of patients but may also occur following other types of cardiac operations. The diagnosis may be difficult to establish and equally difficult to exclude. Serial changes in electrocardiograms showing new Q waves and/or loss of R waves over precordial leads are generally accepted as evidence of new infarctions, particularly if there is an associated increase in myocardial-specific serum enzymes (CPK-MB, HBD, LDH, CPK, SGOT). Higher enzyme rises increase the likelihood that an infection has occurred; however, small transient increases immediately after operation are not indicative of infarction. Similarly, transient S–T segment changes and inverted T waves on the electrocardiogram may not indicate a myocardial infarction. Myocardial imaging techniques using radioisotopes are not now sufficiently sensitive to detect small infarctions.

POSTPERICARDIOTOMY SYNDROME

A syndrome characterized by fever, increased atypical leukocytes, chest pain, and a pericardial friction rub may occur one to four weeks after open cardiac surgery. The etiology of the syndrome is not definitely

ı, but it is probably due to intraoperative infection with common
s and subsequent production of antiheart antibodies. The syndrome is most likely to occur in patients who require the most extensive
trauma to the myocardium. Occasionally patients develop pericardial
effusion that requires paracentesis after confirmation of the diagnosis by
echocardiography. Acetylsalicylic acid (0.3 to 0.6 gm four to six times per
day with food) for four to six weeks usually produces symptomatic relief.
Occasionally patients require a course of steroids.

PULMONARY PROBLEMS

Routine pulmonary care attempts to prevent respiratory complications that are common after open heart surgery. Congested lungs are
more susceptible to atelectasis and infection than normal lungs, and a
variety of serious mishaps can occur to intubated patients who are
receiving mechanical ventilatory support. Continuous vigilance, periodic chest roentgenograms, and measurement of arterial blood gases are
essential to prevent serious postoperative respiratory complications.

Vomitus or slack tongue can obstruct the airway in an extubated,
heavily sedated, or semiconscious patient. Blood or mucus can obstruct
the endotracheal tube of intubated patients. Airways of mechanically
ventilated patients may become disconnected or develop leaks so that
alveolar ventilation is inadequate. The tip of the endotracheal tube may
extend below the tracheal carina so that only one lung is ventilated.

Atelectasis is common after heart surgery, and if atelectasis persists
the airway becomes colonized with bacterial pathogens, and pneumonia
may develop. Atelectasis is usually detected by chest roentgenograms;
pneumonia is diagnosed by chest roentgenograms, positive sputum
cultures, and clinical signs of fever and purulent airway secretions.
Adequate humidification, positive end-expiratory airway pressure, aspiration of airway secretions, frequent changes in position, and regular,
thorough, and vigorous chest physiotherapy are the most effective
preventive and therapeutic measures for atelectasis. Pneumonia is
similarly treated with the addition of antibiotics. Antibiotics are initially
chosen on the basis of a gram stain of the sputum; later results of sputum
cultures and antibiotic sensitivities determine the choice of antibiotics.

Tension pneumothorax is unusual after open heart surgery, but
partial pneumothorax occurs commonly. Small (< 10 per cent) stable
pneumothorax does not require treatment; larger pneumothoraces
should be aspirated. If the pneumothorax recurs, a chest tube should be
inserted and attached to suction and water seal drainage for two to five
days. Accumulations of blood or fluid within the hemithorax should be
aspirated; some patients require a chest tube for recurrent pleural
effusion. Small pleural effusions can sometimes be effectively treated by
diuretics.

Sometimes patients require prolonged respiratory support. The degree of respiratory support can be varied almost infinitely by changing inspired oxygen concentrations, end-expiratory pressures, and the number of mandatory ventilations delivered by the respirator during spontaneous ventilation. These patients require intubation either by endotracheal tube or tracheostomy. Polyvinyl endotracheal tubes are well tolerated for weeks if cuff pressures are carefully controlled to prevent tracheal ischemia and necrosis and if secretions can be adequately controlled. Alternatively, a tracheostomy may be indicated if prolonged respiratory support is anticipated. Gradual withdrawal of respiratory support is coupled with measures to improve pulmonary function, control heart failure, and augment strength and nutrition. These patients often benefit from intravenous hyperalimentation or nasogastric tube feeding.

BLEEDING

Heparin, which inhibits the coagulation cascade at several points, is used to prevent blood from clotting during cardiopulmonary bypass. Although protamine in adequate doses (1.3 mg per each mg heparin) reverses the heparin effect, bleeding times are generally prolonged in most patients after cardiopulmonary bypass. The principal cause is loss and dilution of platelets by surface contact with the extracorporeal system and a loss of function of many of the platelets that remain. Although Factors V and VIII are decreased slightly during cardiopulmonary bypass (particularly in cyanotic, polycythemic patients), the major causes of nonsurgical bleeding after open heart surgery are incomplete reversal of the effect of heparin and deficiency in platelet numbers and function.

Careful wound hemostasis is mandatory after open heart surgery, and the wound is not closed until the field is dry. This may prolong operating time and require the use of platelet transfusions and one or two units of fresh frozen plasma in the operating room.

Chest drainage is measured hourly (more often if necessary), and the amount is replaced by intravenous blood or colloid to maintain satisfactory cardiac filling pressures and cardiac output. Chest tubes are stripped often to prevent obstruction by clot and development of pericardial tamponade. If bleeding persists (> 5 ml per kg body weight during the first hour), blood is sent for measurement of prothrombin time, partial thromboplastin time, fibrinogen, and platelet count. An activated coagulation time or protamine titration test performed at the bedside helps to determine whether or not additional protamine is needed to reverse heparin. Any discovered coagulation deficiencies are usually treated by either fresh frozen plasma or platelet concentrates or both. In some patients positive end-expiratory airway pressure (PEEP) at 5 to 15 cm H_2O and infusion of vasodilators to reduce mean systemic arterial pressure to 60 to 70 torr may reduce mediastinal bleeding and promote hemostasis. Epsilonaminocaproic acid, an inhibitor of fibrinolysis, is seldom needed to control bleeding after heart surgery and should not be used unless fibrinolysis is demonstrated.

Bleeding that exceeds 10 ml per kg the first hour after operation or 5 ml per kg for each of the next three hours is an indication for reexploration of the wound and search for specific bleeding points. Surgical bleeding is found in approximately one-half of the patients who return to the operating room; in many of the others, no specific bleeding points are found, but often reexploration reduces the amount of bleeding to within safe guidelines.

Transfusions of homologous blood, plasma, packed erythrocytes, platelet concentrates, and Factor VIII concentrates carry a risk of serum hepatitis. The risk is increased by using pooled blood fractions and decreased by using frozen plasma fractions. Most surgeons are assiduously conservative about administering blood during open heart surgery; minimal use of blood and blood products postoperatively is the best prevention against serum hepatitis.

RENAL PROBLEMS

Renal failure following open heart surgery (serum creatinine > 2.5 mg per dl) occurs in approximately 7 per cent of adult patients and is more common in older patients and in those with low cardiac output, oliguria, or renal dysfunction preoperatively. Low cardiac output is thought to be the primary cause of renal failure after open heart surgery. Measures that elevate cardiac output generally improve renal blood flow; however, epinephrine in doses over approximately 1.5 μg per kg per min and dopamine over 12 μg per kg per min cause renal vasoconstriction and reduce cortical renal blood flow. Hemoglobinuria, generally associated with prolonged cardiopulmonary bypass, does not usually contribute to renal failure if a high volume of alkaline urine output can be maintained until the hemoglobin has cleared.

The use of diuretics and mannitol to protect against subsequent development of acute tubular necrosis (ATN) has never been clearly established in cardiac surgical patients. These drugs are usually given during or immediately after operation in patients with low cardiac output to test whether or not the kidneys can produce urine. High urine volumes in the immediate postoperative period do not rule out the possibility that either polyuric or oliguric ATN will develop. The diagnosis is made most easily by serial measurements of serum creatinine and urine volumes. Urine volumes less than 4 ml per kg per day or a rising serum creatinine to over 5.0 mg per dl indicate severe oliguric acute tubular necrosis. A rising serum creatinine associated with large urine output and with a urine osmolarity nearly identical to serum osmolarity indicates polyuric acute tubular necrosis.

If urine output exceeds 0.5 ml per kg per hr after cardiac surgery and cardiac output is 2.4 l per m² per min or more, renal function is probably adequate. Serum creatinine and BUN values should be followed to monitor renal function and/or the development of prerenal azotemia. If urine volumes are unusually high (> 2.0 ml per kg per hr), the possibility of polyuric ATN arises. Serum creatinine and potassium should be monitored, and urine should be analyzed for casts, protein, sodium, and osmolarity. The presence of casts, a high concentration of sodium, and osmolarity nearly identical to serum is consistent with polyuric ATN. If the serum creatinine rises on serial determinations, urine losses of fluid and electrolytes should be replaced volume for volume by appropriate intravenous crystalloids. Serum potassium and bicarbonate concentrations should be monitored. The prognosis of patients with polyuric ATN is much more favorable than those with oliguric ATN.

Urine outputs < 0.5 ml per kg per hr suggest the possibility of oliguric ATN. Infusion of mannitol (0.5 to 1.0 gm per kg) and furosemide (1 to 5 mg per kg) may increase urine output to over 1.0 ml per kg per hr and indicates that renal function is present. Persistent oliguria for three consecutive hours with casts, elevated urine sodium, and fixed osmolarity approximately equal to serum osmolarity establishes the diagnosis of oliguric ATN.

Treatment of oliguric ATN in postoperative cardiac surgical patients is directed toward maintaining fluid and electrolyte balance and preventing further renal injury. Measures to augment cardiac output also improve renal blood flow, but if tubular necrosis has occurred, increased renal blood flow does not hasten recovery. All drugs that are excreted by the kidney are stopped, or the dosage is reduced. Nephrotoxic drugs are stopped. Extrarenal fluid losses should be replaced, but only 200 ml per m² per day should be given to replace insensible losses. If the patient is ventilated with humidified gases, the lungs may actually absorb water. The number of intravenous catheters should be reduced to one or two, using "heparin-locked" catheters if necessary. The Foley catheter should be removed and the urine should be cultured.

Serum potassium, sodium bicarbonate, creatinine, and BUN measurements should be monitored at least daily. Serum potassium should be monitored every four hours if over 4.5 mEq per l and hourly if over 5.5 mEq per l. The electrocardiogram may indicate high serum potassium by high, pointed T waves and a widened QRS complex.

Elevations of serum potassium must be treated immediately. Be sure that no potassium is present in administered fluids or medications. Kayexalate ion exchange resin (20 to 35 gm in 250 ml 25 per cent sorbitol for adults) may be given by enema, which should be retained for at least 45 minutes. Alternatively, the Kayexalate can be given in 50 ml 25 per cent sorbitol by nasogastric tube. If serum potassium exceeds 6 mEq per l or if the electrocardiogram shows spiked T waves and a widened QRS, calcium gluconate 0.5 gm is given intravenously. If serum potassium exceeds 6.5 mEq per l or if cardiac arrhythmias develop, give NaHCO₃

(44.5 mEq), 50 ml of 50 per cent glucose, and 10 units of regular insulin (for adults) intravenously over a 15-minute period.

Peritoneal dialysis is indicated to control complications of uremia, hyperkalemia, acidosis, or excessive fluid accumulation. Peritoneal dialysis is started in lethargic patients with a BUN > 100 mg per dl or serum creatinine > 8 mg per dl or in all patients with a BUN > 125 mg per dl or serum creatinine > 10 mg per dl. Pulmonary edema or uncontrolled elevations of left atrial or pulmonary wedge pressure or serum sodium < 130 mEq per l indicates water retention. Hemodialysis should not be carried out unless the cardiac index exceeds 2.8 l per m² per min.

Oliguric ATN has a poor prognosis; most patients with serum creatinine levels > 5.0 mg per dl die of sepsis with or without failure of other organ systems. Every effort must be made to prevent sepsis in patients with oliguric ATN; the only survivors are those in whom renal function returns to normal or near normal before septicemia develops.

INFECTION

Wound infections are uncommon after open heart surgery. Any drainage from the wound should be cultured, and if skin edges become erythematous and swollen, the skin and subcutaneous tissues should be opened and packed. Frequent dressing allows the wound to develop healthy granulation tissue and close secondarily.

If the infection extends to the sternum and the sternal edges are slightly separated or drainage originates from beneath the sternum, the patient should be returned to the operating room for irrigation, débridement, and reclosure of the wound. Any sternal osteomyelitis should be debrided, and necrotic tissue should be lifted away. The wound should be irrigated copiously with dilute aqueous Betadine solution. All pockets of pus or serum should be evacuated. Extraneous foreign material, such as pacemaker wires, should be removed; however, sometimes foreign material, such as aortotomy sutures and Teflon felt, must remain. Two or more chest tubes should be inserted into the mediastinum for drainage. Additionally, one or more plastic tubes should be left in place so that the space beneath the sternum can be continuously irrigated at 50 to 100 ml per hr with dilute Betadine solution (1 part Betadine to 20 parts saline) for 7 to 10 days. The sternum should be closed tightly with wire mattress sutures. The muscle layer over the sternum can be closed, but generally the subcutaneous tissues and skin are not closed. The sternal wires may require tightening in subsequent days to keep the sternal edges tightly approximated. Appropriate antibiotics are given parenterally before and during reclosure and are continued until the wound is solidly healed and the patient is afebrile. After 7 to 10 days of irrigation, all catheters and drainage tubes are removed.

During this period the patient should have adequate nutrition supplemented by intravenous hyperalimentation if necessary. If the infection is promptly recognized and treated by reoperation, chances of a successful outcome improve. Unrecognized, invasive and indolent infections involving exposed coronary grafts, great vessels, or the heart itself may result in vascular-cutaneous fistulas, which are generally fatal.

Bacteremia after open heart surgery is generally detected by one or more positive blood cultures (obtained daily as long as arterial and central venous catheters are in place). Fever and leukocytosis may or may not be present but develop in addition to hypotension, tachycardia, low cardiac output, and oliguria if septicemia occurs. In infants septicemia generally causes a profound thrombocytopenia. Diffuse intravascular coagulation may occur coincidentally. Petechial hemorrhages and splenomegaly may or may not be present and are generally signs of subacute or chronic infection with endocarditis.

Vascular catheters should be removed or changed to new locations as soon as bacteremia is detected or after four days in place, whichever comes first. Tips of the catheters should be cultured. Multiple blood cultures should be obtained before antibiotics are changed or started. Although infectious disease experts frequently deplore the use of parenteral antibiotic therapy before the identity of the bloodstream organism is known, occasionally such treatment is lifesaving if acute septicemia with circulatory depression occurs. Every effort must be made to culture the organism before changing antibiotics. Once the organism is cultured, antibiotics may be changed again in order to eradicate the infection before organisms can establish colonies within the heart at suture lines, prosthetic valves, grafts, or patches. If multiple cultures indicate septicemia, parenteral antibiotics should be continued for four to six weeks. During this period the patient should be carefully followed for signs of endocarditis. Serial echocardiograms may be helpful. Changing murmurs, deterioration of circulatory hemodynamics, fever, positive blood cultures, unexplained leukocytosis, splenomegaly, and petechial hemorrhages suggest uncontrolled infection, which may require reoperation with removal and replacement of the infected prosthesis, patch, or graft.

CENTRAL NERVOUS SYSTEM DYSFUNCTION

Serious injuries to the central nervous system (CNS) occur in 1 to 4 per cent of patients after open heart operations. Embolic injuries, particularly those due to air embolism, are the most common perioperative CNS injuries. Thrombi, muscle fragments, fat, atherosclerotic debris, and calcium are other sources of operative cerebral emboli. Air emboli usually produce only transient injuries unless massive embolism has occurred. Air trapped in the heart or great vessels may embolize after bypass is terminated, or air may enter the arterial line during cardiopulmonary bypass.

Patients with preexisting carotid occlusive disease are at risk to postoperative cerebrovascular accidents. Anoxic injury to the brain may occur as a result of cessation of the circulation, failure to oxygenate the blood during bypass, or rarely in association with deep hypothermia and circulatory arrest. Bleeding into the brain during bypass is rare.

Neurologic deficits become apparent after recovery from anesthesia and removal of pharmacologic paralyzing agents. If the patient awakens, weakness or paralysis of muscle groups is readily apparent. Patients who remain comatose after operation have a poor prognosis, and many do not regain consciousness. The diagnosis of CNS injury is made by physical examination. A lumbar puncture is seldom useful; however, computerized tomography of the brain is very helpful in localizing lesions and in evaluating recovery.

Measures to decrease cerebral swelling are helpful in preventing extension of the brain injury during the early postoperative period. In unconscious patients, intracranial pressure should be monitored continuously using an intracranial bolt. Mannitol, diuretics, and steroids are given to reduce cerebral swelling. In addition, $PaCO_2$ should be kept low and hypoxia should be avoided. Systemic anticoagulants are not recommended after brain infarction because of the possibility of converting an ischemic infarct into an extended hemorrhagic infarct. Unconscious patients require intubation and ventilatory support during at least the first few days after open heart surgery.

Occasionally, patients develop seizures following open heart surgery. Emboli are the probable cause of most postoperative seizures, but seizures may occur in patients with fluid overload and electrolyte imbalance. A previous cerebral injury (healed scar) may serve as a focus for postoperative seizures. Postoperative seizures are more common after heart surgery in infants and young children than in older individuals. Sometimes seizures are the result of a major anoxic or embolic brain injury. Seizures should be stopped by barbiturates (phenobarbital) or Valium given intravenously, and if possible, the cause of the seizure should be determined. Diphenylhydantoin is added to help prevent recurrent seizures. Rarely pharmacologic paralysis may be required to control seizure activity.

Behavioral problems are common after open heart surgery and occur more frequently in patients who require prolonged intensive care than in those who recover quickly. Agitation, irritability, and combativeness require the use of sedatives (Valium or Haldol) and sometimes physical restraints. Depression, which more commonly occurs several days after operation, usually responds to reassurance and increasing the patient's activities. Drugs are seldom required. Some patients may develop severe depression or frank psychosis; these patients require the help of a consulting psychiatrist. Most behavioral difficulties after open heart surgery are temporary.

REFERENCES

Abel, R. M., Buckley, M. J., Austen, W. G., Barnett, G. O., Beck, C. H., and Fischer, J. E.: Etiology, incidence and prognosis of renal failure following cardiac operations. J. Thorac. Cardiovasc. Surg., 71:323, 1976.

Braunwald, E., Sonnenblick, E. H., and Ross, J., Jr.: Contraction of the normal heart. In Braunwald, E. (ed.): Heart Disease. Philadelphia, W. B. Saunders Co., 1980, p. 413.

Edmunds, L. H., Jr., and Alexander, J. A.: Effect of cardiopulmonary bypass on the lungs. In Fishman, A. P. (ed.): Pulmonary Diseases and Disorders. New York, McGraw-Hill Book Co., 1980, p. 1728.

Edmunds, L. H., Jr., and Stephenson, L. W.: Cardiopulmonary bypass for open heart surgery. In Glenn, W. W. L., Liebow, A. A., and Lindskog, B. S. (eds.): Thoracic and Cardiovascular Surgery with Related Pathology, 4th ed. New York, Appleton-Century-Crofts, 1982.

Harker, L. A., Malpass, T. W., Bronson, A. G., Hessel, E. A., II, and Slichter, S. J.: Mechanism of abnormal bleeding in patients undergoing cardiopulmonary bypass: Acquired transient platelet dysfunction associated with selective granule release. Blood, 56:824, 1980.

Kolkka, R., and Hilberman, M.: Neurologic dysfunction following cardiac operation with low-flow, low-pressure cardiopulmonary bypass. J. Thorac. Cardiovasc. Surg., 79:432, 1980.

Thurer, R. J., Bognolo, D., Vargas, A., Isch, J. H., and Kaiser, G. A.: The management of mediastinal infection following cardiac surgery. J. Thorac. Cardiovasc. Surg., 68:962, 1974.

21

Stomach and Duodenum

JAMES C. THOMPSON

We operate on the stomach and duodenum most often for complications of peptic ulcer, for carcinoma, for hiatal hernia with reflux esophagitis, for hemorrhagic gastritis, and for trauma. The incidence of duodenal ulcer and of gastric carcinoma has lessened over the last several decades, and stress ulceration appears to require operation less often than a decade ago. However, operations on the upper gastrointestinal tract continue to be among the most commonly performed abdominal surgical procedures.

PREOPERATIVE CONSIDERATIONS

Important among the principles of surgery is that the stomach should be emptied prior to induction of anesthesia; otherwise, there is the risk of vomiting with sudden, often fatal aspiration of gastric contents. It is the surgeon's responsibility either to get the stomach completely empty or to consult with the anesthesiologist prior to induction of anesthesia in order to avert this catastrophe. Aspiration is almost always avoidable, and when it occurs, it is usually the result of omission of standard precautionary measures.

The stomach is usually considered to be sterile because of its high acid content. There often are abundant bacteria in the duodenum, particularly in the third and fourth portions, and in patients with low or absent gastric acidity, the stomach itself may contain many bacteria. Standard preoperative methods for intestinal antisepsis should be utilized in patients with low gastric acid or in patients in whom there may be a fistula between the stomach and colon.

It is probably no longer necessary or desirable to perform gastric secretory analysis routinely on all duodenal ulcer patients before operation. On the other hand, if a surgeon should adopt a new operative treatment for duodenal ulcer (for example, should he or she begin to treat patients utilizing selective proximal vagotomy), comparison of preoperative and postoperative gastric secretory levels may provide the only method of evaluation of the adequacy of the newly adopted operative technique. We should all know that it is not possible to make a diagnosis of duodenal ulcer by gastric analysis, but very low secretory values (for example, a *maximal* acid output of less than 12 mEq per hr) makes the diagnosis of duodenal ulcer unlikely. The upper limit of normal for acid output under basal conditions is 4 mEq per hr for women and 6 mEq per hr for men; the upper limits for maximal acid output after stimulation with histamine, betazole (Histalog), pentagastrin, or insulin is 30 mEq per hr for women or 40 mEq per hr for men.

PREOPERATIVE PREPARATION

ROUTINE ELECTIVE PROCEDURES

The evening meal on the day before operation should be a light one, and the patient should be fasted overnight. We usually do not insert a nasogastric tube before anesthesia is induced. After induction, the anesthesiologist should pass a No. 18 French double-lumen tube through the nose into the stomach. As soon as the surgeon opens the abdominal cavity, he or she should check the position of the tip of the tube; it is often at the esophagogastric junction and, therefore, does not function to decompress the stomach.

PATIENTS WHO ARE BLEEDING

Patients with massive upper gastrointestinal hemorrhage may require exercise of great skills in diagnosis and treatment. It is *sometimes* dangerous, especially in patients with diminished cardiopulmonary reserves, to give blood transfusions rapidly, but if a patient has lost a great deal of blood rapidly, he or she can safely receive rapid replacement. Large catheters should be placed in large central veins for rapid blood transfusion and for measurement of central venous pressure. If there is any question about the adequacy of blood replacement or if the surgeon suspects the possibility of cardiopulmonary insufficiency, preoperative insertion of a Swan-Ganz catheter may be helpful. These catheters often give rise to trouble (tricuspid valve injury and vegetations, small pulmonary emboli) if left in too long. They should be promptly removed after operation if not strictly needed.

A nasogastric tube should be placed in order to try to empty the stomach and, if the patient has not vomited blood, to determine whether there is blood in the proximal gut. Insertion of an Ewald tube may be helpful in aspirating clots from the stomach because of its larger diameter than the usual nasogastric tube. Hematemesis or bloody gastric aspirate signifies that the source of bleeding is proximal to the ligament of Treitz. A Foley catheter should be placed in the bladder in order to monitor the patient's urinary output. If the patient is hypovolemic, resuscitation may begin with administration of Ringer's lactate solution until blood becomes available. If the patient is hypotensive, it is helpful to administer oxygen by face mask. The majority of patients with upper gastrointestinal hemorrhage will stop bleeding spontaneously; a few, however, will persist and will require immediate operation.

After appropriate resuscitative measures are under way, an accurate diagnosis of the cause of bleeding must be secured. This usually is not difficult. The history and physical examination will be helpful in determining whether or not patients are alcoholic or have hepatic dysfunction or have bled before. Emergency fiberoptic endoscopy is the salient diagnostic maneuver. We studied 195 patients with massive upper gastrointestinal bleeding and found that 26 per cent were bleeding from a duodenal ulcer, 18 per cent from hemorrhagic gastritis, 15 per cent from esophageal varices, 10 per cent from gastric ulcer, and 8 per cent from Mallory-Weiss tears of the esophagogastric mucosa (Villar et al., 1977). If for any reason the patient has not had endoscopy before operation or if the diagnosis was not made correctly, it is often helpful to perform fiberoptic endoscopy per os during the operative procedure. This avoids long gastrotomy or duodenotomy incisions to locate sites of bleeding.

If the patient is bleeding from varices, temporary cessation of hemorrhage may be achieved by the intravenous administration of vasopressin (Pitressin), which diminishes the flow in the superior mesenteric artery and lowers portal pressure. The initial infusion of 20 units of vasopressin in 5 per cent dextrose in water takes 20 minutes. It may be helpful to repeat the infusion, but tachyphylaxis is common, and repeated infusions are often less and less effective. Further temporary control of variceal hemorrhage may be achieved with the Sengstaken-Blakemore tube. This device is dangerous to use and should be placed only by those who are experienced with it or who have carefully informed themselves about the proper technique for insertion and maintenance (Conn and Simpson, 1967). If the bleeding is caused by diffuse gastritis or an acute stress ulcer, irrigation with iced saline mixed with antacids may be helpful. It is worthwhile to consider routine prophylactic antacid treatments in patients in the intensive care unit who are at risk for the development of stress ulceration. One to two ounces of antacids are instilled into the stomach, and the nasogastric tube is clamped for 1½ hours. Suction is then applied for one-half hour, and the process is repeated continuously around the clock. The pH of the gastric aspirate should be maintained at >5. The dose of antacid is adjusted to achieve that goal. Spontaneous cessation of bleeding is common, and since we have learned to treat the underlying causes (sepsis, hypoxia, and low-flow states) more vigorously, the incidence of stress ulcer bleeding requiring operation has dropped dramatically in the last 10 years. Intra-arterial infusion of vasopressin (Athanasoulis et al., 1974) is occasionally of help, but rebleeding is frequent.

Nasogastric aspiration should be maintained to remove acid-peptic juice and to get out as much blood as possible. The stomach is often filled by a large, nearly solid clot that resists attempts at aspiration. If the patient is to be operated upon as an emergency, the endotracheal tube may be placed safely under local anesthesia with the patient awake. Then, if he aspirates, he can cough.

If the patient should lose massive quantities of blood, clotting elements may be diluted sufficiently to compromise normal mechanisms for coagulation. In such instances, it may be necessary to administer fresh frozen plasma, platelet concentrates, or fresh blood after the administration of two or three liters of banked blood. The surgeon must check on continued availability of blood. Shortage of the patient's specific type may tip the scale toward earlier operative intervention.

PERFORATION

The diagnosis of perforation of the stomach or duodenum can usually be made on clinical and radiologic evidence, but if there is doubt and if there is no free air under the diaphragm, diagnosis can be confirmed by fiberoptic endoscopy. This is necessary only on very rare occasions. If the perforation is more than several hours old, there may be considerable local sequestration ("third spacing") of extracellular fluid, and the patient may become hypovolemic. The surgeon should anticipate that induction of anesthesia may cause loss of vasoconstrictor reflexes, which may in turn cause the patient to lapse into shock. The patient's preoperative blood volume may be estimated by measurement of central venous pressure; if there is a deficit, correction should be achieved with lactated Ringer's solution. We believe that antibiotics should be given preoperatively as a routine prophylaxis.

GASTRIC OUTLET OBSTRUCTION

The great variability of symptoms that occur in response to nearly complete pyloric obstruction may obscure the diagnosis of the underlying lesion. If obstruction occurs rapidly, there is often dramatic vomiting with great loss of fluid and electrolytes. More often, however, obstruction is insidious, and the stomach dilates and hypertrophies in response. Patients may manifest overflow regurgitation of brackish fluid. Once the obstruction is discovered, the stomach should be emptied as quickly as possible. Emptying is best accomplished by vigorous irrigation and aspiration with a large bore tube (Ewald or other). Proper emptying of accumulated debris may take great perseverance; it should be accomplished as soon as possible. While this is being done, fluid and electrolyte losses may be replaced. With classic pyloric obstruction, the patient may have a hypochloremic, hypokalemic alkalosis. The hypochloremia and hypokalemia are the result of direct loss of H^+ and Cl^- by vomiting; gastric juice has a relatively low concentration of K^+, and the hypokalemia is due chiefly to renal substitution of K^+ for H^+. In the majority of instances, it is possible to correct the electrolyte imbalance by intravenous administration of saline and potassium chloride. In rare instances, it may be necessary to give HCl intravenously (Thompson, 1981).

After the stomach is emptied, gastroscopy should be performed prior to radiographic studies of the stomach. It is often difficult to differentiate benign from malignant pyloric obstruction; multiple gastric biopsies often provide the answer.

Surgical correction of pyloric obstruction is never an emergency, and the stomach should be emptied and subjected to continuous nasogastric aspiration to minimize edema and allow restoration of muscle tone. The degree of gastric outlet obstruction can be estimated by means of the saline load test, which is conducted in a fasting patient whose stomach has been completely emptied. A No. 18 nasogastric tube is placed in the stomach, and 750 ml of 0.9 per cent sodium chloride solution is instilled at room temperature. The tube should be clamped for 30 minutes, after which the stomach should be aspirated; if more than 400 ml is retained, obstruction appears certain (retention of more than 200 ml is abnormal).

Although there is no emergency indication for operation, excessive delay in restoration of gastrointestinal continuity must be avoided. These delays often occur because the correct diagnosis is not suspected or because attempts at emptying the stomach are insufficiently vigorous. The average interval between hospital admission and operation is unnecessarily long in patients with pyloric obstruction.

Occasionally patients with long-term pyloric obstruction develop a degree of gastritis sufficient to destroy most of the parietal cells, and the acid output may be low or even absent. In such cases, it may be wise to instill a nonabsorbable antibiotic such as kanamycin or erythromycin base into the stomach on the day before operation. Systemic administration of antibiotics such as the cephalosporins may also be helpful.

MASSIVE HYPERSECRETION

Occasionally patients with duodenal ulcer disease will develop critical situations in which they secrete massive quantities (greater than 3 liters per day) of gastric juice. This is sometimes seen in patients with pyloric outlet obstruction and otherwise uncomplicated duodenal ulcer. It is commonly found in patients with the Zollinger-Ellison (Z-E) syndrome. If the basal acid output is greater than 15 mEq per hr, the Zollinger-Ellison syndrome should be suspected. It is often possible to dramatically reduce the acid hypersecretion with large doses of atropine or, preferably, by intravenous infusion of the H_2-blocking agent cimetidine in dosages up to 600 mg every six hours.

In any patient with massive hypersecretion, blood samples should be obtained for measurement of serum gastrin; any fasting value greater than 200 is suspicious, and if the patient hypersecretes acid and has a serum gastrin level greater than 400, the diagnosis of the Z-E syndrome is most likely. Diagnosis can be confirmed by the means of testing the effect on serum gastrin of the challenge of calcium and secretin infusions (Thompson et al., 1975).

If gastrin studies suggest that the patient may have a gastrinoma, attempts should be made to locate the tumor by means of selective celiac and superior mesenteric arteriography.

Should serum gastrin be measured in each patient with a duodenal ulcer? This depends upon the ease with which the measurement can be obtained. We do believe that gastrin levels should be obtained in the following patients: (1) in any patient in whom the Zollinger-Ellison syndrome is suspected and specifically in patients with recurrent peptic ulcers or recurrent peptic ulcer symptoms after an acid-reducing operation, (2) in patients with a duodenal ulcer and massive hypersecretion of acid (>15 mEq per hr basal), (3) in patients with duodenal ulcer and diarrhea, (4) in patients with duodenal ulcer and hypercalcemia, (5) in ulcer patients with relatives who have the Zollinger-Ellison syndrome or the multiple endocrine adenoma I syndrome, (6) in patients who have postbulbar or jejunal peptic ulcers, (7) in patients whose upper gastrointestinal radiologic studies are suggestive of the Zollinger-Ellison syndrome, (8) in patients under 20 years of age with duodenal ulcers, and (9) in postoperative patients in whom inadvertent exclusion of antral mucosa is suspected. We now obtain serum gastrin measurements in any duodenal ulcer patient who is regarded as a candidate for operation.

NUTRITIONAL PROBLEMS

Patients with prolonged gastric outlet obstruction or with gastric carcinoma are often malnourished, and some may be in advanced states of catabolism. Such nutritional deficiencies can be corrected most efficiently by total parenteral nutrition, which may be administered for 5 to 10 days prior to operation. It is usually not necessary to establish by formal laboratory study that the patient has achieved a positive nitrogen balance before operation. This transformation can usually be appreciated clinically by weight gain and by general appearance. The surgeon must guard against the possibility that the weight gain may be due to edema. It is usually not a good plan to institute total parenteral nutrition immediately before operation. Patients vary in their adaptation, and it is preferable to allow sufficient time (four to six days) for adaptation to and assimilation of intravenous nutrition. For a more complete discussion of parenteral and enteral therapy, see Chapters 4 and 5.

POSTOPERATIVE CARE

The most common early postoperative problems after operations on the stomach and duodenum are respiratory, and proper attention should be taken to prevent and to treat postoperative atelectasis.

NASOGASTRIC SUCTION

The stomach should be decompressed routinely after operation by means of a nasogastric tube. We do not believe that the extra risk of making an opening into the stomach is justified by the putative advantages of gastrostomy decompression. There have been several fatal complications of simple postoperative gastrostomy drainage. Nasogastric tubes are certainly not innocuous, but in our opinion are less likely to contribute directly to major complications.

Decompression of the stomach should be maintained until the gut is functioning. This may occur on the day after operation in patients with elective proximal gastric vagotomy; patients who have had prolonged pyloric obstruction may require one or two weeks before they regain sufficient gastric tone to empty the stomach. We often remove the nasogastric tube and replace it in four to six hours to check gastric residual. If more than 200 ml is present, we leave the tube in place and resume aspiration.

Nasogastric tubes require attention. They should never be connected to high-vacuum wall suction, as the great negative pressure may damage the gastric mucosa and lead to hemorrhage. Tubes should be connected to intermittent low-pressure suction devices, and they should be irrigated frequently to insure patency.

VAGOTOMY WITHOUT RESECTION

Performance of both truncal and selective proximal vagotomy requires dissection under the left leaf of the diaphragm, which is often followed by atelectasis of the left lower lobe. Serious abdominal complications are rare after both procedures. Leaks may occur from pyloroplasty or gastroenterostomy or, very rarely, from the denuded lesser curvature after selective proximal vagotomy. Development of signs of sepsis should always raise the possibility of a leak.

Adequacy of vagotomy can be measured by postoperative secretory studies. We used the Hollander test in the past, but we no longer do so

(Thompson, 1981). The reasons for this change in attitude are as follows: gastric secretory tests are of little actual value in the diagnosis of recurrent ulcer per se, and insulin tests are no better than any other in separating patients with recurrence from those without recurrence; the notion that insulin-stimulated acid secretion is mediated only by the vagus is unproved. Since antrectomy alone may result in a negative Hollander test, the entire anatomic significance of these tests must be reassessed. As few as 60 per cent of patients with recurrent ulcer have a positive Hollander response. Ten per cent of patients with a positive Hollander test and 2 per cent with a negative test develop recurrence. Because the insulin test is difficult to interpret and is dangerous (there have been several deaths reported) and because it provides no better discrimination than does any other standard secretory test, we have replaced it with determination of maximal acid output using betazole (Histalog) or pentagastrin. Neither serum gastrin levels nor acid secretory measurements appear to have any predictive value for ulcer recurrence in any single patient. Postoperative results from different surgical procedures for duodenal ulcer seem to be remarkably similar (Thompson, 1974). The chief differences are a higher rate of ulcer recurrence after truncal vagotomy and a near freedom from all undesirable sequelae in the early experience after selective proximal vagotomy.

Repair of Esophageal Hiatal Hernia

These patients usually require no special postoperative attention except that care must be taken in insure that the stomach does not become distended. Some fundoplication procedures make vomiting or belching difficult. The nasogastric tube should not be removed until full bowel function has resumed, and the tube should be replaced to check for gastric residual within four to six hours.

Gastric Resection

Early postoperative complications may include bleeding, especially from the anastomotic suture line. This may be properly evaluated by fiberoptic endoscopy. The bleeding may or may not stop spontaneously.

The nasogastric tube should be removed when bowel function has resumed. Initial postoperative feedings should be clear liquids. If the patient can tolerate clear liquids, he or she can tolerate a full diet, and it is usually not necessary or advisable to order the changes from full liquids to a soft diet to a regular diet. It is important that high carbohydrate loads be avoided in the early postoperative stage in order not to establish a pattern of dumping. Some patients with gastric resection, particularly after removal of a large portion of the stomach, may develop late nutritional complications (weight loss, steatorrhea, and calcium or iron deficiencies).

If the patient should become septic after gastrectomy or if bile-stained material should drain from the wound, there may be a leak at either the duodenal stump or at the Billroth I or II anastomosis. The patient's fluid balance should be carefully checked, antibiotics administered, and early operative repair instituted. It is important to provide for adequate drainage after repair of the leak.

In gastric resections involving the proximal stomach, leaks at the esophagogastrostomy are common. It is wise to drain these anastomoses. If the patient should become febrile, patency of the anastomosis can be tested radiographically by use of a water-soluble contrast medium. Small leaks may heal spontaneously; large leaks require repair and often extensive reconstruction.

TOTAL GASTRECTOMY

Total gastrectomy is performed for extensive gastric neoplasms, for the Zollinger-Ellison syndrome, or rarely for diffuse hemorrhagic gastritis. Prognosis varies depending upon the indication for operation; postoperative complications are common when the operation is done for carcinoma or hemorrhagic gastritis and rare when done for the Zollinger-Ellison syndrome. The best anastomosis in our hands is an end-to-end esophagojejunostomy Roux-en-Y. Various substitute pouches can be constructed in patients with gastric carcinoma, but we believe that they are usually unnecessary. The poor nutritional results usually associated with total gastrectomy are usually due to one of two causes: progression of neoplastic disease or bile reflux esophagitis. Use of the Roux-en-Y esophagojejunostomy with a 30 cm jejunal limb prevents bile reflux. Our nutritional results have been good if the patient did not have residual cancer.

We leave a nasojejunal tube in place for seven or eight days, and after removal, we check the anastomosis by barium swallow on about the ninth or tenth day. If all is well, we initiate small liquid feedings and rapidly progress to a six-meal regular diet. For reasons that are not clear, significant dumping symptoms are uncommon. These patients have lost the entire mass of parietal cells (which secrete intrinsic factor), and therefore, they will require periodic regular administration (every three to four months) of Vitamin B_{12}. These patients may also require additional supplementation with iron.

REFERENCES

Athanasoulis, C. A., Baum, S., Waltman, A., Ring, E. J., Imbembo, A., and Salm, T. J.: Control of acute gastric mucosal hemorrhage: Intra-arterial infusion of posterior pituitary extracts. N. Engl. J. Med., 290:597, 1974.

Conn, H. O., and Simpson, J. A.: Excessive mortality associated with balloon tamponade of bleeding varices. J.A.M.A., 202:587, 1967.

Thompson, J. C.: Standard versus experimental surgical procedures in the treatment of duodenal ulcers. Tex. Med., 70:51, 1974.

Thompson, J. C.: Stomach and Duodenum. In Sabiston, D. C. (ed.): Davis-Christopher's *Textbook of Surgery*, 12th ed. Philadelphia, W. B. Saunders Co., 1981, pp. 896–976.

Thompson, J. C., Reeder, D. D., Villar, H. V., and Fender, H. R.: Natural history and experience with diagnosis and treatment of the Zollinger-Ellison syndrome. Surg. Gynecol. Obstet., 140:721, 1975.

Villar, H. H., Fender, H. R., Watson, L. C., and Thompson, J. C.: Emergency diagnosis of upper gastrointestinal bleeding by fiberoptic endoscopy. Ann. Surg., 185:367, 1977.

22

The Liver and Portal Vein

W. DEAN WARREN
WILLIAM J. MILLIKAN, JR.

Patients with surgical problems related to the liver and portal vein usually present with (1) jaundice, (2) hepatic mass, (3) trauma, or (4) a complication of portal hypertension.

JAUNDICE (Algorithm 1, Table 22–1)

Evaluation of jaundice has become more precise with the development of improved techniques of upper gastrointestinal and biliary endoscopy. However, careful history, physical examination, and scrutiny of "standard liver function tests" (Table 22–2) collectively represent the first step of the algorithm for evaluation of jaundice.

Obstructive or surgical jaundice is due to partial or complete blockage of the biliary ducts at any point from the ampulla of Vater to the cholangioles. The most frequent cause is common duct stones, but carcinoma of the pancreas, duodenum, or common or hepatocellular ducts may be indistinguishable from calculus disease on initial evaluation. Pancreatitis is frequently recognized as a cause of obstructive jaundice, and intrahepatic lesions (metastatic disease, granulomas) may present in similar fashion. Obstructive jaundice is characterized by an elevated direct bilirubin, increased alkaline phosphatase, and normal or slightly elevated levels of serum glutamic-oxaloacetic transaminase (SGOT). Serum cholesterol may be normal or elevated, and prothrombin time may be prolonged because of malabsorption of vitamin K.

Further evaluation of obstructive jaundice is required prior to operative intervention if there is doubt as to the cause of the obstructing lesion. In this era of spiraling medical costs and aggressive peer review, it is equally unjustified to subject the young woman with recurrent right upper quadrant colicky pain and two nonvisualizing oral cholecystograms to endoscopic retrograde choledochopancreatography (ERCP) as

Table 22–1. Algorithm 1: Jaundice (Total Bilirubin 3.5)

History and physical examination
Standard liver function tests

OBSTRUCTIVE JAUNDICE

Increased direct bilirubin and alkaline phosphatase; SGOT and prothrombin time normal or slightly deranged

ERCP
Echo
Skinny (Shiba) needle cholangiography

Biliary disease

Pancreatic disease
Cyst or mass

Arteriogram

Avascular mass

Vascular mass

HEPATOCELLULAR JAUNDICE

Total bilirubin elevated with direct and indirect fractions split; alkaline phosphatase and prothrombin time normal or slightly deranged; SGOT elevated

Percutaneous liver biopsy

Diagnosis

HEMOLYTIC JAUNDICE

Indirect bilirubin elevated; SGOT, alkaline phosphatase and prothrombin time normal

Reticulocyte count
Serum-free hemoglobin
Haptoglobin
Sickle cell prep
Hemoglobin electrophoresis

Diagnosis

Table 22–2. Normal Values for Hepatic Function Tests

Test	Normal Value
Serum albumin	3.5–5.0 gm/100 ml
Total protein	5.0–6.5 gm/100 ml
Albumin/globulin	1.5–3.5 gm/100 ml
Cholesterol	100–250 mg/100 ml
Alkaline phosphatase:	
Bodansky	1.5–4.0 units
King-Armstrong	3–13 units
Shinohara-Jones-Brock	1.8 × Bodansky units
Serum glutamic-oxaloacetic transaminase (SGOT)	40 units
Serum glutamic-pyruvic transaminase (SGPT)	45 units
Bromsulphalein retention	0–6% at 45 minutes
Prothrombin time	90–100%
Fibrinogen	200–400 mg/100 ml
Blood "ammonia"	40–60 μg/100 ml
Serum bilirubin:	
Total	Less than 1.5 mg/100 ml
Direct	Less than 0.3 mg/100 ml
Indirect	Less than 1.2 mg/100 ml
Urinary bilirubin	0
Urobilinogen (urine)	0.2–3.0 mg/24 hours

(Modified from Schwartz, S. I.: Surgical Diseases of the Liver. New York, McGraw-Hill, 1964.)

it is to operate upon the 55-year-old male with weight loss and obstructive jaundice without an attempt to define the anatomy of the biliary and pancreatic duct systems.

A total serum bilirubin greater than 3.0 mg per 100 ml usually precludes oral or intravenous cholangiography. ERCP and transhepatic (Shiba needle) cholangiography are both valuable adjuncts for evaluating obstructive jaundice. ERCP is valuable when clinical suspicion implicates the pancreas as the cause of obstruction, but if the common bile duct is completely blocked, ERCP may be unable to define common and hepatic duct anatomy. If primary common duct obstruction is suspected, percutaneous transhepatic or transjugular cholangiography may better define stones or anatomic obstruction than will ERCP. The clinical situation in which both are required is uncommon, and routine combined use is to be condemned because of significant potential morbidity inherent in each procedure.

Beta mode ultrasonography (echo) is a noninvasive test that may eliminate the need for either ERCP or transhepatic cholangiography (Bradley and Clements, 1974). In experienced hands, echo can define choledocholithiasis and the dimensions of an obstructed biliary system. Ultrasonography can often determine whether a peripancreatic mass is solid or cystic. Beta ultrasonography in combination with either ERCP or transhepatic cholangiography should define the point of blockade in obstructive jaundice. If beta ultrasonography and ERCP or transhepatic cholangiography define an intrahepatic point of obstruction, percutaneous biopsy may provide exact diagnosis and alter anticipated surgical therapy, as in the case of metastatic cancer and granulomatous disorders (sarcoid, tuberculosis).

Percutaneous biopsy is also definitive in patients with hepato-cellular jaundice characterized by an elevated bilirubin, elevated SGOT, and normal alkaline phosphatase. The most common cause of primary hepatocellular jaundice is serum hepatitis, which infrequently dictates either surgical consultation or biopsy. Persistence of elevated SGOT and jaundice signals chronic active hepatitis (Mistilis and Lam, 1972), which requires biopsy for diagnosis. A not infrequent problem confronting the practicing surgeon is evaluation of the patient with chronic active hepatitis who requires either elective or emergency operation. Steroid therapy may mask chronic indolent hepatic activity, and elective surgical therapy requires preoperative liver biopsy to define the most opportune time for operation. Emergency operation, like elective operation, requires careful management of steroid therapy and anticipation of postoperative hepatic decompensation.

Alcoholic hepatitis also requires percutaneous biopsy for diagnosis and definition of activity. Elective operation and operation that would otherwise be considered semiurgent (common duct stone) should be postponed in patients with active alcoholic hepatitis because of the high associated increase in postoperative morbidity. Galambos (1972) has defined the hazard of operation in patients with active alcoholic hepatitis and has shown that the prothrombin time is a valuable longitudinal parameter in following the disease process. Abstinence from ethanol and improved nutrition for three months will usually stabilize alcoholic hepatitis and prepare the patient for operation (see Portal Hyperten-sion).

Hemolytic jaundice, which is discussed in Chapter 27, is character-ized by an elevated indirect bilirubin, normal SGOT and normal serum alkaline phosphatase. Active hemolysis is accompanied by increased amounts of serum-free hemoglobin and reticulocytosis. Patients with primary hematologic or reticuloendothelial system disorders may re-quire splenectomy. Clinical jaundice with hypersplenism secondary to portal hypertension is rare, and splenectomy is relatively contraindicat-ed (see Portal Hypertension).

HEPATIC MASS (Algorithm 2, Table 22–3)

PREOPERATIVE DIAGNOSTIC EVALUATION

Table 22–4 lists the spectrum of pathologic conditions that can present as space-occupying lesions of, or associated with, the liver and defines the need for thorough preoperative evaluation. A careful history and physical examination, standard liver tests, oral cholecystogram, and barium studies of the upper gastrointestinal tract and colon should

Table 22–3. ALGORITHM 2

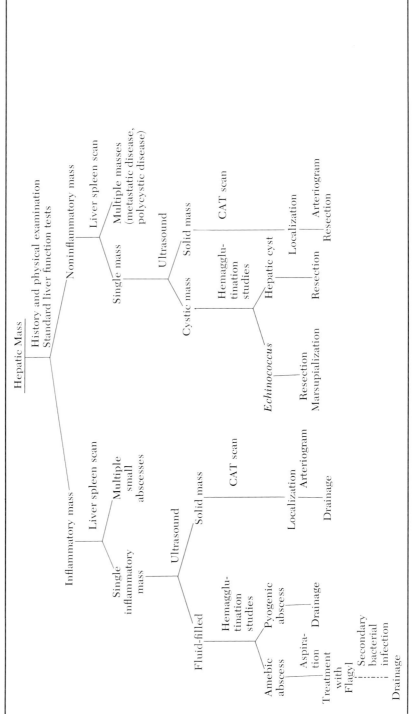

Table 22–4. HEPATIC MASSES

I. Cysts
  A. *Echinococcus*
  B. Solitary cyst
    1. Congenital
    2. Post-traumatic
  C. Polycystic disease
II. Abscesses
  A. Pyogenic abscess (bacterial, fungal, tuberculous)
    1. Single
    2. Multiple
  B. Amebic
III. Benign Neoplasms
  A. Parenchymal tumors
    1. Hepatic cell adenomas (hepatoadenomas)
    2. Bile duct adenomas (cholangioadenomas)
    3. Mixed hepatic cell and bile duct adenomas (cholangiohepatoadenomas)
  B. Vascular tumors
    1. Hemangiomas
    2. Lymphangiomas
  C. Neoplastic cysts
    1. Cystadenoma
    2. Dermoid
    3. Cystic teratoma
  D. Mesenchymal tumors
    1. Fibroma
    2. Lipoma
    3. Leiomyoma
IV. Malignant neoplasms
  A. Carcinoma
    1. Hepatoma
    2. Cholangioma
    3. Mixed and anaplastic
  B. Metastatic
  C. Sarcoma
    1. Hemangioendothelioma
    2. Rhabdomyosarcoma
    3. Leiomyosarcoma
    4. Lymphoma
  D. Malignant teratoma

exclude lesions of the stomach, gallbladder, and hepatic flexure. In addition, history and physical examination should differentiate between an inflammatory and a noninflammatory mass.

In addition to being classified as inflammatory or noninflammatory, masses of the right upper quadrant may be perihepatic or intrahepatic. The liver scintillation scan, utilizing technetium sulphur colloid, which is taken up by the reticuloendothelial cells, will define intrahepatic lesions greater than 2.5 cm in diameter in patients with adequate hepatic function. When coupled with a simultaneous lung scan, technetium liver scan can isolate subphrenic abscess. In patients with pre-existing cirrhosis, technetium uptake is often patchy, and lesions larger than 2.5 cm can be missed. Scintillation scanning with gallium 67 was originally heralded as being superior in the detection of intrahepatic abscesses because the gallium is taken up by hepatocytes and preferentially by cells that line abscess cavities. Experience has raised questions about the degree of accuracy of gallium scans in diagnosis of inflammatory hepatic lesions, but in cirrhotic livers gallium may delineate noninflammatory intrahepatic masses.

Scintillation scanning can demonstrate a space-occupying lesion within or impinging on the liver, and beta ultrasonography usually defines if the lesion is cystic, fluid-filled, or solid. Pancreatic pseudocysts in the head of the pancreas or presenting through the gastrohepatic or gastrocolic ligament can be differentiated from true hepatic lesions by ultrasound. In addition, ultrasound can quantify the thickness and morphology (thin-even vs. thick-shaggy) of the cyst wall, thereby aiding in the differentiation of true cysts from hepatic abscesses.

Hepatic abscesses are of two major classes: pyogenic (bacterial) (Altemeier et al., 1970) and amebic (Powell, 1972). Both single and multiple pyogenic abscesses result from bacterial or fungal hematogenous spread via the portal vein or hepatic artery. The organisms most frequently cultured from single hepatic abscesses are a mixture of aerobic and anaerobic forms *(Streptococcus, Bacterioides)*. The therapy of choice for single pyogenic abscesses is surgical drainage, but surgical drainage for amebic abscesses as primary therapy is contraindicated. This dichotomy of therapeutic modalities defines the importance of further diagnostic studies in patients with hepatic abscess. In the critically ill patient with sepsis uncontrolled by antibiotics, surgical drainage must be instituted immediately. If possible, aspiration of the abscess is initially performed, the contents are cultured (aerobic, anaerobic, fungus), and smears are prepared (Gram stain and A, B, F). If aspiration and Gram stain reveal pyogenic abscess, definitive drainage can be performed immediately. Aspiration of chocolate or anchovy paste–like material from an abscess cavity is not diagnostic of amebic abscess because sterile yellow or green pus is frequently seen.

In patients with intrahepatic abscess in whom drainage is not felt to be emergent, serologic tests for *Entamoeba histolytica* can be performed. The Castle-Lewis hemagglutination test appears more sensitive than the complement fixation or gel diffusion tests. Combined accuracy of serologic tests is greater than 95 per cent in patients with proven amebic abscesses. Tests of stool for parasitic cysts and trophozoites may be performed but are positive in less than 20 per cent of cases. Initial therapy for amebic abscess should be with metronidazole (Flagyl) (250–500 mg by mouth every six hours). Large amebic abscesses may require aspiration and retreatment (Flagyl, Emetine) after initial treatment with Flagyl.

Definitive treatment for large single pyogenic abscesses is surgical drainage; treatment of choice for multiple small abscesses (less than 2 cm) is systemic antibiotics. Unfortunately, multiple small hepatic abscesses frequently complicate major systemic and intra-abdominal infection. An intra-abdominal abscess that fails clinically to respond to drainage should alert the surgeon to an incompletely drained collection or hepatic abscess. Although the mortality of multiple small intrahepatic abscesses is high, supportive therapy should be maintained because small abscesses can coalesce and be drained surgically.

The use of selective hepatic arteriography and computerized axial tomography (CAT scan) in the diagnosis of intrahepatic abscess is infrequently required. In isolated cases in which evaluation with echo and scintillation scans fails to define the lesion as an abscess, arteriography and CAT scan may be helpful. Use of these diagnostic modalities should be reserved for nonemergent evaluation of noninflammatory hepatic tumors.

The most common primary hepatic tumor is hepatoma (Balasegaran, 1975); the most common malignancy in the liver is metastatic disease. This fact defines the need to eliminate other organ systems as the source of a single (or multiple) hepatic tumor mass. Prior to consideration of possible resection, barium studies of the entire gastrointestinal tract must be performed, and colon endoscopy (colonoscopy) must be utilized if the cecum or other areas of the colon are not clearly defined.

Beta ultrasonography should be performed to separate solid tumors from cysts. If the intrahepatic mass is thin-walled and fluid-filled, serologic tests for *Echinococcus* (such as the hemagglutination test or immunoelectrophoresis) can be performed by commercial laboratories or the Center for Disease Control in Atlanta, Georgia. Most hydatid cysts are asymptomatic and require no surgical intervention. If the cyst is symptomatic or resection is required because of imminent or potential rupture, aspiration should be performed before operation with instillation of formalin or hydrogen peroxide to prevent spillage of viable scoleces during definitive extirpation.

If beta ultrasonography demonstrates that the hepatic mass is solid and no other source of primary malignancy can be found, selective hepatic and superior mesenteric arteriography should be performed to define the vascular supply of the tumor. The arterial phase of the study may also show additional metastatic tumor blushes unidentified by liver scan. It is also important to document the venous filling phase of the superior mesenteric arteriogram to ascertain whether or not the tumor has obstructed portal venous flow.

Computerized axial tomography (CAT scan) is currently being evaluated as an additional diagnostic tool in the evaluation of intrahepatic masses. The study may prove to be a valuable addition to current diagnostic tools of scintillation scanning, beta ultrasonography, and arteriography.

The majority of hepatomas appear in patients older than 40 years of age. During the last 10 years, the increasing frequency of hepatic adenomas in young females taking oral contraceptives has been documented (Edmonson, 1976). There is good evidence that spontaneous regression of these adenomas will occur if the exogenous estrogens are withdrawn. In this patient population, observation is justified only if liver biopsy documenting adenomas has been obtained.

Table 22–5. Clinical and Laboratory Classification of Hepatic Function

CLASS	A	B	C
Functional impairment	Minimal	Moderate	Severe
Serum bilirubin (mg/100 ml)	<2.0	2.0–3.0	>3.0
Serum albumin (gm/100 ml)	>3.5	3.0–3.5	<3.0
Ascites	None	Easily controlled	Poorly controlled
Neurologic disorders	None	Minimal	Moderate to severe
Nutrition	Excellent	Good	Poor, wasted

(Modified from Stone, H. H.: Preoperative and postoperative care. Surg. Clin. North Am., 57(2):409, 1977.)

Alpha fetal protein is a serum globulin often elevated (greater than 70 per cent of the time) in patients with primary hepatoma, but its absence in no way excludes the diagnosis or dictates that further preoperative studies, such as percutaneous liver biopsy, should not be performed.

PREOPERATIVE PREPARATION

The principles of preoperative preparation for hepatic resections include concepts used to prepare any patient for a major operative procedure plus two major additions: hepatic function and state of nutrition.

Stone (1977) has utilized the Child classification (Table 22–5) in patients requiring hepatic resection and has shown that postoperative mortality and morbidity can be a function of the preoperative state (Table 22–6). Assuming the concept to be valid, all attempts should be made to improve the patient's liver function and nutritional status. Class A patients, as exemplified by noncirrhotic young females with adenomas,

Table 22–6. Basic Liver Function and Operability

Class A	No limitations Normal response to all operations Normal ability of liver to regenerate
Class B	Some limitation of liver function Altered response to all operations, but tolerated well if prepared preoperatively Limited ability to regenerate new hepatic parenchyma so that all sizable liver resections are contraindicated
Class C	Severe limitation of liver function Poor response to all operations regardless of preparatory efforts Liver resection, no matter what the size, is contraindicated

(Modified from Stone, H. H.: Preoperative and postoperative care. Surg. Clin. North Am., 57(2):409, 1977.)

may require no additional preoperative therapy. Enteral or parenteral alimentation, in addition to blood transfusions, fresh-frozen plasma, and vitamin K supplementation, should be used in Class B and C patients in an attempt to improve both liver function and nutritional status. Stone (1977) has emphasized the importance of improving the Child classification by stating that hepatic resection is contraindicated in Class C patients except in life-threatening circumstances.

POSTOPERATIVE CARE

The principles of postoperative care include those utilized during preoperative preparation with three important additions necessitated by the alterations in hepatic physiology caused by hepatic resection:

1. Hepatic resection causes splanchnic sequestration and decreases effective plasma and red blood cell volume. Resection of less than 30 per cent of hepatic mass can cause significant hypovolemia, and resection of greater than 30 per cent will require additional blood transfusions in the immediate postoperative period (Table 22–7). Resection of 60 per cent or greater of the hepatic mass will cause marked splanchnic sequestration, and hypovolemic shock will ensue if additional blood is not given. Sequestration begins during the surgical procedure but usually characterizes the immediate postoperative period (four to eight hours). All patients should have central venous pressure or Swan-Ganz pulmonary wedge pressure determined hourly for the first 24 postoperative hours.

2. Hepatic resection causes hypoglycemia and increased demand for exogenous glucose. Hepatic resection is one of the few operative

Table 22–7. SEQUESTRATION FOLLOWING HEPATIC RESECTION

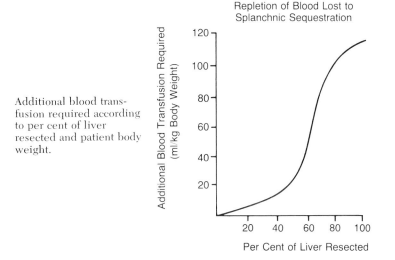

Additional blood transfusion required according to per cent of liver resected and patient body weight.

Table 22–8. GLUCOSE NEED FOLLOWING HEPATIC RESECTION

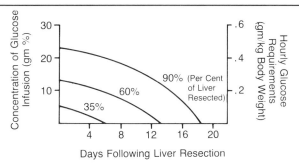

Concentration of glucose and duration of infusion according to massiveness of liver resected.

procedures that elicits marked hypoglycemia requiring greater than 50 gm glucose in the first 24 postoperative hours. Although the mechanism is poorly understood, the degree of hypoglycemia roughly parallels the extent of resection. Patient response is variable, but an estimate of grams of glucose per hour per kg body weight can be made from Table 22–8. Thus, a 50 kg patient with a 50 per cent hepatic resection could require 11 gm of glucose per hour or 40 ml of 25 per cent glucose solution per hour during the first postoperative day. A satisfactory protocol for maintaining the glucose level utilizes a concentrated 25 per cent glucose infusion through a central venous catheter while monitoring urine sugars every two hours (1 to 2+) and blood sugars every four to six hours (150 to 200 mg per 100 ml). Special care is required in patients treated with intravenous hyperalimentation before operation who have increased endogenous insulin capacity. The hypoglycemic response to hepatic resection may be prolonged and may require additional glucose support for two to three weeks.

Table 22–9. FIRST DAY ALBUMIN REQUIREMENTS FOLLOWING HEPATIC RESECTION

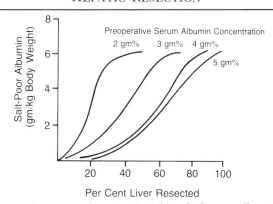

First day albumin requirements as based on initial level of serum albumin and percentage of liver substance resected.

Table 22–10. CONTINUED NEED FOR ALBUMIN REPLACEMENT
FOLLOWING HEPATIC RESECTION

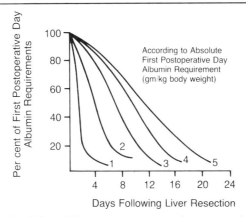

Predictability of the need to continue albumin supplements.

3. Hepatic resection causes decreased albumin production and hypoalbuminemia. In addition to blood transfusions and additional glucose, albumin must be given following hepatic resection. Table 22–9 provides a guideline for albumin requirements to maintain preoperative albumin levels and an adequate capillary osmotic pressure. Although patient response is variable, the 50 kg patient with a preoperative albumin of 3.0 gm per 100 ml who has a 50 per cent resection will require more than 250 gm of salt-poor albumin during the first postoperative day. The requirement for additional albumin may be prolonged, and the amount needed is often a function of early postoperative requirements (Table 22–10). Thus, the patient who required 250 gm of salt-poor albumin to maintain a preoperative level of 3.0 gm per 100 ml on the first postoperative day may require 150 gm on the eighth postoperative day.

In addition to treating the metabolic consequences of hepatic resection, maintenance of electrolyte balance, nutrition, and clotting factors is required. Dilutional hyponatremia and metabolic alkalosis often require sodium restriction and potassium supplementation.

Compulsive care of drains is required to minimize infection. Although no prospective randomized studies are available, most authorities use prophylactic antibiotics (cephalosporin) in patients requiring hepatic resection.

HEPATIC TRAUMA

The liver is the most frequently injured solid organ associated with blunt and penetrating trauma. Penetrating injuries of the abdomen present less of a diagnostic dilemma than blunt trauma because the majority of penetrating injuries are explored rapidly after stabilization of the patient.

Blunt trauma presents a greater diagnostic challenge, as the trend in recent years has been to observe such cases in hopes of decreasing the number of unnecessary negative laparotomies. Proponents of routine exploration following blunt trauma of the abdomen point out the increased morbidity associated with "waiting" when intra-abdominal injuries of the colon are involved.

Peritoneal lavage can minimize this "waiting" period while simultaneously decreasing the number of negative laparotomies. One thousand ml of balanced salt solution is introduced through an 18 gauge plastic catheter in the midline, 3 cm below the umbilicus, after the bladder is emptied with a Foley catheter. With this reservoir to minimize injury to viscera or major vascular structures, the 18 gauge catheter is withdrawn and a peritoneal dialysis catheter used to infuse an additional 1000 ml of salt solution within the abdominal cavity. The salt solution is then gravity drained and examined grossly and microscopically for red and white blood cells while amylase content is quantified. Gross blood, greater than 100,000 red blood cells per high-power field, greater than 500 white blood cells per high-power field, or an elevated amylase content are all generally considered indications for exploration. Exact numbers are less important than the visible appearance of blood in the lavage fluid.

Most hepatic injuries will cause hemoperitoneum but do not require hepatic resection. These are managed intraoperatively with simple drainage in combination with omental pack or suture ligation and present no unique problem to postoperative management. Ten per cent of liver injuries require some degree of hepatic resection and demand attention to maintenance of red blood cell volume, serum albumin, and glucose as described previously (under Hepatic Masses).

Injuries to the portal vein or hepatic artery may cause splenic sequestration or hepatic failure in the postoperative state. Sustained patency of repaired portal veins is very low, and sudden splanchnic sequestration in the postoperative period must be anticipated and blood volume must be replenished fully as required. Injury with or without repair of the hepatic artery is usually well tolerated but may be followed by some degree of hepatic decompensation.

The high mortality and morbidity rate associated with hepatic injury is often related to concomitant injuries of major vascular structures, the biliary tree, and hollow viscera. The hepatic mass has a tremendous regenerative capacity, and death secondary to hepatic failure after trauma is rare.

PORTAL HYPERTENSION

The three potential surgical problems that are sequelae of portal hypertension are (1) bleeding from gastroesophageal or ectopic varices, (2) massive ascites, and (3) hypersplenism.

BLEEDING VARICES: PREOPERATIVE DIAGNOSTIC EVALUATION

Upper gastrointestinal bleeding from gastroesophageal varices is a surgical diagnostic emergency, and endoscopy should be performed immediately to rule out gastritis, cancer, and peptic ulcer disease. Although history and physical examination will incriminate varices in patients with Laennec's cirrhosis, variceal bleeding may be unsuspected in patients with postnecrotic cirrhosis, chronic active hepatitis, extrahepatic portal vein thrombosis, schistosomiasis, and splenic vein thrombosis.

Once endoscopy determines that the upper gastrointestinal bleeding is from varices, all efforts should be made to stop the bleeding nonoperatively because of the severe mortality and morbidity that accompany emergency operations. Emergency operation should also be avoided in portal hypertensive patients bleeding from ectopic varices, which are most frequently found in previous operative sites, such as after appendectomy or previous pelvic surgery. Bleeding from ectopic varices usually presents as melena or massive hematochezia, mimicking diverticular bleeding. Preoperative diagnosis requires a high index of suspicion and can be made during the venous phase of the superior mesenteric arteriogram. Treatment of choice for ectopic varices, as in the case of gastroesophageal varices, depends upon the nature and location of the varices and the status of the general portal circulation.

The two goals of preoperative evaluation and preparation in patients bleeding from gastroesophageal varices are (1) stopping the bleeding in order to convert an emergency to a semiemergent or elective operation (resuscitation) and (2) quantifying and stabilizing the hepatic disease while improving nutritional status.

RESUSCITATION

Once the diagnosis of bleeding from gastroesophageal varices is made by endoscopy, the patient is admitted to an intensive care unit, a central venous pressure or Swan-Ganz pulmonary artery wedge catheter is placed in position, and a Foley catheter is used to measure urine output.

At this point, patients with bleeding varices can be divided into three categories: (1) patients who stop bleeding spontaneously, (2) patients who continue to bleed slowly, and (3) patients who continue to bleed massively with persistent hypotension and oliguria. Algorithm 3 (Table 22–11) presents the treatment plan for each group of patients.

Group 3 patients who continue to bleed massively upon admission to the intensive care unit fortunately represent the fewest number but unfortunately often have the more advanced hepatic disease with jaundice, ascites, and marked abnormalities in clotting factors. In this population of patients (Child's Class C), emergency shunt carries the highest mortality and morbidity, and an attempt should be made to stop bleeding promptly without operation.

Table 22–11. ALGORITHM 3.

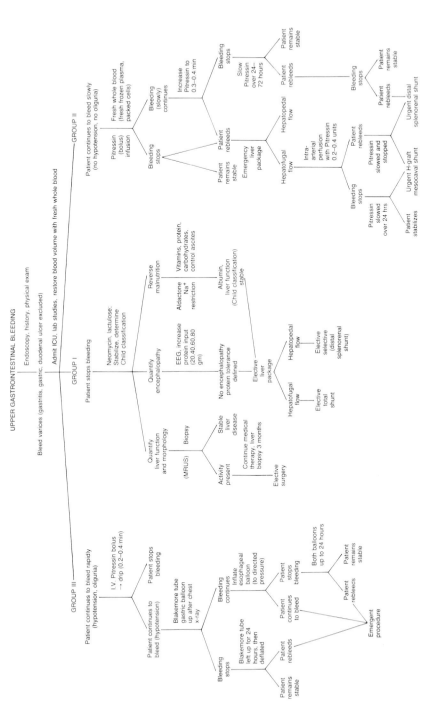

UPPER GASTROINTESTINAL BLEEDING

Endoscopy, history, physical exam

Bleed varices (gastritis, gastric, duodenal ulcer excluded)

Admit ICU, lab studies, restore blood volume with fresh whole blood

While volume is being replaced with fresh whole blood or packed cells and fresh frozen plasma, intravenous vasopressin (Pitressin) therapy is initiated, first in bolus form (20 units over 20 minutes), then as a constant infusion (0.2 to 0.4 units per minute in 5 per cent dextrose in water). Type-specific whole blood may be used while other blood is being cross-matched.

If the patient responds to intravenous Pitressin and bleeding stops or slows significantly, the Pitressin is continued and the patient becomes a Group 2 patient (see Algorithm 3). If bleeding with hypotension and oliguria continues in spite of intravenous Pitressin, a Blakemore tube is used. Although the Blakemore tube can be a life-saving device, it is a potentially lethal weapon and requires great care in placement.

The Blakemore tube is passed into the stomach through the nares, and proper placement is verified by injecting 50 ml of air while auscultating over the epigastrium. If the tip of the tube is in the stomach, 50 ml of air are used to inflate the gastric balloon partially, and a chest roentgenogram is taken immediately to verify balloon position. If the balloon is in the stomach, it is inflated with 300 to 500 ml of air and held with minimal tension against the gastroesophageal junction by fastening the proximal end of the tube to the facemask of a football helmet.

If the chest roentgenogram shows the partially inflated balloon above the gastroesophageal junction, the balloon is deflated, and the tip of the Blakemore tube is repositioned to lie within the stomach. A gastric balloon inflated with 500 ml of air inside the esophagus will tear the esophagus and cause mediastinitis and usually death.

Inflation of the gastric balloon will stop bleeding in many Group 3 patients. The tube is left inflated for 24 hours and then the tension is released. Most patients will remain stable, the tube is removed after 24 hours, and the patient is now considered to be in Group 1 or 2 (see Algorithm 3).

If inflation of the gastric balloon does not stop the bleeding, the esophageal balloon is inflated in series with a manometer to 15 to 40 mm Hg pressure.* A small (No. 12) nasogastric tube must be placed between the esophageal balloon and the esophagus wall to collect secretions. Inflation of the esophageal balloon will stop bleeding in most patients who fail to respond to the gastric balloon. If bleeding stops, the esophageal and gastric balloons are kept inflated for 24 and 30 hours, respectively. When the balloons are deflated, many patients will remain stable and be reclassified to Group 1 or 2 (see Algorithm 3). If bleeding remains brisk after inflation of both gastric and esophageal balloons, and hypotension and oliguria continue in spite of blood transfusions, emergency portasystemic decompression is required. The procedure of choice is usually mesocaval (Drapanas, 1972) or portacaval interposition

---

*Pressure will depend upon the design of the esophageal balloon and varies according to manufacturer's design. Follow the directions accompanying the double balloon tube.

H-graft shunt for three reasons: (1) Either procedure is technically feasible under emergency conditions, and operating time is short; (2) Ascites is usually prominent, and side-to-side total shunt ameliorates postoperative ascites; and (3) If severe postoperative encephalopathy occurs, the H-graft mesocaval or H-graft portacaval shunt can be closed easily and does not prohibit the construction of a selective shunt.

Whereas preoperative diagnosis, evaluation, and operation in Group 3 patients is compressed into a few hours, Group 2 patients, who continue to bleed slowly, usually undergo operation in a matter of days or weeks. The majority of Group 2 patients stop bleeding with either the bolus or infusion of Pitressin and are reclassified to Group 1 category (see Algorithm 3). If slow bleeding persists during intravenous Pitressin therapy and requires continued blood transfusions, emergency superior mesenteric arteriography is performed, and intra-arterial infusion of Pitressin is begun (0.2 to 0.4 units per minute). If the patient remains stable, venous phase studies are performed to determine the presence of hepatopetal or hepatofugal flow. If the patient has hepatopetal flow and remains stable, selective splenic arteriography with venous phase, left renal venography, and hepatic vein wedge pressure determination are performed to define anatomic eligibility for distal splenorenal shunt.

Most Group 2 patients will stop bleeding with either intravenous or intra-arterial Pitressin. If bleeding is controlled with Pitressin, the infusion is tapered over 48 hours, and the catheter is removed at the end of 36 hours. As with all chronic intra-arterial or intravenous catheters, meticulous care must be taken to minimize the chance of infection. Sudden resumption of bleeding during arterial perfusion usually means the catheter has slipped out of the superior mesenteric artery. Patients usually continue to pass stool during arterial infusion, and abdominal distention and absence of bowel sounds are usually due to ileus. The development of abdominal pain or tenderness requires that Pitressin infusion be slowed or stopped.

All Group 1 and 2 patients should have blood drawn for standard liver function studies and clotting parameters immediately upon their admission. Child classification (see Table 22–3) should be determined within 24 hours of admission. The prothrombin time and its response to administration of vitamin K and fresh frozen plasma is of special importance because, in nonjaundiced patients, its prolongation and failure to respond may be the only clues to the presence of alcoholic hepatitis. Neomycin and Lactulose are begun in Group 1 and 2 patients upon admission to decrease the pH of the colonic contents and lower the ammonia production in the enterohepatic circulation.

In patients who stabilize and stop bleeding within 24 hours of admission to the hospital, the resuscitative phase of the preoperative evaluation is complete. The second phase or goal has two aspects: (1) to quantify, stabilize, and improve hepatic function and encephalopathy and (2) to reverse malnutrition and control ascites.

QUANTIFICATION OF LIVER FUNCTION

Standard liver functions are valuable in initial evaluation of a patient with bleeding varices secondary to portal hypertension and can be used prognostically to predict the patient's response to shunt procedures. However, standard liver function tests are insufficient to evaluate stable patients who have recently bled and received transfusions. The maximal rate of urea synthesis (MRUS) (Rudman et al., 1973) is a quantitative study that measures the capacity of the hepatocyte mass to convert amino acid protein to urea and has been shown by Rudman to stratify further cirrhotic patients of Child's Class A and B. Cirrhotic patients with good MRUS have greater hepatic reserve and have a lower incidence of hepatic encephalopathy than patients with low MRUS.

Most physicians are unable to test the MRUS. This reinforces the need to plan elective surgery at the most opportune time, which may require several weeks or even months of careful medical management. For this reason, scrutiny of the preoperative liver biopsy is essential. In alcoholic patients and in patients with chronic hepatitis, marked activity represents a relative contraindication to surgery. Fortunately, abstinence from ethanol and improved nutrition will stabilize and reverse alcoholic hepatitis, and steroids and immunotherapy may improve chronic active hepatitis.

Hepatic encephalopathy is the most frequently forgotten preoperative sign in patients with cirrhosis, which probably reflects lack of a readily obtainable quantitative means of study. The problem is real, however, because treatment for hepatic encephalopathy with protein restriction can potentiate existing malnutrition and prevent or prolong improvement in Child's classification.

Patients with history or evidence of encephalopathy require electroencephalography as soon as possible after cessation of bleeding. If the EEG is normal while the patient receives a 20-gm protein diet, the diet may be increased slowly in 20-gm increments to 60 or 80 gm of protein per day as long as serial electroencephalograms remain normal. This regimen of titrating the patient's dietary protein against the electroencephalogram is safe because EEG abnormalities will be manifest before clinical symptoms develop (Parsons-Smith et al., 1957). Further, by giving a patient the best nutrition, progression to higher Child's classification is accelerated and patient compliance is improved.

CONTROL OF ASCITES

Increased protein content also makes dietary sodium restriction, required for control of ascites, more tolerable for the patient. Although the mechanism of ascites formation in cirrhotics is not completely understood, its control prior to and following operation is mandatory. Sodium is limited to 1 to 2 gm (44 to 88 mEq) in the diet, and spironolactone (Aldactone) alone or in combination with thiazides or "loop" diuretics (furosemide [Lasix]) usually will provide satisfactory natriuresis. It should be emphasized that gentle mobilization of ascites is preferred over rapid diuresis because hypovolemia and azotemia may predispose to the hepatorenal syndrome.

In some patients, however, ascites may be very resistant to standard diuretic regimens, and intermittent use of a "cocktail" composed of rapid intravenous infusion of 500 ml of plasma or 100 gm of salt-poor albumin followed by intravenous mannitol (50 gm) and Lasix (80 mg) usually promotes a rapid mobilization of salt and water. The diuresis is often followed by several days of relatively decreased effective plasma volume and oliguria while the patient reaches equilibrium. Care must be taken not to be overly aggressive with the "cocktail" at the expense of the glomerular filtration rate. Frequent determinations of blood urea nitrogen and creatinine clearance in conjunction with daily weights provide a simple method of monitoring ascites.

Although improvement of nutrition, quantification of encephalopathy, and control of ascites are important, the single most important preoperative test for determination of the operation of choice is visceral angiography. A prospective randomized study has shown that the most important deterrent to postoperative encephalopathy is preservation of hepatopetal flow. For this reason, if the venous phase of the preoperative superior mesenteric arteriogram or venous phase of the splenic arteriogram reveals hepatopetal flow, our procedure of choice is selective trans-splenic decompression (distal splenorenal shunt).

The presence of hepatofugal flow before surgery or nonvisualization of the portal vein during the venous phase studies is an indication for nonselective or total shunt. As stated before, side-to-side portasystemic (including H-graft) shunts have the advantage of protecting against postoperative ascites.

When it is determined which surgical procedure is indicated, final preparation for operation should include measures to insure effective plasma volume at induction of anesthesia and the use of prophylactic antibiotics and steroids. Although there is no prospective randomized study to prove the efficacy of prophylactic antibiotics in shunt surgery, extrapolation from peripheral vascular studies justifies starting cephalosporin before operation and continuing antibiotics for three days after operation. In the experimental animal, high-dose steroids (dexamethasone [Decadron] 3 mg per kg body weight per 24 hours) stabilizes hepatocyte lysosomes and may lessen the chance of postshunt hepatic failure. Decadron is administered before the operative procedure is begun and is discontinued 36 hours postoperatively.

POSTOPERATIVE CARE

Principles of postoperative care are based on a continuation of concepts utilized during the preoperative evaluation and preparation for operation. Cirrhosis is characterized by secondary aldosteronism, which is heightened by the traumatic response to injury. For this reason, sodium restriction is instituted at the beginning of operation while maintaining effective plasma with salt-poor albumin. Utilizing this regimen of 5 per cent dextrose in water (30 ml per kg body weight per 24 hours) and salt-poor albumin (2.0 gm salt-poor albumin per kg body weight per 24 hours) for the first five postoperative days minimizes development of ascites. Most patients are started on a full liquid diet (1 gm sodium, 40 gm protein) by the third postoperative day. Prolonged ileus is treated with patience and peripheral intravenous alimentation.

Aldactone (100 to 150 mg per 24 hours) is begun with the diet; no other medicines are used routinely except lactulose in patients who have poor protein tolerance and brittle encephalopathy before operation.

Ascites accumulation following distal splenorenal shunt is common but mild, and usually is no problem to the patient's management if the principles outlined previously are employed. The exception to this rule is chylous ascites. Approximately 5 per cent of patients treated by distal splenorenal shunt have developed persistent ascites characterized by high levels of triglycerides. Patients with chylous ascites are self-defined in the second or third postoperative week (or much later) with ascites that is refractory to aggressive diuretic therapy. In this situation, diagnostic paracentesis is performed, and if the ascitic fluid is milky-white, the patient is slowly drained of the ascites while effective circulating volume is concomitantly maintained with infusions of salt-poor albumin. Reaccumulation of chylous ascites may or may not occur. Treatment with a low fat diet supplemented with medium-chain triglycerides has been helpful in several patients. The LeVeen valve has also been utilized in a small number of patients and has been helpful.

Mild upper gastrointestinal bleeding is common in the immediate postoperative period after distal splenorenal shunt and may require additional blood transfusions. Endoscopy usually reveals gastritis, which may be related to the gastric devascularization accompanying the trans-splenic decompression procedure. Our prospective randomized study has shown that the recurrent variceal bleeding rate is no higher after distal splenorenal shunt than in patients treated by total shunt. The presence of varices after distal shunt reinforces the need for subsequent arteriography to document shunt patency in the immediate postoperative period.

Hypersplenism, characterized by leukopenia and thrombocytopenia, is common in patients with portal hypertension, but is incriminated infrequently as a source of bleeding. Splenectomy for hypersplenism in patients with portal hypertension is rarely if ever indicated and precludes distal splenorenal shunt.

SUMMARY

Preoperative evaluation and preparation of patients with surgical problems of the liver and portal vein require appreciation of the spectrum of disease processes that present as jaundice, hepatic mass, and upper gastrointestinal bleeding. The use of algorithms allows a logical approach to evaluation and preoperative preparation while minimizing errors of omission. Successful postoperative care incorporates the principles of preoperative preparation while anticipating the pathophysiologic changes elicited by the surgical procedure.

ACKNOWLEDGMENT   *The authors would like to acknowledge technical assistance from H. Harlan Stone, M.D.; R. B. Smith, III, M.D.; V. Watson; A. Watson; and P. D. Genovese, M.D.*

REFERENCES

Altemeier, W. A., Schowengerdt, C. G., and Whiteley, D. H.: Abscesses of the liver: Surgical considerations. Arch. Surg., 101:258, 1970.

Balasegaran, M.: Management of primary liver cell carcinoma. Am. J. Surg., 130:33, 1975.

Bradley, E. L., III, and Clements, J. L.: Implications of diagnostic ultrasound in the surgical management of pancreatic disease. Am. J. Surg., 127:163, 1974.

Drapanas, T.: Interposition mesocaval shunt for treatment of portal hypertension. Ann. Surg., 176(4):435, 1972.

Edmondson, H. A., Henderson, B., and Benton, B.: Liver cell adenomas associated with use of oral contraceptives. N. Engl. J. Med., 294(9):470, 1976.

Galambos, J. T.: Alcoholic hepatitis, its therapy and prognosis. In Popper, H., and Schaffner, F. (eds.): Progress in Liver Disease, Vol. IV. New York, Grune and Stratton, 1972, p. 567.

Mistilis, S. P., and Lam, K. C.: Treatment of chronic hepatitis. In Popper, H., and Schaffner, F. (eds.): Progress in Liver Disease, Vol. IV. New York, Grune and Stratton, 1972, p. 419.

Parsons-Smith, B. G., Summerskill, W. H. J., Dawson, A. M., et al.: The electroencephalogram in liver disease. Lancet, November 2, 1957.

Powell, S. J.: Latest developments in the treatment of amebiasis. Adv. Pharmacol. Chemother., 10:91, 1972.

Rudman, D., Fulco, T. J., Galambos, J. T., et al.: Maximal rate of excretion and synthesis of urea in normal and cirrhotic subjects. J. Clin. Invest., 52:2241, 1973.

Stone, H. H.: Pre- and post-operative care: Symposium on Hepatic Surgery. Surg. Clin. North Am., 57(2), 1977.

23

The Biliary Tract and Exocrine Pancreas

R. SCOTT JONES
WILLIAM C. MEYERS

In the past several years we have witnessed development of improved diagnostic methods, permitting increased accuracy of anatomic diagnosis in patients with biliary and pancreatic problems. The development of transhepatic cholangiography, endoscopic retrograde cholangiopancreatography, ultrasound scanning, and computerized axial tomography has permitted greater precision in the diagnosis of biliary and pancreatic disease.

In spite of these advances, there are numerous unsolved problems, particularly regarding the recognition and treatment of inflammatory and neoplastic disorders of the pancreas. There is a continuing need for improved clinical skills in the management of biliary disorders.

PREOPERATIVE CARE

Chronic Calculous Cholecystitis

A typical history of a patient with chronic calculous cholecystitis includes recurrent attacks of right upper quadrant abdominal pain usually associated with nausea. The pain may be referred to the tip of the scapula or to the right shoulder. A history of jaundice characterized by yellow skin or sclera, dark urine, light stools, or pruritus should be sought in a patient with symptoms of cholelithiasis. Physical examination is usually normal in patients with chronic calculous cholecystitis. Evaluation of the patient should include a hematocrit, leukocyte count with differential, and liver function tests consisting of serum bilirubin, alkaline phosphatase, GOT, GPT, cholesterol, and albumin concentrations. Ten per cent of patients with gallstones will have radiopaque stones demonstrable on plain roentgenograms of the abdomen.

Definitive diagnosis of cholelithiasis has generally been made by cholecystography following the oral administration of iopanoic acid (Telepaque) or tyropanoate sodium (Bilopaque) tablets. If the patient ingests the tablets, absorbs them, has a gallbladder, and liver excretory function is adequate, three general outcomes are possible. (1) The gallbladder may visualize and appear to be normal, a finding that usually excludes the diagnosis of cholelithiasis. (2) The gallbladder may visualize and contain radiolucent defects, confirming cholelithiasis, except in the rare patient with a tumor of the gallbladder. (3) If the gallbladder fails to visualize 10 to 15 hours following administration of the contrast agent, the procedure is repeated, and if subsequent examination fails to disclose a gallbladder, there is a 95 per cent probability that the patient has significant gallbladder disease, usually cholelithiasis. Recently, ultrasound examination has been added to the techniques for detecting gallstones. This test is particularly helpful in jaundiced patients or in those who have nonvisualizing gallbladders. Ultrasound is becoming very accurate in the diagnosis of gallstones. There are a small number of patients who have the typical symptoms of cholelithiasis but in whom gallstones are not demonstrable by oral cholecystography. Examination of fluid aspirated from the patient's duodenum following the intravenous administration of cholecystokinin to empty the gallbladder may yield evidence of cholesterol crystals, indicating that the patient has the underlying abnormality for the development of gallstones and may indeed have cholesterosis of the gallbladder or tiny stones in the gallbladder lumen. The finding of cholesterol crystals in biliary drainage has the same implication as the finding of gallstones.

Elective cholecystectomy is recommended for those patients who have gallstones, particularly if they experience pain attacks. Controversy exists regarding the surgical management of asymptomatic gallstones. We generally agree with those who favor elective cholecystectomy in patients, especially diabetics, with asymptomatic cholelithiasis unless there are prevailing factors that prevent safe, elective surgery. Recent studies demonstrate that the oral administration of chenodeoxycholic acid in human beings will increase biliary bile salt concentration and decrease biliary cholesterol concentration to permit dissolution of cholesterol gallstones. A large cooperative study evaluated scientifically the efficacy and safety of chenodeoxycholic acid in the treatment of gallstones. The drug is safe and dissolved stones in 15 per cent of patients treated.

Since gallstones are extremely common in our population (8 per cent incidence in the Framingham study), it is possible that a patient could have gallstones concomitant with another serious disorder. The surgeon should consider the possibility of coexisting diseases, such as peptic ulcer, carcinoma of the pancreas, and other abdominal problems, when evaluating patients with cholelithiasis.

ACUTE CHOLECYSTITIS

Typically the patient with acute cholecystitis complains of severe right upper quadrant abdominal pain, frequently with radiation to the tip of the right scapula or shoulder. Nausea often accompanies the pain and may be followed by vomiting. Right upper quadrant abdominal tenderness and in some cases guarding and rebound tenderness are generally elicited during physical examination. The gallbladder may be palpable in advanced cases. The differential diagnosis of acute cholecystitis includes acute pancreatitis, acute peptic ulcer with penetration or perforation, pneumonia, hepatitis, and urinary tract infection. Following a complete history and physical examination, hematocrit, leukocyte count with differential, serum electrolyte measurements, EKG, liver function tests, and serum amylase determinations are carried out in addition to blood type and crossmatch. A specimen for urinalysis should be collected immediately and two hours later for urinary amylase determination. The remainder of the preliminary work-up should include roentgenographic examinations of the abdomen and chest. Plain films of the abdomen may be very helpful in aiding detection of radiopaque gallstones and/or gas in the biliary system or gallbladder. Interstitial gas in the region of the gallbladder suggests the diagnosis of emphysematous cholecystitis. Previous documentation of gallstones simplifies the diagnostic work-up and management of the patient.

Because ultrasound examination is safe and rapid, it is being employed with increasing frequency in patients with acute cholecystitis and has proved very helpful in this instance. In addition, the HIDA scan is an extremely helpful test in evaluating patients suspected of having acute cholecystitis. The HIDA scan is safe, rapid, and effective, supporting or refuting the diagnosis of acute cholecystitis in over 95 per cent of cases.

The management of the patient with acute cholecystitis depends to some extent upon when in the course of the illness he or she is evaluated and also the progression and severity of the disease. For example, many patients with gallstones may have episodes of severe right upper quadrant pain, nausea, and vomiting, which subside spontaneously after a period of a few hours. They may not develop fever, signs of peritonitis, or leukocytosis. In such instances, the cholelithiasis should be documented, and arrangements should be made for elective definitive management of their disease. Other patients, however, may progress from the syndrome of simple biliary colic to develop fever, leukocytosis, direct and rebound tenderness, and guarding. Such patients are best managed by a regimen including nasogastric suction to relieve vomiting, restoration of fluid and electrolyte balance, administration of antibiotics, and early scheduled cholecystectomy. If such a patient has elevated serum and urinary levels of amylase, the differential diagnosis between acute cholecystitis and acute pancreatitis becomes a problem, and, in general, operation is deferred as long as the values are returning to normal and other clinical parameters are improving. Elderly patients with acute cholecystitis may have minimal clinical findings despite severe gallbladder abnormalities. They, of course, require additional preoperative and postoperative attention to cardiac, renal, and pulmonary disorders when they exist.

Although acute cholecystitis is associated with a 95 per cent incidence of gallstones impacted in the cystic duct, the disorder can develop in the absence of gallstones. Acalculous cholecystitis characteristically occurs following major surgical procedures or severe trauma, and in some series the mortality rate associated with this disorder approaches 50 per cent. The diagnosis is frequently difficult to make because the disease develops in patients with coexisting complicated problems. Cholecystitis should be suspected in any patient who develops right upper quadrant pain, tenderness, and guarding after prolonged fasting, numerous blood transfusions, major surgery, or trauma.

The patient with sickle cell anemia may present special clinical problems in diagnosis and management. Signs and symptoms simulating cholecystitis with upper abdominal pain, nausea, vomiting, fever, and leukocytosis may occur with sickle cell crisis. Jaundice may also occur with sickle cell crisis and with acute cholecystitis. If the jaundice is due to hemolysis, oral cholecystography may still provide helpful information. If the diagnosis is acute cholecystitis and surgical treatment is planned, preoperative exchange transfusion to reduce the proportion of hemoglobin S is recommended by some authorities. Before elective cholecystectomy, hypertransfusion begun several weeks before surgery is generally recommended. Transfusion to a normal hematocrit can be harmful because the increased blood viscosity may increase the possibility of vascular thrombosis. Other precautions to consider when operating upon patients with sickle cell anemia include avoidance of hypoxia, acidosis, hypothermia, stasis, and dehydration.

As part of the preoperative preparation of a patient with acute cholecystitis, the surgeon should make arrangements to perform intraoperative cholangiography, particularly if there have been elevations of amylase, bilirubin, or alkaline phosphatase. The incidence of common duct stones in patients with acute cholecystitis is approximately 15 per cent, and choledocholithiasis should be diagnosed definitively at the time of cholecystectomy. The majority of patients with acute cholecystitis who are operated upon can be managed most effectively by cholecystectomy. Cholecystostomy should be considered in those cases in which marked inflammatory changes around the gallbladder prevent recognition of adjacent structures or in patients who have other severe diseases accompanying the acute cholecystitis.

SUPPURATIVE CHOLANGITIS

The syndrome of abdominal pain, right upper quadrant tenderness, jaundice, fever, and chills suggests the diagnosis of suppurative cholangitis. If this condition progresses, the patient usually experiences bacteremia, hypotension, tachycardia, oliguria, and profound shock. Suppurative cholangitis only occurs with obstruction of the bile ducts. The most common causes of obstruction leading to cholangitis are gallstones and biliary stricture. In some cases it may be difficult, if not impossible, to differentiate between the findings accompanying empyema of the gallbladder and acute suppurative cholangitis. Any patient who develops acute suppurative cholangitis should receive prompt and vigorous resuscitation with intravenous fluids and administration of gentamicin and clindamycin or other appropriate combinations of antibiotics. Parenteral administration of vitamin K or fresh frozen plasma is often indicated to correct a prolonged prothrombin time. When the patient's hypotension, tachycardia, and oliguria have been reversed or corrected, urgent operation is indicated because suppurative cholangitis cannot be treated optimally by conservative means alone. The basis for successful management of suppurative cholangitis is prompt relief of biliary obstruction. Percutaneous transhepatic cannulation of the obstructed bile ducts will often decompress the ducts enough to permit control of cholecystitis and to allow operation to be done electively at a later time. Transhepatic intubation may be very important, especially in elderly poor-risk patients. In addition, endoscopic papillotomy with extraction of common duct stones may be life-saving in elderly patients with septic cholangitis due to common duct stones.

JAUNDICE

Hemolysis, hepatocellular disease, or bile duct obstruction may cause jaundice. The principal objective of the surgeon in evaluating a jaundiced patient is to determine the existence of extrahepatic obstruction. The history frequently is very important in this assessment. Unrelenting jaundice with the absence of chills and fever strongly suggests a malignant neoplasm. Intermittent jaundice, particularly with chills and fever, suggests choledocholithiasis or biliary stricture. The tumors that commonly produce obstructive jaundice are carcinoma of the head of the pancreas, carcinoma of the ampulla of Vater, and carcinoma of the bile ducts. During physical examination of a patient with jaundice, one should pay particular attention to the presence of surgical scars, indicating that prior operations have been performed. In addition, the presence of abdominal masses may indicate the presence of a neoplasm, and one occasionally can palpate a carcinoma of the pancreas. Moreover, the classic finding of a distended gallbladder in the presence of jaundice (Courvoisier's sign) is important. Palpable masses in the liver suggest primary or metastatic liver tumors. Occult blood in the stool has been found in 75 per cent of jaundiced patients with carcinoma of the ampulla of Vater on multiple testing.

In general, most patients with jaundice, particularly those whose liver function tests suggest obstruction, will require roentgenographic evaluation. Plain films of the abdomen may disclose gallstones or soft tissue masses. An upper GI series may reveal evidence of enlargement of the head of the pancreas by inflammation or tumor. An intraluminal mass seen in the second portion of the duodenum is strongly suggestive of carcinoma of the ampulla of Vater. All patients with occult blood in the stool and evidence of a mass in the second portion of the duodenum on upper GI series should have duodenoscopy because preoperative endoscopic biopsy confirmation of carcinoma of the ampulla of Vater greatly facilitates the intraoperative management of such a lesion. Liver scans may help in evaluating jaundiced patients, particularly if there is a filling defect suggesting either neoplasm or abscess.

Upper abdominal ultrasound examination is a helpful, noninvasive method of initial evaluation of jaundiced patients (Fig. 23–1). In addition to providing evidence of cholelithiasis, ultrasonography may indicate dilated bile ducts. If there is ultrasound evidence of dilated intrahepatic ducts and other studies support biliary obstruction, one should proceed either to Chiba ("skinny") needle percutaneous transhepatic cholangiography (PTC) or to endoscopic retrograde cholangiopancreatography (ERCP). The choice between these two techniques is determined by several factors, and guidelines are still being established as experience with these techniques continues to improve (Table 23–1). In general, if one suspects an abnormality of the terminal bile duct or desires information about the pancreatic ducts, ERCP is the more appropriate procedure

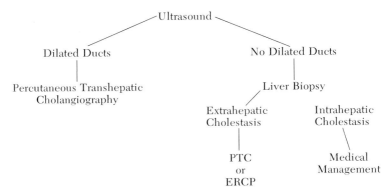

Figure 23–1. Use of ultrasound for diagnosis of jaundice. Ultrasound may be used as a screening technique for the diagnosis of jaundice. This diagram is a general scheme for utilization of ultrasound for jaundiced patients.

Table 23–1. GUIDELINES FOR USE OF TRANSHEPATIC
VERSUS RETROGRADE CHOLANGIOGRAPHY

PTC	ERCP
Roux-Y limb	Impaired hemostasis
Inexperienced endoscopist	Postoperative jaundice
Acute pancreatitis	Gallbladder nonvisualization
History of biliary tract surgery	Sepsis
Probable extrahepatic cholestasis	Necessary to define distal common duct lesion
	Primary pancreatic problem
	Endoscopy of stomach and duodenum also indicated
	Probable intrahepatic cholestasis

Percutaneous transhepatic cholangiography (PTC) and endoscopic retrograde cholangiopancreatography (ERCP) are useful and often complementary procedures for the evaluation of jaundiced patients. Utilization of either depends to a large degree upon available expertise. Above are some general guidelines concerning initial selection of one procedure over the other when jaundice is present. PTC is technically easier in the patient with a Roux-Y limb or Billroth II gastrectomy. Some authorities feel that ERCP is contraindicated in acute pancreatitis. PTC generally is more likely to be successful when extrahepatic biliary obstruction exists. ERCP, on the other hand, is generally preferred when impaired hemostasis or infection exist, for distal common duct or nonacute pancreatic pathology, or with nondilated biliary radicles.

to use. If there has been prior biliary surgery and stricture is the likely diagnosis, then transhepatic cholangiography is preferable as the initial invasive procedure. If there are no dilated ducts indicated on ultrasound examination, percutaneous needle biopsy of the liver may be the most helpful next test. Biopsy with the Menghini needle has been demonstrated to be safe and reliable and may reveal evidence of hepatitis or intrahepatic cholestasis. If, on the other hand, liver biopsy reveals evidence of bile plugs, ductal dilatation, or cholangitis, cholangiography with a Chiba needle or ERCP should again be considered. Clearly, all patients do not require all of these studies. For example, an elderly patient with a persistent serum bilirubin level in the range of 25 mg per ml and with a palpable gallbladder could be handled satisfactorily by early laparotomy to establish the diagnosis.

Before operating upon a patient with obstructive jaundice, it is important to correct nutritional deficits and anemia and to be certain that prothrombin and partial thromboplastin times are normal to avoid hemorrhagic complications.

CANCER OF THE BILIARY SYSTEM

Ductal cancers occur infrequently relative to the prevalent incidence of cancer of the pancreas and may occur in any portion of the ductal system. The principal sign of bile duct malignancy is jaundice. The anatomic site of the tumor is usually established by either ERCP or

PTC. Because the diagnosis may be difficult both from the anatomic and pathologic standpoints, many patients with such tumors may have had one or more operations before the diagnosis is established. Cancers near the confluence of the right and left hepatic ducts are particularly difficult to recognize and should be suspected in any patient who has a normal or small common bile duct at laparotomy for obstructive jaundice. Excision of proximal bile duct cancers is the best treatment and should be done if possible. In most cases significant palliation may be obtained by inserting a tube stent through the tumor. Cancers of the distal portion of the extrahepatic ductal system are managed best by excision. Pancreatico-duodenectomy when possible offers the best chance for cure.

Cancer of the ampulla of Vater can be diagnosed by endoscopy (see Jaundice). Pancreaticoduodenectomy offers the best chance for cure in such cases.

Cancer of the gallbladder is not often diagnosed preoperatively and is usually discovered as a cause of obstructive jaundice at laparotomy. Occasionally cancer of the gallbladder is discovered coincidentally during cholecystectomy for cholelithiasis.

CHRONIC PANCREATITIS

Chronic pancreatitis can produce several syndromes. One syndrome, sometimes referred to as chronic relapsing pancreatitis, is characterized by intermittent episodes of acute pancreatitis with relatively normal intervening periods. A diagnosis that should be considered in patients with such a syndrome is cholelithiasis, because in the majority of such cases, cholecystectomy will prevent further attacks. In other cases of relapsing pancreatitis, specific etiologies cannot always be determined; however, the condition may be associated with metabolic abnormalities such as hyperparathyroidism or aminoaciduria.

The most common syndrome of chronic pancreatitis is characterized by chronic unrelenting abdominal pain. This illness is most commonly due to chronic alcoholism, although it may be idiopathic. Typical symptoms include severe upper abdominal pain radiating to the back, and as the disease progresses, symptoms of pancreatic endocrine insufficiency become manifest by hyperglycemia and glycosuria. Pancreatic exocrine insufficiency causes steatorrhea and weight loss. Plain roentgenograms of the abdomen in patients with chronic pancreatitis often disclose pancreatic calcifications. Barium studies may reveal deformity of the stomach or duodenum. Most patients with chronic pancreatitis are best managed conservatively with enzyme replacement, low-fat diet, hypoglycemic agents, and analgesics. A few patients cannot be handled satisfactorily in this manner and may require a surgical procedure. Retrograde endoscopic pancreatography may be helpful in assessing the status of the pancreatic ducts. If the duct of Wirsung is dilated, palliation of pain can be often achieved by providing drainage of the dilated ductal system. Pancreaticojejunostomy has the advantage that it may relieve pain without interfering further with pancreatic function. In the preoperative preparation, particular attention must be directed toward correction of malnutrition, if present, by administration of supplemental enzymes or in some cases by intravenous hyperalimentation.

ACUTE PANCREATITIS

One of the initial preoperative problems in the patient with acute pancreatitis is establishing the diagnosis. The classic syndrome of acute pancreatitis follows ingestion of alcohol, and the syndrome is characterized by severe abdominal pain radiating to the back, nausea, vomiting, and signs of paralytic ileus. Physical findings include tenderness, guarding, and in many cases the presence of an upper abdominal mass. The differential diagnosis includes acute cholecystitis, perforated ulcer, and strangulated small bowel obstruction. The laboratory tests that help establish a diagnosis of pancreatitis include elevated levels of serum and urinary amylase. Although elevated amylase concentrations may occur in cholelithiasis, perforated ulcer, and strangulated obstruction, the levels are usually higher in acute pancreatitis. The patients with acute pancreatitis may also exhibit hypocalcemia, hyperlipidemia, roentgenographic evidence of a retrogastric mass, enlargement of the head of the pancreas, and edema of the second portion of the duodenum. Absence of intestinal obstruction also helps to corroborate the diagnosis. Other concurrent radiographic findings include left pleural effusion and unilateral or bilateral pulmonary infiltrates.

The principles in the management of acute pancreatitis consist of nasogastric suction and administration of intravenous fluids. Many patients require large volumes of water to replace losses into the pancreas, the retroperitoneal area, and peritoneal cavity. Vital signs, urinary output, central venous pressure, hematocrit, arterial blood gases, plain abdominal and chest roentgenograms, electrolytes, and serum calcium should be carefully monitored. The relief of pain by large doses of narcotics or, in some cases, by epidural anesthesia improves the patient's comfort and pulmonary ventilation. One prospective randomized trial has indicated that antibiotics are not effective in altering the natural history of pancreatitis. However, the cases in that study were relatively mild. We generally do not employ antibiotics initially; however, if the patient exhibits fever, a rising white blood cell count, or a positive blood culture, we administer appropriate antibiotics.

Since most patients with acute pancreatitis can be managed satisfactorily with conservative measures, we have generally favored that approach. Whether and when to operate on patients with acute pancreatitis remains a topic of controversy. One indication for operation is diagnostic uncertainty. Surgical intervention should also be contemplated if there is evidence of peripancreatic infection or if common duct stones are suspected. Peritoneal lavage has been demonstrated to prolong survival of dogs with acute pancreatitis in the laboratory. However, whether or not lavage alters morbidity and mortality of human patients is uncertain. Factors that have been shown to be of prognostic significance at the time of hospitalization in patients with acute pancreatitis are age greater than 55 years, blood glucose level greater than 200 mg per ml, lactate dehydrogenase (LDH) greater than 350 IU per liter, serum glutamic-oxyloacetic transaminase (SGOT) greater than 250 units, or white blood cell count greater than 16,000. During the initial 48 hours, a BUN increase greater than 5 per cent, hematocrit decrease greater than 10 per cent, serum calcium level less than 8 mg per ml, base excess greater than 4 mEq per liter, or fluid sequestration greater than 6 liters are important indices. Patients with five or more of the preceding factors have a greater than 50 per cent mortality.

PANCREATIC ABSCESS

Approximately 10 per cent of patients experiencing an attack of acute pancreatitis develop a major pancreatic infection. Such a diagnosis is indicated by high fever, leukocytosis, and positive blood cultures with radiographic and ultrasound evidence of a pancreatic mass. Surgical exploration is mandatory treatment of this complication, with débridement of devitalized tissue and establishment of wide drainage of retroperitoneal area with Penrose drains as well as sump drains. There is evidence to suggest that laparotomy early in the course of acute pancreatitis may foster the development of a major pancreatic infection, which is one reason that careful judgment must be employed in planning operations on patients with acute pancreatitis.

PSEUDOCYSTS

The most common cause of a pancreatic pseudocyst is acute alcoholic pancreatitis. A recent study demonstrated that about one-half of patients with acute pancreatitis develop ultrasound evidence of a pancreatic pseudocyst with spontaneous resolution of a large number of such pseudocysts. If a pseudocyst develops, it is generally preferable to treat the patient conservatively until such time as further decrease in size of the pseudocyst cannot be documented by either physical or ultrasound examination. A period of several weeks' observation is usually required for this determination. If a patient has a persistent cyst, a palpable abdominal mass, unrelenting pain, and consistently elevated amylase levels, the pseudocyst should be treated operatively, preferably by internal drainage.

Cancer of the Pancreas

Most patients with cancer of the head of the pancreas develop obstructive jaundice, a symptom that leads to the diagnosis (see Jaundice). Most patients with cancer of the head of the pancreas are operated upon to establish the diagnosis, to relieve the jaundice, and, in infrequent cases, to remove the tumor. Many patients with cancer of the head of the pancreas experience great weight loss, which may be due to anorexia with decreased caloric intake or possibly to malabsorption resulting from obstructed bile and pancreatic ducts. If a patient with marked weight loss exhibits hypoproteinemia, anemia, or anergy to skin tests, a period of enteral or parenteral nourishment should precede operation, particularly if a major resection is contemplated.

Carcinoma of the body or tail of the pancreas is a difficult diagnosis to establish. The patients usually experience upper abdominal pain with radiation to the back and weight loss. Plain abdominal roentgenograms are rarely helpful. In some advanced cases, invasion of the third or fourth portion of the duodenum will be noted on upper GI series. Selective superior mesenteric and celiac arteriography is frequently helpful in the diagnosis of cancer of the body of the pancreas when it reveals cuffing or narrowing of peripancreatic arteries. Computerized axial tomography promises to be helpful in diagnosing pancreatic cancer. Percutaneous fine-needle aspiration of the pancreas for cytodiagnosis is safe and may permit a preoperative diagnosis of pancreatic cancer in many cases.

POSTOPERATIVE CARE

Cholecystectomy

In general, most patients undergoing cholecystectomy will not require a nasogastric tube for more than one day, if at all. Oral intake, however, should be withheld until there is evidence of return of intestinal function manifested by passage of flatus. The patient should be out of bed on the first postoperative day primarily to improve pulmonary ventilation. One of the frequent complications of cholecystectomy is right lower lobe atelectasis. This can be minimized by postoperative physical therapy or optimally by early ambulation. On the day of operation, the patient should be monitored carefully for evidence of postoperative hemorrhage. This can be done best by hematocrit determination, careful recording of the patient's vital signs, and inspection for wound drainage. For the first 24 hours postoperatively, the patient should receive intravenous fluids and by the second day should be able to take fluids by mouth. It is common to insert Penrose drains into the gallbladder fossa following cholecystectomy. When drainage decreases, drains should be advanced daily until they have been removed after about the third advancement. Some surgeons do not use drains following simple and uncomplicated cholecystectomy.

OPERATIONS ON THE BILE DUCTS

Following common duct exploration, most surgeons insert a T tube. The T tube inserted after choledochotomy for common duct stones may be managed by dependent drainage until the drainage around the Penrose drains ceases. Then the T tube may be clamped, usually on the third to the fifth postoperative day. In general, a postoperative T tube cholangiogram is performed on the seventh to tenth postoperative day, and if such an examination is normal we will remove the T tube between the tenth and the fourteenth postoperative days. There are circumstances in which it may be desirable to leave the T tube for longer periods of time. For example, if a repair of a common duct abnormality has been carried out, most surgeons favor leaving the tube for several weeks longer. If the postoperative cholangiogram is equivocal, one may choose to leave the T tube in place when the patient is discharged and repeat the study at a subsequent time. It is generally our practice to administer systemic antibiotics before and one day following the T tube cholangiogram to minimize the possibility of cholangitis and bacteremia. Usually the Penrose drains inserted following choledochotomy can be managed in a manner similar to that following uncomplicated cholecystectomy. Occasionally, patients will have tubes inserted into the biliary system that are intended to remain for a long period of time, for the management of strictures and tumors. These tubes are best managed by careful wound hygiene and daily tube irrigation.

POSTOPERATIVE BILIARY FISTULA

Although copious bile drainage from Penrose drains following operations on the common bile duct only occasionally occurs, it is a disconcerting problem. Large volumes of bile can drain through needle holes and between sutures in the bile duct. If there are no other symptoms, conservative management and observation should be employed. In most cases, such biliary drainage is not due to serious mechanical problems. However, following a presumed simple cholecystectomy, large drainage of bile from the wound has ominous implications, and this may mean gross leakage from the cystic duct. It is possible that a small bile duct may have been transected and not recognized. Large volumes of bile emanating from the drain site may also result from an unrecognized common duct injury. This complication should also be managed conservatively, particularly if the patient does not develop jaundice and if there is no evidence of infection. Cholangiography may help in the evaluation of bile leakage.

Jaundice

The development of jaundice following a biliary operation is likewise a troublesome sign. Occasionally patients have coexisting hepatocellular disease, and this may be aggravated by the surgical procedure. In the absence of documented hepatocellular disease or extensive intraoperative blood transfusion, one must assume that postoperative jaundice is due to extrahepatic obstruction, particularly if the jaundice is associated with elevated serum alkaline phosphatase levels. With rising serum bilirubin and alkaline phosphatase concentrations, one must establish whether an obstruction exists and then provide satisfactory drainage of bile, preferably into the alimentary tract to prevent cholangitis, liver damage, or both.

Retained Common Duct Stones

Retained common duct stones following common duct exploration for cholelithiasis may occur in 3 to 5 per cent of cases. Obviously the best approach to this problem is careful common duct exploration and meticulous evaluation of the duct by intraoperative cholangiography to avoid missing common duct stones. However, recognition of the retained common duct stone and its management require careful judgment. In general, if a retained common duct stone is recognized, particularly if it is distal to the T tube, nothing should be done for four to six weeks to permit a satisfactory fibrous tract to develop between the skin and the common duct around the T tube. Also, with the T tube clamped and bile flowing through the distal bile duct, there is a possibility that a small stone may pass spontaneously into the duodenum. The tube should remain clamped provided the patient does not develop pain, fever, or jaundice. Fortunately, greater than 90 per cent of retained stones can be removed with a Dormia stone basket passed via the T tube tract. Patients in whom the stone cannot be retrieved by basket extraction generally require a second surgical procedure.

Pancreatic Operations

In the majority of cases, a pancreatic fistula will close spontaneously. However, until such closure occurs, there are several problems that require attention. High-output pancreatic fistulas may cause serious nutritional problems. If the external drainage of pancreatic secretion is sufficient to deprive the duodenum of normal pancreatic enzyme concentrations, maldigestion and malabsorption can occur. In addition, pancreatic juice contains a large amount of protein in the form of pancreatic enzymes. External losses of protein may contribute significantly to the patient's malnutrition. Intravenous hyperalimentation minimizes the effects of malabsorption, restores body protein, and also permits decreased pancreatic secretion, thereby reducing further protein loss. Water and bicarbonate losses are easily corrected by intravenous therapy.

The skin irritation of patients with pure pancreatic fistulas is fortunately largely due to severe skin maceration and not skin digestion. The trypsinogen is generally not activated because it does not come into contact with duodenal or jejunal mucosa, where the activating enzyme enterokinase is secreted. However, when proximal small intestinal fistulas occur and trypsinogen does become activated, skin digestion becomes a serious problem. In recent years, the techniques for application of karaya-seal appliances have improved greatly the nursing care of patients with external pancreatic and intestinal fistulas. These appliances usually permit adequate collection of the drainage, sparing the skin of the devastating effects of activated digestive enzymes. Sump drains also can be adapted to these appliances to facilitate drainage.

The total or near total diversion of pancreatic juice from the duodenum is an ulcerogenic problem because alkalinization of the duodenum by the pancreas is important in preventing duodenal ulcerations. Therefore, patients with large-volume external pancreatic fistulas should be regarded as being at risk for the development of acute peptic ulcer, and measures should be taken to reduce acid secretion from the stomach.

Adequate drainage of chronic pancreatic fistulas must be maintained in order to prevent infection. Premature cutaneous closure of the fistula tract can be prevented by maintaining a rubber tube in the opening of the fistula.

HEMORRHAGE

Because of the abundant and multiple sources of blood supply to the pancreas and to the retroperitoneal area, one of the frequent complications of pancreatic surgery is postoperative hemorrhage. This occurs most frequently in the presence of pancreatic fistula or peripancreatic infection. When hemorrhage occurs following pancreatic operations, it often requires urgent laparotomy with careful suture of the bleeding areas with nonabsorbable sutures. Bleeding from a pancreatic pseudocyst usually necessitates external drainage of the cyst in addition to careful suture of the bleeding point.

DIABETES

Diabetes occurring following pancreatic surgery is normally due to inadequate insulin secretion and usually requires exogenous insulin for control. About two-thirds of patients undergoing 80 to 95 per cent pancreatectomy become insulin-dependent diabetics. The insulin requirement varies considerably, but generally the postpancreatectomy diabetic requires less insulin than a juvenile onset diabetic. Insulin requirements, which may initially be about 20 units per day, often increase slightly in the months following pancreatectomy, perhaps due to scarring or progressive disease in the remnant of the gland. The chronic pancreatitis patient is especially prone to hypoglycemic attacks because of unpredictability of dietary starch absorption, other dietary factors, and fluctuating insulin requirements. Diabetic ketoacidosis is relatively unusual. Moderate to high carbohydrate ingestion, therefore, is frequently indicated.

Exocrine Insufficiency

Pancreatic exocrine insufficiency occurs more often after pancreatic duodenectomy than after distal pancreatic resection owing to more severely altered pancreatic secretory mechanisms. Management requires unpredictably large quantities of pancreatic enzyme supplements such as pancrelipase (Cotazym) or pancreatin (Viokase) along with antacids to minimize destruction of the lipase. Most patients respond to between 4 and 12 gm of enzyme taken in divided doses one hour before and with each meal. Patients may continue to lose weight for a variety of reasons, including poor patient cooperation and inactivation of lipase in the duodenum. Dietary supplementation with medium-chain triglycerides (MCT) may be tried. MCT is prepared commercially from coconut oil and has several absorptive advantages over the usual delivery long-chain triglycerides.

CONCLUSION

Preoperative and postoperative care of patients with diseases of the biliary tract and pancreas vary considerably depending on the underlying diagnosis, urgency of the condition, and presence or absence of complicating factors. A general approach to some of the more common problems has been presented in this chapter.

REFERENCES

Carey, L. C. (ed.): The Pancreas. St. Louis, The C. V. Mosby Co., 1953, pp. 153–240.
Conn, H., Redeker, A., and Zimmon, D.: Editorial: ERCP vs PTC. Gastroenterology, 71(3):520, 1976.
Flye, M. W., and Silver, D.: Biliary tract disorders and sickle cell disease. Surgery, 72:361, 1972.

Hinshaw, D. B.: Acute obstructive suppurative cholangitis. Surg. Clin. North Am., 53(5):1089, 1973.

Ottinger, L. W.: Acute cholecystitis in the postoperative period. Ann. Surg., 184:162, 1976.

Ranson, J. H. C., Rifkind, M., and Turner, J. W.: Prognostic signs and nonoperative peritoneal lavage in acute pancreatitis. Surg. Gynecol. Obstet., 143:209, 1976.

Way, L. W., and Dunphy, J. E.: Biliary tract. In Dunphy, J. E., and Way, L. W. (eds.): Current Surgical Diagnosis and Treatment, 3rd ed. Los Altos, Lange, 1977, p. 525.

Wenckert, A., and Robertson, B.: The natural course of gallstone disease. Gastroenterology, 50:376, 1966.

Winship, D.: Clinical conference on pancreatitis: Pancreatic pseudocysts and their complications. Gastroenterology, 73(3):593, 1977.

Zimmerman, M. J.: The differential diagnosis of jaundice. Med. Clin. North Am., 52(6):1417, 1968.

24

The Small Intestine

M. D. TILSON
H. K. WRIGHT

Emergency operations on the small intestine are usually undertaken for one or more of the following reasons: obstruction, perforation, bleeding, or infarction. Elective operations on the small intestine are performed based on a variety of indications, including complications of Crohn's disease, radiation enteritis, tumors, and morbid obesity. General considerations in postoperative management, such as intravenous fluid therapy and gastrointestinal decompression during paralytic ileus, will be discussed in this chapter, as well as complex problems following small intestinal surgery, such as fistulization, short-gut syndrome, and blind loop syndrome.

PREOPERATIVE CONSIDERATIONS WITH EMERGENCY INDICATIONS FOR SURGERY

INTESTINAL OBSTRUCTION

Most obstructions of the small intestine in the adult are caused by either adhesions or hernias. Adhesions and hernias are also the most frequent causes of obstructions that progress to strangulation or gangrene of the involved intestine. Other causes of intestinal obstruction include Crohn's disease, intussusception, volvulus, foreign bodies, gallstones (as in gallstone ileus), tumors, and other inflammatory disorders. Paralytic ileus may simulate mechanical intestinal obstruction with vomiting and distention. However, the characteristic radiologic finding in ileus (air throughout the entire gastrointestinal tract) and the absence of bowel sounds on abdominal auscultation, as well as the clinical history, should make the proper diagnosis evident.

Presently, the major cause of mortality in patients with intestinal obstruction is delay in the diagnosis of strangulation, followed by

459

secondary sepsis. Death from dehydration should be avoided in the present era of fluid and electrolyte management, and death from aspiration pneumonitis is usually avoided by early gastrointestinal intubation and decompression. Nevertheless, respiratory complications and fluid imbalances are always potential hazards and will be discussed in some detail.

Early Diagnosis

Patients with proximal jejunal obstruction present with nausea, copious vomiting, and epigastric pain. Distention may be minimal. Patients with more distal obstruction present with nausea, vomiting (which may become feculent as bacteria proliferate in the lumen), colic (spasmodic crampy pain occurring every few minutes as the obstructed bowel attempts to propel its contents past the obstruction), and progressive distention of the abdomen. Bowel sounds are hyperactive early in the course of obstruction, but the passage of stool and flatus ceases.

Flat and upright roentgenograms of the abdomen should be obtained promptly if obstruction is suspected. The findings are usually characteristic: The bowel is distended and shows air fluid levels, but there is usually no air in the colon unless sigmoidoscopy has been performed. Some surgeons find it helpful to instill some contrast material through the nasogastric tube to delineate the obstruction, but in general such a study can be avoided in most patients unless it is particularly important to rule out paralytic ileus. Occasionally a barium enema is helpful in the adult to rule out obstruction of the colon (after a distal lesion has been excluded by sigmoidoscopy). Plain films of the abdomen are not helpful in ruling out strangulation, because the radiologic differential diagnosis is unreliable and the radiographic signs of strangulation, such as free air following perforation or air in the bowel wall, appear late. A presumptive diagnosis of strangulation should be made sooner on the basis of clinical acumen.

When strangulation occurs, the pain increases in intensity and may become continuous. Increasing abdominal tenderness develops and may become localized with signs of peritoneal irritation such as guarding and involuntary spasm. Fever and leukocytosis with a left shift in the differential should arouse suspicion that strangulation is occurring. The serum amylase may rise, suggesting an inappropriate diagnosis of pancreatitis; however, in strangulation obstruction, the rise in serum amylase usually is not as high as in pancreatitis.

In general, the old rule of never letting the sun rise or set on an intestinal obstruction continues to be sound practical advice. After appropriate fluid resuscitation and medical stabilization, a prompt and early operation is the best insurance against progression to strangulation with its greatly increased risk of mortality. In high-risk patients, the surgeon must balance the probability of strangulation against the advantages that may be gained by a longer period of medical stabilization (for example, to correct a diabetic ketoacidosis). There are a few exceptions to these general principles. First, patients known to have Crohn's disease rarely develop strangulating obstruction, so that management by intubation and observation is usually sound practice. Second, patients with multiple recurrent obstructions and several previous operations may be managed conservatively for a period of time if there are no signs or symptoms of strangulation. Third, obstruction in the postoperative period may be handled expectantly if the surgeon feels quite sure that there are no signs of strangulation. Fourth, the patient with known abdominal carcinomatosis usually does not obtain lasting relief from operations for partial obstruction, and considerable judgment must be exercised before deciding to operate.

Fluid Resuscitation and Management

Several liters of extracellular fluid rich in electrolytes may be lost by the patient in the first 24 hours of a small bowel obstruction, particularly if the obstruction is in the proximal small intestine. These losses occur both by vomiting and by sequestration of fluid in the distended and obstructed intestine and its walls. As the volume of extracellular fluid contracts and the red cell mass remains stable, the hematocrit begins to rise and serves as a rough estimate of the volume of fluid lost. Subsequent shifts of interstitial fluid to maintain circulating blood volume result in loss of skin turgor, dry mucous membranes, and other signs of advanced dehydration. These matters are discussed in more detail in Chapter 3. Although studies of unidirectional ion fluxes indicate that absorption of fluid and electrolytes from the obstructed intestine continues at near normal rates until intraluminal pressures reach three or four times normal, secretion of fluid and electrolytes into the intestine proceeds at a much more rapid pace than normal. This cycle is self-perpetuating, since the greater the level of intraluminal pressure in the obstructed segment, the more stimulus there is for increased gastrointestinal secretion. With a closed loop segment in which there are two sites of obstruction, this vicious cycle eventually raises the tension in the wall of the bowel to exceed capillary pressure; strangulation then occurs, and gangrene develops. As bacterial metabolism contributes gases to the closed loop, the partial pressure of nitrogen falls, creating a gradient for nitrogen diffusion into the closed loop from the blood. This shift in gases also perpetuates the vicious cycle of closed loop obstruction.

Fluid resuscitation requires intravenous infusion through a large-diameter cannula. Simultaneously, blood should be drawn for determination of BUN, sodium, potassium, chloride, bicarbonate, hematocrit, white blood cell count, differential count, blood sugar, prothrombin time, partial thromboplastin time, blood typing, and amylase. If the site of obstruction is very proximal, the fluid lost may resemble gastric juice, leading to a hypochloremic, hypokalemic alkalosis. This type of loss should be replaced with normal saline and supplemental potassium. If the obstruction is low, as is the usual case, infusion of a balanced salt solution such as Ringer's lactate replaces more closely the fluid lost. Potassium need not be given in large amounts in the first 24 to 48 hours, and then only after adequate renal function is insured. Arterial blood gas measurements also help to define the severity of acid-base derangement and to plan proper resuscitation.

The rate at which the appropriate fluids are infused is determined largely on clinical grounds. Pulse rate, blood pressure, and urine output should be followed carefully. If a low intestinal obstruction has been present for 24 hours, it should be anticipated that a minimum of 2 or 3 liters of fluid will be required for replacement. If a high intestinal obstruction has been present for 24 hours, the patient may be in shock and may require infusion of several liters of an electrolyte solution as initial replacement. Deficits may be replaced rapidly in patients who are otherwise healthy, but one must proceed more slowly in patients with cardiac or pulmonary disease and borderline or frank congestive heart failure. In complicated cases with borderline cardiac insufficiency, a Swan-Ganz catheter to monitor left atrial pressure will yield more information than central venous pressure measurements alone. Blood transfusion may also be appropriate in some patients, particularly those with strangulation and loss of red blood cells into gangrenous bowel.

Sepsis

As stated previously, the major cause of death in patients with obstruction arises from strangulation of the bowel and ensuing sepsis. Bacteria proliferate exuberantly in closed loops, and the combination of bacteria in addition to products of red blood cell decomposition and other necrotic debris produces toxins that are extraordinarily lethal. Occasionally it is necessary to resuscitate some of these patients from septic shock with very large volumes of fluid. Broad-spectrum antibiotics should be started immediately whenever strangulation is even remotely suspected. We presently use a combination of cephalothin (Keflin), gentamicin, and clindamycin.

Decompression

The final step to be initiated very promptly is decompression of the gastrointestinal tract by intubation. An ordinary nasogastric tube should be passed immediately to empty the stomach and to minimize the possibility of aspiration. As abdominal distention is reduced, there is less pressure on the diaphragm and less compromise of ventilation. When the stomach is empty, vomiting and aspiration of infected fluid into the lungs is less likely. Even with a nasogastric tube in place, we prefer induction of anesthesia by awake or "crash" intubation to minimize the danger of aspiration.

Long tubes, such as the Miller-Abbott or Kantor tubes, may not empty the stomach and are not recommended preoperatively for the ordinary patient. However, a long tube may be useful in the group of patients described previously for whom nonoperative management is often preferable. Passage of long intestinal tubes is facilitated by positioning the balloon at the pylorus under fluoroscopy and putting the patient right side down.

The passage of a long tube into the duodenum preoperatively may also be helpful in selected patients with long-standing low intestinal obstruction. At the time of operation, the balloon may be manually advanced to decompress the intestine prior to wound closure and to stent the bowel in a position with no acute angulation. Occasionally we have used a long tube inserted through a jejunostomy at the time of operation for these purposes, especially if a prolonged postoperative ileus is anticipated. Insertion of a gastrostomy tube may also be appropriate under these circumstances, particularly in patients with chronic pulmonary disease.

PERFORATION FROM TRAUMA OR DISEASE

Almost without exception, the previous principles dealing with obstruction apply to perforations of the intestine. Sepsis is the primary cause of mortality; accordingly, early diagnosis and early institution of a systemic antibiotic regimen is important. Similarly, prompt decompression by nasogastric intubation reduces spillage of intestinal contents into the peritoneal cavity and reduces the danger of aspiration pneumonitis. With penetrating abdominal stab wounds, it is our practice to examine the tract carefully in the emergency room under local anesthesia if needed and to take patients with wounds that obviously violate the peritoneal cavity to the operating room for early exploration. However, it is not always possible to identify a stab wound of the abdominal wall that penetrates into the peritoneal cavity, and such patients must be observed closely for the next 24 hours. Blunt trauma is managed conservatively unless there is evidence of intraperitoneal bleeding or peritonitis. In such suspicious cases, a peritoneal tap or lavage may be helpful.

Free perforation of the small bowel into the peritoneal cavity due to primary bowel disease is rare, but it is seen occasionally in patients with typhoid fever, Meckel's diverticulum, idiopathic ulceration of the ileum, and other uncommon disorders. As in strangulation obstruction, signs of peritonitis compel prompt operation. Pain (which may be generalized), guarding, muscle spasm, ileus, and leukocytosis point the way to the operating room. Free air on an upright roentgenogram of the abdomen is sometimes seen. Perforations of the small bowel also occur in Crohn's disease and are usually sealed off and localized so that generalized abdominal findings are unusual. These perforations usually result in internal or external fistulas, which may warrant elective but not emergency operations. However, if the inflammatory process does not subside promptly on antibiotics, operation may be required.

BLEEDING

Bleeding from the small intestine usually presents as melena, although bright red blood may be seen when the bleeding is massive. Presentation as hematemesis is unusual. The diagnosis usually is made by exclusion of the more common causes of colonic and gastroduodenal hemorrhage. When a Meckel's diverticulum, tumor, or vascular malformation is suspected as the cause of acute small bowel bleeding, selective mesenteric arteriography may be the most rewarding diagnostic study. A scan with ^{99}Tc pertechnitate may localize heterotopic gastric mucosa in a Meckel's diverticulum.

Preoperative preparation follows the guidelines discussed elsewhere for patients bleeding from the more common lesions of the gastrointestinal tract.

INFARCTION

Most symptoms of intestinal infarction are similar to those of strangulation. However, the diagnosis is more difficult because the clinical signs may develop insidiously and without obvious clinical features of obstruction such as abdominal distention. Some cases are associated with occlusion of the superior mesenteric artery by either an embolus or a thrombus. Emboli arise from a mural thrombus in the heart or a fibrillating left atrium. The superior mesenteric artery is vulnerable to embolization because of its moderately large size and its direction of origin paralleling the aorta. An embolus often presents with sudden onset of pain and rapid development of other symptoms because of the absence of a chronic stimulus for collateral circulation, while the symptoms from a thrombosis may unfold more slowly. Thrombosis occurs in situ superimposed on chronic atherosclerotic narrowing of the artery. Some patients with thrombosis have had premonitory symptoms of abdominal angina.

Nonocclusive intestinal infarctions almost always occur in a critically ill patient on digitalis with low cardiac output. Digitalis is a mesenteric vasoconstrictor; when cardiac output is redistributed in low flow states, blood flow to the intestine may fall below minimal required levels. A primary venous thrombosis with infarction may be seen in women on contraceptive pills or in patients with hypercoagulable states of various etiologies. Finally, the small bowel blood supply may be compromised in patients with acute dissecting aneurysms of the aorta.

An acute occlusion of the mesenteric blood supply initiates a period of intense vasospasm and also spasm of the muscular layers of the bowel. The bowel tends to empty, and early abdominal radiographic studies show little gas. Bloody diarrhea or nasogastric aspirates positive for occult blood should arouse suspicion of an infarction.

After a few hours, the initial vasospasm relents. The bowel becomes cyanotic, mottled, congested, and pregangrenous. On abdominal roentgenographic examination, air-fluid levels are present in distended loops of bowel, and the bowel wall may appear thickened with edema. When these findings seem to end abruptly proximal to the splenic flexure, an acute occlusion of the superior mesenteric artery is very likely. A barium enema may show "thumbprints" indicative of submucosal hemorrhages when the colon is ischemic. Intramural gas in the bowel wall is a late grave sign.

Severe abdominal pain in an elderly patient with minimal physical findings is so characteristic of mesenteric infarction that this clinical picture in and of itself should arouse suspicion. Signs of dehydration develop, and there is usually a pronounced shift to the left in the white blood cell differential count. If the surgeon waits for signs of peritonitis to develop, the opportunity to salvage some of these patients may be lost. The onset of peritoneal symptoms may not occur until the entire small intestine is gangrenous and septic shock is imminent.

When there is suspicion of a mesenteric vascular accident, arteriography should be performed without delay. The diagnosis of occlusive disease is usually obvious. However, if a nonocclusive ischemic event seems likely with patent but vasospastic mesenteric vessels, treatment may be instituted with the selective arterial infusion of a potent vasodilator like glucagon. However, the primary task of management of nonocclusive ischemic episodes should be to improve the overall low flow state by increasing cardiac output. Unfortunately, this is frequently very difficult to accomplish.

Operative intervention for occlusive ischemic disease should be undertaken as soon as the patient is reasonably stable, and considerable judgment is required in the operating room. Sometimes revascularization can be accomplished with salvage of much of the small intestine. Anastomoses after resections may fail because of marginal blood supply, and additional bowel may demarcate after the first operation. For these reasons, a "second look" operation within the following 24 hours is considered advisable.

PREOPERATIVE CONSIDERATIONS IN ELECTIVE INDICATIONS FOR SURGERY

CROHN'S DISEASE

Sometimes emergency operations must be performed for acute complications of Crohn's disease, such as bleeding, perforation, or abscess formation. However, most operations can be carried out electively after the problems of malnutrition and infection have been treated and the patient is in the best possible condition.

Occasionally a patient with signs and symptoms consistent with appendicitis may be found to have only intense inflammation of the ileum at the time of operation. The surgeon is advised to perform an appendectomy if the cecum appears normal.

The usual elective indication for operation in Crohn's disease is fistulization or obstruction that does not respond to conservative management. Initially, a nonoperative conservative strategy is recommended in acute obstruction due to Crohn's disease. Strangulation is rare, and the obstruction is often relieved as the edema subsides during decompression of the bowel and treatment with steroids. A policy of early operation and repeated major resection may lead to a crippling short-gut syndrome that should almost always be avoidable even in patients with extensive Crohn's disease of the small bowel. Necessary resections should remove only the obstruction or fistula itself, and attempts should be made to preserve as much bowel as possible.

The nutritional status of these chronically ill patients is likely to be very poor. Anemia is common because of occult blood loss, iron deficiency, and destruction of the ileal mucosa with its capacity for vitamin B_{12} absorption. Diarrhea is also common because of bile salt malabsorption. Chronic sepsis is also common secondary to fistulization and abscess formation. The metabolic cost of sepsis superimposed on chronic malnutrition is enormous. Abscesses should be drained when localized, and antibiotics should be given as indicated. As sepsis is controlled, further gains in the nutritional status of the patient may be possible. The mainstays of hospital management in preparation for operation are parenteral nutrition in patients with chronic obstruction and oral or intravenous hyperalimentation in patients with fistulas. A period of "rest" for the bowel may also help to initiate regression in the inflammatory changes.

Since lesions of Crohn's disease may occur from the mouth to the anus, gastrointestinal radiopaque studies should be obtained from above and below. Skip areas may be identified that enable the surgeon to consider various alternatives in preoperative planning. The "string sign" of the distal ileum on barium enema is a hallmark for making the diagnosis. An intravenous pyelogram should also be done to assess involvement of the right ureter in inflammatory processes.

Preoperative bowel preparation with antibiotics is advisable, since operations commonly include ileo-right colectomy with anastomosis to the colon. Prophylactic systemic antibiotics should be administered. Supplemental steroids should be given if the patient has been treated within the previous 12 months with steroid preparations.

Postoperatively, it is advisable to reduce steroid administration to maintenance levels within 10 days. Often postoperative complications such as sepsis are masked at high steroid levels and do not become apparent until much later in the postoperative course compared with the usual surgical patient. Delayed wound healing may be a major problem in these patients and has been ascribed to the disease process itself plus steroid administration. This problem is less frequent now that surgeons pay more attention to the preoperative nutritional state of the patient.

INTESTINAL BYPASS PROCEDURES

Until recently, jejunoileal bypass procedures for morbid obesity were the standard against which all other experimental techniques such as gastric bypass or gastric stapling procedures were measured. However, prospective studies of jejunoileal bypass now indicate that the risk of major postoperative complications in the long run probably exceeds the benefits of significant weight loss. Accordingly, many medical centers treating morbid obesity surgically now are using intestinal bypass procedures only for patients not suitable for gastric procedures.

Important preoperative considerations with obese patients are assessments of motivation, nutritional condition, and medical risk for operation. The overall planning optimally involves a team including an internist and a psychiatrist. There must be a serious commitment by the physicians and the patient to long-term follow-up. The definition of "morbid obesity" should be strict, namely body weight over twice ideal weight for at least five years and refractory to aggressive institutionalized dietary management. The development of diabetes or hypertension while a patient is morbidly obese are other findings that warrant consideration for bypass surgery. However, it should be emphasized that operations for morbid obesity should be done only in highly selected cases and then probably only in hospitals capable of undertaking major long-term prospective metabolic studies of such patients.

When used, the operation has produced a functioning small intestinal segment composed of approximately 12 inches of jejunum and 4 to 10 inches of distal ileum. Immediate postoperative complications have occurred in approximately one-fourth of these morbidly obese patients, usually as wound infections or thrombophlebitis with occasional embolism. This early complication rate would be acceptable if not followed by major long-term problems. However, the weight loss, which in two-thirds of these patients approaches 40 per cent of preoperative weight in the first year and a half, is often accompanied by several major metabolic problems. There may be significant body protein loss in addition to the fat loss, which accounts for most of the weight loss. Indeed, this probably occurs in 50 per cent of the patients and requires close postoperative follow-up to prevent major nutritional deficiencies from developing. Electrolyte losses from diarrhea also require dietary supplementation, particularly potassium administration, as outlined in the discussion of the short-gut syndrome in this chapter.

Liver failure has occurred after jejunoileal bypasses, most often in patients with excessive early weight loss, and may require reversing the bypass on an emergency basis. Bypass enteritis, pneumatosis cystoides intestinalis, and pneumoperitoneum have been mentioned in a number of reports. Intussusception of the bypassed limb has also occurred. Perhaps the most disturbing complication of all has been the development of oxylate stones in over 10 per cent of patients in some series. The determination of urinary oxylate after surgery has not been of prognostic value, since almost all such patients have elevated urinary oxylate for several months after the procedure. This complication to date has been reversible only by taking down the bypass. Since taking down the bypass is almost invariably followed by rapid weight gain back to the preoperative morbid obesity level, several centers now advocate performing gastric bypass or gastric stapling at the time of takedown, with excellent prevention of weight gain.

TUMORS

Tumors of the small intestine are uncommon but may present with occult bleeding, partial obstruction, or intussusception. A very carefully done small intestinal barium series may demonstrate some tumors. Selective mesenteric arteriography may also localize tumors in the small bowel.

Benign tumors are more common than malignant tumors, leiomyomas being the most common of all. Hamartomas of Peutz-Jeghers syndrome and hemangiomas of Osler-Weber-Rendu disease are associated with cutaneous manifestations. Carcinomas are the leading malignant tumors and usually present with partial obstruction. However, they are extremely rare in contrast to carcinomas of the stomach and large intestine.

Carcinoid tumors have a misleading name, since they are often malignant; about one-third of carcinoids found in the ileum have already produced metastases. With one exception, carcinoid syndrome due to release of serotonin and other vasoactive amines indicates hepatic metastasis. This exception occurs with carcinoid tumors of the ovary where the venous effluent bypasses the portal circulation directly into the systemic venous blood. In the carcinoid syndrome, the output of urinary 5-hydroxyindoleacetic acid is usually increased severalfold. In addition to the usual symptoms, nutritional symptoms related to niacin deficiency may develop because of tumor metabolism of tryptophan and its diversion from normal pathways.

RADIATION ENTERITIS

Irradiation produces acute and chronic injury to the bowel. Acute injury is due to damage to the mucosa with its large population of rapidly replicating cells in the crypts. This injury may result in bloody diarrhea, which should be managed conservatively. Chronic injury results from vasculitis, endothelial proliferation, chronic intestinal ischemia, and eventual fibrosis. There is a sharp increase in the incidence of radiation enteritis when the patient is irradiated at doses of 4500 to 6000 rads. Fortunately, these cases are becoming less common as techniques of irradiation therapy have become more sophisticated and lower dose irradiation is combined with chemotherapy and/or immunotherapy in new treatment protocols.

A conservative strategy should be followed as in Crohn's disease, but operation may be required for obstruction, fistulization, or hemorrhage. The surgeon should operate only to relieve severe symptoms, and a bypass of badly damaged bowel or a proximal colostomy may be performed if a resection does not appear feasible. The intestine near the point of obstruction or fistulization may grossly appear normal, but in many cases radiation vasculitis is present that precludes normal healing. Anastomoses should be avoided in such patients unless the surgeon is sure that the bowel being sutured is free of radiation injury.

GENERAL CONSIDERATIONS FOR POSTOPERATIVE CARE

FLUID MANAGEMENT

In addition to following the usual clinical guidelines based on pulse rate, blood pressure, urine output, and general appearance, it is advisable to balance intake and output meticulously on a daily basis. When an extended period of intravenous fluid therapy is anticipated, daily weights should be recorded and followed, especially when daily output measurements are imprecise. Regular blood urea nitrogen and serum electrolyte determinations are also useful. When losses are large and the patient is unstable, monitoring left atrial pressure with a Swan-Ganz catheter is subject to less error than central venous pressure. When copious amounts of gastrointestinal fluids are lost, determining the electrolyte composition of the fluids will provide a guideline for replacement. Intestinal losses should always be considered as losses of extracellular fluid and should be replaced with balanced salt solution. If sodium-free or sodium-poor solutions are used, dilutional hyponatremia will result.

DECOMPRESSION AND ILEUS

After operations on the small intestine, a period of disorganized propulsive activity called ileus may occur. Decompression of the gastrointestinal tract by a nasogastric tube is then necessary to prevent vomiting and aspiration into the lungs and to protect the anastomosis.

Actually, normal small bowel function usually returns early in the postoperative period, and the small intestine will absorb nutrients delivered by local infusion even while the stomach is still atonic. The passage of flatus or stool is a signal that the stomach as well as the colon has resumed peristaltic activity, at which time the nasogastric tube may be removed. The return of bowel sounds alone is a less reliable guide.

Prolongation of postoperative ileus for more than three or four days is often a sign that something is amiss: serum electrolyte concentrations should be measured to rule out severe hypokalemia and hypocalcemia. A search should be made for intra-abdominal infection. If more than two liters of fluid are aspirated daily, a distal obstruction should be suspected. Strangulation is very rare, because early adhesions are soft and filmy (unlike dense fibrous adhesions several months later). Consequently, most early postoperative obstructions can be managed conservatively. The most difficult question to answer is how long to wait before recommending reoperation. We are conservative on this point, but considerable judgment and experience are required in making the decisions whether and when to intercede operatively.

PULMONARY CARE

Respiratory complications are common after small bowel surgery because of the limited excursion of the diaphragm associated with bowel distention and abdominal pain. Adequate decompression of the gastrointestinal tract and vigorous pulmonary care (coughing, ambulation, and deep breathing) are the best preventive measures against atelectasis commonly seen after intestinal surgery.

NUTRITION

Attention to nutrition is of paramount concern in patients with complicated postoperative courses. Nutrition is discussed in other sections of this chapter and also in other chapters of this manual (Chaps. 4 and 5). In general, hyperosmolar intravenous feeding should be started if the patient cannot take food by mouth within 7 to 10 days after intestinal surgery.

MANAGEMENT OF OTHER POSTOPERATIVE PROBLEMS

FISTULAS

Development of a small intestinal fistula is a major complication in the postoperative course that still carries a significant mortality. Most fistulas occur as complications of intestinal anastomoses, but they may also occur after drainage of intra-abdominal abscesses and difficult enterolysis procedures. Fistulas also occur spontaneously in diseases of the small bowel, such as Crohn's disease or irradiation enteritis.

The development of a fistula is usually obvious. After several days of fever and abdominal pain, the fistula declares itself as external drainage through the wound or a drain site. Immediate confirmation may be obtained by the oral administration of charcoal or a dye (such as methylene blue), but the odor and characteristics of the discharge usually leave little doubt as to the nature of the drainage. A fistulagram with water-soluble contrast medium and barium studies from below and above may further define the site and extent of fistulization.

Isolation and collection of the fistula drainage are essential for measurement and replacement of fluid losses and for patient comfort. Satisfactory receptacles with karaya gum or other adhesives are commercially available. However, collection is especially difficult when there are multiple draining tracts through the abdominal wall and through incisions that have separated. The use of sump drains may be helpful in the management of these problems.

Small bowel drainage is rich in enzymes that digest the abdominal wall and excoriate the skin. Aluminum paste protects the skin somewhat. Karaya powder may also be used to build up protective margins around the fistula, and sometimes a template can be cut from a large ileostomy bag to fit the border. A soft suction catheter can sometimes be used to intubate the proximal end of a fistula. A collecting catheter may also be placed in a dependent portion of the wound, and another catheter may be used to irrigate the wound with buffered saline. Positioning the patient on a Stryker frame has even been used to obtain control of the drainage.

Initial management of a fistula usually includes nasogastric aspiration and cessation of oral intake. Fluid replacement is based on the site and quantity of drainage. Proximal jejunal fistulas require more extensive management than distal ones because of greater losses of fluid and electrolytes. Daily weight, frequent electrolyte determinations, and careful charting of intake and output serve as guides for replacement therapy.

Deterioration of nutritional status is inevitable without parenteral therapy in patients with high intestinal fistulas because of the loss of proteins through the fistula and the inability of the patient to eat. An accelerated catabolic state accentuated by sepsis results in poor wound healing, muscle wasting, and deterioration of host resistance. However, if as much as four feet of proximal bowel are intact, a trial of nutrition by gavage with a low-residue elemental diet may be undertaken. Usually parenteral nutrition must be employed to overcome the loss of body nitrogen. Although it has often been recommended that sepsis should be controlled before inserting a central venous catheter for parenteral nutrition, we have become more aggressive in this regard and believe that an effort to control the catabolic state should be initiated simultaneously.

Patients with fistulas are often septic and may have multiple intra-abdominal abscesses. Clinical examination, contrast studies, liver-lung scan, gallium scan, and fluoroscopy of the diaphragm may help to localize a collection that can be drained.

Spontaneous healing may occur if there is no distal obstruction and if there has not been a major disruption in the continuity of the bowel. Most lateral intestinal fistulas at anastomoses will close. Spontaneous healing is less likely in patients with residual chronic disease of the bowel, such as Crohn's disease, ischemia, or metastatic carcinoma. High-output proximal fistulas may be difficult to close. If significant reduction in the volume of fistula drainage has not occurred within three or four weeks with control of intra-abdominal infection and maintenance of nutrition by intravenous hyperalimentation, surgical reexploration is indicated. Distal ileal fistulas do not affect nutrition so adversely, and a longer period of conservative management can be tried. The use of elemental diets to decrease fluid delivery to the fistula can be useful in these cases. At operation, bypass or exteriorization of the fistula often entails less risk than a primary resection and anastomosis.

Pseudomembranous Enterocolitis

Pseudomembranous enterocolitis is an ulcerating and diffuse process occurring in the colon and/or small bowel that is commonly associated with overgrowth of *Staphylococcus aureus* and is attributed to broad-spectrum antibiotic administration. A number of antibiotics have been implicated, but the common denominator is usually a severely ill patient with a low flow state. In other words, the clinical setting is similar to that of nonocclusive intestinal ischemia. The primary therapeutic effort should be similar to that previously discussed: expand effective circulating volume and improve general perfusion.

BLIND LOOP SYNDROME

The term "blind loop syndrome" refers to a broad spectrum of digestive disturbances that result from the overgrowth of bacteria in the small intestine. Many prefer the term "contaminated small bowel syndrome" in referring to this group of disturbances, since any abnormality in the mechanisms that regulate the bacterial flora of the intestine may have the same pathophysiologic consequences. For example, disturbances of motility in diseases like diabetes mellitus predispose to an increase in bacterial flora. There are also several causes of bacterial overgrowth in surgical patients without true anatomic blind loops. Examples include gastrojejunocolic and other fistulas, strictures, and contamination of the small intestine from a diseased biliary tract.

Anemia and steatorrhea are the two most common clinical presentations. More recently it has been recognized that some patients with bacterial overgrowth have severe panmalabsorption and deliberating malnutrition. The mechanisms of protein and carbohydrate malabsorption are less well understood than the causes of fat malabsorption but may be related to direct competition of the flora with the host for nutrients or to toxic effects of bacterial metabolism.

STEATORRHEA

Normal absorption of fat depends upon the normal metabolism of bile salts. The bile salts (cholic and chenodeoxycholic) synthesized by the liver from cholesterol are conjugated by the liver to taurine or glycine and are excreted in the bile. The conjugated bile salts form micelles and are essential for the solubilization phase of fat absorption.

Certain bacteria, such as *Bacteroides,* that proliferate in blind loops can enzymatically cleave taurine or glycine from the bile acid molecule, liberating free bile acids. Several disturbances ensue. First, free bile acids do not form micellar solutions efficiently. Since the dietary lipid then cannot be solubilized in a micellar phase, malabsorption of fat results. Second, the normal enterohepatic circulation is short-circuited. Under normal conditions, the conjugated bile acids are present in critical micellar concentrations in the jejunum, where 95 per cent of all fat absorption takes place. The jejunum does not have an efficient active transport mechanism for the absorption of conjugated bile acids, so a critical concentration of bile acids is maintained until the chyme reaches the ileum, where sites for active transport absorb the bile acids and return them to the liver. Free bile acids, however, may be absorbed directly from the jejunum by passive nonionic diffusion. Thus, instead of a normal ileohepatic circulation of bile salts, there may be an abnormal jejunohepatic short circuit. Third, there is some evidence that free bile acids may have a direct toxic effect on the absorptive surface of the bowel, adding to the malabsorption.

ANEMIA

Megaloblastic anemia is common in the blind loop syndrome, and it is the result of B_{12} deficiency. A Schilling test in these patients demonstrates that the absorption of B_{12} is not corrected by an intrinsic factor as in the case of pernicious anemia. However, after a course of antibiotic therapy, the Schilling test usually becomes normal, indicating that bacterial overgrowth is responsible for malabsorption of the vitamin. Most evidence suggests that bacteria can metabolize vitamin B_{12} and thus compete directly for this essential nutrient with the host.

Diagnosis

The history of diseases or previous surgical procedures associated with the blind loop syndrome is usually the initial clue to the diagnosis. In patients who have had previous operations, one of the first steps is to review the operative record for a clue to the possible presence of a blind loop (for example, a side-to-side anastomosis). Routine contrast studies of the GI tract are essential. The presence of steatorrhea should be documented by a quantitative 24- to 72-hour stool fat test. Urinary 5-hydroxyindoleacetic acid is usually elevated, reflecting abnormal bacterial metabolism of tryptophan. A small bowel biopsy may be necessary to rule out common causes of steatorrhea such as sprue, although the mucosa usually appears normal by routine microscopy in blind loop syndrome. Quantitative cultures of jejunal chyme indicating 10^7 or 10^8 organisms per milliliter (normal 10^3) are virtually diagnostic, especially if combined with low levels of conjugated bile salts in the same chyme. A trial of antibiotic therapy with tetracycline usually results in clinical improvement as well as a reduction in fecal excretion. A recent innovation in the diagnosis of bacterial overgrowth is a breath analyzer test, which is based on the administration of isotope-labeled conjugated bile salts by mouth and the identification of radioactive CO_2 in expired air. Another new breath test screens for the presence of hydrogen in expired air; only excessive numbers of intestinal bacteria can produce measurable hydrogen.

Treatment

Patients with anatomic blind loops or other lesions amenable to direct surgical revision (such as strictures and fistulas) are cured by an appropriate operation. Some patients with abnormalities of motility or with extensive small intestinal diverticulosis must be managed medically, and antibiotics must be given for prolonged periods of time.

SHORT-GUT SYNDROME

A syndrome of malnutrition, steatorrhea, and acidic diarrhea follows massive small bowel resection. The postoperative course of the patient is determined by the length and site of the resected gut as well as by the nature of the underlying disease process. In general, a 70 per cent small bowel resection can be tolerated fairly well if the terminal ileum and ileocecal valve can be preserved. If these structures are resected, nutrition can be severely impaired by a 50 to 60 per cent resection.

Effect of Resection of the Ileum

The ileum is a more useful residual remnant than the jejunum, even though the jejunum normally serves as the site of most food absorption. By the same token, resection of the ileum is tolerated less well than resection of the jejunum, because important active transport sites for vitamin B_{12} and bile salts are selectively localized in the ileum. Pernicious anemia eventually appears after a delay of two to five years when body stores of B_{12} are exhausted. The effects of loss of active bile salt absorption are more immediate.

The process by which the ileum recovers the bile salts from the chyme for the enterohepatic circulation is so efficient that only a low level of synthesis of new bile salts by the liver is required daily. After ileal resection, bile salts are lost in the stool, and the bile salt pool is depleted more rapidly than the liver can increase its rate of synthesis. This depletion of bile salts results in failure of the solubilization phase of fat absorption. Steatorrhea then occurs, although the usual site of fat absorption in the jejunum remains undisturbed.

Both the fatty acids and the bile salts that escape absorption in the small intestine stimulate secretion by the colonic mucosa and may produce diarrhea on this basis alone. This phenomenon has been referred to as the "castor oil effect" of ileal resection (castor oil is a poorly absorbed triglyceride of ricinoleic acid and when hydrolyzed induces diarrhea as a result of the irritant property of its fatty acid component).

Gastric Hypersecretion

Gastric hypersecretion after massive small bowel resection is common. There are three effects of this outpouring of acid juice into the small intestine:

1. The proximal intestinal mucosa is injured by the acid delivered to it from the stomach, and absorption of all foods is impaired. Indeed, the damage may be so severe that net secretion of fluid takes place into the bowel and augments the diarrhea.

2. Inactivation of lipase and trypsin occurs because of the low intraluminal pH. Maldigestion of fat and proteins may follow.

3. The high solute load of gastric juice may exceed the transport capacity of the remaining remnant, and diarrhea can again result. This effect is particularly pronounced after massive resections, since the amount of hypersecretion appears to be proportional to the extent of the resection. Interestingly, this phenomenon is not seen after intestinal bypass operations, suggesting that hypersecretion after massive resections is related to loss of an inhibitor of gastric secretion that was produced by the missing gut.

Renal Stones

Urinary stones of calcium oxalate are common because of an increase in oxalate absorption from the colon. This condition is termed intestinal hyperoxaluria. It probably develops because there is insufficient calcium in the stool to keep the oxalate relatively insoluble, since calcium is bound to excess free fatty acids as soaps.

Intestinal Adaptation

Intestinal adaptation begins promptly after a massive resection to make up for the lost intestine. Morphologically, compensatory hypertrophy develops and the villi grow longer. Functionally, the intestine increases its absorptive capacity for water, sodium, sugars, and amino acids. Much research in both animals and humans indicates the following general conclusions about adaptation:

1. The gut remnant will hypertrophy if the patient can be maintained in a relatively normal nutritional state for a finite period of time after massive resection. This may require a year or more.

2. Provision of nutrients both to the gut lumen and to the patient by parenteral means appears to facilitate this process.

3. Certain localized transport processes probably cannot be replaced by adaptation, and permanent substitution therapy may be required.

Clinical Course

Because of gradual adaptation, the clinical course of patients after a massive resection goes through several stages.

Stage 1 is characterized by an initial period of massive diarrhea requiring intensive replacement of fluid and electrolyte deficits. Diarrhea exceeds 2 to 2.5 liters each day. Feeding is by total parenteral means. This stage will usually last from one to three months. All electrolytes should be monitored closely during this phase, including calcium, magnesium, and zinc.

Stage 2 is the period of adaptation during which oral intake is gradually initiated and increased. This stage may last for a few months to over a year.

In *Stage 3*, maximal adaptation is achieved, and a relatively normal home existence is regained. Some patients never reach this stage of oral nutrition, but encouraging progress has been made in making the transition to life at home with continuing parenteral nutrition.

TREATMENT

The emphasis of treatment depends upon the clinical stage of recovery as outlined in Table 24–1.

Table 24–1. TREATMENT AFTER ILEAL RESECTION BASED ON STAGE OF RECOVERY

STAGE	SIGNS	TREATMENT
First stage	Diarrhea exceeds 7–8 bowel movements per day or more than 2.5 liters per day	a. Intravenous fluids only b. Control diarrhea medically c. Maintain fluid and electrolyte balance d. Total parenteral nutrition
Second stage	Diarrhea less than 2 liters per day on oral intake	a. Continue intravenous hyperalimentation if oral calorie intake higher than 1800 calories per day accentuates diarrhea b. Start oral fluids to maintain fluid and electrolyte volume, consider oral hyperalimentation, add carbohydrates and proteins, medium chain triglycerides (no fats)
Third stage	Stabilization of diarrhea on fat-free diet	a. Add fat b. Let weight adjust to gut length c. Consider adjunctive surgical procedures to control gastric hypersecretion and motility

Stage 1

Nothing is gained by premature oral feeding. Instead, electrolyte and fluid losses usually are made worse. Consequently, there is every reason not to feed patients for several weeks after massive resections. Intravenous hyperalimentation will insure that all essential nutritional, electrolyte, and fluid needs are met without oral intake. Accordingly, nothing should be given by mouth while diarrhea exceeds 2.5 liters per day or seven to eight bowel movements per day with the patient on intravenous fluids alone. Details of parenteral nutrition are discussed in Chapter 5.

Intramuscular codeine is the best drug for severe diarrhea. Although it can be given orally if more than three feet of small bowel remain, usually it escapes absorption early in the course of recovery after more massive resections. Codeine must be given in doses as high as 64 mg every three or four hours to be effective during the first two or three weeks. Paregoric (5 to 10 ml every two to four hours) and Kaopectate (180 to 240 ml per day) usually are ineffective when diarrhea exceeds 2 liters a day. They should be substituted for codeine later, when the number of semisolid bowel movements falls below five to seven per day. Diphenoxylate with atropine (Lomotil), which is less effective than codeine, is a better drug to use in the late stages of recovery.

Stage 2

Oral fluids should be started when the diarrhea is less than 2 to 2.5 liters per day. Hypotonic balanced salt solutions should be given first, followed by skim milk. Whole milk should be avoided because of its fat content. The primary goal in feeding short-gut patients is to deliver more and more calories without potentiating the diarrhea. The concentration of solutions should not exceed isotonicity at first and usually cannot be raised more above 400 to 450 mOsm per kg for several weeks. At these concentrations, it is impossible to provide for the patient's entire nutritional needs by mouth. Unfortunately, amino acids, hydrolysates, boiled skim milk, sugar solutions, and other combinations are quite unpalatable at these dilute concentrations. Dilute elemental diets may be delivered slowly by gastric gavage through a fine, nonirritating, soft nasogastric tube, but the physician must be alert for any signs of aspiration. Intravenous supplementation should be continued to provide adequate calories until the volume of diarrhea falls below 2 liters per day on moderately hypertonic elemental diets. Trial and error and control of output then will indicate when to increase and to enrich the diet. Carbohydrates as cooked starches should be tried first, since they are almost always absorbed well even from small remnants of bowel. When carbohydrates are well tolerated at the 50 to 100 gm per day level, protein may be added to the oral diet. The vitamins usually are well absorbed and may be given orally during this phase; one exception is vitamin B_{12} after resection of the ileum. Monthly injections of cyanocobalamin 100 μg are necessary. Hypoprothrombinemia is encountered occasionally, but it is due to development of liver disease (fatty liver) and not to impaired absorption. Vitamins K, D, and A may be given in supplemental doses, because they are fat-soluble and will be lost in the stool when steatorrhea is severe. Serum folate levels should be carefully monitored to avoid anemia.

Once the patient is stabilized on oral intake of carbohydrate and protein with electrolyte and water balance maintained primarily by the oral route, a significant amount of fat can be added to the diet. Medium chain triglycerides can be tried first, particularly in patients who have had very massive resections. Then fat can be added in 25 gm increments, maintaining each level of dietary fat intake for at least a week before increasing further. Stool fat can be measured and should not exceed 50 per cent of intake. An increase in steatorrhea above the 25 gm per day level is poorly tolerated because of increasing diarrhea, foul bowel movements, and depletion of calcium and magnesium. If this level must be accepted, the supplementary feeding of 3 to 5 gm of calcium carbonate and parenteral magnesium salts should be used in order to replace the secondary losses of these cations.

Because bile acids reaching the colon stimulate secretion and produce loose stools, cholestyramine may reduce the diarrhea of short-gut patients by binding bile acids that cannot be reabsorbed, even if this treatment results in reduced fat absorption. However, patients with resected segments of ileum greater than 100 cm in length rarely have a good response. Thus, cholestyramine may be helpful primarily for patients with diarrhea associated with ileal resections of short and intermediate lengths.

Stage 3

After approximately three months of treating patients with 70 to 80 per cent resections, and after 6 to 18 months for more severe cases, stabilization of diarrhea and fat absorption usually occurs. Xylose absorption returns to normal. The increasing serum lipids, cholesterol, carotenes, and vitamin A levels reflect improved fat absorption. The dietary fat can be increased gradually to near normal levels over this period.

Low dietary oxalate is recommended for life to prevent renal stones, and supplemental calcium may be helpful. Regular maintenance with vitamin B_{12} may be necessary, along with oral supplementation of the fat-soluble vitamins (A, D, and K). Oral cholestyramine should be continued if it was helpful in the earlier trials for limited ileal resection. Peptic ulceration is not often a problem in the remote postoperative period, and antacid therapy may eventually be discontinued.

25

Alimentary Tract Stomas

MARVIN L. CORMAN

While the technical aspects of creating a satisfactory stoma are extremely important, they will not be discussed in this chapter; several excellent textbooks are available that describe the various surgical procedures (Goligher, 1980; Hill, 1976; Turnbull and Weakley, 1967). In addition to a properly timed, competently performed operation, rehabilitation of a patient with an ostomy requires preoperative and postoperative education.

Patients who undergo an operation with a resultant stoma are confronted with a little-understood, artificial container for human waste. The individual may feel that he has compromised his dignity and the quality of his life. Myths and misunderstandings further prejudice the patient's attitude. Many patients may even be unsure as to whether they have a colostomy or an ileostomy.

It is mandatory for any surgeon who performs ostomy procedures to be involved with preoperative counseling and to have a working knowledge of ostomy management.

PREOPERATIVE PREPARATION OF THE OSTOMY PATIENT

COLOSTOMY

The most common indication for performing a permanent colostomy is carcinoma of the rectum. The surgeon must consider not only the patient's concerns about mortality but also the fear of being deformed. Many patients, in fact, fear the prospect of the colostomy more than the operation or the cancer itself.

After the patient realizes that an operation is necessary and that creation of a colostomy stoma is indicated, two questions should be asked: Do you know what a colostomy is, and do you know anyone who has had a colostomy? Answers to these questions often reveal a remark-

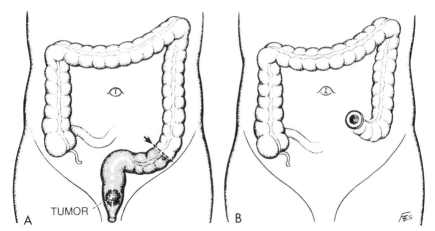

Figure 25–1. Anatomy of the colon showing the rectal cancer and the operative procedure.

able ignorance, prejudice, and fear. If the patient knows of someone who leads a fulfilled and nonrestricted life with a colostomy, the surgeon's job becomes easier.

Once the patient's general knowledge of the subject has been established, the specific relevant aspects of the operation can be explained. It is important for the patient to understand why intestinal continuity cannot be reestablished and why the stoma must be exteriorized on the abdominal wall. It must be emphasized that the ultimate purpose of the procedure is to cure the patient of malignancy. A drawing made by the surgeon at the bedside can serve as a useful aid in explaining the nature of the procedure (Fig. 25–1). It is also helpful to give the patient informative literature, such as that which is available through the United Ostomy Association.*

The enterostomal therapist can be of great help to the patient and to the surgeon by spending unhurried time and by sharing his or her expertise and experience with the patient. This nurse therapist should be consulted as early as possible in the course of the patient's management. While most of the formal teaching is carried out after the operation, the emotional preparation of the patient and the selection of the site for the stoma must be accomplished beforehand. Several books can also be utilized to aid the surgeon in this regard (Mahoney, 1976; Yukovich and Grubb, 1973; Walker, 1976).

The importance of proper placement of the stoma and proper maturation technique cannot be overestimated. Ease or difficulty in management of the stoma may mean the difference between a normal lifestyle and one that is severely limited. Proper location of the stoma

---

*United Ostomy Association, 2001 West Beverly Boulevard, Los Angeles, California 90057

can prevent future complications such as prolapse, parastomal hernia, skin problems, and poor appliance adhesion. Areas that frequently interfere with appliances are the groin, waistline, costal margins, umbilicus, skin folds, and scars. It is advisable to leave a 5 cm margin of smooth skin around the stoma. The stoma should always be placed at the summit of the infraumbilical bulge and within the rectus muscle (Fig. 25–2). If the stoma is brought out lateral to the rectus, in time herniation will occur.

Another factor to consider is the patient's preference for clothing style, especially where the belt is worn, because stomas should be placed below the waist and preferably below the belt line. Patients should be able to wear their clothes, carry out their work, and manage their activities without encumbrance. This can be accomplished only by giving careful thought and attention to the location of the stoma.

In addition to permanent colostomy after abdominoperineal resection for carcinoma of the rectum, a colostomy (either permanent or temporary) may be indicated for benign colonic obstruction or perforation, diverticulitis, anal fistula, Crohn's disease, congenital anomalies, anal incontinence, and trauma. When an emergency arises, by taking a few extra moments in the operating room prior to making the incision

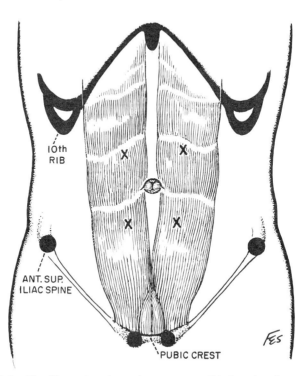

Figure 25–2. The illustration shows the proper possible locations for a stoma (marked by Xs). Note that the stoma should always be brought through the split rectus muscle and that care should be taken to avoid the bony promontories.

and by marking a potential site for the placement of a stoma, future difficulties may be avoided. Even when a transverse colostomy is contemplated, an effort should be made preoperatively to identify the proper site for its creation (that is, away from the rib margin and through the split rectus muscle).

ILEOSTOMY

An ileostomy is usually advised for inflammatory bowel disease — ulcerative colitis or Crohn's disease. Ideally, the patient should be well informed about the need for an ileostomy long before the operation is required. It is even reasonable to give informative brochures to a patient who has colitis some time before anticipated surgery. It is usually of great benefit to acquaint the patient with someone of comparable age, sex, and socioeconomic status who has an ileostomy and is well adjusted to it so that the patient can be reassured that a normal lifestyle is possible. Unfortunately, some patients do not receive adequate preoperative counseling, either because the physician fails to mention the possibility of an ileostomy during the course of treatment of the condition or because the patient requires urgent surgical intervention, such as may be necessary for hemorrhage, toxic megacolon, perforation, or sepsis. Under these circumstances, the patient may always believe that the operation was performed too precipitously and that perhaps a more vigorous approach to medical management might have avoided or at least deferred the need for a stoma until a later time.

Preoperative consideration of the placement of the stoma is mandatory. The site chosen must be free of eschar, especially if the eschar is irregular rather than flat and smooth. The stoma should not be near a bony promontory, such as the iliac spine or the rib margin. Like the colostomy, it should be exteriorized through the split rectus muscle. The patient may actually wear the appliance before operation and note areas where subsequent appliance management may become difficult — for example, the presence of skin folds, the location of the waistline, and the usual position of pants or belt. If the appliance is not available, potential problem areas can be pinpointed before operation in patients undergoing elective operations by placing a faceplate on the abdomen and having the patient lie down, sit up, ambulate, and stand. The site chosen should be identified with markings, such as a scratch on the skin or an ink tattoo, that cannot be erased. In an emergency, a sterile metal disk can be used to mark the site when the patient is in the operating room. One disadvantage of delaying determination of the site of the stoma until the time of operation is that abdominal skin folds may not be apparent when the patient is lying down.

A recent innovation in ostomy surgery is the technique of the Kock continent ileostomy (Kock, 1971). Patients are now inquiring about the appropriateness of this procedure for their own needs. The advantages of the lack of an appliance, a flush stoma, and a stoma placed low on the abdominal wall are tempting enticements for the patient and surgeon. While reports have been encouraging (Goligher, 1976; Gelernt et al., 1977; Beahrs, 1975; Beart et al., 1979), the Kock procedure continues to be associated with a high incidence of complications. The procedure may be relegated to one of historic interest only, or at most applied to the unusual situation if the newer sphincter-saving approaches are proved successful (e.g., Parks et al., 1980).

ILEAL CONDUIT

The preoperative preparation and location of the stoma are similar for patients who need an ileal conduit for urinary diversion to those discussed for patients who require an ileostomy. An additional concern in male patients undergoing cystectomy for bladder cancer is that they will be impotent after operation. This is another important indication for preoperative counseling and support. The appliance equipment is somewhat different and will be discussed later in this chapter under Postoperative Care.

COMMENT

A general principle of preoperative preparation is that the patient must be able to care for the stoma and manage the appliance without help. If the patient has severe rheumatoid arthritis, has a visual impairment, or is mentally retarded or senile, it may be physically impossible for that individual to care for a stoma. Accordingly, one must solicit support from the family or a visiting nurses' association, or institutionalization in a nursing facility may be required. Under these circumstances consideration should be given to alternative approaches to ostomy.

POSTOPERATIVE CARE

An enterostomal therapist can help immensely during the initial postoperative period when concerns about skin care, stomal appearance, and appliance management are frequent.

COLOSTOMY

Following establishment of a sigmoid colostomy, the appliance selected is usually a simple, transparent, drainable, adhesive bag (Fig.

25–3). This permits ready visualization of the stoma and allows the contents to be emptied without the need for frequent changes of the appliance.

It is practically impossible to be completely familiar with all ostomy equipment (a partial list of manufacturers and a glossary of terms are available at the end of this chapter). Therefore, two or three different products should be selected that will allow adequate management of most problems.

Procedure for Application of Disposable Appliance

1. Empty the contents and remove the appliance, using adhesive solvent if necessary.
2. Cleanse the skin with warm water and dry the area.
3. Measure the stoma and either cut out a disk or select an appliance with an appropriate-sized opening approximately ⅛ inch larger than the stoma.
4. Spray a skin preparation around the stoma and allow to dry.
5. With the hand in the opened bag, place the opening squarely over the stoma. During the immediate postoperative period when the patient is not ambulatory, place the bag on sideways for ease of drainage. Press the adhesive disk firmly against the skin to avoid wrinkles.
6. Insert a deodorant (optional) into the bag.
7. Close the open end of the bag securely.

The steps are similar for patients with ileostomies and urinary conduits; however, the appliances are slightly different.

Irrigating the Colostomy. Whether the colostomy should be ir-

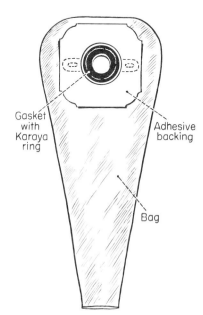

Gasket with Karaya ring

Adhesive backing

Bag

Figure 25–3. An open-ended colostomy (ileostomy) appliance.

rigated or allowed to function spontaneously is a decision that the patient and surgeon must make. Most patients tend to return to the bowel habits they had before operation, usually within 6 to 12 weeks. In other words, if they defecated every morning after breakfast, the colostomy will probably continue to function on that schedule. Under these circumstances, irrigating may be unnecessary, and such patients can frequently avoid an appliance for the rest of the day or merely use a small dressing or Stomacap. A closed-ended "security pouch" can also be used.

Conversely, if a patient had irregular bowel function preoperatively, the colostomy will probably act irregularly postoperatively. These patients are often happier with irrigation. However, under no circumstances should the patient be *told* to irrigate the colostomy. The technique should be learned, but the decision as to whether to utilize irrigation should be left to the individual.

Procedure for Irrigating. A nipple, cone, or catheter is inserted into the stoma. The cone tip is now being used more frequently for colostomy irrigations than the catheter because not only is there less chance of perforating the bowel, but it also provides a dam to prevent backflow. If the catheter is used, the patient should be taught to insert it without exerting any force. Furthermore, it should only be inserted four inches. The colon does not need to be washed out; the bowel is merely stimulated with the irrigant to produce evacuation. Usually one quart of warm water is used in the reservoir and is suspended from a hook so that the bottom of the bag is at shoulder height when the patient is seated. When the irrigation is completed, the patient usually waits approximately 15 minutes on the toilet to allow drainage. The collecting sleeve can then be closed while the patient tends to other activities. After approximately 45 minutes, the irrigant usually will have been expelled. Over a period of time the patient may require irrigations only every 48 hours or even every 72 hours. Some patients may never be able to irrigate completely and may require a pouch all the time. Under these circumstances it is difficult to justify the time and effort expended to perform this task.

ILEOSTOMY

The major difference between an ileostomy and a colostomy appliance is that some form of protective ring must be used around the ileostomy stoma because of the corrosive nature of the effluent. Preserving the integrity of the skin is of greatest concern in the postoperative period. Meticulous attention to skin care must begin with the first application of the skin barrier and placement of the pouch in the operating room.

A *skin barrier* is a porous material with adhering qualities that is applied directly to the skin to afford protection from contents of the colon or ileum. The pouch is put on top of the barrier. In contrast to the skin barrier, a *skin protective agent*, such as Skin Prep or Skin Gel, provides a clear dressing that coats the skin. Generally, protective agents are used when tapelike products contact the skin in order to protect the epithelium from irritation. Distinction must be made between a skin barrier and a protective agent; patients with ileostomies should never use a protective agent in place of a skin barrier. There are a number of skin barriers available on the market. These include karaya products, Stomahesive, Hollihesive, ReliaSeal, and Crixiline. A skin barrier should be placed in the operating room immediately after the procedure. The inner diameter should be cut to fit snugly around the base of the stoma. The outer aspect should be rounded and made slightly smaller than the adhesive portion of a soft-backed, disposable clear pouch. The skin must be completely dry before applying any skin barrier.

The pouch should be changed on the first postoperative day. This enables inspection of the base of the stoma, cleansing of the peristomal skin, and utilization of a larger opening if the stoma is edematous. Appliance changes should continue every other day or three times a week until the patient leaves the hospital. During the first six to eight days after surgery, a disposable soft-backed pouch will be required in addition to an appropriate skin barrier. By the seventh or eighth day, the stoma should be remeasured because the edema will usually have resolved, although it usually takes four to six weeks for the stoma to shrink to its final size.

Two types of pouches are available — disposable and reusable. Disposable pouches come with an adhesive or microporous tape backing and in some cases with a soft plastic faceplate and belt tabs (Fig. 25–3). A number of such commonly used products include the Hollister, United Surgical, Marlen, ColoPlast/Bard, and Nu-Hope pouches. They are lightweight, easy to apply, and very effective choices for the firm abdomen not requiring a more rigid faceplate for peristomal support. In addition, no assembly is required.

The disadvantages of the disposable system include shorter wearing time, increased cost, and limitation to certain body configurations. A faceplate with a firm base provides better peristomal support, particularly in a patient with a "flabby" abdomen. A disposable pouch *always* requires a skin barrier to enhance the wearing time and to provide adequate skin protection.

Reusable or "permanent" appliances are available in one or two pieces, depending on whether the faceplate is detachable (Fig. 25–4). A faceplate for any appliance must always have a means of attaching it to the body, regardless of the type of skin barrier employed. This is usually accomplished by the use of precut double-faced adhesive seals. The inner diameter of an adhesive disc must equal exactly the inner diameter of the faceplate.

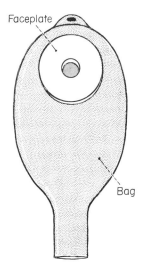

Faceplate

Bag

Figure 25–4. Reusable appliance. Faceplate may be attached (one piece) or detachable (two piece).

A one-piece appliance may be preferred by patients with arthritis affecting the use of the hands, those who have poor eyesight or who are blind, active youngsters who need a secure pouch construction with ease of application, patients with a neurologic deficit, and those with flush stomas. The choice of the one-piece appliance may also be simply personal preference.

The main advantages of the two-piece system are cost-effectiveness and durability. An elastic (O-ring) around the neck of the pouch holds the appliance to the faceplate. The placement of a double-faced adhesive disc to the back of the faceplate is the same as that with the one-piece appliance. Generally, the firmer the abdomen, the softer and flatter should be the faceplate.

In addition to the reusable system, many patients have a supply of disposable pouches available for an emergency, for rapid change, or for camping and traveling. It is important for these patients to be aware of the availability of both systems.

Procedure for Application of Reusable Appliance

1. Mount the faceplate on the pouch (if a two-piece appliance) and apply the O-ring.
2. Prepare the skin.
3. Apply the double-faced adhesive disk to the back of the faceplate.
4. Place the karaya washer around the stoma and expose the other side of the double-faced adhesive disk.
5. Seat the appliance around the stoma using the guidestrip.

With a well-positioned stoma of adequate length, a properly applied reusable pouch should remain in place without leakage and without skin injury for four to seven days. One may also shower or bathe with the pouch in place.

To remove the pouch when a protective skin shield is being used,

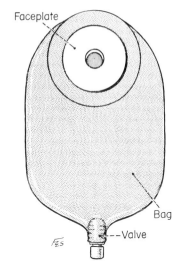

Figure 25–5. An ileal conduit appliance.

simply pull it away from the skin. If an adhesive cement is used, drip the solvent with a pipette between the skin and the faceplate as it is lifted off. All solvent should then be washed off the skin.

ILEAL CONDUIT

As mentioned earlier, the appliance is slightly different for urinary ostomies (Fig. 25–5), but the principles are basically the same. However, because urine dissolves karaya, this material cannot be used in an appliance. Alternatives include Stomahesive, ReliaSeal, or Colly-Seals.

Procedure for Application of Appliance

1. Cleanse the skin and apply skin preparation.
2. Use the appropriate protective disk.
3. Apply the pouch with the double-faced adhesive centered over the stoma.
4. Tape the faceplate on all sides.
5. During sleep it is necessary to employ a night drainage system.

COMPLICATIONS

Management of stoma complications — stenosis, prolapse, fistula, hernia, and abscess — are not within the scope of this chapter; discussions of these problems can be gleaned from the references (Goligher, 1976; Mahoney, 1976; Turnbull and Weakley, 1967; Corman et al., 1976).

MANUFACTURERS' PRODUCTS*

COMPANY	PRODUCT(S)
Atlantic Surgical Co., Inc. 1834 Lansdowne Ave. Merrick, LI, NY 11566 (516) 868-4545	Appliances Adhesive foam pads Stoma paper guidestrips Karaya powder
Coloplast/Bard, Inc. Berkeley Heights, NJ 07922 (201) 277-8000	Disposable pouches
Davol, Inc. Box D Providence, RI 02901 (401) 463-7000	Appliances ReliaSeal
Duke Labs, Inc. PO Box 529 South Norwalk, CT 06856 (203) 838-4737	Double-faced adhesive
Thomas Fazio Labs PO Box 35 Assonet, MA 02702 (617) 823-0753	Appliances Karaya powder
Ferndale Labs and Surgical, Inc. 780 West Eight-Mile Road Ferndale, MI 48220 (313) 548-0900	Deodorant tablets
John F. Greer Co. 530 E. 12th St. Oakland, CA 94606 (415) 465-4162	Appliances
Hollister, Inc. 211 East Chicago Ave. Chicago, IL 60611 (312) 680-1000	Disposable appliances Karaya washers, karaya paste Skin gel
Eli Lilly and Co. 307 E. McCarty Indianapolis, IN 46285 (317) 261-2000	Oral deodorant (bismuth subcarbonate)
Marlen Manufacturing and Development Co. 5150 Richmond Rd. Bedford, OH 44146 (216) 292-7060	Appliances Stoma paper guidestrips Karaya powder
Marsan Manufacturing Co., Inc. Packer Dr. Wausau, WI 54401 (715) 842-3391	Appliances
Mason Labs PO Box 334 Horsham, PA 19044 (215) 675-6044	Colly-Seals Colly-Seal appliances

MANUFACTURERS' PRODUCTS* *(Continued)*

COMPANY	PRODUCT(S)
3M Medical Products Div. 3M Center St. Paul, MN 55101 (612) 733-1110	Double-faced adhesive Adhesive foam pads Micropore paper tape
Nu-Hope Labs, Inc. 2900 Rowena Ave. Los Angeles, CA 90039 (213) 666-5248	Appliances
The Parthenon Co., Inc. 3311 West 2400 South Salt Lake City, UT 84119 (801) 355-7630	Deodorant tablets Devrom oral deodorant (bismuth subgallate)
The Perma-Type Co., Inc. PO Box 448 Farmington, CT 06032 (203) 677-7388	Appliances Karaya powder Fresh tabs
Perry Products 3803 East Lake St. Minneapolis, MN 55406 (612) 722-4783	Nonadhesive appliances
H. W. Rutzen and Son 345 West Irving Park Rd. Chicago, IL 60618	Appliances
Rystan Co. Dept. OQ, 470 Mamaroneck Ave. White Plains, NY 10605 (914) 761-0044	Derifil deodorant and tablets
E. R. Squibb and Sons, Inc. Professional Services Department Princeton, NJ 08540 (609) 921-4006	Kenalog spray Mycostatin powder Stomahesive
Torbot Co. 1185 Jefferson Blvd. Warwick, RI 02886 (401) 739-2241	Appliances
United Surgical Corp. 11775 Starkey Rd. Largo, FL 33540 (813) 392-1261	Appliances Adhesive foam pads Stoma paper guidestrips Bismuth subgallate Banish Skin prep Uri-Kleen

*This product list was prepared for the convenience of the reader and does not imply endorsement by the author, editors, publisher, or the American College of Surgeons.

GLOSSARY

TERM	DEFINITION
Faceplate	The mount that attaches to the pouch and is secured to the skin; the mounting ring or disk
Pouch	The bag
O-ring	An elastic rubber ring that secures the pouch to the faceplate in two-piece appliances
Double-faced adhesive disks	Paper, fiber, or cloth disks with adhesive on both sides to secure the appliance to the skin
Cement	A chemical that glues the faceplate to the skin; it must be removed with a solvent
Solvent	A chemical to cleanse the skin of adhesive or cement
Karaya washer	A protective ring placed around the stoma but of smaller opening than the faceplate so that the stoma and peristomal skin are protected
Stoma guidestrip	A soluble paper that is used to guide the appliance over the stoma
Skin preparation	Protective dressing that coats the skin

CONCLUSIONS

It is imperative that the ostomy patient be prepared adequately for adjustment to a new body image and lifestyle before the operation. The patient having an ileostomy often adjusts to this change more readily than the patient having a colostomy. The ileostomy patient's altered route for elimination allows that individual to pursue educational, social, vocational, and recreational goals that were not possible before because of his or her illness. However, the creation of a stoma because of cancer is often very difficult for the patient to accept. The reasons for this are the relatively short duration and the usually minimal symptoms of illness. For these patients, the cure may indeed seem worse than the disease.

To the patient, the most important part of the operation is the stoma. The surgeon should take as much care in the location and the creation of a satisfactory stoma as he or she does in securing adequate hemostasis. Successful rehabilitation requires a team effort.

REFERENCES

Beahrs, O. H.: Use of ileal reservoir following proctocolectomy. Surg. Gynecol. Obstet., 141:363, 1975.

Beart, R. W., Jr., Beahrs, O. H., Kelly, K. A., Dozois, R. R., and Wolf, S. A.: The continent ileostomy, a viable alternative. Mayo Clin. Proc., 54:643, 1979.

Corman, M. L., Veidenheimer, M. C., and Coller, J. A.: Ileostomy complications: Prevention and treatment. Contemp. Surg., 8:36, 1976.

Gelernt, I. M., Bauer, J. J., and Kreel, I.: The reservoir ileostomy: Early experience with 54 patients. Ann. Surg., *185*:179, 1977.

Goligher, J. C.: Present status of the continent ileostomy: Experience at the General Infirmary, Leeds. Dis. Colon Rectum, *19*:195, 1976.

Goligher, J. C.: Surgery of the Anus, Rectum and Colon, 4th ed. London, Balliere, Tindall, 1980.

Hill, G. L.: Ileostomy: Surgery, Physiology and Management. New York, Grune & Stratton, 1976.

Kock, N. G.: Ileostomy without external appliances: A survey of 25 patients provided with intra-abdominal intestinal reservoir. Ann. Surg., *173*:545, 1971.

Mahoney, J. M.: Guide to Ostomy Nursing Care. Boston, Little, Brown & Co., 1976.

Parks, A. G., Nicholls, R. J., and Belliveau, P.: Proctocolectomy with ileal reservoir and anal anastomosis. Br. J. Surg., *67*:533, 1980.

Turnbull, R. B., and Weakley, F. L.: Atlas of Intestinal Stomas. St. Louis, The C. V. Mosby Co., 1967.

Vukovich, V. C., and Grubb, R. D.: Care of the Ostomy Patient, 2nd ed. St. Louis, The C. V. Mosby Co., 1973.

Walker, F. C.: Modern Stoma Care. New York, Longman, 1976.

26

The Colon and Rectum

WARD O. GRIFFEN, Jr.

Many different operative procedures are performed on the colon and rectum. Whether performed electively, urgently, or as an emergency, they all have one thing in common: the exposure of incised tissue to contamination by colonic contents. Thus, reduction of bacterial content in the colon, particularly in the elective situation, is of paramount importance. Combatting potential or evident sepsis in the patient characterizes much of the preoperative and postoperative care.

Patients with colonic disease, however, also have unique problems. Often they are elderly and show the spectrum of diseases that commonly afflict this age group. Whether the colonic lesion produces obstruction, perforation, or toxic megacolon, the patient will have hypovolemia because of significant third space loss. The competent ileocecal valve in a patient with an obstructing lesion of the left colon presents a particular problem. The need for a temporary or permanent ostomy, interference with urinary tract function, postoperative sexual dysfunction, and the implications of cancer are all situations that need to be discussed thoroughly with the patient undergoing colon or rectal surgical procedures.

ELECTIVE OPERATIVE PROCEDURES ON THE COLON

PREOPERATIVE PREPARATION

General Features

Once the patient has agreed to colon resection or another colonic procedure, careful evaluation of the patient's other organ systems must be performed. The status of the heart with regard to rhythm and pumping function must be ascertained. If atrial fibrillation or congestive failure is present, the patient will require digitalis and stabilization before undergoing a major colonic resection. Pulmonary function can usually be evaluated adequately by history and a few simple maneuvers at the bedside. If doubt exists about the functional capacity of the lungs, baseline arterial blood gas determinations may alert one to specific problems that may be improved preoperatively by asking the patient to stop smoking, and by providing pulmonary physiotherapy and/or bronchodilators. Rarely is chronic obstructive airway disease a contraindication to operations on the colon, but it is important to recognize its existence preoperatively in order to insure better postoperative care.

Urinary tract problems are important to ascertain and correct preoperatively for two reasons. The finding of an elevated BUN or serum creatinine must be evaluated and corrected or improved before an operation is undertaken, simply to be assured that the patient will likely tolerate such a major procedure with minimal risk of renal embarrassment. If there is microscopic hematuria or any suspicion of urinary involvement by the colonic lesion, an intravenous pyelogram (IVP), cystogram, cystoscopy, or other appropriate tests should be performed preoperatively. If it appears there may be significant ureteral involvement by the disease in the colon, such as diverticulitis, it may be necessary to insert ureteral catheters preoperatively to help identify the ureters intraoperatively.

Other blood indices are necessary to obtain and evaluate. A fasting or random blood sugar may detect diabetes mellitus, which must be under control before the patient undergoes an operation. Since many of these patients are in the older age group, they may already be taking medication for a variety of ailments. The various oral diuretic agents are the greatest offenders in this area, since most of them act by increasing urinary excretion of potassium. Serum potassium concentration may not reflect actual total body potassium, and potassium deficiency can produce significant myocardial problems when a general anesthetic is given. If a patient has been receiving an oral diuretic and if his or her renal function is adequate, he or she should receive preoperative intravenous fluids containing potassium regardless of the serum potassium level. Obviously if the serum potassium level is low, supplemental potassium *above maintenance requirements* must be given before an operation is undertaken. Anemia is often seen with colonic malignancies, especially lesions of the right colon, and must be corrected prior to the operation. Packed red cell or whole blood transfusions given several days before the planned procedure provide for a more stable cardiovascular situation than waiting until a few hours before operation to administer blood or having to give blood during the operation.

A Foley catheter is usually not inserted until after the patient is anesthetized. In some instances when accurate monitoring of intake and output is desired preoperatively, the urinary catheter may be inserted the evening prior to the operation. Also, a central venous pressure line may be inserted prior to the operation to monitor the patient who exhibits marginal circulatory reserve. Skin shaving (if done at all) is performed immediately before the procedure, usually in the operating room. If nasogastric suction is necessary, and it is used more or less routinely except for left hemicolectomy, the tube is not inserted until anesthesia has been accomplished. Arterial catheterization is usually not needed except in those patients who may require frequent blood gas determinations in the postoperative period. If ureteral catheterization is necessary to aid in intraoperative identification of the ureters, this may be done after general anesthesia has been induced.

Colonic Factors

The preparation of the colon for patients who are to undergo an operation on the colon falls into two categories: (1) mechanical cleansing and (2) reduction of fecal bacteria. There is virtually unanimous agreement that preoperative mechanical preparation of the colon is essential for the performance of elective procedures on that portion of the gastrointestinal tract. The controversy that exists in this area revolves around the use of clear liquids versus elemental diets to reduce colonic fecal content and electrolyte solutions given by mouth in large quantities versus several enemas given in association with a cathartic administered per os. While controversy raged for a considerable period of time during the midportion of this century regarding the use of oral and systemic antibiotics in patients undergoing colonic operations, the controversy now has decreased to one of technique, i.e., which antibiotics to use, how often, when to start them, and when to discontinue their use, rather than a controversy about the concept of "sterilization of the bowel." Regardless of the variations on the theme, mechanical preparation and antibiotic reduction of bacterial content seem warranted in all operations in which the colon is to be opened or transected, and this preparation requires 48 to 72 hours preoperatively.

Preparation of the patient who is to undergo a colonic procedure is given in Table 26–1. Basically it consists of beginning a low-residue diet (clear liquids) three days before the operation is scheduled. A strong cathartic is given on that day unless the patient has received considerable catharsis in preparation for radiologic studies of the colon. Two days prior to the scheduled operation, enemas are given. Although the usual routine is to request enemas until clear, the nursing personnel differ greatly in their definitions of clear returns so that the number of enemas given to a single patient may vary from 3 to 15. In addition, significant electrolyte disturbances and metabolic derangements have been reported following long-term intestinal preparation. Therefore, it seems reasonable to order a specific number of enemas, and four or five enemas, depending upon the amount of feces or barium retained by a patient, provide adequate mechanical emptying of the colon in 95 per cent of the patients. Gentle oral laxatives are also given on the day preceding the operation. Clear liquids are continued until midnight. Supplemental intravenous fluids are begun on the evening preceding the operation.

Table 26–1. PREOPERATIVE PREPARATION OF PATIENTS FOR ELECTIVE COLON SURGERY PROCEDURES

Day 1 — Low-residue diet
        Castor oil (flavored) 45–60 ml

Day 2 — Low-residue diet
        Magnesium sulfate, 30 ml of 50% solution, p.o. A.M. and P.M.
        Saline enemas (4 or 5 depending on colon contents)

Day 3 — Clear liquids
        Magnesium sulfate in A.M.
        Neomycin 1 gm ⎫
                          ⎬ 1 P.M., 2 P.M., 6 P.M., and 8 P.M.
        Erythromycin 1 gm ⎭
        Intravenous fluids begun at 9 P.M. containing antibiotics and appropriate electrolyte composition

Day 4 — Operation

Neomycin and erythromycin by mouth are begun in the afternoon of the day preceding the operation, and administration of systemic antibiotics is begun on the evening preceding the operation. No enemas are given on the day preceding the operation because we have found that enemas given that soon prior to an operation often lead to a colon that is distended with a considerable amount of gas and some residual fluid.

Prophylactic Anticoagulation

Probably one of the most important advances in the care of the surgical patient has been the evaluation and prophylaxis of postoperative pulmonary embolism. This is particularly true in the patient undergoing colonic resection, both because of the magnitude of the operative procedures and the age group of the patients involved. A major factor in the prevention of postoperative pulmonary embolism is the use of small doses of heparin given subcutaneously, the so-called miniheparin regimen. Unless the patient is bleeding significantly, miniheparin is given to the patient upon admission to the hospital and is continued throughout hospitalization. The usual dosage is 5000 units (50 mg) of heparin subcutaneously every 12 hours. If a patient is quite obese, i.e., 25 kg or more above his or her ideal weight, the dose of mini-heparin may be increased to 5000 units subcutaneously every eight hours. The usual dosage regimen can be given at 6 A.M. and 6 P.M. each day so that the patient receives a dose of mini-heparin about two hours prior to a scheduled 8 A.M. operation.

POSTOPERATIVE CARE

General Features

The postoperative course in a patient who has undergone an elective procedure on the colon should be uncomplicated. The usual factors involved in the postoperative care of such patients are no different than those considered for any patient who has had a major abdominal procedure. Nasogastric suction is used for the prevention of intestinal distention. This is usually accomplished through a No. 18 sump-type nasogastric tube, which is placed at the time of the operation. The position of the tube can be checked during the operation, and of course in order to be effective in the prevention of intestinal distention, it must be patent and functioning. Other forms of gastrointestinal decompression are not as useful in the management of patients undergoing colonic operations. In particular, cecostomy should be condemned both because of the various difficulties associated with another colotomy and drainage catheter and because it is an ineffective means of decompressing the colon. The use of gastrostomy may be complicated by occasional leaking or bleeding as well as the possibility of a postoperative hernia. Frequently, nasogastric decompression is not necessary in operations on the left colon, including left hemicolectomy and low anterior resection.

Other postoperative complications that are seen after colon resections but that are not peculiar to these intra-abdominal operations include wound infection, pneumonia, urinary tract infection, occasional bleeding from the suture line, and mechanical bowel obstruction. The latter complication is not only rare but also difficult to diagnose in the postoperative period in any patient who has had an abdominal procedure.

The standard care of a patient who has had a colon operation, therefore, includes administration of intravenous fluids as long as nasogastric decompression is needed or as long as the patient is maintained without adequate oral intake. In general, the appearance of bowel sounds is *not* a suitable criterion for effective intestinal peristalsis. Indeed, a bowel movement may occur in the first day or two, but even this is not necessarily evidence of the return of normal peristalsis. In general, nasogastric suction is required for three or four days after which a 24-hour period without nasogastric suction but also without oral intake is required. The patient may then be fed and rapidly progressed to a regular diet as tolerated. Early ambulation, beginning the evening of the operation or certainly by the morning after, is the rule. While the patient is in bed, the legs are kept elevated at approximately 30 degrees, and active leg exercises are encouraged. Elastic stockings or elastic bandage wraps are not used, although intermittent pump elastic stockings may prove beneficial. If a miniheparin regimen has been started preoperatively, it is continued in the postoperative period.

Significant complications that occur with somewhat increased frequency following operations on the colon include septic problems of the wound, intra-abdominal spaces, and the pelvis, which are usually secondary to a leaking anastomosis after a left hemicolectomy. Less common complications include intestinal obstruction, urinary tract problems, and, rarely, bleeding.

Sepsis

A patient undergoing colon resection will often have an elevation of temperature postoperatively to 39°C. The obvious maneuvers on physical examination must include those used for detection of pulmonary problems, urinary tract infection, and other "extracolonic" reasons for fever. Abdominal examination in these patients is essential for the detection of wound infections, intra-abdominal abscesses, or an anastomotic leak with or without pelvic abscess. If the colon is opened during the operative procedure and leakage of a great deal of fecal contents occurs, it is my practice to close the fascia of the incision but to pack the wound open with povidone-iodine–soaked gauze and to allow the wound to close by secondary intention. If, on the other hand, the wound has been closed primarily, the usual signs of infection in the wound include increased tenderness, local redness and swelling, or increasing induration.

Prolonged ileus or the inability of the patient to tolerate any length of time without nagogastric suction indicates a lack of effective intestinal peristalsis postoperatively and may be the harbinger of an intra-abdominal abscess. In this instance, an acute abdominal series or three-way films that include a supine and upright examination of the abdomen in conjunction with a chest roentgenogram may be helpful in pinpointing an intra-abdominal abscess. Unfortunately, such abscesses are sometimes difficult to locate by means of radiologic examination and are not obvious on physical examination in the patient with continuing fever or prolonged ileus. A number of newer techniques have been devised for the detection of intra-abdominal sepsis and include ultrasonography, computerized axial tomographic scanning, and gallium scans. The first two techniques can be performed fairly expeditiously but still are only 70 to 75 per cent accurate. The gallium scanning technique requires approximately 48 hours to complete and is approximately as accurate as the other two methods.

Leakage from the anastomosis of small bowel to large bowel following a right colectomy is relatively rare. On the other hand, leakage from a colocolostomy following a left colectomy or low anterior resection probably occurs more often than is suspected. In a prospective study in which all patients undergoing low anterior resection had a radiopaque enema in the immediate postoperative period, Goligher et al. (1970) found an overall incidence of anastomotic leak of 69 per cent. In the majority of instances the leaks were minor and were associated only with a postoperative fever; there was no indication to perform any additional surgical procedure. However, major anastomotic leaks requiring surgical intervention occur in about 5 per cent of such patients. They seem to occur despite the variety of anastomotic techniques that are used. I personally prefer a two-layer closure consisting of interrupted nonabsorbable suture of the seromuscular outer layer and a running absorbable suture of the mucosal layer. The outer layer is an inverting one. If the leak from the anastomosis is causing significant systemic sepsis or is massive, then the patient must undergo another operation. The choices are (1) a proximal colostomy that must divert the fecal stream and that can be fashioned either as a loop colostomy or an end colostomy with a mucous fistula or (2) separation of the entire anastomosis with inversion of the rectal segment and exteriorization of the proximal segment as an end colostomy. The concept of "protecting" a low anterior anastomosis by performing a proximal diverting colostomy is popular but usually unwarranted. If the surgeon is sufficiently concerned about any anastomosis in that area, he or she should either repeat the anastomosis or turn in the rectal stump and bring out an end colostomy. If the poorly constructed anastomosis is allowed to remain in situ, it will probably leak and perhaps stricture, whereas the colostomy, usually a loop colostomy, may not divert. Since in this instance the patient ends up with a colostomy anyway, it would seem that an end colostomy is preferable because it presents an easier nursing problem.

Intestinal Obstruction

This complication is not only rare but also difficult to diagnose when it occurs in the immediate postoperative period. It is most frequently due to entrapment of a loop of bowel in a space that could not be adequately closed, for example, the pelvic floor following a left colectomy or around a colostomy. Occasionally it is due to adhesive bands. Every attempt must be made to close mesenteric defects: the procedure of choice is to suture the mesentery of colostomies to the peritoneum rather than leave even wide spaces around a colostomy. Differentiating intestinal obstruction from paralytic ileus can only be done by persistence in clinical evaluation and the use of serial roentgenographic examinations. If the patient has sepsis and mechanical bowel obstruction, then determining whether there is strangulation of the bowel becomes an exceedingly difficult problem. In general, abdominal tenderness postoperatively should decrease progressively as the patient recovers. Persistence of generalized tenderness, development of localized tenderness, or an increase in abdominal tenderness, development of localized tenderness, or an increase in abdominal tenderness in association with continued distention of the bowel either clinically or radiologically should make one suspicious of bowel obstruction. If, in addition to these signs, fever, instability of blood pressure, and an elevated leukocyte count are also seen, strangulating obstruction must be considered. Whenever there is a high suspicion of obstruction, reoperation is preferable to a "wait and see" policy.

Urinary Tract Problems

Urinary retention is a common complication in patients undergoing colonic surgery requiring pelvic dissection. It is more common in the male, especially one who has had any problem with prostatic enlargement. In fact, if the patient who requires a colonic operation has a significant degree of urinary tract obstruction on the basis of prostatic enlargement, he should be evaluated for an operation on the prostate gland prior to his colonic resection if possible. If this is not feasible, it may be necessary to provide for suprapubic urinary bladder drainage at the time of the colon resection in order to avoid long-term indwelling urethral catheterization. Most patients undergoing colonic resection already have a Foley catheter in place, and it is usually necessary for the catheter to remain in place for four or five days. Care must be taken to insure that it is functioning at all times in order to avoid overdistention of the bladder, and the usual catheter care of periodic irrigation and avoidance of introduction of bacteria is necessary in order to reduce the incidence of urinary tract infection.

Bleeding

Infrequently a patient undergoing colonic resection may have rectal bleeding postoperatively. Our experience suggests that the use of a continuous mucosal suture reduces the likelihood of this complication to a great extent. Nevertheless, when bleeding does occur, the source must be located. If the anastomosis is low enough, sigmoidoscopy can be used to visualize the site of bleeding and even allow coagulation of the bleeding site via the sigmoidoscope. Colonoscopy can be performed in the patient with a more proximal anastomosis, and the bleeding site can also be controlled by electrocautery via the colonoscope. If the hemorrhage is too massive to permit adequate visualization by means of a scope, arteriography may demonstrate the bleeding site, which can then be controlled by embolization with blood clot or Gelfoam. If all of these measures fail, reoperation may be necessary.

URGENT OR EMERGENT PROCEDURES ON THE COLON

PREOPERATIVE PREPARATION

General Features

The problems for which a patient must undergo an emergency colon procedure include obstruction, perforation, or massive bleeding. Under these circumstances there is no time for a prolonged thorough preparation of the colon or complete evaluation of the patient. Nevertheless, rapid evaluation and as much correction of the existing preoperative problems as is possible are the keys to successful management of these patients. Uncontrolled diabetes, congestive heart failure, and renal and pulmonary insufficiency must be ruled out or rapidly corrected preoperatively. Electrolyte derangements should be repaired.

All patients who are to undergo an urgent or emergency colon resection should receive parenteral antibiotics in order to minimize infection secondary to coliform organisms as well as anaerobic bacilli. My own preference is for a cephalosporin and an aminoglycoside given intravenously every six hours. Dosages should be altered for patients with renal insufficiency. In the presence of colonic obstruction or perforation, unless a contraindication exists, all patients should receive subcutaneous heparin, 5000 units preoperatively and every 12 hours postoperatively, as prophylaxis against thromboembolic disease.

Specific Problems

Whether patients have obstruction, perforation, or bleeding, they will be hypovolemic. In the latter instance, this is due to blood loss, and blood replacement is imperative before an operative procedure. If preoperative angiographic localization of the bleeding site is possible, not only may angiography be used for locating the bleeding site, but also the procedure can be therapeutic in that embolization of the small artery may cause the bleeding to cease abruptly and convert an emergency situation to an elective problem. Obstruction and perforation, particularly if the latter has resulted in significant peritonitis, invariably lead to hypovolemia by a third space loss. Preoperative replacement of this functionally lost fluid is essential for reducing postoperative morbidity and mortality. If specific electrolyte deficits are noted, they must be corrected, but often these patients simply show increased serum electrolytes and a slight increase in BUN, indicating dehydration. The patients should receive a balanced electrolyte solution such as Ringer's lactate, depending upon their cardiac status, and should be managed similarly to individuals suffering from multiple traumatic injuries. A central venous pressure line is inserted in order to estimate satisfactory restoration of blood volume, and a Foley catheter is inserted to monitor urinary output. Unless the patient is exsanguinating or the sepsis from the peritonitis is overwhelming, the surgeon usually can invest up to 12 hours in applying supportive measures before proceeding with the operation. It is time well spent.

A unique problem in patients with lesions of the left colon is the phenomenon of a closed loop obstruction. If the sigmoid carcinoma or diverticular disease produces complete obstruction at that level in a patient with a competent ileocecal valve that prevents retrograde flow into the ileum, the colon may distend quite rapidly. Nasogastric suction is imperative to prevent further introduction of air into the small bowel. The preoperative evaluation and general supportive measures must be accomplished quickly in order to avoid the catastrophe of cecal perforation. Once the diameter of the cecum has reached 12 cm or larger, a vent in the form of a colostomy somewhere between the obstructing lesion and the ileocecal valve must be accomplished quickly. Obviously the risks in such a patient or in the individual who is hemorrhaging are greater than in those urgent situations in which some preoperative support can be given.

ELECTIVE PROCEDURES ON THE RECTUM

PREOPERATIVE PREPARATION

The features of preoperative care of patients who are to undergo a procedure on the rectum, be it a total proctocolectomy, an abdomino-perineal resection, or transsacral, transanal, or transsphincteric removal of a lesion of the rectum, are identical to those of the patients undergoing an elective procedure on the colon. The status of their general health should be thoroughly evaluated. Mechanical and antibiotic preparation of the colon should be accomplished, and parenteral antibiotics and prophylactic minidose heparin should be instituted as described before. Foley catheterization is essential to the performance of a procedure on the rectum, particularly if a proctectomy is to be done,

Specific Features

The most important factor in the preoperative preparation of a patient undergoing a procedure on the rectum is a thorough discussion with the patient and the family about the consequences of the operation. Although some sort of ostomy may be necessary when operating on the colon, removal of the rectum invariably involves the creation of an ostomy, and the patient must be advised and informed of all of the problems associated with an ostomy. The surgeon should discuss this matter with the patient first. It is then wise to bring in for preoperative counseling an enterostomal therapist or a member of the local ostomy club for further discussions. If neither of these is available, the surgeon may want to ask one of his or her patients who is known to have a colostomy or ileostomy to see the patient preoperatively. The development of enterostomal therapy has been a great advance in the management of patients requiring an ostomy. Enterostomal therapists are available for preoperative counseling, which can often be given in much more thorough detail than a physician can give. Having met with the patient preoperatively, they can provide superb care in the postoperative period to help the patient in the difficult immediate postoperative transition period. Adequate time spent on the preoperative discussion about the ostomy leads to a satisfied and well-adjusted patient postoperatively. (See Chapter 25 for a more detailed discussion of colostomy and ileostomy.)

The other discussion that must be held with the patient who is facing removal of the rectum involves the genital tract. Males undergoing rectal resection for carcinoma must be informed of the possibility of postoperative impotence; females of childbearing age undergoing rectal resection for whatever lesion, but particularly for a lesion of the anterior wall of the rectum, should be asked to give permission for a hysterectomy if it seems indicated by the operative findings. Thus, sterilization of the patient must be discussed before the procedure is undertaken.

POSTOPERATIVE CARE

The usual postoperative care of patients undergoing resection of the rectum parallels that of the patient who has a colon resection. Nasogastric suction is usually required for three or four days until bowel sounds return and the ostomy begins to function. The urinary catheter may be required for as long as 10 days since the bladder has often lost some of its posterior support and upon falling posteriorly tends to kink the urethra, preventing proper urine evacuation. Additionally, interruption of some nerve pathways to the bladder may produce altered function of detrusion of urine for at least 10 days or longer. Intravenous fluid therapy is usually required for five or six days, and antibiotics are given systemically for two days postoperatively. Miniheparin therapy is continued until the patient is fully ambulatory.

The significant complications that occur following colon operations are also seen after resection of the rectum and include sepsis and intestinal obstruction. The latter complication is seen with somewhat increased frequency because of the presence of an ostomy. Many surgeons advocate keeping the space lateral to the colostomy wide open, but I prefer to close that space in order to prevent a potential volvulus, which can lead to mechanical obstruction of the bowel and even gangrene with perforation. Intestinal obstruction can also occur if defects in the reperitonealized pelvic floor should occur.

A unique problem in the postoperative care of the patient who has undergone proctectomy is management of the perineal space. In situations in which removal of the rectum has been performed for noninflammatory bowel disease, such as carcinoma of the rectum or familial polyposis, it is preferable to obtain meticulous hemostasis in the perineal wound and close it primarily, bringing out a sump suction catheter through a lateral stab wound. If the resection has been performed for inflammatory bowel disease, and particularly if the colon or rectum has been disrupted at any time during the procedure with spillage of fecal contents, the perineal wound should be packed open and allowed to heal by secondary intention. I prefer to use povidone-iodine–soaked Kerlix gauze or vaginal packs, which can then be removed at the time of the first sitz bath, approximately 48 hours postoperatively. Sitz baths are then continued as long as there is more than minimal drainage from the perineal wound. This may occur for as long as three months, and occasionally the perineal wound that has been left open following resection of the rectum for inflammatory bowel disease drains for years and may require secondary operations, such as saucerization of the wound and even resection of the coccyx.

In general, I prefer to mature colostomies and ileostomies in the operating room. This means bringing out approximately 8 cm of ileum and turning the end on itself in order to fashion a mucosa-to-skin closure that covers the serosal surfaces. In contrast, a colostomy is brought out to the surface of the skin where a mucocutaneous junction can be fashioned without having a great deal of the colon mucosa protruding from the stoma site. Temporary ostomy bags are glued to the skin surrounding the stoma and are changed postoperatively as necessary.

OPERATIONS ON THE ANORECTUM

The surgical management of hemorrhoids and other problems of the anorectum is an important consideration for all general surgeons. Anyone who has had the opportunity to perform anorectal procedures on patients realizes that the operation itself is rewarding and the patients are most grateful. Obviously much of the gratitude is the result of relieving the patient of a very uncomfortable situation, but much of it comes from the proper conduct of the operative experience.

PREOPERATIVE PREPARATION

Many patients with complaints referable to the anorectal area are locally uncomfortable. To subject them to a harsh laxative and multiple enemas is to invite dissatisfaction with the procedure no matter how skillfully it is performed. The colon need not be empty for the procedure to be successful, so a single enema may be delayed until appropriate anesthesia is obtained. On the other hand, if discomfort is not great, an enema may be given on the night before the scheduled procedure.

Before any surgical operation on the anorectum is undertaken, the general condition of the patient must be assessed and any abnormalities must be corrected. Many acute problems, such as thrombosis of a hemorrhoid, significant diarrhea, or marked cellulitis, can and should be controlled preoperatively. Occasionally an emergency procedure may be necessary. Regardless of whether the operation is being performed urgently or electively, vigorous instrumentation of the anus should await adequate anesthesia. Nevertheless, all efforts should be directed at assuring the surgeon that *benign* anorectal disease is the cause of the patient's problems and not some other entity, particularly a malignancy.

POSTOPERATIVE CARE

In the surgical therapy of anorectal diseases, the postoperative care is often the mark of a good surgeon rather than the operation that was carried out or how skillfully it was performed. Pain is the paramount problem, and anxiety referable to the first bowel movement is the second consideration. Both of these can be combated by appropriate analgesia.

The current enthusiasm for closed hemorrhoidectomy as an elective procedure has reduced the need for analgesia. When anal and perianal wounds need to be left open because of sepsis or emergency procedures for extensive thrombosis or gangrene, adequate analgesia is usually obtained by morphine or meperidine (Demerol). Local anesthesia, vigorous packing of the anus or frequent digital examination of the surgical site is not necessary and, in fact, may be harmful; for example, local abscesses may occur after the injection of an anesthetic agent in or near the surgical site.

Stool softeners may be useful, and some surgeons use a gentle laxative on the second or third day. I rely on bulk laxatives predominantly, having begun the patient on the regimen preoperatively. The patient gets out of bed on the evening of the operation and usually may go home 36 or 48 hours postoperatvely. If the patient voids immediately before the operation and very little fluid is administered, postoperative catheterization of the patient is rarely necessary.

Complications of operations on the anus include bleeding, local abscesses, anal stenosis, and incontinence. All of these have been reduced considerably with the increasing use of closed hemorrhoidectomy. If the wound must be left open, small mucosal bleeders can usually be controlled by electrocautery at the time of the operation. A small pack of Gelfoam soaked in a topical local anesthetic or placement of a sheet of Oxycel on the open areas will prevent postoperative bleeding. Frequent rectal examinations or anal dilatation is mentioned simply to condemn them. Inspection and gentle palpation of the operative site is all that is necessary, and this approach also lessens the occurrence of anal stenosis and perhaps abscess formation as well. Incontinence and anal stenosis are more often due to an improper operation rather than a complication to be expected in a finite percentage of patients. Incontinence occurs when the external sphincter is damaged and not repaired, and anal stenosis occurs when too much tissue is excised. The technique of closing the wound completely following hemorrhoidectomy almost guarantees excision of a limited amount of tissue.

SUMMARY

Thorough preoperative evaluation of the general health status to the extent possible is essential in the management of patients with disorders of the colon and rectum. Mechanical cleansing procedures and reduction of bacterial flora are of paramount importance to the safety and success of major operative procedures in the colorectum. Intraoperative attention to established technical principles will minimize the incidence of postoperative complications such as wound infection, sepsis, hernia, bowel obstruction, volvulus, hemorrhage, prolonged ileus, urinary retention, and impotence. The management of ostomies, perineal wounds, and the anorectum postoperatively requires dedication and skill if optimal results are to be obtained.

REFERENCES

Goligher, J. C., Graham, N. G., and DeDombal, F. T.: Anastomotic dehiscence after anterior resection of rectum and sigmoid. Br. J. Surg., 57:109, 1970.

Nichols, R. L., Broido, P., Condon, R. E., Gorbach, S. L., and Nyhus, L. M.: Effect of preoperative neomycin-erythromycin intestinal preparation on the incidence of infectious complications following colon surgery. Ann. Surg., 178:453, 1973.

Trinkle, J. K., Fisher, L. J., Ketcham, A. S., and Berlin, N. I.: The metabolic effects of preoperative intestinal preparation. Surg. Gynecol. Obstet., 118:739, 1964.

27

The Spleen

SEYMOUR I. SCHWARTZ

The spleen is an organ that receives surgical consideration for a wide variety of reasons. Trauma may necessitate removal or repair; hematologic disorders may be managed therapeutically or diagnostically by splenectomy, and, rarely, splenic cysts, tumors, or abscesses require surgical intervention. Some preoperative and postoperative principles concerning the spleen pertain to all patients, but many are brought into focus by the basic hematologic disorders for which splenectomy is performed.

GENERAL CONSIDERATIONS

Unless there is a hematologic abnormality, patients require no specific preoperative preparation. Antibiotics should not be instituted unless there is a specific indication. The usual preoperative medications are administered. Nasogastric decompression of the stomach obviates intraoperative gastric distention, which may compromise ligation and division of the short gastric blood vessels. Since this is an intraoperative consideration, it is reasonable to have the anesthesiologist insert the tube after the patient has been anesthetized and intubated endotracheally and then to remove the tube at the end of the operative procedure.

The splenic bed is not drained routinely, since drainage does not decrease the incidence of postoperative subphrenic abscesses. However, Penrose drains are generally employed for patients with myelofibrosis who have abundant collaterals to and from the spleen and in patients who have an increased risk of postoperative bleeding. If injury to the tail of the pancreas is suspected, a sump drain is employed to control pancreatic secretion. Although some clinicians have incriminated drainage of the splenic bed as a source of increased postoperative infection, this has not been documented by others or by our experience.

Following splenectomy or splenic repair, the immediate postoperative complication of greatest concern is hemorrhage. Although a hemostatic defect may be the source of hemorrhage or may play a significant role in its development, more often early reoperation is required to correct surgically remedial bleeding. In the overwhelming majority of patients, bleeding is related to not establishing adequate hemostasis at the time of original operation. Evacuation of a clot, which in itself will contribute to continued bleeding from disrupted small vessels and control of specific bleeding sites, should stop the hemorrhage. In very rare instances, diffuse bleeding associated with splenectomy may be related to pathologic local fibrinolysis as a consequence of trauma to the tail of the pancreas. In this unusual situation, only epsilon aminocaproic acid (EACA), used cautiously, may be effective in stopping the bleeding.

The patient with a predisposition to bleeding who undergoes splenectomy requires special attention to accomplish local hemostasis. With proper replacement therapy in those with deficiencies in coagulation factors or platelets, intraoperative bleeding should be minimal. Unanticipated bleeding at the time of operation may be due to (1) ineffective local hemostasis, (2) a previously present but unidentified hemostatic defect, (3) induced intravascular coagulation or fibrinolysis, (4) complications of blood transfusion, or (5) sepsis.

Chemical agents have been employed to control bleeding. Some are vasoconstrictive; others have properties that increase their bulk and aid in plugging disrupted vessels. Epinephrine applied topically induces vasoconstriction, but extensive use of this agent can result in significant absorption and adverse systemic effects. The most widely used commercially available products facilitating hemostasis during an operation are gelatin foam (Gelfoam), oxidized cellulose (Oxycel), and oxidized regenerator cellulose (Surgicel). Each acts to transmit pressure against the wound surface, and the interstices provide a scaffold on which the clot can organize. More recently, collagen has been used to induce hemostasis. Local application of micronized collagen to wounds or blood vessels may provide hemostasis, even in the presence of significant clotting defects.

Cold packs promote hemostasis by inducing vascular spasm and increasing endothelial adhesiveness. Electrocautery using a direct current between 20 and 100 milliamperes has been applied to control diffuse bleeding from large surface areas. Body cooling has also been used to control bleeding, but generalized hypothermia is of little value, because in order to reduce the blood flow to visceral organs, systemic temperature must be lowered to less than 35°C, and shivering and/or ventricular fibrillation may be encountered. In addition, thrombocytopenia may be a serious consequence of generalized cooling.

The most common complication following splenectomy is left lower lobe atelectasis, which is the most frequent cause of temperature elevation in the early postoperative course. Prevention of this complication may be accomplished by deep breathing exercises and the use of blow bottles or an incentive spirometer.

Fistulas related to surgical trauma to the tail of the pancreas rarely occur and almost always close spontaneously. Insertion of a catheter to control the secretions is helpful in reducing skin irritation.

Postsplenectomy hematologic changes are to be anticipated. Howell-Jolly bodies or nuclear remnants in the red blood cells occur in all patients who have been splenectomized, regardless of the cause (Lipson et al., 1959). The absence of Howell-Jolly bodies after careful inspection of the blood smear is the best indicator of residual splenic tissue. Target cells, cells with fine-inclusions (stippled red cells), and acanthocytes (red cells with an irregular spine), are also common findings in the peripheral blood smear. Neutrophilia, eosinophilia, lymphocytosis, and monocytosis are more variable in their occurrence and duration following splenectomy.

Modest thrombocytosis (increased platelet counts) often occurs after splenectomy, while profound elevations are extremely rare. If the platelet count is less than 1×10^6 per mm^3 and there is no evidence of thrombosis, usually no therapy is required. The blood concentration of platelets in asymptomatic patients that requires treatment is debatable, and many physicians do not treat such patients prophylactically even if the counts approach 2×10^6 per mm^3. We prefer to initiate therapy with acetylsalicylic acid (300 mg per day), and if the platelet count continues to increase, alkylating agents such as busulfan or chlorambucil may be used. Plateletpheresis can be used for short periods of time if urgent indications are present.

If thrombosis occurs, heparin therapy, employing an intravenous regimen, is indicated. Therapeutic doses of heparin and antiplatelet drugs such as aspirin or dipyridamole should not be used simultaneously, as the risk of hemorrhage is too great.

There has been an increasing concern regarding the potential for overwhelming sepsis following splenectomy for patients of all ages, particularly in children, but the data are not firm, and controlled studies in large populations have not been performed (Singer, 1973). It is probable that the risk of fatal sepsis is slightly increased in splenectomized individuals, but the absolute incidence in the adult is so low that it would have little bearing on the decision to do a splenectomy if otherwise indicated. It is essential to be aware of this association in a splenectomized patient who presents with septic shock, and large doses of antibiotics directed at encapsulated bacteria (*Diplococcus pneumoniae* and *Hemophilus influenzae*) should be initiated immediately.

Splenectomy in children under four years of age unquestionably increases the risk of severe infections caused by these bacteria. If splenectomy cannot be delayed or avoided, oral penicillin prophylaxis is indicated at least until puberty is reached. Recently, splenectomized children have received polyvalent pneumococcal vaccine as prophylaxis. Sufficient data are not available for final evaluation of this approach, which ignores other bacteria already implicated as causes of disseminated infection in splenectomized children.

SPECIFIC CONSIDERATIONS

TRAUMA

In view of the increasing concern for the long-term potential for overwhelming infection in children, a trend toward surgical conservatism has evolved. Contributing to the regimen of surgical conservatism has been the use of the splenic scan, with technetium sulfur colloid and splenic arteriogram, both of which aid in defining the extent and site of splenic rupture. In patients with paracentesis demonstrating blood, watchful waiting and the administration of up to four units of blood have been employed. The majority of children in one significant series (Weinstein et al., 1979) required no operation, and splenic bleeding spontaneously ceased. In children explored for splenic bleeding, the application of micronized collagen and omental tamponade has been a successful alternative to splenectomy, and in some, hemisplenectomy with the same measures applied to the raw surface has been successful. When the splenic parenchyma is lacerated during an operative procedure, it is now appropriate to attempt repair rather than to proceed directly to removing the entire organ.

Table 27–1. HEMATOLOGIC DISORDERS
AMENABLE TO SPLENECTOMY

Hemolytic anemias
Hereditary spherocytosis
Hereditary elliptocytosis
Hereditary nonspherocytic hemolytic anemia
Thalassemia
Sickle cell disease
Idiopathic autoimmune hemolytic anemia
Idiopathic thrombocytopenic purpura
Thrombotic thrombocytopenic purpura
Primary hypersplenism
Secondary hypersplenism
Myeloid metaplasia
Hodgkin's disease, lymphosarcoma, leukemia
Miscellaneous disorders
Felty's syndrome
Sarcoidosis
Gaucher's disease
Niemann-Pick's disease
Fanconi's syndrome
Porphyria erythropoietica
Spontaneous rupture

HEMATOLOGIC DISORDERS (Table 27–1) (Schwartz et al., 1971)

Sickle Cell Syndromes

Patients with these disorders rarely require splenic surgery, since the thrombosis that occurs usually results in autosplenectomy. In unusual circumstances, splenectomy may be indicated for an enlarged spleen and a hypersplenic state. The other situation that may necessitate splenic operation in these patients is the development of a splenic abscess requiring splenectomy or drainage. Subjects with homozygous sickle cell disease, sickle hemoglobin, or other hemoglobin abnormalities such as sickle hemoglobin C, are subject to increased risks of vaso-occlusive or thrombotic crises during or shortly after the administration of a general anesthetic or an operation. Subjects with sickle cell trait also may have an increased risk, but this is much lower than those with the disease.

Treatment with antibiotics for any concomitant infection, good hydration, and oxygenation, and the prevention of acidosis are the keystones of successful management. Partial exchange transfusion to reduce the proportion of red cells with sickle hemoglobin and to raise the hemoglobin mass to acceptable levels (about 11 gm per 100 ml) is the mainstay of preoperative management. Hypothermia during the procedure should be avoided because it promotes sickling, and spinal anesthesia imposes a risk by causing peripheral vascular pooling. Similarly, obstruction of limb flow by improper positioning on the operating table should be avoided. When operating upon a patient with sickle cell disease, it is usually appropriate to remove the appendix in order to reduce the difficulty of diagnosing future episodes of abdominal pain.

Other Anemias

Hereditary spherocytosis is the congenital anemia that is most commonly managed by splenectomy. The operation should be delayed until the patient is at least four years of age in order to reduce the risk of infection, and postoperatively, antibiotics are continued prophylactically through puberty. As is the case with all hemolytic anemias, preoperative evaluation should include cholecystography, and intraoperatively the gallbladder should be palpated for calculi. If stones are present, concomitant cholecystectomy is indicated.

Splenectomy should be considered for patients with thalassemia major or intermedia or with unstable hemoglobin Koln when (1) the spleen is moderately or markedly enlarged, (2) anemia is severe, (3) excessive transfusion requirements are present, or (4) leukopenia or thrombocytopenia suggests that hypersplenism accompanies the hemolytic anemia. The spleen may also reach a size that creates mechanical problems or may undergo focal infarctions. Patients with these chronic anemias tolerate a low hemoglobin mass well, and the preoperative hemoglobin level need be raised only to approximately 11 gm per 100 ml to optimize oxygen transport. Thalassemics have an increased propensity to infection, and all children with thalassemia subjected to splenectomy should receive prophylactic antibiotics through puberty.

Patients with immune hemolytic anemias may be advised to have a splenectomy. This procedure is rarely beneficial in diseases associated with cold antibodies and is unnecessary in drug-induced disease. In patients with warm antibodies or immune hemolytic anemias unrelated to drug usage, splenectomy should be considered in the following circumstances: patients who do not respond to high-dose glucocorticoid treatment within six weeks, patients who respond but require dose levels that are intolerable, and patients with contraindications to steroid therapy, such as peptic ulcer or brittle diabetes mellitus.

In these, as in all patients who receive steroids for a long period of time, a preoperative boost is indicated, and glucocorticoids should be administered intravenously during the operation and throughout the early postoperative period. If splenectomy has a favorable effect, which is apparent soon after the operation, rapid discontinuance of steroids can be carried out, since six to eight weeks of preoperative therapy will not result in prolonged adrenal suppression. Particularly in these patients, but also in other anemic patients who have received multiple transfusions, antibody formation may make crossmatching of blood difficult, and time must be allowed preoperatively for this possibility.

Thrombocytopenia

Splenectomy should be performed in patients with idiopathic thrombocytopenic purpura (ITP) who have not responded to glucocorticoid therapy (40 mg per m²) within six weeks or who have responded initially and then have become thrombocytopenic when the dosage is reduced. In glucocorticoid-responsive patients in whom thrombocytopenia recurs when the hormone is tapered, increased doses should be given prior to the operation to improve the platelet concentration. Rarely, intracranial bleeding or profound gastrointestinal hemorrhage may require intensive glucocorticoid treatment and emergency splenectomy.

The indications for splenectomy in thrombocytopenic patients with systemic lupus erythematosus (SLE) are the same as those for ITP, and the preparation is similar. In patients with thrombotic thrombocytopenic purpura (TTP), rapid preparation with glucocorticoids and emergency splenectomy has provided the best results.

Platelet transfusions are *not* administered prior to splenectomy in patients with accelerated splenic disruption of platelets, such as ITP, SLE, TTP, and hypersplenism. The large young platelets in such subjects are hemostatically more effective, and hemostasis may be maintained with many fewer platelets. Moreover, immediately after clamping the splenic pedicle, the platelet count begins to rise, and hemostasis is improved. These patients rarely require platelet transfusion during the operative procedure, but if intraoperative bleeding is excessive and hemostasis appears inadequate, 10 to 20 platelet packs should be administered after the spleen is removed. Therefore, platelet packs should be available for any patient with a reduced platelet count who is to undergo splenectomy. Postoperatively, glucocorticoids can be discontinued rapidly after a sustained rise in the platelet count becomes apparent.

Other Hypersplenisms

Hypersplenism as a result of partial hypertension rarely constitutes an indication for splenectomy. Patients with idiopathic hypersplenism, i.e., an enlarged spleen and cytopenia in the presence of a normal or hypercellular marrow and without evidence of an underlying disease, are helped by splenectomy. If cytopenia persists or recurs after splenectomy in these and other patients, residual accessory spleens or autotransplanted splenic tissue may be implicated. This may be investigated by careful examination of the peripheral blood smear for the absence or disappearance of the usual postsplenectomy changes in red cells and the use of technetium sulfur colloid or radiochromium-labeled, heat-treated red cells to locate residual splenic tissue.

Myelofibrosis

Splenectomy should be considered in patients with this disorder when the spleen is so large that it causes abdominal discomfort or digestive complaints and when multiple symptomatic splenic infarctions have occurred. The hematologic indications are anemia resulting in increasing transfusion requirements, leukopenia resulting in infection, and, rarely, thrombocytopenia causing ecchymosis and/or purpura. There is no evidence that the spleen is a significant hematopoietic organ in these patients, and, therefore, adverse hematologic effects are not anticipated following splenectomy (Schwartz, 1975).

Myelofibrotic patients are the most difficult to treat in reference to their preoperative preparation, intraoperative management, and postoperative therapy. A high complication rate, primarily related to thrombosis and bleeding, has been reported. These complications can be decreased markedly by preoperative treatment to reduce the erythremia and thrombocytosis if either is present. Phlebotomy, chemotherapy with busulfan or chlorambucil, and radioactive phosphorus may be used as required in individual cases. The longer the interval during which the red cell mass and platelet count is normal prior to the operation, the less the risk of hemorrhage and thrombosis.

In view of experience (Gordon et al, 1978) with several patients who developed thrombosis of the splenic vein extending into the portal and superior mesenteric veins after splenectomy, a circumstance that is extremely rare following splenectomy for trauma or other hematologic diseases, we have recently adopted the protocol of preparing these patients with acetylsalicylic acid and low-dose heparin (5000 mg twice a day) and continuing these drugs for one week postoperatively. Since the institution of this regimen, we have not noted the preceding pathologic consequences, and the patients have had no bleeding problems. As mentioned previously, if large venous collaterals are encountered during the procedure, drains are left in the subphrenic space in contradistinction to our usual policy for splenectomy.

Leukemias and Lymphomas

There is little evidence that splenectomy significantly alters the effects of chemotherapy during either the responsive or accelerated phase of chronic myelogenous leukemia (CML). Splenectomy has proved useful in patients with chronic lymphatic leukemia (CLL) and lymphomas with symptomatic splenomegaly or severe cytopenia when residual marrow function is present.

Splenectomy is now performed frequently in patients with Hodgkin's disease and, less often, Hodgkin's lymphoma, as part of the staging to determine the extent of the disease prior to establishing the use and extent of radiotherapy and chemotherapy. The case for surgical staging of Hodgkin's disease is based on the inaccuracy of definition of disease below the diaphragm when clinical evaluation and radiographic assessment are used alone. Presently, most centers are staging Hodgkin's disease in patients who clinically are in the I and II categories, and in some in the clinical IIIA category (asymptomatic patients). An exception to this generalization is the patient in the IA category in whom the pathology demonstrates lymphocyte predominance, since this rarely metastasizes below the diaphragm. The case for staging is enhanced by the fact that radiation therapy can be reduced, the incidence of left lower lobe pneumonitis is reduced, and left renal nephritis is reduced. Another advantage is the avoidance of hypersplenism late in the course of the disease and the improved hematologic tolerance during total lymph node irradiation and myelosuppressive chemotherapy. Percutaneous and peritoneoscopic-directed liver biopsies are alternatives to staging of non-Hodgkin's lymphoma. The yield of staging procedures is highest in patients with nodular lymphomas and is lowest in patients with histiocytic lymphomas, and it is generally concluded that the presence of disseminated disease can be detected in the majority of patients with non-Hodgkin's lymphoma without performing a staging laparotomy.

These patients require little in the way of specific preoperative therapy. Transfusion in patients with CLL and lymphosarcomas should be warmed because these patients may have associated cryoglobulinemia. If postoperative radiotherapy is anticipated for patients, silver clips should be applied to the splenic pedicle to aid in defining the field of treatment.

The question of increased sepsis after staging laparotomy has been raised, and the largest series of reported cases (Donaldson et al., 1976) noted no relationship between splenectomy and sepsis. Therefore, except for the usual prophylaxis in the pediatric patient, antibiotics are not recommended.

MISCELLANEOUS INDICATIONS

In patients with Felty's syndrome (rheumatoid arthritis, splenomegaly, and neutropenia), improvement in the white blood cell count and reduction in the incidence of recurrent infection are to be anticipated. Similarly, splenectomy corrects the hematologic abnormalities associated with sarcoidosis and Gaucher's disease. No specific preoperative and postoperative management maneuvers are required for these patients.

REFERENCES

Donaldson, S. S., Glatstein, E., Vosti, K. L., Wilbur, J. R., Rosenberg, S. A., and Kaplan, H. S.: Serious bacterial infections in pediatric Hodgkin's disease: Relative risks of radiotherapy, chemotherapy and splenectomy. Proc. Am. Soc. Clin. Oncol., 17:252, 1976.

Gordon, D. H., Schaffner, D., Bennett, J. M., and Schwartz, S. I.: Postsplenectomy thrombocytosis: Its association with mesenteric, portal, and/or renal thrombosis in patients with myeloproliferative disorders. Arch. Surg., 113:713, 1978.

Lipson, R. L., Bayrd, G. P., and Watkins, C. H.: The post-splenectomy blood picture. Am. J. Clin. Pathol., 32:526, 1959.

Schwartz, S. I.: Myeloproliferative disorders. Ann. Surg., 182:464, 1975.

Schwartz, S. I., Adams, J. T., and Bauman, A. W.: Splenectomy for hematologic disorders. Curr. Probl. Surg., May, 1971.

Singer, D. B.: Post-splenectomy sepsis: In Rosenberg, H. S., and Bolande, R. P. (eds.): Perspectives in Pediatric Pathology. Chicago, Year Book Medical Pub., 1973, pp. 285–312.

Weinstein, M. E., Govin, G. C., Rice, C. L., and Virgilio, R. W.: Splenorrhaphy for splenic trauma. J. Trauma, 19(9):692, 1979.

28

The Vascular System

LAZAR J. GREENFIELD
ROBERT W. BARNES

This chapter addresses our approach to the perioperative evaluation and management of peripheral arterial diseases. In this discussion, peripheral arterial disease refers to occlusive or aneurysmal disorders of the extrathoracic aorta and its major branches: the major arteries of the extremities, the abdominal visceral arteries, the major vessels of the aortic arch, and the extracranial cerebrovascular arteries of the neck. The unique principles of preoperative, intraoperative, and postoperative evaluation, monitoring, and management of patients undergoing elective and emergent vascular surgical procedures will be emphasized. The chapter will also acquaint the reader with the principles and appropriate application of the noninvasive peripheral vascular laboratory studies that have exerted an increasing influence in vascular surgery in the interval since publication of the last edition of this manual.

PREOPERATIVE EVALUATION

HISTORY

The history obtained from the patient remains the single most important body of information to guide the surgeon in managing the patient with suspected peripheral arterial disease and should systematically answer the following three general questions: (1) Is vascular disease the cause of the patient's symptoms? (2) What is the physiologic effect of the lesion? (3) What is the operative risk?

Claudication, or leg pain with exercise relieved by rest, should define the presence of peripheral arterial disease and should be distinguished from the atypical leg pain (pseudoclaudication) associated with musculoskeletal or neurospinal disorders. Vascular rest pain of the foot, which may be relieved by dependency (a sign of advanced arterial

517

insufficiency) should not be confused with nocturnal leg (calf) cramps, which represent a benign condition unrelated to arterial disease. The history should indicate the physiologic impairment induced by arterial disease, information that cannot be obtained from the arteriogram. The patient's functional impairment is the criterion that dictates whether or not the patient will require operation, and, thus, whether or not arteriography is indicated. Physiologic impairment may be categorized as follows, in descending order of clinical and operative significance: (1) life-threatening lesion (ruptured aneurysm); (2) limb-threatening lesion (rest pain, tissue necrosis); (3) self-care–threatening lesion (advanced claudication); (4) occupation-threatening lesion (claudication); (5) recreationg-threatening lesion (claudication); and (6) asymptomatic lesion (abdominal aortic aneurysm, carotid bruit).

The first three categories of physiologic impairment are indications for emergent or urgent operation. The latter three categories of functional deficit are reasons for elective operation in patients who represent a satisfactory operative risk. Operative risk is determined from a careful history of the presence and severity of associated pulmonary, cardiac, renal, cerebral, and malignant disease. Such disorders may preclude operation or may modify the type of operation if the latter is necessary (extra-anatomic bypass procedures as opposed to intra-abdominal reconstruction).

PHYSICAL EXAMINATION

Inspection. Only signs of advanced arterial occlusive disease are evident on an inspection of the extremity, including tissue necrosis (gangrene or ischemic ulceration), trophic changes (hair loss on toes, thickened nails, and skin atrophy), and elevation pallor with dependent rubor of the foot. A unique form of tissue ischemia is the "blue-toe syndrome," involving digit cyanosis or necrosis in the presence of palpable distal pulses. Such local ischemia is usually the result of an embolus of atheromatous or thrombotic debris from a proximal ulcerated atherosclerotic plaque. This sign should lead to a careful search for vascular bruits. Arteriography should be performed to identify an operable lesion in order to prevent repeated progressive embolization and limb loss. Inspection should also lead to a search for abscesses, particularly in diabetes mellitus, which require prompt incision and drainage prior to arterial reconstruction. However, other forms of local débridement or limited distal amputations should be *avoided* prior to arterial reconstruction in order to prevent extension of tissue necrosis in the presence of advanced arterial occlusive disease.

Palpation. Determination of limb coolness is of diagnostic value only when there is asymmetry of temperature at similar levels of the two extremities. Symmetrical coolness of the hands and feet reflect peripheral vasoconstriction and may not be signs of arterial occlusive disease.

Hypoesthesia and muscle paresis are signs of advanced arterial insufficiency but are not contraindications to expeditious revascularization. However, muscle rigor is an ominous sign and a relative contraindication to vascular reconstruction (because of the threat of cardiac or renal dysfunction from the toxic products of myonecrosis following revascularization). Assessment of pulses is based on the following:

0 — absent pulse (defines proximal arterial occlusion)

1+ — reduced pulse (implies proximal arterial stenosis or occlusion with excellent collateral circulation)

2+ — normal pulse

Auscultation. Vascular bruits define the presence and location of arterial stenosis. In the neck, it is important to distinguish the carotid bifurcation bruit from bruits in the common carotid artery lower in the neck, supraclavicular bruits over the subclavian arteries, and murmurs radiating from the thorax (aortic valve or arch vessels). In addition to listening for common femoral artery bruits in the groin, auscultation should be carried out over the renal arteries (in each hypochondrium and in each flank), abdominal aorta, the common and external iliac arteries, the superficial femoral artery in the thigh, and the popliteal arteries behind the knee. Mild arterial stenosis may not produce a bruit at rest but may be detected by auscultation for bruits following exercise.

VASCULAR LABORATORY

Goals. The noninvasive peripheral vascular laboratory provides objective, diagnostic information for the following purposes:

CONFIRM DIAGNOSIS. The laboratory study permits confirmation of the diagnosis in patients with suspected peripheral vascular disease and resolves ambiguity of clinical manifestations in patients with atypical symptoms (pseudoclaudication and night cramps).

QUANTIFY PHYSIOLOGIC IMPAIRMENT. The laboratory provides quantification of the functional derangement of the circulation at rest and following stress, information that is not available from the arteriogram.

DETECT ASYMPTOMATIC DISEASE. High-risk patients may be prospectively screened for asymptomatic disease, such as carotid occlusive disease or postoperative deep vein thrombosis.

PREDICT THERAPEUTIC OUTCOME. The laboratory evidence is of particular value to the vascular surgeon in predicting the success of aortoiliac reconstruction, femoropopliteal bypass, sympathectomy, or healing at a given level of amputation.

MONITOR THERAPY. Noninvasive techniques permit monitoring of the success of intraoperative reconstructions and the detection of operative complications prior to closure of incisions.

PATIENT FOLLOW-UP. Repeated noninvasive diagnostic studies

permit objective follow-up of the natural history of, or the influence of medical or surgical therapy on, peripheral arterial disease.

NONINVASIVE TECHNIQUES

A description of the methods used in the noninvasive peripheral vascular laboratory is beyond the scope of this manual. However, an understanding of the general principles and appropriate applications is important in the preoperative, intraoperative, and postoperative management of the patient. The two most useful instruments for the surgeon are the Doppler ultrasonic velocity detector and the plethysmograph. The Doppler detector is a relatively inexpensive and versatile instrument for the evaluation of peripheral arterial, cerebrovascular, and venous disease. Although in experienced hands the instrument is the most useful of the available vascular techniques, the method requires considerable experience before maximal accuracy is achieved. Nevertheless, the device may be used by the physician and also by a nurse, technician, or other paramedical personnel. The plethysmograph is useful to record pulse waves or blood flow graphically in various regions of the body. Several plethysmographic techniques have been developed, including water, air, impedance, strain gauge, and photopulse devices. The authors employ the latter two devices, which permit assessment of peripheral arterial, cerebrovascular, and venous disease. Plethysmographs are more expensive than Doppler devices, but their application generally requires less experience and subjective interpretation on the part of the technician.

The data from the vascular laboratory studies usually fall into one of the following two categories: (1) pulse waveform analysis or (2) limb blood pressures.

Pulse waveform analysis generally involves qualitative evaluation of the amplitude and shape of the cyclic pulsations associated with each heart beat. The pulse wave may be arterial blood flow velocity (as recorded with the Doppler velocity detector) or limb volume pulsation (recorded with a plethysmograph). Peripheral arterial occlusive disease progressively dampens the pulse waveform in proportion to the degree of circulatory impairment.

Quantification of the presence and location of arterial occlusive disease is most simply performed by the measurement of segmental limb systolic blood pressures at the proximal thigh, above the knee, below the knee, and at ankle level. All pressures must be referenced to the arm systolic blood pressure. Normally, the segmental leg blood pressure should equal or exceed that of the arm. In the presence of arterial occlusive disease, the segmental limb blood pressures will be below that of the arm by an amount proportional to the degree of circulatory impairment. In advanced arterial occlusive disease (rest pain or tissue necrosis) and in patients with diabetes mellitus, measurement of toe systolic pressures by plethysmography is important. Leg segmental pressures are measured at rest and following treadmill exercise or temporary limb ischemia (reactive hyperemia) in order to quantify the functional impairment.

ARTERIOGRAPHY

The decision to perform arteriography in the patient with peripheral arterial occlusive disease rests upon the decision to undertake arterial reconstruction. The arteriogram is not indicated to establish the diagnosis, which is evident from the clinical examination and the confirming noninvasive laboratory studies. However, arteriography remains the cornerstone for guiding the planned operation, because the procedure defines the reconstructability of the arterial occlusive process. In addition, the arteriogram may reveal unsuspected lesions that may influence surgical management (such aneurysms and renal arterial stenosis). There are many angiographic techniques, and their description is beyond the scope of this manual. The particular technique selected is dependent upon the experience and preference of the radiologist or surgeon performing the procedure. Of critical importance in obtaining adequate preoperative arterial studies is effective communication between the operating surgeon and the radiologist regarding the objectives and specific information desired from the study.

SPECIFIC PROCEDURES

Aortoiliac Reconstruction

The surgeon is concerned with four problems associated with aortoiliac disease: (1) the significance of the aortoiliac bruit; (2) the etiology of impotence (vascular, neurogenic, or psychogenic); (3) the presence of associated conditions requiring correction prior to, or at the time of, major aortoiliac reconstruction; and (4) the likelihood of success of aortoiliac reconstruction in the patient with multisegmental arterial occlusive disease.

A reduced femoral pulse and a loud aortoiliac bruit signify stenosis of hemodynamic significance. A bruit in the presence of a normal femoral pulse requires further assessment to clarify the significance of the lesion. If the femoral pulse is reduced or obliterated following exercise, the stenosis is of hemodynamic significance. A low proximal thigh pressure (below the systolic pressure of the arm) reflects significant aortoiliac stenosis. Finally, alterations in common femoral artery flow velocity as assessed by Doppler ultrasound (loss of reversed flow in diastole and attenuation of systolic flow velocity) are sensitive indicators of the degree of aortoiliac stenosis.

Impotence is assessed by careful history and laboratory evaluation.

Psychogenic impotence is inferred if the patient has a normal morning erection (a reflex associated with the distended urinary bladder). Neurogenic impotence is implied if the penile systolic blood pressure (assessed by plethysmography or Doppler ultrasound) is normal. Vascular impotence is suggested by a low penile systolic pressure (below the mean systemic blood pressure).

Associated arterial occlusive disease must be evaluated prior to aortoiliac reconstruction if suggested by the history or physical or laboratory examinations. Cerebrovascular and coronary artery disease may require correction prior to aortoiliac revascularization. Contrast arteriography may reveal renovascular or visceral arterial lesions that may need correction at the time of aortoiliac reconstruction.

The vascular laboratory provides hemodynamic information of predictive value in identifying the patients who may not receive sufficient relief of symptoms following aortoiliac reconstruction alone in the presence of multisegmental arterial occlusive disease. Such patients tend to have a higher proximal thigh systolic blood pressure and two or more abnormal segmental limb pressure gradients distal to the aortoiliac segment.

Abdominal Aortic Aneurysmectomy

The diagnosis of abdominal aortic aneurysm is usually made by physical examination. An excretory urogram is obtained to assess renal function, determine the course of the ureters, screen for possible renovascular disease in associated hypertension, and detect the rare but important horseshoe kidney. Abdominal ultrasound B-scan is obtained to resolve diagnostic ambiguity about a small aneurysm vs. the tortuous aorta, particularly in the obese patient, to determine the size and extent of the abdominal aneurysm, and to follow the growth rate in patients who are candidates for observation of the aneurysm. Contrast arteriography is performed in the following circumstances: (1) to evaluate associated peripheral arterial occlusive disease, (2) to identify renal arterial lesions in patients with significant hypertension, (3) to evaluate patients with suspected thoracoabdominal aortic aneurysms, and (4) to assess the patency of the mesenteric arteries in suspected insufficiency.

Femoropopliteal (Femorotibial) Reconstruction

The surgeon must address the following four problems in patients who are candidates for femoropopliteal or more distal reconstruction: (1) insuring adequate arterial inflow, (2) insuring adequate arterial outflow, (3) selecting the optimal graft material, and (4) predicting the outcome of operation.

The methods to evaluate disease of the aortoiliac segment have been discussed previously. Assessment of arterial outflow includes determination of segmental leg blood pressures and evaluation of contrast arteriograms, which should be performed to visualize the tibioperoneal vessels and the circulation of the foot. Current reconstructive procedures are designed to bypass all arterial occlusions and stenoses, even to the level of the foot. Autogenous saphenous vein is the conduit of choice for femoropopliteal or femorotibial bypass procedures. In the absence of suitable autogenous vein, the authors currently favor expanded polytetrafluoroethylene, which has been successfully used below the knee, even to the foot. However, careful long-term follow-up studies are necessary to determine whether this prosthesis is a suitable alternative to autogenous saphenous vein in the absence of the latter.

Although an unobtainable or very low (less than 20 per cent of the arm) ankle systolic pressure suggests a poor prognosis for femoropopliteal or femorotibial reconstruction, all suitable candidates for this procedure should undergo arteriography to evaluate the potential for reconstruction. If preoperative arteriography does not define the distal runoff circulation, an attempt should be made to determine the presence of a Doppler arterial signal in one of the pedal arteries. The presence of such a signal suggests patency of the vessel at that location and should prompt the surgeon to consider operative exploration and intraoperative arteriography to identify a patent distal circulation suitable for femorotibial bypass.

Carotid Endarterectomy

Arteriography is recommended for all patients with symptoms or signs of cerebrovascular insufficiency. Operation is indicated for patients with the following findings: (1) hemispheric transient ischemic attacks or amaurosis fugax, (2) hemispheric stroke with significant or complete recovery, (3) vertebrobasilar insufficiency associated with significant carotid stenosis, and (4) nonlateralizing or global symptoms and significant carotid stenosis.

Carotid endarterectomy is performed electively for patients with transient ischemic attacks and a stable stroke with recovery. Operation is delayed four to six weeks following a recent stroke with recovery. Urgent operation is advised for crescendo transient ischemic attacks and for sudden disappearance of a bruit or carotid thrombosis at the time of arteriography in the absence of stroke. Contraindications to operation include the following: (1) progressive stroke, (2) completed stroke (without significant recovery), (3) internal carotid occlusion (except for external carotid endarterectomy for stenosis in the presence of persisting transient ischemic attacks), (4) intracranial disease of greater severity than extracranial disease, and (5) other severe generalized medical disorders.

The surgical management of asymptomatic carotid disease (with or without bruit) remains controversial. A prospective randomized study is planned to clarify this problem. The authors employ noninvasive diagnostic screening techniques (Doppler ultrasound and plethysmography) to determine the hemodynamic significance of the asymptomatic carotid bruit. Selected patients with abnormal cerebrovascular screening tests are evaluated by arteriography, and carotid endarterectomy is recommended for severe stenosis.

Renovascular Reconstruction

A work-up for renovascular hypertension is recommended for patients in the following categories: (1) sudden worsening of long-standing hypertension, (2) sudden development of severe hypertension, (3) the young patient, and (4) a history compatible with renal infarction (embolus or trauma).

The preoperative evaluation should include routine tests of renal function, rapid-sequence excretory urography, renal vein renin assays, and renal arteriography. Split renal function tests are not routinely performed but may be helpful in quantifying the amount of residual renal functional mass in a small ischemic kidney. Operation is recommended for patients of suitable risk in the following categories: (1) severe hypertension uncontrolled by medication, (2) the young patient with severe hypertension, (3) deterioration of renal function, and (4) the patient with severe hypertension who requires concomitant aortoiliac reconstruction for peripheral occlusive disease.

Operation is not advised for patients over 70 years of age, patients with severe generalized atherosclerotic occlusive disease, and poor risk patients with other systemic disease.

Sympathectomy

Lumbar sympathectomy is of limited value for the patient with peripheral arterial occlusive disease. The operation is recommended as a sole means of therapy only in patients with advanced arterial occlusive disease that is not amenable to reconstructive procedures and that results in early foot ischemia, rest pain, or minimal tissue necrosis. The procedure offers no benefit for claudication alone. The efficacy of the procedure may be predicted by noninvasive laboratory testing. The amplitude of digit volume pulsation (determined by plethysmography) normally decreases in response to a deep breath if sympathetic tone is intact. Absence of digit pulse attenuation in response to a deep breath signifies loss of sympathetic tone, which is particularly common in diabetes mellitus patients. The amplitude of plethysmographic pulsation increases during foot reactive hyperemia in response to temporary (three-minute) ischemia induced by a toe pneumatic cuff. Absence of any increment in toe pulse amplitude during reactive hyperemia is absolute evidence of maximal vasodilatation and is a contraindication to lumbar sympathectomy. Lumbar sympathectomy is also not recommended as a routine concomitant procedure during peripheral arterial revascularization. Although foot vasodilatation may be increased following concomitant lumbar sympathectomy, particularly with aortoiliac reconstruction, a randomized prospective study has failed to show any additional benefit of lumbar sympathectomy over the improvement following revascularization alone. Femoropopliteal or femorotibial reconstruction for advanced arterial occlusive disease should result in postoperative foot hyperemia, and the resultant vasodilatation is maximal and not increased by the addition of lumbar sympathectomy.

Amputation

Digit or limb amputation is reserved for the patient with rest pain or tissue necrosis associated with nonreconstructable peripheral occlusive disease. The goal of amputation is to preserve maximal limb length while insuring healing at the selected site of amputation. Noninvasive laboratory evaluation provides hemodynamic information of predictive value in determining the most distal level of probable amputation wound healing. A toe systolic pressure of 50 mm Hg or greater in the nondiabetic and 70 mm Hg or greater in the diabetic is compatible with healing of a digit or transmetatarsal amputation. A below-knee systolic pressure of 70 mm Hg or greater is usually associated with healing of an amputation at that level. However, healing is possible with pressures lower than 70 mm Hg, and a below-knee amputation should always be attempted, if possible, provided an audible Doppler arterial signal is heard in the popliteal fossa. Preoperative counseling and evaluation by the rehabilitation medicine service is an important step in the management of the prospective amputee.

PREOPERATIVE PREPARATION

BOWEL PREPARATION

Prior to aortoiliac reconstruction or other intra-abdominal revascularization procedures, a thorough mechanical bowel preparation is carried out. Oral cathartics and enemas are administered three days preoperatively. A low-residue diet is prescribed, with clear liquids on the day prior to operation. No enemas are administered for 24 hours prior to operation. Antibiotic bowel preparation is unnecessary.

MONITORING CATHETERS

A central venous catheter is inserted on the evening prior to the operation in patients undergoing aortoiliac reconstruction. In patients with a history of congestive heart failure or significant cardiac or pulmonary disease, a balloon-tipped pulmonary artery catheter is inserted for intraoperative and postoperative monitoring of pulmonary artery wedge pressures. A radial or brachial artery monitoring catheter is inserted in the operating room in patients undergoing carotid endarterectomy, major aortoiliac reconstruction, and in patients with a history of significant cardiopulmonary disease. A nasogastric tube and urinary drainage catheter are inserted after induction of anesthesia. The urinary catheter is connected to a graduated receptacle for frequent timed measurements of urinary output during and after operation.

PREOPERATIVE HYDRATION

In all patients undergoing major arterial reconstruction, one liter of balanced crystalloid solution is infused intravenously during the period of no oral intake on the night prior to operation.

PREOPERATIVE MEDICATIONS

Preoperative medications are given as determined by the preference of the anesthesiologist. Of importance is the avoidance of narcotics or other agents capable of producing hypotension in patients who are to undergo carotid endarterectomy. Prophylactic antibiotics, usually a cephalosporin, are administered eight and two hours prior to operation.

SKIN PREPARATION

The patient is instructed to bathe with germicidal soap twice daily for three days prior to operation. Shaving of the operative area is performed in the operating room to avoid the frequent development of furunculosis that develops following shaving on the day prior to operation.

INTRAOPERATIVE CARE

ANESTHESIA

General anesthesia is administered for patients undergoing carotid endarterectomy and aortoiliac reconstruction or other intra-abdominal procedures. General or spinal (or epidural) anesthesia is suitable for patients undergoing femoropopliteal reconstruction or amputation. Local anesthesia is satisfactory for femoral thrombectomy. Patients undergoing carotid endarterectomy must have their blood pressure

THE VASCULAR SYSTEM / 527

under meticulous control with avoidance of hypotension, using vaso-pressors (metaraminol or phenylephrine), if necessary. Marked hyper-tension is controlled by intravenous nitroprusside. Normothermic and normocarbic anesthesia is preferred for carotid endarterectomy. Ade-quate oxygenation is insured by periodic determination of arterial oxygen tension. Frequent communication between surgeon and anes-thesiologist is necessary to insure adequate management of cardiac, pulmonary, and renal function during major vascular reconstruction. Appropriate monitoring of central venous pressure, arterial pressure, pulmonary artery wedge pressure, and urinary output permits optimal management of fluid balance in patients with significant cardiopulmo-nary or renal disease.

Heparin

Prior to clamping of the arteries during major arterial reconstruction, heparin, 100 units per kg of body weight, is administered intravenously. Additional heparin, 50 units per kg, is administered each hour during arterial interruption. The systemic heparin effect is not reversed at the conclusion of the procedure unless excessive bleeding is noted. Patients who undergo operation for ruptured abdominal aortic aneurysm are not given systemic heparin but are managed with regional intra-arterial injection of 20 ml of saline containing heparin, 10 units per ml. A similar solution of heparinized saline is used to irrigate the opened arterial segments. Prophylactic low-dose subcutaneous heparin is not used for prophylaxis of postoperative deep vein thrombosis.

Antibiotics

Intravenous cephalosporin antibiotic is administered every four hours during operation. The operative wounds are irrigated repeatedly with a saline solution containing 1 per cent neomycin.

Operative Technique

Meticulous operative technique with avoidance of excessive tissue trauma and maintenance of careful hemostasis is standard for vascular surgical procedures. Although operative exposure may be accomplished expeditiously, the period of specific vascular reconstruction (endarterec-tomy or bypass) should not be hurried. The use of ocular loupes (2.5 × magnification with wide-angle lenses) facilitates performance of recon-struction of small vessels, including femorotibial bypass procedures, renovascular reconstruction, and carotid endarterectomy.

NONINVASIVE VASCULAR MONITORING

Ankle Blood Pressure. Patients undergoing aortofemoral recon-struction or profundaplasty are assessed by intraoperative monitoring of ankle blood pressures using Doppler ultrasound. Ankle blood pressures, as referenced to arm pressure, are measured after induction of anesthe-sia, after arterial reconstruction, and before closure of operative wounds. The pressures are measured beneath the drapes, outside the sterile operative field. If the ankle:arm pressure index does not improve by at least 10 per cent, arteriography is performed to rule out a thrombotic or embolic arterial complication. If such complications do not exist and the patient has multisegmental arterial occlusive disease, consideration should be given to immediate additional distal arterial reconstruction to avoid an unsatisfactory postoperative result. Patients who have a signifi-cant improvement in ankle systolic blood pressure (greater than 10 per cent increase in ankle:arm pressure index) are significantly improved in the late postoperative period. Patients who have no improvement or deterioration of ankle blood pressure following aortofemoral reconstruc-tion (in the absence of a complication or severe vasoconstriction) show no significant improvement in the follow-up period.

Sterile Doppler Probe. Arterial flow velocity signals are obtained with a sterile Doppler probe at the sites of arterial reconstruction following femoropopliteal or femorotibial bypass procedures, renal reconstruction, and carotid endarterectomy. In addition, a periorbital Doppler examination, outside the sterile operative field, is performed prior to wound closure following carotid endarterectomy. Persistent abnormalities of ophthalmic artery flow are an indication for operative arteriography to exclude a technical misadventure.

Electromagnetic Flowmetery. As an alternative to Doppler ultra-sonic evaluation, an electromagnetic flowmeter is employed to assess resting blood flow through reconstructed arterial segments. An impor-tant evaluation of the integrity of arterial reconstruction is the assess-ment of the increase in blood flow during vasodilatation induced by intra-arterial injection of 30 mg of papaverine. The hyperemic blood flow should be at least twice the resting value in successful arterial re-construction.

INTRAOPERATIVE ARTERIOGRAPHY

The integrity of femoropopliteal or femorotibial reconstruction is assessed by routine operative arteriography. Arteriograms are also ob-tained following femoral thromboembolectomy. Contrast arteriography is performed after aortofemoral, renal, or carotid reconstructions only if noninvasive monitoring suggests a vascular complication.

Specific Procedures

Carotid Endarterectomy. The authors employ selective shunting for cerebral protection during arterial clamping for carotid endarterectomy. The need for an indwelling shunt is determined by measurement of carotid back (stump) pressure. A shunt is employed if the back pressure is less than 40 mm Hg. Monitoring of the electroencephalogram during operation is an excellent alternative for determining the need for a shunt. The most important variable in prevention of postoperative neurologic deficit is meticulous operative technique, with avoidance of undue manipulation of carotid bifurcation prior to clamping, careful unhurried endarterectomy with removal of all residual debris, and careful closure of the arteriotomy. The period of clamping should be of no concern even in the absence of a shunt. The results of carotid endarterectomy without a shunt or with selective shunting techniques compare favorably with reported series in which a shunt is used routinely.

Aortoiliac Reconstruction. An open endarterectomy is performed for localized atherosclerotic disease that does not extend into the external iliac arteries. A knitted Dacron prosthesis is employed for aortofemoral bypass procedures for extensive atherosclerotic disease. The peritoneum is opened over the right side of the infrarenal abdominal aorta; unnecessary dissection over the aortic bifurcation is avoided to prevent postoperative impotence. If the inferior mesenteric artery must be sacrificed, care is taken to avoid injury to the ascending left colic branch to minimize the chance of postoperative colonic ischemia. If colon ischemia is suspected intraoperatively, a sterile Doppler probe is used to determine the presence or absence of arterial flow signals in the antimesenteric border of the colon. If marked ischemia is present, reimplantation of the inferior mesenteric artery with an excised button of aorta is performed to the aortic prosthesis. Declamping of the aorta is performed gradually to avoid hypotension.

Femoropopliteal (Femorotibial) Reconstruction. The autogenous saphenous vein is excised with care to avoid clamping injury of the vein. Blood flow through the vein is maintained until immediately prior to starting the anastomosis. The vein is gently distended with cold heparinized blood to avoid excessive endothelial injury. The anastomoses are carried out with continuous sutures of fine polypropylene. A bypass prosthesis, polytetrafluoroethylene, is used in the absence of a suitable autogenous vein. All significant femoropopliteal or tibial disease is bypassed even if the distal anastomosis must be made at the ankle. Ocular loupes facilitate the careful performance of each anastomosis.

Amputation. Successful amputation requires the same general operative technique as employed in arterial reconstruction. Whenever possible, local foot amputations or below-knee amputations are performed to preserve the functional integrity of the knee joint. In below-knee amputations, long posterior flaps are employed, excising the deep posterior compartment muscles. Although a randomized study failed to demonstrate an advantage to immediate rigid prosthesis over soft elastic dressings, the rigid plaster permits earlier maturation of the stump for accelerated rehabilitation.

POSTOPERATIVE CARE

GENERAL MEASURES

Patients undergoing major arterial reconstruction are monitored in an intensive care unit until a stable and satisfactory postoperative status is achieved. Intravenous fluids, including blood, plasma expanders, crystalloid solutions, and free water, are employed using conventional guidelines of blood pressure and urine output and, in indicated circumstances, central venous pressure, pulmonary artery wedge pressure, and cardiac output determinations, depending upon the complexity of the case. Diligent pulmonary care is essential. Gastrointestinal decompression following intra-abdominal procedures is carried out until bowel function returns. Early ambulation is encouraged after all major peripheral arterial reconstructive procedures unless patient debility or postoperative complications are present. Prophylactic antibiotics are continued for three days after operation. Anticoagulants are not employed. Antiplatelet agents (aspirin, 0.3 gm twice weekly, and dipyridamole, 50 mg four times a day) are routinely employed following carotid endarterectomy, and occasionally after other procedures in which the risk of postoperative thrombosis is considered excessive.

NONINVASIVE MONITORING

Limb temperature, color, and pedal pulses are repeatedly assessed (every hour) in the immediate postoperative period. Because of the fallibility of pulse detection and the fact that patients with multisegmental arterial occlusive disease may not have palpable pedal pulses postoperatively, noninvasive measurements of ankle systolic blood pressures by Doppler ultrasound are performed as a routine part of postoperative nursing care. The ankle pressures are always referenced to the arm systolic pressure (ankle:arm pressure index); deterioration of the ankle pressure index suggests an arterial occlusive complication and may be an early sign of the need for operative reexploration.

COMPLICATIONS

Thrombosis, Embolism. Postoperative occlusion of the reconstructed arterial segment may be detected by loss of pulses, development of signs of ischemia, or a deterioration of the ankle pressure index. All arterial occlusive complications should be considered for immediate reoperation, with the exception of the occurrence of a stroke following carotid endarterectomy. There is no evidence that immediate reoperation for a severe neurologic deficit is efficacious, although early reoperation may be considered when a mild neurologic deficit is present or when there is evidence of postoperative carotid occlusion as determined by noninvasive diagnostic studies.

Hemorrhage. Persistent postoperative bleeding demands operative reexploration except in instances of mild wound hematoma or generalized bleeding diathesis. A groin wound hematoma should not be opened unless it is large, and then it should be evacuated under meticulous sterile conditions in the operating room. The wound should be reapproximated in layers after thorough irrigation with antibiotic solution.

Infection. Infected superficial wounds should be adequately drained. If wound infection in the groin extends to a limb of the aortofemoral prosthesis, the prosthesis will probably require removal. However, focal groin wound infections that do not involve a collection of fluid around the prosthesis may be treated by local wound dressings saturated in organic iodine solution, with frequent changes as often as necessary to avoid collection of exudate. If excision of the prosthesis is required, arterial reconstruction via extra-anatomic bypass (axillofemoral bypass) may be required. A wound infection complicated by bleeding from the suture line of a prosthesis is always an indication for removal of the prosthesis. Infection involving an autogenous vein may be treated by local wound care unless suture line bleeding develops, which necessitates ligation of the affected arterial segment and removal of the graft.

Colon Ischemia. If diarrhea occurs in the immediate postoperative period with or without blood in the stool, colon ischemia must be suspected and sigmoidoscopy should be performed. If colon ischemia or infarction is noted, oral intake is avoided and systemic antibiotics are administered. The majority of such patients will heal their lesions without stricture. If stricture develops, colostomy and segmental colon resection may be required. If signs of colon perforation develop, immediate operation and colostomy must be carried out with removal of the necrotic segment of colon. Avoidance of postoperative hypotension is important in order to minimize the risk of colon ischemia.

Neurologic Deficits. Immediate or delayed neurologic deficit, either transient or permanent, is the most serious complication following carotid endarterectomy. The usual cause is embolic debris from the site of carotid endarterectomy, either prior to or after release of the clamps. Such emboli, which can be minimized by meticulous operative technique, are probably more common than cerebral ischemia during the period of carotid clamping. The latter complication can be avoided by appropriate use of an indwelling shunt in patients who require such cerebral protection. Unfortunately, the use of a shunt is attended by occasional complications of atheromatous or air emboli. The most common neurologic deficit following aortoiliac reconstruction is neurogenic impotence. This complication occurs as a result of transection of sympathetic nerves anterior to the terminal aorta and its bifurcation, particularly over the origin of the left common iliac artery. Careful placement of incisions and avoidance of unnecessary dissection will reduce the risk of iatrogenic impotence. A rare but catastrophic complication of aortoiliac reconstruction or abdominal aortic aneurysmectomy is postoperative paraplegia as a result of interruption of a major lumbar arterial supply of the anterior spinal artery.

Other Complications. The most common postoperative complications following vascular reconstruction are those that are common to other major surgical procedures, including cardiac, pulmonary, and renal dysfunctions. Their prevention and treatment require the usual perioperative care necessary for all major surgical procedures.

EMERGENCY PROCEDURES

Ruptured Abdominal Aortic Aneurysm

Preoperative Management. The major goal in the preoperative care of a patient with a ruptured abdominal aortic aneurysm is the expeditious transfer of the patient to the operating room. Only a minimal number of preoperative procedures should be carried out, including the insertion of large-bore intravenous lines and the submission of a blood specimen to obtain type-specific blood. Unless the patient is in shock, excess fluid administration must be avoided to minimize aggravation of a contained retroperitoneal hematoma. Other diagnostic studies, including radiography, particularly arteriography, must be avoided. Much of the emergent preoperative preparation, such as insertion of additional intravenous lines, electrocardiographic monitoring, a Foley catheter, and possibly an arterial catheter, can be carried out in the operating room.

Intraoperative Management. The abdomen should be shaved, prepared, and draped prior to induction of anesthesia. Anesthetic induction should be as gentle and rapid as possible to avoid straining by the patient and possible aggravation of bleeding. The abdomen should be entered rapidly through a long midline incision. Immediate control of the aortic rupture is best carried out by manual compression of the suprarenal aorta by the first assistant. Blind clamping of the aorta through the hematoma must be avoided to prevent injury to the renal vein or artery or tearing of the inferior vena cava. If the neck of the aneurysm cannot be readily identified, the aneurysm itself may be incised rapidly and the thumb of the operating surgeon inserted immediately into the neck of the aneurysm. A Foley catheter (30 ml bag) can be inserted for control of bleeding from the aorta, with similar catheters controlling each iliac artery. The neck of the aneurysm can then be identified by direct exposure with subsequent placement of a vascular clamp on the infrarenal aorta. Regional heparinization of each iliac artery is accomplished by infusion with 20 ml of heparinized saline solution. Urinary output is maintained using appropriate fluid replacement and diuretics, if necessary. Minimal dissection is performed, and the arterial reconstruction is accomplished with a Dacron prosthesis, using a tube graft if possible.

ACUTE ARTERIAL THROMBOSIS OR EMBOLISM

Preoperative Management. Acute arterial occlusion is manifested by one or more of the classical findings of pain, pallor, paresthesia, paresis, coldness, and lack of a pulse in the extremity. The two most common causes of acute arterial occlusion are embolism, usually from cardiac disease, and thrombosis superimposed on an underlying atherosclerotic plaque. It is important to differentiate the two conditions, if possible, because the operative management may differ for the two conditions. Arterial embolus is suggested by a history of sudden pain in the extremity, absence of a history of antecedent claudication, the presence of cardiac arrhythmia (atrial fibrillation), mitral stenosis, or prior myocardial infarction, and the presence of intact peripheral pulses in the uninvolved extremity. Arterial thrombosis is characterized by gradual onset of numbness of an extremity, a history of antecedent claudication, absence of cardiac disease, and the presence of bruits or pulse deficits in the contralateral extremity. Arteriography is helpful in the patient with suspected arterial thrombosis in order to plan possible arterial reconstruction. However, arteriography is unnecessary in the patient with suspected arterial embolism and should be avoided in patients with marked ischemia requiring immediate revascularization for limb salvage. Heparin therapy, 100 units per kg body weight intravenously, should be administered as soon as possible in order to avoid extension of thrombosis and to prevent additional embolism

Operative Management. Arterial revascularization is indicated in all patients with acute arterial occlusion unless satisfactory collateral circulation is present in a high-risk patient or unless irreversible ischemia is present. A contraindication to revascularization, in addition to advanced gangrene, is the presence of muscle rigor with inability to force extension of the affected muscle. Revascularization of such a limb may result in fatal cardiac or renal dysfunction as a result of the systemic effects of toxic metabolites from myonecrosis.

Most patients with acute arterial occlusion of the lower extremity are initially approached by exploration of the common femoral artery, which may be accomplished under local anesthesia, unless arterial reconstruction for chronic arterial occlusive disease is anticipated.

Thrombectomy using a balloon catheter (Fogarty) should be performed, preferably within six hours of arterial occlusion. However, it is important to realize that delayed thrombectomy, even days or weeks after occlusion, may be possible provided that the limb is viable. Introperative assessment of adequacy of inflow and outflow may be carried out by noninvasive vascular monitoring and by operative arteriography. Major arterial reconstruction may be necessary in patients with arterial thrombosis superimposed upon underlying arterial occlusive disease. The necessity for such procedures must be anticipated when preparing and draping the patient. Aortoiliac reconstruction must be considered for good risk patients, and axillofemoral and femoral-femoral bypass procedures should be considered in patients of poor operative risk.

Postoperative Management. Systemic heparinization should be initiated 12 hours postoperatively if the patient has suffered an arterial embolus. A search for and treatment of cardiac disease should be carried out in the postoperative period. Continued anticoagulation is recommended with oral sodium warfarin if a persisting cardiac source of recurrent embolus is present. In patients who have undergone revascularization for marked ischemia, the surgeon should be alert to the development of postoperative compartment compression requiring fasciotomy, as dictated by clinical signs and/or determination of compartment muscle pressure or blood flow.

ARTERIAL TRAUMA

Preoperative Management. The usual measures of resuscitation, including attention to airway, control of bleeding, and treatment of shock, require the usual priority. Rapid control of hemorrhage must be carried out with direct pressure. The surgeon should know the rapid methods of approach to major vessels, particularly branches of the aortic arch in the chest and neck. Such vascular injuries may require immediate thoracotomy or mediastinotomy in the emergency room to prevent exsanguination. Arteriography is performed in instances of diagnostic ambiguity if arterial or venous injury is suspected in the absence of obvious major hemorrhage. The preoperative measures should be accomplished with dispatch in order that the patient can be transported to the operating room immediately. Prophylactic antibiotics are administered along with tetanus prophylaxis.

Operative Management. Arterial repair may require simple closure, resection and end-to-end anastomosis, resection and vein graft interposition, or bypass of the injured arterial segment. Prosthetic material should be avoided except in repair of injury to large arterial segments. In the presence of gross contamination, particularly with intestinal contents, ligation of the injured artery may be necessary. If limb viability is threatened, an extra-anatomic bypass may be necessary. Some venous injuries may be managed by ligation, but critical venous segments, particularly the popliteal vein, should be repaired to avoid massive venous congestion and possible venous gangrene postoperatively.

SUMMARY

The most critical variables in successful elective or emergent peripheral arterial reconstruction are the appropriate selection and careful preoperative and postoperative management of the patient. A detailed history and thorough physical examination remain the most important guides to the detection of the specific vascular problem and decision for operative management of the patient. The vascular laboratory provides valuable noninvasive objective information to confirm the diagnosis, resolve diagnostic ambiguity, quantify physiologic impairment, and predict and monitor the results of medical and surgical therapy. Arteriography is reserved for the patient who is a candidate for operation in order to define the reconstructability of the arterial occlusive disease. In addition, noninvasive techniques and arteriography provide important intraoperative information about the success of arterial reconstruction and the presence of operative complications. Intelligent attention to preoperative, intraoperative, and postoperative care will minimize the complications and increase the likelihood of successful revascularization of peripheral arterial disease.

29

Surgery of the Thyroid Gland

EDWIN L. KAPLAN

In recent years, thyroidectomy has become a very safe operation when performed by experienced neck surgeons. However, the procedure is not without occasional serious problems, even in the best surgical hands. Colcock and King, for example, reported that no deaths occurred in 1246 consecutive operations; however, significant postoperative complications, such as tetany and recurrent laryngeal nerve injury, occurred in a small percentage of patients.

In order to achieve such an enviable record, a surgeon must have both an excellent knowledge of the anatomy of the neck and superb technical skill. It is of equal importance that he or she have a sound understanding of the pathophysiology of the diseases of the thyroid; he or she must properly prepare the patient for operation; and, finally, must be cognizant of the potential postoperative complications and be prepared to treat them appropriately.

PREOPERATIVE EVALUATION

HISTORY AND PHYSICAL EXAMINATION

A careful, thorough history and physical examination are of great importance. They aid the examiner in evaluating the patient's physiologic thyroid status, in differentiating between benign and malignant nodules, and, finally, in assessing the patient's operative risk. For example, in evaluating a patient with a thyroid nodule, perhaps the most important information to establish is whether there has been a history of low-dose irradiation exposure to the neck, since the risk of thyroid cancer is much greater for such individuals. A history of medullary thyroid carcinoma in a family member also places the individual at a much higher risk for also having a similar carcinoma.

THYROID FUNCTION TESTS

Many of the commonly used thyroid function tests are listed in Table 29–1. Each is a direct or indirect assessment of thyroxine and tri-iodothyronine secretion from the thyroid gland. In past years, the measurement of basal metabolic rate (BMR) and protein bound iodine (PBI) were the most commonly utilized assessments. More recently these tests have been replaced by measurements of serum total thyroxine (TT_4), serum tri-iodothyronine (T_3), and by the resin T_3 uptake (RT_3U) test, which provide more specific and accurate information. The calculation of the free thyroxine index (FTI, also called the T_7 test)° is very important, since it corrects for elevations in TT_4 that are found during pregnancy or estrogen therapy that are due to an increase in thyroxine-binding globulin in these states. Currently, the FTI is the best and most effective test of serum thyroid hormone that is routinely available. It correlates closely with the circulating free thyroxine concentration, the physiologically important fraction of thyroxine. Unfortunately, it is dif-

---

°Free thyroxine index (FTI) = $T_4 \times \dfrac{\text{patient's } RT_3U}{\text{control } RT_3U}$

Table 29–1. THYROID FUNCTION TESTS

TEST	NORMAL RANGE	COMMENTS
Serum thyroxine (T_4 or TT_4)	4.9–12.0 μg%	Radioimmunoassay (RIA)
Serum tri-iodothyronine (T_3)	100–200 ng/100 ml	Usually RIA
Resin T_3 uptake (RT_3U)	Varies with lab 20–30%	Indirect assessment of unsaturated thyroxine-binding globulin capacity (TBG)
Free thyroxine index (FTI)	Varies with lab 6.4–10.5 μg%	Combines T_4 and RT_3U
Radioactive iodine uptake (RAIU)	Varies with lab 10–30%	Range depends on iodine intake in the diet
Serum TSH	Varies with lab 0–8 or 15 μU/ml	RIA
Basal metabolic rate (BMR)	−10 to +10%	Rarely done
Thyroxine-binding globulin capacity (TBG)	12–20 μg T_4/100 ml ±1.8 μg	Electrophoresis or RIA
TRH stimulation test	Peak TSH 10–30 μU/ml at 20–30 min	Elevated response in hypothyroidism if pituitary is normal. Basal TSH increased. Decreased response in thyrotoxicosis and hypopituitary hypothyroidism. Basal TSH decreased.

ficult to measure the free thyroxine concentration, but the FTI or T_7 gives the closest approximation of this value. In general, we measure both the serum TT_4 and FTI as routine screening tests. An elevation of FTI correlates with hyperthyroidism, and a decrease in FTI correlates with a hypothyroid state.

The thyroid uptake of a tracer dose of radioactive iodine (^{131}I or ^{125}I) or of radioactive technetium (^{99m}Tc) as pertechnitate are also useful measurements of thyroid function. However, both of these measurements are greatly influenced by the amount of iodine in the patient's diet—the greater the iodine in the diet, the lower the uptake. Thus, the patient's uptake must always be compared with control values of normal patients. We generally reserve this test for patients who are going to receive radioactive iodine for therapy of Graves' disease. Finally, the measurement of serum TSH (thyroid stimulating hormone from the anterior pituitary) is an excellent indirect measurement of thyroid function, because it is elevated in hypothyroid states and normal or low in thyrotoxicosis.

The thyrotropin-releasing hormone (TRH) stimulation test is a means of testing the responsiveness of the pituitary. TRH is administered and the output of TSH is measured in the blood.

Specific Diagnostic Serum Tests

Autoimmunity

The presence of circulating antithyroglobulin antibodies (TGHA) and/or antimicrosomal antibodies (MCHA) in the serum correlates very well with the presence of chronic lymphocytic thyroiditis (Hashimoto's thyroiditis). Many patients with Graves' disease also have positive antithyroid antibodies. Long-acting thyroid stimulator (LATS), an abnormal gamma globulin that stimulates the thyroid of a test animal, is also found in many patients with Graves' disease. Recently, thyroid stimulating immunoglobulins (TSI) can be measured and are found in the serum of many individuals with Graves' disease.

Tumor Markers

Elevated plasma *calcitonin* concentrations are found in patients with medullary carcinoma of the thyroid and its precursor, C cell hyperplasia. Measurement of this peptide is very effective as a screening test in high-risk populations.

High levels of circulating *thyroglobulin* have been found in some patients with papillary or follicular thyroid cancers. Unfortunately, these elevations are most commonly found in patients with widely spread metastatic cancer. Elevated thyroglobulin values after total thyroidectomy mean that metastases are present.

THYROID SCANS

Thyroid scans are used to demonstrate visually the anatomic features of the thyroid gland. They localize areas of increased or decreased accumulation of isotope within the gland and may aid in diagnosis of metastatic areas outside of the thyroid as well, especially after the thyroid gland has been removed. Single nodules may be "cold," "warm," or "hot." None of these characteristics defines the histopathology of the lesion; however, a cold nodule is more likely to be a carcinoma.

Originally, radioiodine-131 (^{131}I) was routinely used for scanning, since it is trapped and bound by the thyroid. However, because of the recent demonstration that low-dose, external irradiation to the neck may later lead to thyroid cancer, ^{131}I is less commonly used, as it results in 50 to 100 rads of radiation exposure to the thyroid (Table 29–2). Instead, either iodine-123 (^{123}I) or technetium-99M as pertechnitate ($Na^{99m}TcO_4$), which is also trapped by the thyroid, should be used, since each delivers a much lower dose of radiation to the thyroid.

^{75}Selenomethionine scans have been utilized in patients preoperatively by some investigators to identify which "cold" nodules are carcinomas. A thyroid nodule that is cold on iodine or technetium scan but hot on selenomethionine scan is more likely to be a carcinoma. However, we have had little experience with this technique.

ULTRASOUND SCANS

B-mode ultrasonography has been helpful in the preoperative evaluation of thyroid nodules. Its main value is in differentiating cystic from solid nodules, since cystic lesions of the thyroid are much more commonly benign than their solid counterparts.

Table 29–2. ABSORBED RADIOACTIVITY FROM THYROID SCANNING AGENTS

NUCLIDE	AVERAGE DOSE OF ACTIVITY ADMINISTERED, μC	MAXIMAL THYROID ABSORBED DOSE, RADS	TOTAL BODY ABSORBED DOSE, RADS	CRITICAL ORGAN ABSORBED DOSE, RADS
^{131}I	50	50	0.040	Thyroid
^{125}I	50	50	0.030	Thyroid
^{123}I	300	4.5	0.030	Thyroid
Pertechnitate-99m ($Na^{99}mTcO_4$)	2500	1.0	0.030	Stomach (±1 rad)
Selenomethionine-75 (^{75}Se)	250	2.2	2.2	Kidney (14 rads)

(From DeGroot, L. J., and Stanbury, J. B.: The Thyroid and Its Diseases. New York, John Wiley and Sons, 1975.)

Needle Biopsy of the Thyroid

Both aspiration biopsy for cytology and needle biopsy using a Vim-Silverman needle to obtain a core of tissue have been utilized to distinguish benign from malignant thyroid nodules. The risk of these procedures is small, and a great deal of information can be obtained from such a procedure. However, errors exist both in sampling (i.e., missing the nodule) and in interpretation of the small amount of tissue that is obtained. The risk of possibly spreading malignant cells along the needle tract is minimal. We have become more enthusiastic about these techniques in recent years. The acceptance of needle aspiration with cytology is growing in this country.

Evaluation of Vocal Cord Function

Prior to each thyroid operation, in addition to obtaining a complete blood count, urinalysis, chest roentgenogram, and electrocardiogram, vocal cord function should be evaluated by indirect laryngoscopy. This simple test is very important, since vocal cord paralysis may already be present as a result of either invasion of the recurrent laryngeal nerve by tumor or damage to the nerve at a prior operation. At times, a unilateral vocal cord paralysis may be present without causing a significant change in the quality of the patient's speaking voice, especially if the vocal cord is fixed in the midline. Obviously, when a unilateral cord paralysis is present, the surgeon must exercise great caution when the contralateral thyroid lobe is subjected to operation.

PREPARATION FOR OPERATION

Prior to either a thyroid or nonthyroid operative procedure, it is very important that the patient be in a euthyroid state. While minor deviations from normal do not cause great difficulty, gross hypothyroidism or hyperthyroidism leads to both excessive postoperative morbidity and mortality. These disorders must be recognized preoperatively and treated effectively before an elective operation is performed. If an emergency operation is necessary for such a patient, corrective treatment should be started preoperatively and continued postoperatively. Expert anesthesia management is mandatory in such cases if severe complications are to be minimized.

Hypothyroidism

Chronic hypothyroidism may occur insidiously after radioactive iodine therapy, thyroid resection, or ingestion of goitrous drugs (primary hypothyroidism). It may also occur because of some deficiency in the pituitary gland or hypothalamus. However, the most common cause is thought to be the end state of a long-term autoimmune process similar or identical to Hashimoto's thyroiditis.

Myxedema is the term applied to the most severe expression of chronic hypothyroidism. Patients with myxedema suffer from a severe hypometabolic state and, furthermore, manifest myxedematous (mucopolysaccharide) filtrations of most organs of the body, especially in the skin and muscle. The common symptoms and signs of chronic hypothyroidism are listed in Table 29–3.

Table 29–3. INCIDENCE OF SYMPTOMS AND
SIGNS IN HYPOTHYROIDISM

	PERCENTAGE OF 77 PATIENTS
Weakness	99
Dry skin	97
Coarse skin	97
Lethargy	91
Slow speech	91
Edema of eyelids	90
Sensation of cold	89
Decreased sweating	89
Cold skin	83
Thick tongue	82
Edema of face	79
Coarseness of hair	76
Cardiac enlargement (radiographic)	68
Pallor of skin	67
Impaired memory	66
Constipation	61
Gain in weight	59
Loss of hair	57
Pallor of lips	57
Dyspnea	55
Peripheral edema	55
Hoarseness	52
Anorexia	45
Nervousness	35
Menorrhagia	32
Palpitations	31
Deafness	30
Poor heart sounds	30
Precordial pain	25
Poor vision	24
Fundus oculi changes	20
Dysmenorrhea	18
Loss of weight	13
Atrophic tongue	12
Emotional instability	11
Choking sensation	9
Increased fineness of hair	9
Cyanosis	7
Dysphagia	3

(From Means, J. H., and Lerman, J.: Symptomatology of myxedema: Its relation to metabolic levels, time intervals, and rations of thyroid. Arch. Intern. Med., 55:1, 1935.)

Operative Risk

Patients with long-standing, severe hypothyroidism with or without myxedema are extremely poor operative risks. These individuals are exquisitely sensitive to anesthetic agents. They are very susceptible to hypotension because they lack the appropriate sympathetic responsiveness. Recovery from anesthesia is slow because normal metabolism of the anesthetic agents is diminished. Furthermore, they are quite sensitive to small doses of opiates and similar drugs, which may produce severe respiratory depression.

Many organ systems are deranged in these patients, and they frequently manifest generalized nervous system depression. Their cardiac output is low, and they may present with pericardial effusion. Pulmonary function is often abnormal, and these patients clear secretions from their lungs poorly. Thus, they are very likely to develop respiratory infections. Patients with hypothyroidism also suffer from gaseous distention and may present with generalized dilatation of the colon or with ascites. Postoperatively, ileus may be quite prolonged. Their adrenal response to stress is sluggish at times and may be inadequate. Patients with severe hypothyroidism may also have coagulation abnormalities and may bleed excessively at the time of operation; however, these disorders revert to normal after appropriate treatment. Hypercholesterolemia and increased plasma triglycerides and β-lipoproteins are commonly seen in these patients, and some investigators believe that generalized atherosclerosis is accelerated as well. Finally, the ultimate expression of the lowered metabolism due to thyroid hormone deficit is myxedema coma, which has a very high mortality even with the provision of optimal therapy.

Patients with mild forms of hypothyroidism are more difficult to diagnose definitively. They are often fatigued, experience an increased need for sleep, demonstrate a hypersensitivity to cold, weight gain, menorrhagia, constipation, hoarseness, or, rarely, excessive bleeding at operation. They also have an increased operative risk when compared with normal patients, although the risk is not as serious as it is in those with frank myxedema. Thus, it is imperative that patients with hypothyroidism be clinically recognized; optimally, operation should be delayed until their physiologic thyroid status is returned to normal.

Laboratory Diagnosis

Patients with hypothyroidism demonstrate characteristic laboratory abnormalities. The BMR is low — usually minus 30 per cent to 45 per cent in severe cases. The serum TT_4 and FTI levels are low. The result of the resin T_3 test is also low because of an undersaturation of plasma thyroid hormone-binding sites by endogenous hormone. The serum cholesterol is generally elevated in primary hypothyroidism.

The measurement of an elevated level of plasma TSH is perhaps the most sensitive indicator of most cases of hypothyroidism. In even mild cases, the TSH level will be greater than 10 μU per ml. Furthermore, the response of plasma TSH to the administration of thyrotropin-releasing hormone (TRH) is useful in distinguishing primary from secondary hypothyroidism. In primary hypothyroidism, the basal level of TSH is high. Following administration of TRH, the TSH response is greater than in normal subjects. On the other hand, patients with pituitary failure and hypothyroidism have low or absent TSH levels that do not respond to TRH.

Treatment

Mild Hypothyroidism. A patient with mild hypothyroidism rarely presents a difficult therapeutic problem. If elective surgery is contemplated, he or she should be treated first with oral thyroid hormone in the usual replacement doses (desiccated thyroid, 2 grains, or L-thyroxine [Synthroid], 0.15 mg daily). Most individuals will revert to euthyroid within several weeks. An elective operation can be performed with safety soon after this state is achieved. If an emergency operation is necessary, L-thyroxine may be given intravenously in a dose of 100 to 200 μg per day preoperatively; this medication can be continued intravenously after operation until oral medications can be resumed.

Severe Hypothyroidism and Myxedema. Individuals with severe hypothyroidism with or without myxedema fall into a much different category. These patients are in a precarious physiologic condition and are more difficult to manage. They are very sensitive to most drugs and excrete administered fluids and electrolytes very poorly. Furthermore, they are very sensitive to thyroid medications. Hence, correction of their hypothyroid state must be accomplished cautiously because severe angina pectoris, congestive heart failure, aggravated diabetes mellitus, or a psychotic reaction may be precipitated. Cardiac arrest has also occurred when thyroid therapy has been too aggressive.

If elective surgery is necessary for a myxedematous patient with no known heart disease or diabetes, one should begin thyroid therapy with one-fourth to one-half of the expected full replacement dose of thyroid hormone, such as L-thyroxine, 50 to 100 μg a day for two to three weeks. The dose should then be gradually increased if no adverse reactions occur. If the patient has known heart disease, however, the physician must be more cautious; only 25 μg thyroxine should be given as the initial dose. After one to two weeks, if no complications ensue, the amount can be doubled for a similar period of time and so forth. Ideally, the operation should not be performed until several weeks after the patient has regained a euthyroid state.

If an emergency operation is necessary in a patient with severe hypothyroidism or myxedema, this is a much more serious situation.

Preoperatively, small doses of intravenous L-thyroxine, 50 to 100 μg, should be given daily. The patient should be monitored carefully following each dose by an electrocardiogram. If operation is urgently needed, administration must still be undertaken, although the patient is only beginning to return toward a normal thyroid state. In these situations, because of marked hypersensitivity, only small doses of all drugs should be given. If morphine is used, for example, start with only 0.5 mg; this might prove to be sufficient. All other drugs and anesthetic agents should also be reduced to small fractions of their usual doses. Restraint must be used as well in the administration of intravenous fluids. A urine output of 20 ml per hour is sufficient. These patients will *not* withstand extensive surgical procedures. The surgeon should do the smallest and safest effective operation that is possible and should plan for reoperation at a later time when the patient is in a more favorable physiologic state.

Postoperatively, the patient's metabolic status should be slowly corrected by gradually increasing the dose of thyroid medication. Minimal doses of analgesic medication and careful replacement of fluids and electrolytes should be continued. Oral thyroxine can be used instead of an intravenous preparation as soon as oral alimentation is adequate. One should aim to restore the patient to a euthyroid state over a period of four to six weeks. At that time, a maintenance replacement dose of thyroxine can be given.

HYPERTHYROIDISM

Thyrotoxicosis is a condition caused by an accelerated and distorted metabolism in most tissues of the body produced by the action of excess thyroid hormone. It is most commonly found in patients with diffuse toxic goiter (Graves' disease) or in those with a toxic nodular goiter. However, it can be seen in cases of subacute (granulomatous) thyroiditis, radiation injury to the thyroid, toxic thyroid adenomas or carcinomas, and hyperfunctioning thyroid tissue in ectopic locations, as in struma ovarii. Thyrotoxicosis occasionally occurs because of a TSH-secreting pituitary tumor or due to thyroid-stimulating substances secreted from hydatidiform moles, choriocarcinomas, and seminomas. Thyrotoxicosis can also occur from ingesting excessive thyroid hormone or from the administration of exogenous TSH. The common signs and symptoms of hyperthyroidism are listed in Table 29–4.

Graves' disease is the eponym commonly used to denote a disorder that manifests itself as a diffuse goiter with thyrotoxicosis, by a unique type of infiltrative ophthalmopathy resulting in exophthalmos and proptosis, and by a specific dermopathy called pretibial myxedema. It is thought to be a systemic, autoimmune disease, but each patient may not manifest all three parts of the syndrome.

Table 29–4. INCIDENCE OF COMMON SIGNS AND
SYMPTOMS IN THYROTOXIC PATIENTS

SYMPTOMS	THYROTOXIC PATIENTS, %	SIGNS	THYROTOXIC PATIENTS, %
Dyspnea on exertion	81	Goiter	87
Palpitation	75	Diffuse	49
Fatigue	80	Nodular	32
Preference for cold	73	Single adenoma	4
Excessive sweating	68	Exophthalmos	34
Nervousness	59	Lid lag	62
Increased appetite	32	Hyperkinesis	39
Decreased appetite	13	Finger tremor	66
Weight loss	52	Sweating hands	72
Diarrhea	8	Hot hands	76
Scant menses	18	Auricular fibrillation	19
		Regular pulse over 90	68
		Average pulse in beats/min	100

(From Wayne, E. J.: The diagnosis of thyrotoxicosis. Br. Med. J., 1:411, 1954.)

Operative Risk in Thyrotoxicosis

Patients with uncontrolled thyrotoxicosis are extremely poor operative risks. The major difficulties relate to (1) complications associated with the hypermetabolic state and (2) excessive bleeding during operation, especially in cases of diffuse toxic goiter (Graves' disease).

Patients with thyrotoxicosis whose condition is not well controlled are prone to develop an accentuation of all the symptoms and signs of their disease at times of stress, infection, and operation. This is referred to as *thyroid storm* and will be discussed in greater detail later in this chapter.

Fever, tachycardia, and cardiac arrhythmias — paroxysmal atrial tachycardia, atrial fibrillation, or atrial flutter — are not uncommon if a patient with gross thyrotoxicosis who has not been properly prepared undergoes operation. Congestive heart failure may occur, especially if underlying heart disease is present. The greatest danger to such a patient is the rare episode of ventricular tachycardia or fibrillation that occurs because the myocardium is sensitized to the effects of catecholamines. During thyroidectomy, some thyroid hormone is released into the circulation. Thus, fever and cardiac abnormalities may occur at times during operation upon a patient with Graves' disease, even when the gland has been well prepared.

Proper anesthetic management for patients with thyrotoxicosis is important. The former agents, ether and cyclopropane, and any other present-day drugs that further sensitize the myocardium to catecholamines should be avoided. High concentrations of oxygen should be given because of the body's increased oxygen consumption. Finally, larger doses of drugs may be necessary because they are more rapidly metabolized. Digitalis, for example, must be given to the thyrotoxic patient in doses that otherwise would be excessive. The careful use of intravenous propranolol (Inderal) may be very helpful in controlling intraoperative tachycardia and many other cardiac abnormalities.

The second risk of operation for a patient with uncontrolled thyrotoxicosis relates to the potentially excessive amount of blood loss. This is especially true in patients with Graves' disease who have not been properly prepared for operation. These individuals have an increased cardiac output and peripheral vasodilation, which often result in excessive bleeding, even from the skin incision. In addition, the blood flow across the thyroid gland is greatly increased in such patients. This is manifested clinically by the characteristic bruit and thrill that are present over the untreated diffuse goiter of Graves' disease. These signs disappear following effective therapy. Finally, the untreated Graves' gland is soft, and attaining hemostasis may be difficult.

Thus, operating upon an untreated thyrotoxic patient may result in a large blood loss as well as the risk of many dangerous systemic manifestations. With proper preoperative preparation, however, these patients should present no greater operative risks than those that exist for other euthyroid patients.

Laboratory Data

In addition to a careful clinical assessment, laboratory data are very helpful in diagnosing or confirming the diagnosis of thyrotoxicosis. The serum TT_4 and FTI are increased, as is the radioactive uptake of iodine. Patients with normal TT_4 and FTI may occasionally have thyrotoxicosis due to excessive circulating T_3 (so-called "T_3 toxicosis"). Serum TSH is normal or low in thyrotoxicosis. With TRH administration, no rise of serum TSH occurs in these individuals.

Patients with Graves' disease often have circulating antithyroid antibodies. In addition, LATS and other gamma globulin antibodies (thyroid stimulating immunoglobulins) are often present that presumably stimulate the thyroid gland. An exophthalmos-producing substance, possibly secreted by the pituitary, may be related to the infiltrative ophthalmopathy in these patients.

Types of Therapy for Thyrotoxicosis

Three forms of therapy are available for the treatment of thyrotoxicosis: (1) blockage of hormone synthesis by antithyroid drugs, (2) destruction of the thyroid by irradiation, and (3) surgical ablation of the thyroid. Each has advantages and disadvantages.

Antithyroid Drugs. Treatment of patients with Graves' disease or toxic nodular goiter with thiocarbamide drugs, such as propylthiouracil (PTU) and methimazole (Tapazole), is attractive because no operation is required, no harm is done to the parathyroid glands or recurrent laryngeal nerves, and no radiation exposure occurs. It is also probably the least expensive form of therapy. However, the patient must take the medication strictly every eight hours, and frequent visits to a physician are essential. In addition, toxic reactions occur in 4 to 8 per cent of patients. Fever, rash, pruritus, arthralgias, jaundice, and polyserositis may occur. The most serious reactions are neutropenia and agranulocytosis. Additionally, even after taking drugs for one year, only about one-quarter to one-third of individuals with Graves' disease will have a permanent remission if the drugs are stopped. The others will experience recurrent thyrotoxicosis. Thus, in most individuals, a definitive mode of therapy, either radioiodine or surgery, is necessary.

Radioactive Iodine Therapy. The ^{131}I treatment is very effective in treating Graves' disease. It is usually given in doses of about 3 to 8 millicuries [131]I. This is an attractive mode of therapy because no operation is necessary, it is less expensive than thyroidectomy, and the medication can be given to patients who are considered to be poor operative risks. In some clinics, it has become the treatment of choice and has even been given to children. We *strongly disagree* with this philosophy and limit its use to individuals 35 to 40 years of age or older in most instances. Theoretical disadvantages include the uncertainty of potential genetic abnormalities in the offspring, the possibility of future leukemia, and the production of carcinoma of the thyroid many years later as occurs with low-dose external irradiation to the neck. [131]I cannot be given to pregnant women because the fetal thyroid would also be ablated and should only rarely be given if the uptake of iodine by the thyroid is very low, since a very large dose of irradiation would be necessary. Additionally, it has been demonstrated that an increased incidence of hypothyroidism of about 3 per cent per year occurs after ^{131}I therapy, presumably for as long as the patients live. Thus, insidious hypothyroidism may occur many years later in the unwary patient. New low-dose regimens which are being tried show promise of decreasing the incidence of hypothyroidism after treatment. However, in many patients a second or third dose of radioiodine must be given to achieve a euthyroid state.

Patients with toxic nodular goiters may also be treated effectively by radioiodine therapy. However, larger doses of the nuclide are generally needed than in diffuse toxic goiters.

Surgical Treatment. Because of the possible long-term risks of radioiodine therapy, the popularity of thyroidectomy as treatment for Graves' disease is increasing once more. We currently operate on almost all of these patients who are 35 years of age or younger. Older patients who have a nodule of the thyroid or who do not want radioiodine therapy also undergo operation. Subtotal thyroidectomy is the treatment of choice for Graves' disease during pregnancy in individuals who are not controlled by drugs as well as in some children with this disorder.

The major advantage of operation is the rapid reversal of the thyrotoxic state, which permits rapid rehabilitation of the patient. The disadvantages include the need for an operation and for a general anesthetic; a greater expense than the other forms of therapy; possible cosmetic difficulties; and lastly, the complications of operation, especially vocal cord paralysis and hypoparathyroidism. Fortunately, the incidence of each of these complications is low.

Most commonly, a subtotal thyroidectomy for Graves' disease is performed, leaving the posterior portion of each thyroid lobe. An estimated total weight of 8 to 10 gm or less of well-vascularized thyroid tissue is left in situ at the completion of operation; the remaining thyroid gland is resected. Thyroidectomy is effective therapy for toxic nodular goiter and functioning adenomas or carcinomas as well.

Preparation for Operation

Graves' Disease. In 1923, Plummer demonstrated that iodine blocked the release of thyroid hormone in patients with Graves' disease. Administration of iodine for the first time permitted patients with the symptoms of diffuse toxic goiter to be partially or completely controlled prior to operation and to undergo operation without an overwhelming mortality. The next great advance in therapy occurred in 1943, when Astwood introduced the thiocarbamide drugs, such as propylthiouracil (PTU). When these were used with iodine, patients tolerated operation with a much lower morbidity. Finally, the recent introduction of propranolol has made operation for Graves' disease still safer.

In Table 29–5, some of the more common preoperative regimens used to prepare patients with Graves' disease are listed. Our standard protocol consists of treatment with propylthiouracil, 150 to 600 mg orally per day, or Tapazole, 15 to 60 mg orally daily in three or four divided doses until a euthyroid state is obtained. This usually requires at least four to six weeks. Subsequently, iodine, 5 drops orally three times a day as saturated solution of potassium iodide SSKI or Lugol's solution, is given for about 10 days before operation. For faster control, iodine can be added soon after the PTU has been started while the patient is still toxic. The iodine serves to make the thyroid gland firmer and decreases

Table 29–5. PREOPERATIVE TREATMENT
REGIMENS FOR GRAVES' DISEASE*

Iodine alone
PTU + iodine
PTU + thyroxine + iodine
PTU + propranolol + iodine
Propranolol + iodine
Propranolol alone

*Most of our patients are prepared for operation by the use of propylthiouracil (PTU) and iodine, with or without the addition of propranolol.

its vascularity as well. If a patient becomes hypothyroid on this regimen, thyroid hormone can be added. Some surgeons routinely use thyroid hormone with PTU, since they feel that this combination makes the gland smaller and easier to operate upon.

If a patient has severe symptoms of tremor, nervousness, or tachycardia, propranolol, 10 to 40 mg orally four times a day, can be added to the PTU regimen and will generally relieve these symptoms. Once started, propranolol therapy is continued until surgery. We have not experienced complications of myocardial depression during anesthesia at this dosage level. Postoperatively, all PTU and iodine is stopped.

We *do not* favor the use of propranolol alone or with only iodine as the routine preparation for patients with Graves' disease before operation. Despite the rapid action of these treatment programs, we do not think that they are as safe as the PTU and iodine regimen, which restores a euthyroid state. We have utilized these regimens with success in selected patients who are allergic to PTU or iodine, however. If propranolol has been given until operation, it should be continued postoperatively and slowly tapered and stopped over a one- to two-week period, because such patients are still toxic after surgery.

Toxic Nodular Goiter and Toxic Adenoma. If the operation is elective, patients with these disorders should be treated until they are euthyroid with PTU or Tapazole with or without the addition of propranolol. Individuals with toxic nodular goiter are generally older than those with Graves' disease and are subject to arrhythmias and congestive heart failure. Careful preparation and excellent anesthesia are necessary if these elderly patients are to be operated upon safely.

POSTOPERATIVE COMPLICATIONS

The surgeon, house officers, and nurses must be cognizant of the possible complications that may occur following thyroid operations; all complications should be anticipated and treated expeditiously and effectively if they occur. As with all procedures, nausea, vomiting, headache, and some minor difficulty in breathing are common occurrences immediately after operation. Specific complications are discussed next.

HEMORRHAGE AND HEMATOMA

Bleeding may occur from an artery or vein in the thyroid region that has not been effectively ligated or from the site of excision of the thyroid gland following subtotal thyroidectomy, especially for Graves' disease. We generally use a small suction catheter following most thyroid operations and especially after a subtotal thyroidectomy for Graves' disease.

In most cases, these are removed on the morning after operation. Despite usage of these drains, if significant bleeding ensues, a hematoma can still form deep to the strap muscles, which are loosely reapproximated. The greatest danger in such cases is compression of the trachea, respiratory compromise, and possible death.

If respiratory compromise from a hematoma is diagnosed, the wound should be opened without delay, even at the bedside, and the hematoma should be evacuated. This may be a life-saving procedure. Later, the patient can be taken to the operating room if necessary for a more leisurely exploration. It is our practice to keep a sterile tracheostomy pack at the bedside of each patient who has recently undergone thyroidectomy so that proper instruments will be available is necessary. Respiratory compromise is a very rare complication, but it is a very serious one.

RECURRENT LARYNGEAL NERVE INJURY

Damage to the recurrent laryngeal nerve is a dangerous complication as well. If this nerve is injured during operation, the ipsilateral vocal cord becomes paralyzed and can no longer abduct. The voice usually becomes husky and hoarse since, in most cases, the cords no longer approximate one another. Occasionally the cord can be fixed in a midline position, in which case the speaking voice will not be greatly impaired. In other instances, with time, the opposite cord may spontaneously compensate and move across the midline to approximate the paralyzed cord. In this case, a husky voice might become much better in quality.

A recurrent nerve injury may occur because of trauma or rough dissection during operation. In these instances, the vocal cord paralysis may be *transient*, and function may spontaneously return after several months. But if a recurrent nerve is divided at operation, *permanent* vocal cord paralysis will occur. If this situation is recognized at the time of operation, the two ends should be approximated carefully by microsurgical technique. Return of function may occur after several months or longer. If no return of function occurs following a period of six months to one year after nerve injury, Teflon injection into the vocal cords may greatly improve the quality of the patient's speaking voice, since this usually leads to better vocal cord approximation.

Bilateral recurrent nerve injury with bilateral vocal cord paralysis represents a very serious situation. The patient is susceptible to aspiration when swallowing and cannot cough effectively. Furthermore, if the cords are approximated near the midline, the airway may be inadequate, and the patient may be dyspneic at rest or with mild activity. Even if the cords are fixed in the paramedian position, there is a danger that they may move toward the midline with time. Thus, many of the patients require a tracheostomy immediately postoperatively. If no vocal cord function returns, at a later operation one vocal cord can be moved laterally in order to insure an adequate airway. Other reinnervation operations are also being tried.

Bilateral vocal cord paralysis must be avoided. Careful attention should be paid to each recurrent laryngeal nerve if both lobes of the thyroid are operated upon. Each nerve should be identified and then treated gently and with great respect. Fortunately, recurrent nerve injuries occur only infrequently.

SUPERIOR LARYNGEAL NERVE INJURY

Damage to the external branch of the superior laryngeal nerve during operation may occur when the superior thyroid vessels are ligated. This nerve innervates the cricothyroid muscle, which is a general tensor of the vocal cords. Following this injury, the patient cannot sing as well as before and cannot shout or project the voice effectively. Fortunately, in most people there is great improvement of these functions within several months.

HYPOPARATHYROIDISM

Following subtotal or total thyroidectomy or after parathyroid surgery, acute hypoparathyroidism may occur. The symptoms of this disease are primarily due to a significant fall in concentration of the serum calcium ion, the physiologically active form of circulating calcium.

When severe hypocalcemia is present, the patient often becomes tense and anxious. Not uncommonly he or she states that the fingers and toes tingle or "feel asleep," and the area around the mouth is numb. Physical examination reveals that the deep tendon reflexes are usually hyperactive. If the area in front of the patient's ear over the facial nerve is tapped, twitching and contraction of the facial muscles will occur (Chvostek's sign). Initially the response is very subtle, and only a slight, almost imperceptible movement of the upper lateral lip area is seen. As the serum calcium concentration decreases further, this reaction is more readily observable. The presence of significant hypocalcemia may also be clinically determined by the Trousseau sign. A blood pressure cuff applied to the patient's upper arm is inflated to just above systolic pressure for several minutes. A positive test is indicated by carpal spasm; the affected wrist and metacarpophalangeal joints become flexed, while the interphalangeal joints are extended. The hand cannot be voluntarily opened to a normal position because of the spasm. When hypocalcemia is full-blown, carpopedal spasm or tetany often occur spontaneously; both hands and feet may be held involuntarily in a spastic state. Abdominal cramps, urinary frequency, and even intestinal ileus may also occur with severe hypocalcemia.

The greatest risks of hypocalcemia result from two other complications, each of which may be life-threatening. With severe hypocalcemia, *convulsions* may occur, especially in children. Secondly, *laryngeal spasm* may occur, and it results in stridor and inability to breathe effectively. Respiratory death may result if treatment is not instituted immediately.

LABORATORY EVALUATION

Ideally, the serum calcium *ion* concentration should be measured; however, the measurement of this cation is difficult in most laboratories. Therefore, the *total* serum calcium should be determined, which usually is a reflection of parathyroid activity.

Hypoparathyroidism is characterized by a decrease in serum calcium and an increase in serum phosphorus concentrations. The urinary calcium output decreases as the serum calcium level falls and may be used as a rough guide to the serum concentration of this ion. Some physicians follow the urinary calcium concentration postoperatively by a simple method that utilizes Sulkowitch reagent. However, we prefer to measure the serum calcium level frequently (several times daily) and find this repeated maneuver to be a more accurate guide to therapy. The urinary phosphorus output also decreases in hypoparathyroidism as the phosphaturic effect of parathyroid hormone on the renal tubule is diminished. When hypocalcemia exists, a prolongation of the Q-T interval is often evidenced on the electocardiogram.

While patients differ somewhat in their individual responses to a fall in serum calcium concentration, most develop symptoms by the time the serum calcium level reaches 8.0 mg per 100 ml or less. Severe symptoms usually represent a circulating calcium level of 7.5 mg per 100 ml or less in most patients. Some individuals develop symptoms of hypocalcemia at higher levels of serum calcium, which suggests that the *change* in serum calcium concentration rather than the absolute level is most important.

TRANSIENT VERSUS PERMANENT HYPOPARATHYROIDISM

During a total or subtotal thyroidectomy or parathyroidectomy, all parathyroid tissue might be inadvertently removed, irrevocably damaged, or devascularized; each leads to *permanent hypoparathyroidism.* Fortunately, however, most hypoparathyroidism that occurs following thyroidectomy is *transient* and is spontaneously reversed in less than one week.

For the first few postoperative days, it is impossible to determine by laboratory tests whether the hypocalcemia is transient or permanent.

However, in transient hypoparathyroidism, the lowest serum calcium level usually occurs between 24 and 72 hours postoperatively and then begins to rise spontaneously. Usually, the lowest serum calcium concentration is 7.5 mg per 100 ml or greater in these cases. In permanent hypoparathyroidism, on the other hand, the serum calcium concentration falls at the same rate shortly after the operative procedure but remains low thereafter, often decreasing to 7 mg per 100 ml or below if no treatment is instituted.

TREATMENT OF POSTOPERATIVE HYPOCALCEMIA

Since hypocalcemia following thyroidectomy is usually transient, a period of careful observation will suffice for most patients until the serum calcium level returns toward normal. However, during this watchful period, it is imperative that no harmful effects of hypocalcemia occur in the patient. The serum calcium concentration should be determined on the evening following operation and every 12 hours thereafter for several days, then daily until the patient is discharged. Serum phosphorus concentration is measured if hypocalcemia persists.

When mild hypocalcemia occurs, no treatment is needed. However, if the patient becomes symptomatic secondary to the lowered calcium level, 1 gm of calcium gluconate can be given rapidly by intravenous injection. Then 2 gm of calcium gluconate are added to the intravenous fluid regimen and given continuously over each eight-hour period. This is the amount of choice, since it generally relieves all symptoms without greatly raising the serum calcium concentration. Within several days, all calcium therapy can usually be stopped. It must be remembered that calcium chloride and calcium gluconate are not interchangeable ampule for ampule, for each gram of calcium chloride contains about twice as much calcium ion as does calcium gluconate.

For more persistent hypocalcemia, oral calcium is begun at a dose of 1.5 to 2.0 gm of calcium ion per day. In order to provide 1 gm of elemental calcium daily, 4 gm of calcium acetate, 5.5 gm of hydrated calcium chloride, 8 gm of calcium lactate, or 11 gm of calcium gluconate must be administered. Calcium gluconate is the most palatable and is our drug of choice (usually in a liquid form). It is well tolerated by the patient; unfortunately, diarrhea is a major side effect of all of these calcium preparations. Once started, the oral calcium can be tapered and discontinued after several weeks in most patients. It is preferable not to add vitamin D to this regimen early unless it is necessary to raise the serum calcium concentration still further or unless one strongly suspects that permanent hypoparathyroidism has occurred. The addition of vitamin D makes follow-up more difficult, since the effects of these preparations may last for weeks or even several months after they are discontinued. In most patients who are given about 20 gm of calcium gluconate orally daily, the serum calcium level rises sufficiently after several days without the administration of vitamin D.

If *permanent hypoparathyroidism* is suspected, in addition to the oral calcium therapy, the patient should be started on vitamin D_3, 50,000 to 100,000 units per day (1.25 to 2.5 mg per day). Other physicians prefer to use dihydrotachysterol, 0.125 to 1.0 mg per day or 1,25 dihydroxy D, 1 to 2 μg daily. Several days usually pass before the serum calcium begins to rise after vitamin D_3 therapy is begun; however, the rise of this ion is faster after the use of the other preparations. The serum calcium concentration must be measured frequently, since some patients are insensitive to these preparations and require larger doses, while others develop vitamin D intoxication with severe hypercalcemia while receiving relatively small doses. Good control means that the serum calcium level remains within the normal physiologic range.

Serum PTH concentrations should be measured at regular intervals in patients being treated for permanent postoperative hypoparathyroidism. Several patients whom we have seen have been treated unnecessarily with vitamin D therapy for many years because postoperative tetany occurred. If serum PTH levels are in the normal range, vitamin D therapy should be tapered and finally terminated, if possible.

PREVENTION OF PERMANENT HYPOPARATHYROIDISM

To avoid permanent hypoparathyroidism, the surgeon should try to identify the parathyroid glands during thyroid operation and leave at least one gland intact, with an undisturbed vasculature. Furthermore, the inferior thyroid artery should *not* be ligated laterally, since this might completely devascularize the parathyroid glands, especially when the superior thyroid vessels are also ligated. Rather, the small branches of the artery should be individually divided close to the thyroid capsule in order to leave the parathyroid glands with a good blood supply.

At thyroidectomy, if it is recognized that a parathyroid gland has been unintentionally removed or devascularized, it can be minced (following histologic confirmation that it is a parathyroid gland) and implanted into a sternocleidomastoid or arm muscle. This autotransplantation technique is almost universally successful.

THYROID STORM

Thyroid storm is a sudden, life-threatening exacerbation of thyrotoxicosis. It usually follows either an episode of severe infection or operation in a patient with Graves' disease; it also can occur in patients with toxic nodular goiter, but this occurs less frequently. While this was formerly very common in patients who were prepared for operation with iodine alone; today, with proper preoperative preparation, its incidence is far lower. If it does occur, it can be treated much more effectively than previously. In the classic form of thyroid storm, severe fever, tachycardia, tremor, nausea, vomiting, dehydration, delerium, and coma begin several hours postoperatively. Also, congestive heart failure, cardiac arrhythmias, jaundice, and possible adrenal insufficiency are frequently seen. Mortality was reported to be as high as 30 to 50 per cent in former years.

This diagnosis must be made on clinical grounds. The TT_4, FTI, and T_3 are usually elevated, but treatment must be started before results of these studies can be obtained. Treatment requires careful monitoring and excellent nursing care. In general, a primary goal is to slow the pulse and reduce the fever. Most recommended regimens include oxygen, 10 per cent dextrose solutions, sedation, rehydration, digitalization if congestive heart failure is present, and cooling of the patient. In addition, PTU, 150 to 250 mg every six hours, should be given orally. One hour after this drug has been started, iodide should be given either orally or intravenously in a dose of 50 mg twice daily. If there is any suspicion of adrenal insufficiency, hydrocortisone, 100 to 200 mg daily or its equivalent, should be administered. This dose can be tapered as the patient recovers.

Reserpine, 1 to 3 mg intramuscularly every eight hours, or guanethidine, 20 to 50 mg every eight hours, has been used in the past to reduce the restlessness, tremulousness, and tachycardia. Today, the treatment of choice is propranolol. Usual doses are 20 to 80 mg orally every six hours or 0.5 to 2 mg intravenously every four hours. Propranolol reduces the pulse rate and tremor, but it probably does not have a more specific effect on the hypermetabolism of thyrotoxicosis.

THYROID REPLACEMENT THERAPY AFTER OPERATION

After removal of a thyroid nodule or following unilateral thyroid lobectomy, most patients do not require thyroid hormone replacement in order to prevent hypothyroidism. The remaining lobe is almost always sufficient for normal thyroid function. However, following a near-total or total thyroidectomy, all patients require thyroid hormone replacement therapy to restore their hormonal status to normal. Patients with differentiated carcinomas of the thyroid should be treated with thyroid replacement to suppress pituitary TSH even if some thyroid tissue remains after resection. In these cases, we prescribe enough thyroid hormone to suppress TSH to low levels but *do not* attempt to titrate the patient to the maximal tolerance of thyroxine. There is suggestive evidence that thyroid hormone replacement may be helpful following the removal of benign lesions of the thyroid as well. This therapy prevents the remaining part of the gland from forming a goiter in cases of

Table 29-6. DESICCATED THYROID, L-THYROXINE, L-TRI-IODOTHYRONINE–EQUIVALENT DOSAGES

DESICCATED THYROID OR LIOTRIX EQUIVALENT, mg	L-THYROXINE, μg	L-TRI-IODOTHYRONINE, μg
15	25	10
30	50	20
60	100	40
100	150	65
120	200	80
200	300	125
300	500	200

(From DeGroot, L. J., and Stanbury, J. B.: The Thyroid and Its Diseases. New York, John Wiley and Sons, 1975.)

lymphocytic thyroiditis, and it also possibly decreases the occurrence of future nodules after a benign thyroid nodule has been resected.

For thyroid replacement therapy, desiccated thyroid, L-thyroxine (T_4), L-tri-iodothyronine (T_3), or combinations of T_4 and T_3 (liotrix) may be prescribed. Thyroxine and desiccated thyroid have an apparent onset of action in three to five days, and if therapy is withdrawn, diminished activity is noted in seven to ten days. With tri-iodothyronine, results are noted in one to three days, and a deficiency can be recognized in three to five days if the drug is discontinued. T_4 is converted to T_3 in the body; thus, when thyroxine is used, normal levels of circulating T_3 are found as well. The approximate equivalent doses of these various preparations are shown in Table 29-6. Most patients require about two grains of desiccated thyroid hormone or 0.15 to 0.20 mg of L-thyroxine daily to restore physiologic thyroid homeostasis.

REFERENCES

Alvioli, L.: The therapeutic approach to hypoparathyroidism. Am. J. Med., 57:34, 1974.

Astwood, E. B.: Treatment of hyperthyroidism with thiourea and thiouracil. J.A.M.A., 122:78, 1943.

Colcock, B. P., and King, M. L.: The mortality and morbidity of thyroid surgery. Surg. Gynecol. Obstet., 114:131, 1962.

DeGroot, L. J., Frohman, L. A., Kaplan, E. L., and Refetoff, S.: Radiation-Associated Thyroid Carcinoma. New York, Grune and Stratton, 1977.

DeGroot, L. J., and Stanbury, J. B.: The Thyroid and Its Diseases. New York, John Wiley and Sons, 1975.

Kaplan, E. L.: Parathyroid. In Schwartz, S. I. (ed.): Principles of Surgery, 3rd ed. New York, McGraw Hill Book Co., 1980.

Means, J. H., and Lerman, J.: Symptomatology of myxedema: Its relation to metabolic levels, time intervals, and rations of thyroid. Arch. Intern. Med., 55:1, 1935.

Mitchie, W., Hamer-Hodges, D. W., Pegg, C. A. S., Orr, F. G. G., and Bewsher, P. D.: Beta-blockade and partial thyroidectomy for thyrotoxicosis. Lancet, 1:1009, 1974.

Oyama, T.: The Thyroid. In Oyama T. (ed.): Anesthetic Management of Endocrine Disease. Berlin, Springer-Verlag, 1973, pp. 92–106.

Plummer, H. S.: Results of administering iodine to patients having exophthalmic goiter. J.A.M.A., 80:1955, 1923.

Wayne, E. J.: The diagnosis of thyrotoxicosis, Br. Med. J., 1:411, 1954.

30

Disorders of the Parathyroid Glands

SAMUEL A. WELLS, JR.

The parathyroid glands are tiny organs normally located in the neck, two adjacent to each thyroid lobe. They secrete parathyroid hormone (PTH), a polypeptide that primarily affects bone, where it activates resorption, and kidney, where it promotes phosphaturia and an increased tubular reabsorption of calcium. Parathyroid hormone also increases the intestinal absorption of calcium indirectly by increasing the rate of activation of $25(HO)$ vitamin D_3 to $1,25(HO)_2$ vitamin D_3.

Disorders of the parathyroid glands, although relatively infrequent, can be divided into those associated with decreased function (hypoparathyroidism) and those associated with excessive function (hyperparathyroidism). Of these two conditions, the latter is more common and its mode of clinical presentation much more variable. The fundamentals of the diagnosis and treatment of hyperparathyroidism and hypoparathyroidism will be reviewed in this chapter.

HYPERPARATHYROIDISM

For clinical convenience, hyperparathyroidism is divided into primary, secondary, and tertiary types. In primary hyperparathyroidism, there is de novo enlargement of one or more parathyroid glands accompanied by hypersecretion of parathyroid hormone. In secondary hyperparathyroidism, a pathologic process elsewhere in the body, such as chronic renal insufficiency or the gastrointestinal malabsorption of calcium, results in a decrease in the serum calcium concentration. In response, the parathyroid glands enlarge and produce increased amounts of PTH. On occasion, patients with secondary hyperparathyroidism develop autonomous hyperfunction of one or more parathyroid glands. This condition is referred to as tertiary hyperparathyroidism.

PRIMARY HYPERPARATHYROIDISM

The prevalance of primary hyperparathyroidism is approximately one in 1000 persons, and although it was once considered an uncommon disease, it has been diagnosed with greater frequency in recent years. This apparent increased incidence is primarily due to the widespread use of biochemical screening tests (which include determination of the serum calcium concentration) as a part of routine inpatient or outpatient evaluation. Accordingly, an appreciable number of patients with hypercalcemia are detected, many of whom are found to have hyperparathyroidism.

Symptoms

Most patients with primary hyperparathyroidism, especially those diagnosed by biochemical screening, will have few if any symptoms. On careful questioning, however, one often obtains a history of weakness, fatigue, polyuria, or constipation. Unfortunately, if only these symptoms are volunteered, they may not arouse sufficient suspicion to lead to the correct diagnosis. Of patients with hyperparathyroidism who do present with symptoms, approximately 60 per cent have complaints referable to stones in the urinary tract, while 10 to 15 per cent complain of bone pain or fractures. Usually patients with primary hyperparathyroidism can be grouped into one of three categories with little overlap: (1) those with renal or bladder calculi, (2) those with bone disease detectable radiographically (osteitis fibrosa), and (3) those with neither bone disease nor renal disease. Generally, patients with osteitis fibrosa have a shorter duration of symptoms compared with those presenting with renal calculi.

Less commonly, patients present with pancreatitis or epigastric pain due to peptic ulcer disease. Rarely, patients have abnormal mental behavior as the only presenting symptom.

Signs

There are few physical findings that aid in the diagnosis of hyperparathyroidism. Occasionally patients will have band keratopathy of the cornea demonstrable by slit lamp examination. Also, proximal muscle weakness may be demonstrable by neurologic testing. It is most unusual for patients with hyperparathyroidism to have a palpable nodule in the neck attributable to an enlarged parathyroid gland. In such individuals, one should suspect thyroid rather than parathyroid pathology.

Diagnosis and Preoperative Evaluation

The diagnosis of hyperparathyroidism depends primarily on the documentation of an elevated serum calcium concentration. In most laboratories, the normal range of serum calcium is between 8.5 and 10.5 mg per dl. Of the total serum calcium, approximately 45 per cent is bound to protein, primarily albumin. The remaining calcium exists in a free or unfilterable form, approximately 10 per cent of which is complexed with anions such as phosphate or citrate. The serum calcium concentration should always be interpreted in light of the serum protein concentration, as an elevation in the latter results in an increase of the former even though the absolute quantity of the physiologically important ionized calcium does not change. In patients with mild hyperparathyroidism, the serum calcium concentration might not always be above the upper limit of normal. It is important, therefore, if one is suspicious of this disease or if one notices an initial elevated level to perform serial determinations in order to substantiate the validity of the hypercalcemia. A disease entitled "normocalcemic hyperparathyroidism" has been described in certain patients having renal stones but normal serum calcium levels. In clinical studies reporting the operative experience in these cases, however, the documentation of enlarged or abnormal parathyroid glands has been inconsistent, thus emphasizing the fact that the diagnosis of primary hyperparathyroidism should not be entertained unless an elevated serum calcium concentration has been repeatedly documented.

Approximately 40 per cent of patients with hyperparathyroidism will have a low serum phosphate (<2.5 mg per dl). An elevated alkaline phosphatase will be present in about 20 per cent. Individuals with primary hyperparathyroidism frequently have a mild metabolic acidosis characterized by an elevated plasma chloride level and a decreased bicarbonate concentration. The clinical usefulness of determining the relationship of chloride to phosphate has been stressed. A ratio greater than 33 is almost always associated with hyperparathyroidism, whereas patients having hypercalcemia from other causes usually have a ratio less than 30. In approximately 30 per cent of patients, the 24-hour urinary excretion of calcium will be elevated (>300 mg per 24 hr in females and >400 mg per 24 hr in males).

Whereas it is important to determine these biochemical indices, it should be understood that the only abnormality detected may be an elevated serum calcium concentration. Currently there is no single clinical or biochemical test available that allows one to unequivocally establish the diagnosis of hyperparathyroidism in a hypercalcemic patient. The two most helpful laboratory procedures, however, appear to be the determination of plasma parathyroid hormone levels by radioimmunoassay and the measurement of renal nephrogenous cyclic AMP.

Radioimmunoassay of Parathyroid Hormone

Of the radioimmunoassays measuring polypeptide hormones in plasma, the determination of parathyroid hormone (PTH) is among the most difficult. When this radioimmunoassay was first developed, it did not provide a clear separation among patients with hyperparathyroidism, patients with hypercalcemia from other causes, and normal subjects. It is now generally agreed that the most reliable clinical radioimmunoassays are those that utilize an antibody against the carboxyl-terminal fragment of the molecule. The detection of an elevated plasma level of this portion of the hormone, associated with an elevation of the serum calcium concentration, is virtually diagnostic of hyperparathyroidism. Not all patients with hyperparathyroidism, however, have both an elevated PTH level and an elevated serum calcium concentration.

Nephrogenous Cyclic AMP

The interaction of parathyroid hormone with its specific receptor on the kidney cell causes the release of cyclic adenosine monophosphate (cyclic AMP) into the urine. Measurement of this substance excreted in the urine has proved an important discriminant in separating patients with hyperparathyroidism from those with hypercalcemia of other causes. An important modification that increases the specificity of the test has been the determination in urine of the cyclic AMP actually secreted by the kidney (nephrogenous cyclic AMP).

Radiologic Studies

In patients with hyperparathyroidism, certain characteristic changes may be noted on radiologic studies. An intravenous pyelogram may demonstrate nephrolithiasis or nephrocalcinosis. A skeletal survey may reveal subperiosteal resorption of the metacarpals and phalanges and demineralization of the distal ends of the clavicles and the bony calvarium. Brown tumors (osteoclastomas) occasionally are demonstrable in the cortices of the long bones. Of importance is the possibility that other abnormalities of the skeletal system associated with hypercalcemia (such as multiple myeloma, metastatic carcinoma, and Paget's disease) may be ruled out by roentgenographic studies.

Differential Diagnosis

Although many patients who present with hypercalcemia will have hyperparathyroidism, there are several other diseases that cause an elevation of the serum calcium concentration, and these must be excluded before one proceeds with a neck exploration.

The most common cause of hypercalcemia is malignancy. If hypercalcemia occurs in a patient with malignancy, it is usually on the basis of increased bone resorption due to osteolytic metastases. Less commonly, no abnormalities of the skeletal system are evident, and it has been assumed that the hypercalcemia in these patients is due to some humoral factor secreted by the neoplastic cells. It is as yet unclear which specific factors are causative, but several have been proposed: parathyroid hormone (or a similar polypeptide), prostaglandin E_2, and osteoclast activating factor. The hypercalcemia of malignancy occurring in patients without bony involvement has been termed "pseudohyperparathyroidism," and the most common associated neoplasms are carcinomas of the kidney, oat cell carcinoma of the lung, and squamous cell carcinomas of the lung. Hypercalcemia has also been demonstrated to occur as a complication of lymphoma, leukemia, and multiple myeloma.

Uncommonly, patients who have hyperthyroidism develop hypercalcemia. This is presumably due to increased bone turnover caused by the hypermetabolic state. This disease can usually be ruled out by physical examination and by thyroid function tests. Patients with sarcoidosis will occasionally develop hypercalcemia supposedly due to increased gastrointestinal absorption of calcium.

Patients who ingest excessive amounts of vitamin D or vitamin A may develop hypercalcemia. Other patients, almost always those with peptic ulcer disease, may ingest excessive amounts of milk and calcium carbonate. Such patients frequently develop the so-called milk-alkali syndrome with associated hypercalcemia. Lastly, patients who are ingesting thiazide diuretics or chlorthalidone will occasionally develop hypercalcemia. In such patients, the diuretics should be stopped for a period of four to six weeks, and the serum calcium concentration should be reevaluated.

Lastly, there are infrequent causes of hypercalcemia such as addisonian crisis, Paget's disease with immobilization, and idiopathic hypercalcemia of infancy.

All nonparathyroid causes of an elevated serum calcium concentration must be excluded as carefully as possible prior to subjecting patients to neck exploration.

Special Problems Associated with Hyperparathyroidism

Patients who present with nephrolithiasis occasionally have bacteriuria, and this should be treated with appropriate antibiotics prior to neck exploration. If ureteral obstruction secondary to an impacted stone is present or if pyonephrosis has occurred as a result of a renal calculus, then surgical correction of the disorder should usually precede parathyroid surgery. Adequate hydration and periodic observance of the serum calcium concentration are mandatory if these urologic procedures are to be performed first.

Patients who have decreased renal function manifested by elevated serum creatinine level and a reduced creatinine clearance occasionally develop a further increase in the serum creatinine and a transient metabolic acidosis postoperatively. This aggravation of compromised renal function is poorly understood; fortunately, however, it is almost always transient.

Patients occasionally develop an acute arthritis during the immediate postoperative period, and this usually occurs when the serum calcium concentration is at its nadir. The cause of the arthritis is usually pseudogout, and the diagnosis can be made by demonstrating calcium pyrophosphate crystals in the joint fluid. Pseudogout can be treated with phenylbutazone or aspirin.

Although primary hyperparathyroidism is usually an insidious disease most often detected in asymptomatic patients, it can present in a much more virulent form termed hypercalcemic crisis. Patients with this disorder usually present with nausea, vomiting, muscle cramps, extreme lethargy, azotemia, and mental derangement. Characteristically, they are severely dehydrated. The serum calcium concentration is usually in excess of 13 mg per dl, and levels exceeding 20 mg per dl have been reported. The immediate danger of such an elevated serum calcium concentration is a markedly altered nerve conduction with cardiac arrest and coma as possible terminal events. Hypercalcemic crisis is not necessarily a phenomenon uniquely associated with hyperparathyroidism, as it also occurs in patients with other causes of hypercalcemia, especially that due to malignancy. Regardless of the cause of the elevated serum calcium, the clinical situation is a medical emergency, and treatment should be instituted immediately. After the patient has been rendered normocalcemic or nearly so, then attention must be directed to identification and management of the underlying disease process.

The cornerstone of resuscitative therapy in these individuals is parenteral hydration. Saline is the agent of choice, but caution must be taken not to overhydrate patients, especially those with borderline cardiac or renal function. Saline is preferable to glucose because it promotes the renal excretion of calcium. A more potent agent in this regard is sodium sulfate, and the infusion of 1000 ml of an isotonic solution (0.12M) over two hours lowers blood calcium approximately 1 mg per dl. The effect of sodium on the renal excretion of calcium can be enhanced by the adjunctive administration of the diuretic furosemide or ethacrynic acid. Either of these agents can be administered intravenously with sodium, and the result of the combined regimens may be quite dramatic with a drop of several milligrams in the serum calcium concentration occurring within hours after the initiation of therapy. Rarely, calcium chelating agents such as citrate or ethylene diamine tetra-acetic acid (EDTA) are used; however, more suitable therapeutic alternatives are usually available.

Salmon calcitonin has also been useful in the management of hypercalcemia, primarily owing to its potent inhibition of bone resorption. Currently, its greatest clinical use has been in patients with Paget's disease.

Oral inorganic phosphate is most effective and reliable in the prolonged treatment of hypercalcemia. It is especially useful in patients with hypercalcemia due to malignancy in whom chronic control of the serum calcium level is desired. The administration of 2000 mg of phosphorus daily can lower the serum calcium concentration by several mg per dl. This dose may cause gastrointestinal intolerance, however, and only small amounts may be tolerated initially with modest increments thereafter.

The intravenous administration of phosphate salts is hazardous, especially in patients who are azotemic. Deaths have been reported as a complication of this route of administration, and generally it is unwise to resort to this mode of phosphate therapy.

A more potent agent useful in the management of hypercalcemia, especially that refractory to the more conventional therapies mentioned above, is mithramycin. This antitumor agent directly inhibits bone resorption and is particularly indicated in patients with hypercalcemia secondary to malignancy. To be effective, it usually must be administered over several days. It has the adverse side effect of marked thrombocytopenia.

It is important to recognize that primary hyperparathyroidism may occur in a familial pattern. In its simplest form, only hyperparathyroidism is present, and there are no other associated endocrinopathies. However, hyperparathyroidism may be a component of one of the multiple endocrine neoplasia syndromes. Multiple endocrine neoplasia type I is characterized by the concurrence of pancreatic islet cell tumors (most commonly gastrinomas or insulinomas), pituitary adenomas, and multiglandular parathyroid enlargement. Less commonly, patients have thyroid adenomas or adrenocortical adenomas or hyperplasia. The Zollinger-Ellison syndrome may be associated with gastrin-producing pancreatic islet cell tumors. Multiple endocrine neoplasia type IIa is characterized by the association of pheochromocytoma(s), medullary carcinoma of the thyroid gland, and generalized parathyroid enlargement. Each of these syndromes is inherited in a mendelian autosomal dominant pattern such that if a parent has the disease, one-half of the children will develop it. It is, therefore, most important when evaluating patients with primary hyperparathyroidism to rule out the presence of associated disease in other endocrine organs. Also, one should obtain a careful family history in patients presenting with an elevated serum calcium concentration to rule out the presence of hyperparathyroidism or multiple endocrine neoplasia in relatives. In addition, serum calcium determinations may be helpful in screening family members.

Definitive Treatment of Hyperparathyroidism

There has been some controversy regarding the indications for operation in patients suspected of having hyperparathyroidism. In patients with documented disease of the kidneys or skeletal system or in patients with hypertension or hypercalcemia in excess of 11 mg per dl, there is little argument that they should be managed operatively. There are other patients, however, who have only a mildly elevated serum calcium concentration (10.5 to 11 mg per dl) and who are asymptomatic. An argument has been made for following these patients conservatively with evaluation of renal, metabolic, and blood pressure status yearly. If subjects develop either hypertension, a progressively increasing serum calcium concentration, evidence of renal stones or bone disease, or deterioration of renal function, they should undergo neck exploration. In studies evaluating the nonoperative management of patients with minimal elevations in serum calcium concentration, it has been found that an appreciable number (approximately 5–10 per cent per year of follow-up) require neck exploration. Sequential long-term evaluation of these patients has been tedious and generally unsatisfactory. Accordingly, a case can be made for advising patients with minimal hypercalcemia due to hyperparathyroidism to undergo immediate neck exploration.

Preoperative Discussion with the Patient

Prior to operation, the patient should be informed regarding the proposed operative procedure, the expected postoperative course, and the potential complications. The possibility of recurrent or superior laryngeal nerve damage should be explained, as should the remote possibility of an ectopic enlarged parathyroid gland necessitating subsequent reoperation. The expected postoperative development of hypocalcemia with its characteristic symptoms (circumoral tingling and muscle cramps) should be explained. Even though many of the symptoms that develop postoperatively are transient, it is much better to explain them preoperatively.

The night prior to operation, the patient should be mildly sedated and kept without food after midnight. Diazepam, 10 mg IM, is given on call to the operating room, and after arriving there, general anesthesia is induced. The head and chest are elevated about 30°, and the neck is extended and placed on a head ring.

Surgical Management of Hyperparathyroidism

As many as 65 to 70 per cent of patients with primary hyperparathyroidism will be found to have a single enlarged parathyroid gland and three normal-sized parathyroid glands. Such patients can be managed by removing the enlarged parathyroid and obtaining a biopsy of the other three normal glands. Some surgeons have proposed that such patients be managed by 3½ gland subtotal parathyroidectomy, assuming that almost all patients with primary hyperparathyroidism have generalized involvement. This represents a minority opinion, however. Studies from several laboratories have shown that in almost all patients with hyperparathyroidism due to a single enlarged gland, removal of the gland results in a permanent cure.

Of the remaining 30 to 35 per cent of patients with primary hyperparathyroidism, most will have generalized (four gland) parathyroid enlargement, but some will have two or three parathyroid glands enlarged with the remaining gland(s) normal. In patients with two or three enlarged parathyroid glands, it is the general policy to remove the enlarged parathyroid glands only and leave the remaining normal-sized gland(s) in the neck. In those patients having enlargement of all four parathyroid glands, the usual surgical procedure is to remove 3½ glands. A portion of one gland is left in the neck in an attempt to prevent the occurrence of hypocalcemia while avoiding hypercalcemia. In our experience, a suitable alternative to this procedure has been the performance of a total parathyroidectomy accompanied by transplantation of a portion of one gland to a forearm muscle. If the autograft subsequently becomes hyperfunctional and the patient develops hypercalcemia, a portion of the graft can be removed under local anesthesia.

Previously, the histologic characteristics of enlarged parathyroid glands were defined as "adenomas" or "hyperplasia." However, it is clinically more accurate to classify hyperparathyroid patients into those having single gland disease and those with multiple gland disease. The gross appearance of the parathyroid glands at operation and their actual weight and size are the most important factors in determining whether they are normal or abnormal. The decision regarding the surgical management of patients should be made primarily by these factors and only secondarily by histologic characteristics.

Postoperative Management

Usually patients will tolerate clear liquids the evening of the operation or almost certainly by the next morning. Thereafter, they can progress to a regular diet, usually by the second postoperative day. Discomfort is usually minimal, and acetaminophen or oxycodone hydrochloride may be administered orally. The wound sutures can be removed on the third or fourth postoperative day and a light dressing placed to avoid discomfort.

It is important to determine the serum concentrations of calcium, phosphorous, alkaline phosphatase, total protein, albumin, potassium, chloride, sodium, bicarbonate, and creatinine at frequent intervals in the postoperative period. If the operation has been successful and all hyperfunctional parathyroid tissue has been removed, the serum calcium concentration will fall dramatically from preoperative levels, usually reaching a nadir by the second to the fourth postoperative day. When the serum calcium concentration decreases below 8 mg per dl, patients usually develop signs and symptoms of tetany. If bone disease was present preoperatively, one can expect the drop in serum calcium concentration to be more marked and prolonged. Patients must be carefully observed during this period for the presence of a Chvostek's or a Trousseau's sign. Chvostek's sign can be elicited by tapping over the path of the facial nerve anterior to the ear. If hypocalcemia is sufficient to cause nerve irritation, the facial muscles will contract. Approximately 10 per cent of normal subjects have a Chvostek's sign, and attempts to elicit this should be made preoperatively. Trousseau's sign is elicited by inflating a blood pressure cuff on the upper arm and occluding arterial pressure. If hypocalcemia is present, carpal spasms will develop within three minutes. To elicit Trousseau's sign is uncomfortable, and it is usually sufficient only to check for Chvostek's sign. Hypocalcemic patients frequently have muscle cramps, predominantly in the hands, legs, and feet. The sensorium may change so that patients become frightened or depressed. Rarely will the serum calcium concentration fall below 7 mg per dl, and unless patients are moderately symptomatic, they can be managed without calcium replacement. The serum calcium concentration will usually begin to rise by the fourth or fifth postoperative day, and there is then little concern for the need for replacement therapy.

Should the serum calcium concentration fall below 7 mg per dl or persist below 7.5 mg per dl, it may be necessary to administer intravenous calcium. Usually one ampule of calcium gluconate (100 mg elemental calcium) is given over 10 minutes. Patients will experience a warm flush, and the signs and symptoms of hypocalcemia will abate. The serum calcium concentration will become transiently elevated and will remain so for several hours. Patients should be observed and the serum calcium concentration checked the following day. If hypocalcemia and marked symptoms recur, then patients may require more aggressive treatment with large amounts of intravenous calcium (10 ampules of calcium gluconate, 1 gm calcium ion) per 24 hours. If after two to three days of this treatment the hypocalcemia recurs, then patients should be started on vitamin D and calcium replacement therapy orally. Once normocalcemic, they may be discharged and seen two weeks postoperatively for reevaluation of their serum calcium concentration. If it is normal, the calcium and vitamin D can be reduced, and unless hypocalcemia recurs, replacement therapy can be stopped in four weeks. Subsequently, patients should have their serum calcium level determined at yearly intervals.

Rarely, one will note in the immediate postoperative period that the patient is hoarse. This could be due either to mild trauma during intubation or more likely to damage of the recurrent laryngeal nerve or the superior laryngeal nerve. If the patients have been prepared for this preoperatively, they are not alarmed. Almost always the hoarseness is transient and will disappear during the first week postoperatively or shortly thereafter.

SECONDARY HYPERPARATHYROIDISM

This disease most commonly occurs as "renal osteodystrophy" in patients with severe renal disease. The etiology of the disease is uncertain, but the indications for operation are intractable pruritus, severe bone disease, and extraosseous metastatic calcification. At operation, the parathyroid glands are usually markedly enlarged. The indicated surgical procedure is either subtotal (3½ gland) parathyroidectomy or total parathyroidectomy with heterotopic autotransplantation. The serum calcium level falls rapidly, and oral calcium and vitamin D therapy may be required for a long period postoperatively until normocalcemia is established. Often patients are undergoing renal dialysis, and the operative procedure should be coordinated so that the patient is not dialyzed on the day after operation. Even with "regional heparinization," patients receiving dialysis within 24 hours postoperatively frequently develop wound hematomas.

REOPERATION FOR PERSISTENT OR RECURRENT HYPERPARATHYROIDISM

Occasionally the initial neck exploration will be unsuccessful, and the patient will develop recurrent or persistent hypercalcemia in the postoperative period. If the hyperfunctional parathyroid tissue has not been found or if inadequate parathyroid tissue has been resected, such as in unsuspected multiple gland disease, almost certainly a second neck exploration will be indicated. Repeat neck surgery is of much greater difficulty than primary surgery owing to the large amount of scar tissue present. Furthermore, the functional state of the remaining parathyroid glands is often unknown. The reexploration can usually be undertaken as early as two to four weeks postoperatively; however, it is often wise to perform certain tests to aid in localizing the hyperfunctional parathyroid tissue. Two simple procedures that are of low yield but of minimal risk to the patient are a thyroid scan, which might demonstrate a "cold" area within a thyroid lobe, perhaps indicative of an intrathyroidal parathyroid gland, and a barium swallow, which might show an enlarged posterior parathyroid gland indenting the esophagus. Two additional but more complicated procedures are usually of greater help. The first consists of selective thyroid arteriography. By catheterizing the superior and inferior thyroid arteries individually and injecting them with contrast material, one can sometimes demonstrate an enlarged parathyroid gland. When positive, it greatly simplifies the subsequent operation, assuming, of course, that the demonstrated blush is a hyperfunctional parathyroid gland. This test is helpful in about 60 to 70 per cent of patients. Unfortunately, the technique is performed only at selected medical centers and should be undertaken only by an experienced vascular radiologist. The procedure may be associated with serious complications such as transient cortical blindness, transverse myelitis, or a cerebrovascular accident. The second procedure is selective thyroid venous catheterization with sampling for parathyroid hormone determination. This test is almost always performed after the arteriography, since the venous phase of the arteriogram will demonstrate veins for selective catheterization for hormone measurements. Elevated parathyroid hormone levels in veins draining one side of the neck indicate hyperfunctional parathyroid tissue. The demonstration of elevated parathyroid hormone levels on both sides of the neck indicates multiple gland disease. This technique lateralizes the hyperfunctional tissue but does not actually localize the abnormal gland. It is helpful diagnostically in approximately 70 per cent of patients. Computed axial tomographic scan of the neck has been found useful in localizing ectopic parathyroid. This procedure may become more commonly used than invasive ones such as arteriography as experience with it is gained.

As soon as preoperative evaluation and testing have been completed, reexploration is planned. If the possibility of a mediastinal parathyroid gland exists, one must be prepared to perform median sternotomy if the neck exploration is negative. Repeat neck surgery is not only technically difficult but often the parathyroid excised represents the only functional tissue remaining in the neck, and thus the patient is rendered aparathyroid and dependent on vitamin D and calcium replacement therapy for life. As has been recently demonstrated, this dilemma can be avoided by cryopreserving autologous parathyroid tissue and observing the patient in the immediate postoperative period. Should it become obvious that the patient is aparathyroid, a portion of the frozen parathyroid gland can be autografted to the forearm muscle and the eucalcemic state restored.

HYPOPARATHYROIDISM

Patients who develop persistent hypoparathyroidism postoperatively represent difficult management problems. Although the serum calcium concentration can usually be maintained within the normal range, the development of hypercalciuria is frequent. Furthermore, hypercalcemia may develop in the summer months, necessitating changes in vitamin D and oral calcium doses.

Of the vitamin D preparations, USP vitamin D in a dose of 50,000 to 100,000 units per day is most commonly used. It is important to use gelatin capsule preparations, since other, hard capsules are often not absorbed. Vitamin D is fat-soluble, and frequently the patients have persistent effects of this drug several weeks after it is stopped. For short-term use, a more suitable vitamin D preparation is dihydrotachysterol. This is usually given in a maintenance dose of 0.125 mg a day after a loading dose of 0.6 mg for five or six days. Calcium replacement therapy is most commonly given as calcium gluconate wafers, usually in a dose of 20 gm a day. A more effective oral calcium dose is calcium glubionate (Neo-Calglucon syrup), which is administered in 15 ml doses four times a day. In any case, treatment of hypoparathyroidism must be guided by the serum calcium response, and sufficient vitamin D and calcium must be given to achieve (but not exceed) normocalcemia without excessive calciuria.

REFERENCES

Alveryd, A.: Parathyroid glands in thyroid surgery. Acta Chir. Scand. (Suppl.), 389:1, 1968.

Deftos, L. J., and Neer, R.: Medical management of the hypercalcemia of malignancy. Ann. Rev. Med., 25:323, 1974.

Mallette, L. E., Bilezikian, J. P., Heath, D. A., and Aurbach, G. D.: Primary hyperparathyroidism: Clinical and biochemical features. Medicine, 53:127, 1974.

Palmer, F. J., Nelson, J. C., and Bacchus, H.: The chloride-phosphate ratio in hypercalcemia. Ann. Intern. Med., 80:200, 1974.

Purnell, D. C., Scholz, D. A., and Beahrs, O. H.: Hyperparathyroidism due to single gland enlargement. Arch. Surg., 112:369, 1977.

Purnell, D. C., Scholz, D. A., and Smith, L. H.: Diagnosis of primary hyperparathyroidism. Surg. Clin. North Am., 57:543, 1977.

Schneider, A. B., and Sherwood, L. M.: Pathogenesis and management of hypoparathyroidism and other hypocalcemic disorders. Metabolism, 24:871, 1975.

Wells, S. A.: The parathyroid glands. In Sabiston, D. C. (ed.): Davis-Christopher Textbook of Surgery, 12th ed. Philadelphia, W. B. Saunders Co., 1981.

Wells, S. A., and Baylin, S. B.: The multiple endocrine neoplasias. In Sabiston, D. C. (ed.): Davis-Christopher Textbook of Surgery, 11th ed. Philadelphia, W. B. Saunders Co., 1977.

Wells, S. A., Stirman, J. A., and Bolman, R. M.: Parathyroid transplantation. World J. Surg., 1:747, 1977.

31

The Endocrine Pancreas

LARRY C. CAREY
E. CHRISTOPHER ELLISON

PREOPERATIVE AND POSTOPERATIVE CARE OF THE DIABETIC PATIENT

Management of diabetic patients undergoing surgery must be meticulous. The metabolic derangement of diabetes and the high incidence of associated arteriosclerosis predispose these patients to greater operative risk. Persistent and poorly controlled hyperglycemia is associated with ketoacidosis, hyperosmolar coma, intracellular dehydration, electrolyte imbalance, delayed wound healing, and inadequate cellular and humoral responses to infection. Compounded by a high incidence of concomitant cardiac complications, these factors account for an operative morbidity of 16 per cent and an operative mortality of two per cent. In contrast, operation in the nondiabetic population is associated with significant postoperative complications in only approximately five per cent of cases and death in less than one per cent. Safe operation in the diabetic patient requires special attention to prevention or early detection of vascular complications and to regulation of glucose metabolism.

GENERAL APPROACH

Preoperative evaluation requires assessing diabetic control, establishing a baseline of metabolic and cardiac status, and detecting coexisting problems. The patient should be admitted to the hospital one or two days prior to elective operation. Important historical data include the current dose and type of insulin or oral hypoglycemic agent and a history of ketoacidosis or hyperosmolar coma. Particular note is made of past cardiac problems, such as myocardial infarction or angina, and of new cardiovascular symptoms. A complete physical examination is mandatory, with special attention to the cardiopulmonary and peripheral vascular systems. Baseline determinations of fasting blood sugar, electrolytes, bicarbonate, and blood urea nitrogen are essential. Electrocardiogram, urinalysis, and chest roentgenograms should all be obtained. Operation is delayed until aberrations are corrected.

Postoperatively, the patient must be observed for symptomatic as well as silent myocardial infarction and for sepsis, particularly originating from the pulmonary and genitourinary systems.

The major goal of preoperative and postoperative management of the diabetic patient is to establish "a surgical zone" reflecting a steady state of glucose metabolism with the maintenance of blood sugar between 100 mg per 100 ml and 250 mg per 100 ml. A mildly elevated blood sugar and glycosuria are not harmful to the patient, whereas attempts to achieve normal blood glucose levels predispose him or her to hypoglycemia. Successful control of glucose metabolism requires the proper selection of insulin type, a simple and reliable route of insulin administration, and an accurate method of monitoring glucose tolerance. The methods chosen to achieve and maintain a surgical zone vary with the severity of the diabetes and the degree to which the diabetic state is exacerbated by stress-related hormonal changes associated with the primary disease, operation, and postoperative complications.

For most insulin-dependent diabetics undergoing elective surgery, intermediate-acting forms of insulin are preferred. In contrast to the use of regular insulin on a sliding scale, the administration of NPH or lente insulin once or twice daily both preoperatively and postoperatively provides for smooth glucose control and lessens catabolism. However, severe diabetics and those requiring emergency operations often require pronounced increases in the insulin dosage. These patients usually require supplementation of the required dose of intermediate insulin with regular insulin, calculated using blood sugar levels determined at six-hour intervals. The following sliding scale has proved satisfactory in our experience:

Blood Sugar	Regular Insulin
≥ 400 mg/100 ml	15 units
300–400 mg/100 ml	10 units
200–300 mg/100 ml	5 units

Insulin is usually administered subcutaneously. Some surgeons prefer to employ a continuous intravenous infusion of regular insulin, but this method may result in erratic insulin administration due to variable absorption of the drug by the glass and tubing, changing rates of fluid administration, and possible interruption of the infusion by the need for blood or colloid. The subcutaneous route insures reliable absorption and should be employed except in the presence of shock, when poor tissue perfusion prevents reliable subcutaneous absorption. In these cases, intermittent intravenous doses of regular insulin are required.

Before, during, and after operation, glucose tolerance is most reliably monitored by blood glucose determinations. Using measurements of glycosuria and ketonuria as indices of insulin therapy is fraught with error. With the measurement of urine glucose by various methods (Clinitest, Clinistix, Diastix, and Testape), a 23 per cent incidence of falsely high values and a 33 per cent incidence of falsely low values have been observed. The reliability of urine testing is limited by an elevated threshold for renal glucose loss associated with diabetes, shock, dehydration, and bladder dysfunction related to diabetic neuropathy, pain, and narcotic use. In addition, commonly employed drugs alter the results of various testing methods. For example, penicillin G potassium, streptomycin, and cephalosporin cause a positive Clinitest reaction, while ascorbic acid causes falsely low values with Testape and Clinistix. Patients receiving intermediate-acting forms are best monitored by blood glucose measurements at 7:00 A.M. and 3:00 P.M. daily. Severe diabetics and those requiring a supplemental sliding scale of regular insulin should have blood glucose determinations at six-hour intervals.

In summary, the regulation of glucose homeostasis is best accomplished by the daily subcutaneous administration of intermediate-acting insulin monitored by morning and afternoon blood sugar determinations. More frequent glucose monitoring and supplementary regular insulin are required by severe diabetics and those undergoing emergency surgery.

PREOPERATIVE MANAGEMENT

The decision to be made in the preoperative period is what therapeutic alterations, if any, are required to establish and maintain the blood sugar between 100 mg per 100 ml and 250 mg per 100 ml. Prior to elective operation, not only does poor diabetic control necessitate a change in therapy, but also the underlying cause of glucose intolerance must be detected and corrected. Common etiologic factors include lack of patient compliance with prescribed diet or drugs, scar formation at insulin administration sites preventing absorption, stress related to the primary disease, and, most important, unsuspected coexisting problems such as myocardial infarction or infection.

Changes in diabetic therapy are determined by the glucose measurement, using a 7:00 A.M. sample for patients controlled with diet or oral hypoglycemics and a 3:00 P.M. sample for those requiring intermediate insulin. Diabetics with blood sugars less than 250 mg per 100 ml require no variation in therapy, except those patients who receive long-acting oral hypoglycemic agents (i.e., sulfonylureas). These agents should be discontinued preoperatively.

If the blood sugar is between 250 mg per 100 ml and 350 mg per 100 ml, diabetic therapy needs revision. Patients previously managed with diet and oral agents are converted to intermediate insulin the following day. A starting dose of 16 to 20 units of NPH or lente insulin has proved satisfactory. Insulin-dependent diabetics should have the dosage of intermediate insulin increased 10 to 20 per cent the following morning. For example, a patient who has been receiving 50 units of intermediate insulin at 7:00 A.M. with a 3:00 P.M. blood sugar of 300 mg per 100 ml should be given 60 units of long-acting insulin the next day. In all patients, a blood sugar greater than 350 mg per 100 ml necessitates administration of 10 to 20 units of regular insulin immediately, followed by appropriate increments of insulin dosage (as outlined above) the following morning. If the blood sugar is less than 80 mg per 100 ml, glucose is administered. Elective operation is delayed until the surgical zone is established.

The goal of preoperative management of diabetic patients with acute surgical disease is not control of the associated and often profound glucose intolerance but correction of coexisting problems such as hypovolemia and hyperthermia followed by early operative intervention. Delay of surgical treatment related to attempts to regulate glucose may result in increased morbidity and mortality. Safe operation is possible with blood sugar measurements less than 500 mg per 100 ml.

Correction of blood sugar in an emergency situation is best achieved with regular insulin. If the blood sugar is between 350 mg per 100 ml and 500 mg per 100 ml, the patient should receive 25 to 50 units of regular insulin subcutaneously, or intravenously if a shock state exists. For a blood glucose greater than 500 mg per 100 ml, 100 units of regular insulin are given, 50 units subcutaneously and 50 units intravenously, or the total dose is administered intravenously in the presence of vascular collapse. When the patient has diabetic ketoacidosis or hyperosmolar coma, the metabolic derangements must be corrected preoperatively.

OPERATIVE MANAGEMENT

The major intraoperative threat to the well-controlled diabetic is hypoglycemia. To avoid hypoglycemia, two steps are taken. First, a continuous intravenous infusion of 5 per cent dextrose and water or sodium chloride is started the night before operation and continued during the procedure. This is particularly important for patients scheduled for afternoon operations. In addition, the insulin dose is reduced on the day of operation. Medication is withheld from well-controlled patients taking oral hypoglycemic agents on the morning of operation. Patients requiring intermediate insulin alone are given one-half the daily requirement on the day of operation. Patients receiving a mixture of regular and long-acting insulin are decreased to one-half the usual dose.

Excessive hyperglycemia does not present a significant problem in well-controlled diabetics during the surgical procedure. The effect of operative stress on the blood glucose is small, with an average increase of less than 20 mg per 100 ml, or 37 mg per 100 ml for more stressful procedures. To monitor blood sugar, a determination is made at the beginning of the procedure, repeated intraoperatively if the procedure requires more than four hours, and again in the recovery room. Supplemental doses of regular insulin are administered only if the blood sugar is greater than 350 mg per 100 ml.

POSTOPERATIVE MANAGEMENT

Because of humoral responses to stress, it would appear that increased doses of exogenous insulin would be required postoperatively to establish glucose control, to inhibit lipolysis, proteolysis, gluconeogenesis, and ketogenesis, and to maintain an anabolic state. However, operation and anesthesia interrupt or decrease oral caloric intake, and intravenous feeding of 5 per cent dextrose solutions at the usual maintenance rate of 2.5 to 3 liters per 24 hours provides only 500 to 600 calories. Therefore, in order to prevent hypoglycemia, insulin dosages should be reduced in the early postoperative period. Diabetics regulated with diet alone preoperatively require no insulin therapy. Patients previously controlled with an oral hypoglycemic alone rarely require insulin supplementation in the early postoperative period. If needed, regular insulin is administered at six-hour intervals, and the dose is determined by blood sugar measurements. Patients who required conversion to insulin preoperatively and insulin-dependent diabetics are given two-thirds of the preoperative daily requirement of intermediate insulin. Glucose control is monitored by 7:00 A.M. and 3:00 P.M. blood sugar determinations. Adjustments of insulin dosage for the following days are made according to the scheme applied in the preoperative period.

Intravenous feedings are discontinued and preoperative diabetic therapy is resumed when oral intake is possible. Monitoring of blood sugar is continued until a steady state of glucose control is reestablished.

Disruption of glucose tolerance may be the first indication of operative complications, such as infection or an anastomotic leak, and signals the need for a thorough evaluation of the patient. If serious complications ensue, the diabetic state is usually worsened, and oral intake may well be limited. The daily dose of intermediate insulin is then reduced to two-thirds of that previously required, and a sliding scale like that employed for the severe diabetic is used to achieve better glucose control.

At the time of discharge from the hospital, insulin-dependent diabetics should be under-regulated, with blood sugar levels between

100 to 200 mg per 100 ml, because of the known blood sugar–lowering effects of normal activity. Certainly, the status of the patient's diabetic management should be conveyed to the physician who will be caring for him or her on an outpatient basis.

In summary, a flexible approach to the regulation of blood sugar in the diabetic patient should be used before, during, and after operation. Changing insulin requirements resulting from hormonal changes in response to the primary disease, intercurrent problems, the stress of operation, and the patient's ability to eat and ambulate postoperatively demand close attention. Close monitoring of the patient's blood sugar is mandatory to determine changing insulin needs and to individualize therapy.

MANAGEMENT OF UNCONTROLLED DIABETES

Illness in the well-controlled diabetic patient often aggravates the diabetic state, precipitating hyperglycemia, which may progress to either diabetic ketoacidosis or hyperosmolar coma. Diabetic ketoacidosis is characterized by hyperglycemia, dehydration, and metabolic acidosis. Nonketotic hyperosmolar coma is characterized by hyperglycemia without ketosis but with profound dehydration and usually occurs in the older patient. Mortality associated with ketoacidosis is 10 per cent, and that with hyperosmolar coma is 50 per cent, so both of these conditions must be corrected preoperatively.

Either disorder is suspected when a known diabetic develops polydipsia and polyuria associated with some degree of stupor or diminution of mental acuity. The diagnosis is usually not entirely clear from the history and physical examination. Rather, it is established by determination of the blood glucose, serum ketones, arterial blood gases, serum electrolytes, blood urea nitrogen, and creatinine. In diabetic ketoacidosis, the blood sugar is usually between 500 mg per 100 ml and 800 mg per 100 ml, whereas glucose determinations approaching 1000 mg per 100 ml are common in nonketotic hyperosmolar coma. Diabetic ketoacidosis is characterized by high serum ketone levels in addition to ketonuria, both of which are usually absent in hyperosmolar coma. Electrolyte determinations are variable. The serum sodium may be elevated secondary to hypertonic dehydration or may be factitiously depressed owing to the hyperglycemia. Hypokalemia is more characteristic of ketoacidosis but may occur during therapy for hyperosmolar coma. Azotemia is the rule in both disorders, with elevation of blood urea nitrogen in the range of 30 to 40 mg per 100 ml, even in the absence of renal disease.

Once the diagnosis of either entity is established, appropriate studies are obtained to determine the precipitating cause. Intra-abdominal catastrophes, such as acute cholecystitis, mesenteric infarction, and pancreatitis, infection arising from the genitourinary and pulmonary systems, myocardial infarction, and acute pulmonary thromboembolism are examples of conditions that may induce ketoacidosis or hyperosmolar coma.

The surgeon is frequently consulted during this evaluation, since many patients complain of abdominal pain. However, contrary to those with underlying surgical disease, the patient with pure diabetic ketoacidosis invariably has nausea and vomiting preceding the onset of abdominal symptoms. Abdominal examination may be misleading, as many patients display peritoneal irritation, but localized tenderness is usually absent. The patient suspected of having intra-abdominal disease should be admitted to a surgical service and should be observed.

Simultaneously with diagnostic evaluation, therapy for ketoacidosis and hyperosmolar coma is started. Preoperative preparation in both conditions is essentially the same. Special consideration is given to rehydration and correction of the hyperglycemia and the accompanying acid-base and electrolyte imbalance.

Treatment is first directed to monitoring and stabilizing the patient. An adequate intravenous line is placed using aseptic technique. In the presence of a shock state, a central venous line is essential. An indwelling arterial catheter is helpful in patients who require frequent determinations of arterial blood gases. In the unconscious patient or one in shock, an indwelling urinary catheter is necessary to monitor urine production. If the patient is fully awake with stable cardiovascular dynamics, an indwelling bladder catheter is not essential, since urine output can be verified with intermittent catheterization, which lessens the risk of infection. A nasogastric tube is placed in patients with intra-abdominal disease as well as in unconscious patients at risk to develop aspiration pneumonia. Important in this phase of treatment is the initiation and maintenance of a flow sheet for recording urine output, vital signs, and the multiple determinations of blood glucose, arterial blood gases, serum ketones, and electrolytes.

Patients with ketoacidosis or hyperosmolar coma are severely dehydrated, with deficits sometimes approaching seven liters of total body water, and some patients have evidence of vascular collapse. Establishing a urine output of 1 ml per kg per hour and correcting hypotension are required preoperatively. Rehydration is best accomplished with hypotonic fluids, usually one-half normal saline. In the hypotensive patient, normal saline is more appropriate. Plasma expanders have no role in the treatment of diabetic ketoacidosis or hyperosmolar coma. The typical patient requires two to three liters of intravenous fluid during the first two hours of therapy. Subsequent fluid administration rates are adjusted according to urine production and central venous pressure measurements.

The quantity and route of insulin administration is a subject of controversy. Recommended therapy at our institution is the initial administration of 100 units of regular insulin (50 units by intravenous bolus and 50 units subcutaneously) if the blood sugar exceeds 500 mg per 100 ml. Patients with vascular collapse should receive the entire dose intravenously to avoid delayed subcutaneous absorption. If the blood sugar is 350 to 500 mg per 100 ml, a total dose of 50 units of regular insulin is administered, and subsequent insulin requirements are determined by blood sugar measurements at two-hour intervals. When the blood sugar is below 300 mg per 100 ml, insulin administration is curtailed, but glucose determinations are continued to guard against hypoglycemia. At this point, five per cent dextrose may be added to the intravenous fluid regimen. A blood sugar below 500 mg per 100 ml permits safe surgical intervention; however, electrolyte and acid-base disturbances must be corrected prior to operation.

The major electrolyte abnormality in ketoacidosis is hypokalemia, which may approach 5 to 10 mEq per kg but is more commonly 3 to 5 mEq per kg. This deficit is exacerbated by rehydration and insulin therapy. If the initial serum potassium is normal or low, we add 20 to 40 mEq of potassium chloride to each liter of intravenous fluid. Serum potassium should be monitored at two-hour intervals, and the total potassium deficit should be corrected in eight to ten hours. Nonketotic hyperosmolar coma is not characteristically accompanied by hypokalemia, so fluids devoid of potassium are used, and potassium is replaced as indicated by serum determinations at two-hour intervals. Hypernatremia resulting from hypotonic dehydration is common in the hyperosmolar state and is corrected with rehydration.

Metabolic acidosis in both conditions is usually improved with fluid resuscitation and insulin therapy; however, alkali therapy is required for patients with serum bicarbonate levels below 10 mEq per liter and an arterial pH less than 7.1. In these cases, the bicarbonate requirement is determined as follows:

$$\frac{\text{Base deficit} \times \text{Body weight (kg)}}{4} = \text{Bicarbonate requirement (in mEq)}$$

This is administered intravenously as sodium bicarbonate.

Rehydration and correction of the excessive hyperglycemia and associated acid-base and electrolyte imbalance enable the surgeon to operate with maximal safety. Postoperatively, a sliding scale for regular insulin is employed based on blood glucose determinations every four to six hours. As soon as feasible, the patient's premorbid diabetic therapy is reinstituted.

FUNCTIONING TUMORS OF THE ENDOCRINE PANCREAS

Endocrine tumors of the pancreas are best conceptualized as alimentary apudomas. The APUD cells, described by Pearse in 1968, have common cytologic characteristics related to polypeptide and amine synthesis and are widely distributed throughout the body. The apudomas are endocrine tumors that arise from these cells.

APUD cells derive their name from the initial letters of their first three and most important properties: (1) high content of *a*mine, (2) capacity for amine *p*recursor *u*ptake, and (3) the presence of amino acid *d*ecarboxylase. Apudomas are functioning tumors that may be classified pathologically as adenoma, adenomatous hyperplasia, or carcinoma. Biologically, these tumors are characterized by secretion of hormones of the APUD cell series. Apudomas of the alimentary tract are classified as orthoendocrine tumors (i.e., insulinoma, glucagonoma), secreting normal polypeptides or amines of their parent cells; paraendocrine tumors of endocrine glands (i.e., gastrinoma, WDHA), secreting hormones or hormonal agents characteristic of other glands or cells; or as tumors arising from tissues not usually considered endocrine in nature but that secrete humoral agents. Pancreatic apudomas may occur alone or in association with the syndrome of multiple endocrine adenopathy.

Apudomas are less differentiated in function than their parent cells and have a versatile secretory capacity. For example, insulinoma secretes insulin but may also secrete other APUD-related hormones (such as gastrin and secretin). In addition, some paraendocrine tumors are capable of secreting products characteristic of non-APUD cells, such as prostaglandin, histamine, and erythropoietin. This explains the wide variety of clinical symptoms associated with APUD cell tumors.

INSULINOMA

Insulinoma is an orthoendocrine apudoma arising from the B cell of the pancreas, which produces insulin and causes spontaneous hypoglycemia. Although an insulinoma was first discovered in an asymptomatic patient at necropsy by Nicholls in 1902, not until 1921 when Banting and Best isolated insulin was the etiology of the dramatic symptoms associated with these functioning tumors proposed. At this time, diabetics treated with excessive amounts of insulin were recognized to have a symptom complex similar to patients with insulinoma, thus establishing the link between spontaneous hypoglycemia and insulin production. That islet cell tumors could produce clinical symptoms by excess secretory activity was confirmed in 1927 by Wilder and associates, who conclusively demonstrated that hepatic metastases from a B cell tumor contained insulin.

Nearly 1000 cases of insulinoma have been reported in the literature, and the disease is well understood; however, functioning islet cell tumors are uncommon, and the diagnosis is often subtle. Reviews of hospital records and case reports are replete with the tragedy of unrecognized insulinoma. In patients with insulinoma, the episodic and sometimes continuous release of insulin, often at inappropriately low blood glucose levels, produces spontaneous hypoglycemia and the characteristic clinical syndrome. Early symptoms related to the hypoglycemic-induced surge of catecholamines are tremor, restlessness, irritability, weakness, hunger, diaphoresis, tachycardia, and sometimes nausea and vomiting. However, because of the gradual decline of glucose levels in patients with B cell apudomas, these early symptoms often do not occur.

The most common clinical manifestations of insulinoma are episodic disturbances in consciousness and aberrant behavior. Progressive and prolonged hypoglycemic attacks cause neuroglycopenia, resulting in symptoms often thought to be neuropsychiatric, ranging from subtle personality changes and confusion to obtundation and coma. Convulsions may intercede and may be indistinguishable from some forms of epilepsy. Temporary paralysis is associated with severe attacks of hypoglycemia in 5 per cent of the patients with insulinoma, and another 7 per cent incur irreversible central nervous system damage. Death may occur during severe episodes. Between attacks, patients are usually well without distinctive physical findings but may exhibit subtle signs of intellectual deterioration.

Preoperative Assessment

Hypoglycemia in the adult may be nonorganic or organic. Nonorganic causes of hypoglycemia include reactive or functional hypoglycemia associated with gastrectomy or gastroenterostomy, surreptitious administration of insulin or ingestion of sulfonylureas, chronic pancreatitis, chronic adrenal insufficiency, hypopituitarism, ingestion of denatured alcohol, and, rarely, hepatic insufficiency if more than 85 per cent of the liver parenchyma is diseased. Most commonly, hypoglycemia is reactive in origin or associated with early maturity–onset diabetes mellitus. Diagnosis is rarely difficult, as patients typically develop symptoms three to five hours after a meal and do not experience fasting hypoglycemia. In addition, functional hypoglycemia is a nonprogressive disease and usually does not result in loss of consciousness. Factitious hypoglycemia is sometimes difficult to distinguish from insulinoma but is differentiated by demonstrating insulin antibodies and C peptide in the patient's serum.

Organic hypoglycemia is caused by insulinomas and occasionally by tumors arising from retroperitoneal or mediastinal mesenchymal tissues that attain growth to over 1000 gm. These tumors are not likely to be overlooked if the physician is alert to their possible occurrence.

The diagnosis of insulinoma depends upon documentation of fasting hypoglycemia with inappropriately elevated insulin levels. An insulinoma should be suspected in any patient who fulfills Whipple's triad of fast-induced hypoglycemic symptoms with a blood sugar less than 50 mg per 100 ml and relief of the symptoms with administration of glucose. A prolonged fast demonstrating Whipple's triad is the most reliable method for diagnosing insulinoma. Blood glucose determinations should be performed every six hours during the fast or when the patient is symptomatic. Values defining hypoglycemia depend upon both the laboratory method and the sex of the patient. Variations are shown in Table 31–1.

Prolongation of the fast results in a more conclusive test. After 48 hours, two-thirds of the patients with insulin-producing tumors develop symptoms of hypoglycemia relieved by glucose administration. Prolonging the fast to 72 hours and adding exercise at its completion yields positive results in more than 90 per cent of patients.

Simultaneous serum insulin measurements coupled with serum glucose determinations increase the diagnostic accuracy of prolonged fasting. In a patient with insulinoma, radioimmunoassay commonly shows levels above 25 μU per ml. Occasionally absolute insulin concentrations may be in the normal range of 5 to 20 μU per ml, but such values are inappropriate in the presence of hypoglycemia. Therefore, a ratio of the fasting plasma glucose concentration to the simultaneous insulin level is calculated. A value below 2.5 indicates inappropriate hyperinsulinemia and the presence of an insulinoma. The fasting glucose and insulin levels considered diagnostic for insulinoma are presented in Table 31–1.

Further testing is usually not required, but if the diagnosis remains unclear, provocative testing with tolbutamide, glucagon, and L-leucine may be performed and the glucose and insulin responses observed (Table 31–1). These procedures have associated risks and are less reliable than fasting. They should not be performed when the diagnosis is clearly established during prolonged food deprivation.

Tolbutamide infusion is the most helpful of the provocative tests, although diagnostic accuracy is only 50 per cent. One gram of sodium tolbutamide in 20 ml of distilled water is given intravenously over two minutes. Glucose measurements are made every 15 minutes for the first hour and then hourly for the remaining three hours. Insulin determinations are made every ten minutes for the first 30 minutes, then every 30 minutes for two hours.

Tolbutamide induces release of insulin from the pancreatic B cell, causing hypoglycemia, and three aspects of this response must be considered. The extent and rate of fall of the blood sugar do not discriminate between patients with or without insulin-producing tumors. Of greater diagnostic significance is the persistence of the depression of blood sugar for 180 minutes in patients with insulinoma, whereas in normal individuals, blood sugar returns to 70 to 80 per cent of the pretest values in 90 to 180 minutes. Last, the insulin response to tolbutamide is more rapid and the rise is greater in patients with insulin-producing islet cell tumors. Insulin peaks occurring within the first five to 15 minutes with levels of 150 μU per ml strongly suggest insulinoma.

Table 31–1. Diagnostic Tests for Insulinoma*

TEST†	CRITERIA FOR POSITIVE TEST Glucose‡ mg/dl	Insulin§ uU/ml	FALSE POSITIVE	FALSE NEGATIVE	APPROXIMATE FREQUENCY OF POSITIVE TEST IN INSULINOMA‖	COMMENT
Overnight fast (12-hour)	<60	>25	Yes (rare)	Yes	50%	About half have both low glucose–high insulin. Multiple overnight sampling increases frequency of positive tests.
Prolonged fast (24-hour)	Men <55, Women <35	>20, >15	Yes (rare)	Yes	50%	Should be done if overnight plasma glucose > 60 mg/dl. Severe hypoglycemia (without hyperinsulinemia) strongly suggests insulinoma, but other causes must be excluded. False positive tests can occur with insulin injection, rarely with nonpancreatic tumors, and in infants of diabetic mothers.
(48-hour)	Men <50, Women <35	>20, >15	Yes (rare)	Yes	50–75%	
(72-hour)	Men <50, Women	>20	Yes (rare)	Yes	>90%	
Tolbutamide infusion (may be done before prolonged fast)	<66% of fasting level with sustained hypoglycemia	>150	Yes (occasional)	Yes	50%	Severe prolonged hypoglycemia may occur. Contraindicated if FBS 45 mg/dl. False positive tests in alcohol hypoglycemia hepatic glycogen depletion
L-leucine infusion		>100	Yes	Yes	<50%	False positive in adults treated with sulfonylureas and children with leucine sensitivity
Glucagon infusion	None	>130 at any time	Yes (rare)	Yes	80%	Blood glucose initially rises, then falls to pre-test levels. Marked hypoglycemia usually not problem

*By permission, Edward W. Martin, Jr., M.D.

†In the order done by the authors.

‡Serum or plasma glucose (glucose oxidase method) in mg/dl (whole blood is about 15% lower). Criteria for adults.

§Serum or plasma insulin levels are approximate and may require adjustment for individual laboratories.

‖Frequency of both glucose and insulin abnormalities.

When the diagnosis is reasonably secure, selective arteriography of the celiac, superior mesenteric, and hepatic arteries is used to define the position and number of islet cell tumors and to detect the presence of hepatic metastases. Identification of 65 per cent of insulinomas is possible with this technique. Selective catheterization of the splenic vein and tributaries draining the pancreas permits sampling of blood for insulin determination. This has improved preoperative localization. Pancreatic scanning is universally unsuccessful in detecting islet cell tumors.

Management

Preoperative preparation requires adequate hydration, normalization of electrolytes, and avoidance of hypoglycemia. We recommend intravenous infusion of 5 per cent dextrose in 0.45 normal saline or 10 per cent dextrose in 0.45 normal saline commencing the night prior to surgery.

Surgical excision of the tumor is the treatment of choice for insulinoma. Insulinomas are usually single (86 per cent) and may occur in any area of the pancreas. If a tumor is localized in the body or tail of the pancreas, removal of the distal 50 per cent of the gland is required. Tumors of the head of the pancreas are best managed by enucleation, and pancreaticoduodenectomy is rarely necessary. Four per cent of the tumors are ectopic in location, found in descending order of frequency in the hilum of the spleen, wall of the stomach, and small bowel. Local excision suffices in these cases.

In 23 per cent of cases, no tumor is found. A distal pancreatectomy is performed, and the specimen is sectioned in search for islet cell hyperplasia. Persistent or recurrent symptoms postoperatively require reevaluation and, if indicated, exploratory laparotomy and 95 per cent pancreatectomy. In seven per cent of the reported cases, reexploration fails to disclose the tumor. The urgency of locating insulinoma at the first exploration is underscored by the observation that the operative mortality rises from 7 per cent to 18 per cent with reoperation.

In patients with malignant insulinoma and metastases, surgical treatment has little to offer. Isolated malignant tumors should be excised as well as metastases, but recurrences are common.

Intraoperative monitoring of blood sugar is important in the surgical treatment of insulin-producing tumors. Within 30 minutes after tumor excision or blind pancreatic resection, blood sugar levels usually rise sharply if the insulin-producing tissue has been removed. However, this test may be misleading, and postoperative glucose and insulin determinations are needed to confirm the completeness of resection.

Postoperative transient hyperglycemia sometimes requiring insulin therapy is expected but lasts only about three weeks. Nasogastric suction and intravenous hydration are continued until bowel function returns.

After discharge, patients should be seen periodically for blood glucose and insulin determinations and to detect recurrent symptoms or to document metastatic disease. The presence of either requires in-hospital evaluation with fasting and provocative testing as well as arteriography.

Medical management is reserved for patients with metastatic insulinoma and those whose tumor is not found at operation. Both anti-insulin and antineoplastic drugs are employed. Diazoxide and diphenylhydantoin both inhibit insulin release from the pancreas and have been utilized with variable success. Streptozotocin selectively destroys the pancreatic B cell. Whether administered intravenously or intra-arterially, it produces reduced serum insulin concentration in 60 per cent of patients and, reportedly, tumor regression in about 50 per cent of patients. Tretment with this drug is limited because of hepatic, renal, and hematologic toxicity observed in over 50 per cent of cases and the possible carcinogenic properties of streptozotocin. Its administration to rodents has produced both renal and hepatic adenomas. This drug should be used with caution in patients with a long life expectancy. A triple drug regimen consisting of 5-fluorouracil, tubercidin, and streptozotocin may be employed as in the treatment of gastrinoma.

GLUCAGONOMA

A glucagon-secreting islet cell tumor was first described in 1966 by McGavran and his associates. Glucagonoma is an orthoendocrine apudoma of the alpha cells of the pancreas. The hallmark of this disorder is a skin rash and mild diabetes mellitus.

The skin lesions have usually been present for longer than a year. The rash begins as an erythematous area that tends to blister and crust and begins to heal in seven to 14 days. Some lesions are developing while others are healing. Painful glossitis may also be present. The relationship of the hyperglucagonemia to these skin lesions is unknown.

About half the reported cases involve mild adult-onset diabetes mellitus that is not associated with ketoacidosis and usually does not require insulin therapy.

Plasma glucagon legels have been reported to range from 850 to 3500 pg per ml (normal 9 to 120 pg per ml). Successful surgical resection of the tumor is followed by resolution of the hyperglucagonemia, clearing of the skin and mucous membrane lesions, and a return to normoglycemia.

Principles outlined for the surgical treatment of insulinoma are applicable to glucagonoma.

ULCEROGENIC TUMOR

In 1955, Zollinger and Ellison described two patients who exhibited a triad of (1) recurrent fulminant peptic ulceration despite standard acid-reducing gastric operations, (2) gastric acid hypersecretion, and (3) non-beta islet cell tumor of the pancreas. Both patients had a primary ulceration beyond the ligament of Treitz, and one had diarrhea. Within five years, Gregory and Tracy proved that ulcerogenic tumors produce a potent gastric secretagogue subsequently proved to be gastrin. The primary tumor and the metastases were later estimated to elaborate between 35 and 45 times more gastrin than an equivalent weight of porcine antrum. The production of such high levels of extragastric gastrin explained the clinical findings of immense gastric hypersecretion and steatorrhea. There are now almost 1000 cases in the Z-E tumor registry. Although study of these patients has added greatly to knowledge of this disease, many questions remain unanswered.

Preoperative Evaluation

Diagnosis of an ulcerogenic tumor or gastrinoma requires a high degree of suspicion, for this paraendocrine apudoma is present in only a small portion of patients with duodenal ulceration. Commonly, there is a long history of ulcer disease with a higher incidence of complications related to peptic ulcer disease. Gastrointestinal bleeding occurs in almost one-third of the patients, and perforation occurs in approximately one-fourth. Perforation occurs distal to the ligament of Treitz in 10 per cent of the cases. Symptoms not usual in peptic ulcer disease may occur, as in roughly 20 per cent of the patients diarrhea is the initial complaint. Seventy-five per cent of these patients simultaneously or subsequently experience ulcer symptoms.

Patients in whom this syndrome is most likely to be present are (1) patients who have severe ulcer diathesis refractory to intensive antacid therapy and gastric aspiration; (2) patients in whom ulceration recurs after a well-performed standard surgical procedure, although imperfectly performed operations for gastric or duodenal ulcer are the more common cause of recurrence; (3) elderly patients with persistent ulcer symptoms; (4) children or adolescents with ulceration; (5) immediate postpartum patients with massive upper gastrointestinal hemorrhage or perforation; (6) patients who have protracted and unexplained diarrhea, even without symptoms of ulcer disease (5 to 10 per cent); and (7) patients with symptoms of both hyperparathyroidism and upper gastrointestinal ulceration (approximately 25 per cent).

Recurrent ulceration following a standard ulcer operation deserves special attention. It is essential to learn the exact nature of the previous operations to determine whether a physiologically sound procedure was carried out. The original operative notes, laboratory slides, pathology reports, and radiographic studies must be reviewed. All too frequently, a posterior vagus nerve has been overlooked or the gastrojejunostomy stoma has been placed too far from the pylorus, permitting antral distention. Retained antrum must also be considered, although this is becoming increasingly uncommon. Particular attention must be given to drugs prescribed for unrelated conditions such as hypertension or arthritis, including aspirin and aspirin/caffeine–containing drugs. Excessive smoking and coffee ingestion must also be excluded. Other causes of recurrent ulceration may be chronic calcific pancreatitis, extensive small bowel resection, liver disease, and operations to relieve portal hypertension. It is advisable to pursue the diagnostic approach outlined next rather than to repeat resections and explorations.

The diagnosis is established by radiographic studies, gastric analysis, gastrin radioimmunoassay, provocative tests, and endoscopy. Characteristic findings on an upper gastrointestinal series include (1) a large amount of retained fluid in the stomach; (2) giant rugal folds suggesting Menetrier's disease and megaduodenum; (3) unusual ulcer location, such as the second or third portion of the duodenum or beyond the ligament of Treitz, which is pathognomonic in the absence of drug-related disease; and (4) increased transit time.

The gastric analysis, possibly the first clue to an ulcerogenic tumor, is not as significant in establishing the diagnosis as it was a decade ago. However, it remains a good screening test. The aspiration of large volumes of gastric juice rich in hydrochloric acid from an unobstructed stomach signals the presence of an ulcerogenic tumor. Volume averages 100 ml per hour and is not infrequently as much as three to six liters in a 12-hour period. The acid output is fixed in a range greater than 10 mEq per hour, and the acid concentration is 100 mEq per liter or more. Since the gastric glands are being maximally stimulated at all times by the hypergastrinemia, the augmentation of gastrin secretion by the subcutaneous administration of 6 μg per kg of pentagastrin is less than in the normal duodenal ulcer patient. The basal acid output is already 60 per cent or more of the maximal acid output provoked by pentagastrin in two-thirds of the patients.

The mainstay of diagnosis is the gastrin radioimmunoassay developed by McGuigan (1968). Use of this technique has established the diagnosis of the ulcerogenic tumor more frequently and more firmly. The gastrin-producing islet cell tumor is invariably associated with gastrin levels above the normal of 150 per per ml in our laboratory. Gastrin levels greater than 500 pg per ml in combination with the characteristic clinical picture are very suggestive of ulcerogenic tumor and necessitate further evaluation.

However, one elevated gastrin level does not necessarily establish a diagnosis of the Zollinger-Ellison syndrome. To exclude laboratory error, three consecutive fasting gastrin determinations are mandatory. Indeed, as clinical experience with gastrin radioimmunoassay has increased, an ever mounting number of physiologic variations and diseases have been found to be associated with hypergastrinemia. Moderately elevated gastrin levels may be associated with pyloric obstruction or the ingestion of a protein meal. Persistently elevated levels in excess of 250 pg per ml are usually associated with gastrinoma, pernicious anemia, or atrophic gastritis. Hypergastrinemia is also associated with the short bowel syndrome, renal failure, a retained antrum following Billroth II gastric resection, and carcinoma of the body of the stomach associated with achlorhydria. Hyperplasia of the antral G cells may be responsible for elevated gastrin levels. In affected patients there is a doubling of gastrin level following a meal. Gastrin levels in patients with duodenal ulcer disease are variable and may be elevated. The lack of specificity of gastrin radioimmunoassay necessitates the performance of provocative infusion studies when elevated levels of serum gastrin are detected.

The most reliable and sensitive of these tests is the secretin bolus. Prior to administering secretin, skin testing is performed to detect sensitivity to the drug. A dose of 2 units of secretin per kg is administered as a bolus. Samples are taken for gastrin determination at 1, 2, 5, 10, 15, and 30 minutes. This produces a paradoxical rise of serum gastrin levels in excess of 110 pg per ml over basal levels in patients with the ulcerogenic tumor. The gastrin level is depressed in patients with duodenal ulcer, atrophic gastritis, G cell hyperplasia, and retained antrum. This is a simple and safer method than either the calcium or magnesium infusion test to distinguish patients whose gastrin levels and acid studies are inconclusive.

The recognized association between the hypercalcemia of hyperparathyroidism and peptic ulceration has led to the use of calcium infusion in combination with gastric secretory studies and the gastrin radioimmunoassay. The test is performed by giving elemental calcium as calcium gluceptate 15 mg per kg in 500 ml normal saline as a continuous infusion over four hours. Gastrin and calcium levels are measured one, two, three, and four hours after infusion of calcium gluceptate is started and one hour after the infusion is discontinued. Elevation of two to three times the fasting level provides good supporting evidence of tumor.

In patients with hyperparathyroidism or cardiac dysfunction, calcium infusion should be avoided, and elemental magnesium as magnesium sulfate 1.6 mEq per kg in 500 ml normal saline over four hours may be substituted. The test is carried out in the same manner, and similar responses in the presence of gastrinemia are to be expected. This test should not be performed routinely because of attendant central nervous system complications.

As a final diagnostic test, arteriography may be performed but is not significant unless both the celiac and superior mesenteric arteries are cannulated simultaneously. A chest roentgenogram and liver-spleen scan should be performed preoperatively to search for metastatic disease. Transhepatic portal venous sampling for serum gastrin determination has facilitated tumor localization in some centers. CAT scans and echograms are not very sensitive for detecting gastrinomas.

THE ENDOCRINE PANCREAS / **587**

Medical Management of Gastrinoma

Today, with earlier diagnosis, less fulminant forms of the ulcerogenic syndrome are being seen. Thus, the need for emergency surgery has been greatly reduced. This is partially the result of the apparent effectiveness of cimetidine in controlling the gastric hypersecretion associated with gastrinoma. Recent reports indicate that the majority of patients can be managed effectively with cimetidine and antacids.

Once the diagnosis of gastrinoma is made, the patient should be started on a regimen of cimetidine and antacids. The performance of a gastric analysis after cimetidine therapy has begun may be valuable in demonstrating the degree of inhibition of acid secretion. Frequently, these patients will require in excess of 600 mg of cimetidine every six hours, which is twice the standard dose, to control acid production. Treatment with H_2 receptor antagonists only alters acid production; the serum gastrin levels remain elevated, and tumor growth is unaltered. The duration of symptom relief has yet to be established. It appears that the benefits of cimetidine therapy will vary from person to person, and such a program must be individualized and patients followed closely. Most important, this method of treatment should not replace surgical exploration; rather, it should be used as an adjunctive measure to stabilize the patient preoperatively. All patients in whom the diagnosis of gastrinoma is made should undergo laparotomy.

In contrast to the majority of patients with mild symptoms, some have a fulminant ulcer diathesis. Cimetidine and antacids should also be administered to this group. The intravenous administration of 300 to 600 mg of cimetidine at six-hour intervals reduces the volume of gastric juice as well as the acid content, permitting more effective correction of fluid and electrolyte imbalance. Because of the potentially excessive loss of fluids and electrolytes from gastric aspiration or diarrhea, the patient's weight, urine output, electrolytes, and trace elements must be monitored carefully. Continuous nasogastric suction is employed in those with fulminant symptoms in order to protect the acid-sensitive distal gastrointestinal tract, thereby reducing diarrhea. In addition, this provides a method to monitor gastric pH and gastrointestinal losses. The gastric aspirate should be replaced with an equal volume of 0.9 normal saline with 20 mEq KCl per liter. In the patient with nutritional depletion, total parenteral nutrition is indicated to establish a positive nitrogen balance preoperatively.

Operative Treatment of Gastrinoma

Exploratory laparotomy should be performed in all patients. The choice of operation depends on the findings at exploration (Table 31–2).

Table 31–2. GUIDELINES FOR THE SURGICAL MANAGEMENT OF GASTRINOMA

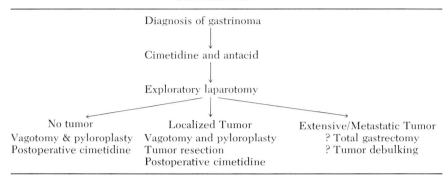

Diagnosis of gastrinoma

Cimetidine and antacid

Exploratory laparotomy

No tumor	Localized Tumor	Extensive/Metastatic Tumor
Vagotomy & pyloroplasty	Vagotomy and pyloroplasty	? Total gastrectomy
Postoperative cimetidine	Tumor resection	? Tumor debulking
	Postoperative cimetidine	

Treatment is directed to the control of the acid production and the control of the tumor, which is frequently malignant but slow-growing. In patients with associated hyperparathyroidism (MEA I), parathyroidectomy should be performed prior to abdominal exploration and surgical control of the gastrinoma. In the past, total gastrectomy was considered to be the method of choice to control the fulminant acid production and is still the preferred method of some surgeons. However, with increasing experience and particularly earlier diagnosis, it is evident that prolonged and comfortable survival is possible with lesser gastric operations. If a lesser gastric operation is performed, it must be made clear that the patient will have to take cimetidine for the rest of his life. In the Z-E tumor registry, Wilson has shown 63 per cent five-year survival following total gastrectomy, compared to 31 per cent for lesser gastric operations. Cimetidine was not employed in these patients. Since the introduction of cimetidine, Zollinger has reported the treatment of seven patients with lesser gastric operations and postoperative H_2 receptor blockade with survival exceeding five years in each case.

Total gastrectomy is certainly indicated for patients who do not wish to take cimetidine for the rest of their lives, for cimetidine failures, and perhaps in those with extensive tumor growth when resection is not possible. When no tumor is found, the minimal operation should be a vagotomy and pyloroplasty. If a tumor is identified, resection should be attempted, as tumor removal seems to improve long-term survival in some recent series.

The question arises whether total gastrectomy is followed by significant tumor regression. At present, there are four cases of gross tumor regression following removal of the stomach. This is not a common occurrence and hence should not be used as a reason to continue to favor total gastrectomy over lesser operations combined with postoperative cimetidine.

The recommendation for resection of gastrinoma is at odds with the information available from the Z-E tumor registry. From past experience, it is clear that the recognition that about two thirds of gastrinomas are multicentric and at least 50 per cent are malignant seems to indicate the futility of attempted resection. Also, there are few accounts of serum gastrin levels returning to normal following an apparently complete excision of the tumor. It appears that no matter how complete the resection, residual microscopic but functional gastrinoma remains. However, Zollinger, in reviewing his 25-year experience, indicates longer survival in patients in whom all gross tumor could be excised. Included were several patients with liver metastases and lymph node metastases. The question of tumor resection is really not resolved. More experience is needed to determine the risk:benefit ratio of tumor extirpation in the management of gastrinoma. However, the improved survival indicated in Zollinger's review certainly justifies a trial.

Postoperative Care

Nasogastric suction is used until intestinal function returns. Measures to secure fluid and electrolyte balance are continued, as is total parenteral nutrition if it was employed preoperatively. As in every postoperative patient, early ambulation and good pulmonary toilet are mandatory. The patient's diet is gradually advanced so that by discharge he or she will be taking six small feedings a day. The patient is encouraged to increase dietary intake to 2000 to 3000 calories per day. Abstinence from cigarettes and coffee is mandatory. Tolerance of dairy products following total gastrectomy is variable, and the patient should be instructed to add them to the diet cautiously.

Following total gastrectomy, monthly vitamin B_{12} injections must be continued throughout the patient's life. At first, patients should be seen at four-week intervals and then at eight-week intervals for the first year to evaluate their weight trends and dietary status.

Serum gastrin levels should be obtained every six months. Provocative tests should be performed yearly or when there is an elevation of the fasting serum gastrin level. In general, patients with progressive disease show modest elevations of serum gastrin with a tendency to double or triple this level following the administration of calcium gluceptate or magnesium. Liver function tests, including alkaline phosphatase and alkaline phosphatase fractionation, should be performed yearly at least.

Radiographic studies are important in the extended postoperative period. Barium studies are repeated every six months for two years and then yearly to carefully evaluate the adequacy of the esophagojejunal stoma. The finding of stenosis mandates dilatation, and if stenosis is severe, transabdominal or transthoracic enlargement of the anastomosis may be necessary. Digestive complaints warrant upper gastrointestinal contrast studies and an oral cholecystogram, as some patients develop cholelithiasis years after total gastrectomy. Any patient who has had hyperparathyroidism or elevated serum calcium should have periodic intravenous pyelograms to detect asymptomatic kidney stones, as well as a bone survey.

If the fasting or stimulated gastrin levels are quite high, indicating progressive disease, a liver-spleen scan followed by hepatic arteriography is indicated. Unexpectedly, the angiogram may show multiple metastases throughout the liver despite only slightly elevated or normal liver function tests and only modest increments of serum gastrin. Patients may tolerate hepatic metastases well and continue to live a normal life. However, the findings of hepatic disease and progressively rising gastrin levels indicate the need for chemotherapy.

Utilizing a combination of tubercidin, 5-fluorouracil, and streptozotocin, the survival of patients with hepatic metastases is 45 per cent at five years. This drug regimen consists of 1.5 mg per kg of tubercidin added to 500 ml of the patient's blood and administered intravenously over four hours. On that same day, 12.5 mg per kg are given intravenously, and this dose is repeated on the second and third days. After one week, streptozotocin 12.5 mg per kg is given every two to three weeks. On the alternate week, a similar dose of 5-fluorouracil is administered. The patient rests for 28 days, and the cycle is repeated every 70 days, starting with tubercidin. Careful attention must be paid to the patient's leukocyte and platelet counts, as well as blood sugar, since hyperglycemia may occur secondary to streptozocin therapy. Response to chemotherapy is followed by repeated fasting gastrin determinations and provocative tests, in addition to yearly arteriography, which is more sensitive than liver-spleen scans in detecting hepatic involvement. A new chemotherapeutic agent, chlorozotocin, seems to be effective in the management of malignant gastrinoma.

DIARRHEOGENIC TUMOR

The syndrome of watery diarrhea, hypokalemia, and achlorhydria was first described by Verner and Morrison. This symptom complex is caused by a paraendocrine apudoma of the pancreas that elaborates one or more polypeptides or other active agents, which affect the entire gastrointestinal tract. The hormone or hormones responsible for this syndrome are unknown, but elevated levels of secretin and vasoactive peptide have been demonstrated in these patients. Jaffe et al. (1977) have observed an associated increase in prostaglandin E.

The classic syndrome is characterized by episodic and recurrent watery diarrhea, sometimes more than six liters per day in volume, hypokalemia, and, in 50 per cent of patients, achlorhydria. In addition, two-thirds of the patients with a diarrheogenic tumor have hypercalcemia, and one-half display hyperglycemia. The diagnosis should be suspected in patients with chronic diarrhea after exclusion of infectious causes, inflammation, and primary bowel tumors, particularly villous adenoma. The key to the tentative diagnosis of the diarrheogenic islet cell tumor is the dangerously low potassium level.

Investigation of recurrent diarrhea begins with radiologic examination of the gastrointestinal tract. Radiographic clues signaling possible tumor are a dilated gallbladder and the presence of dilute barium on a small bowel follow-through. Gastric analysis and radioimmunoassay determinations for excessive polypeptide production, i.e., gastrin, VIP, secretin, GIP, and pancreatic polypeptide, and serum measurements of prostaglandins should be performed. Ultrasonic and arteriographic studies of the pancreas frequently demonstrate the tumor and indicate the necessity for operation.

Operation is delayed until the fluid and electrolyte losses are corrected and renal function returns to normal. Accurate intake and output measurements and daily recording of weight are essential to insure adequate fluid replacement. As much as five to six liters of intravenous fluids and 300 to 400 mEq or more of potassium may be required daily to establish fluid and electrolyte balance. In some patients, the fulminating diarrhea has been partially or temporarily controlled by the administration of steroids or the prostaglandin inhibitor indomethacin.

Operative treatment is removal of the tumor. Superficial lesions are enucleated, while deep-seated lesions require resection of involved pancreas and spleen. Large lymph nodes are excised for frozen section examination for metastatic disease. Hepatic metastases should be enucleated. Since these tumors respond to chemotherapy, heroic measures should be avoided. Careful exploration of the adrenal gland for pheochromocytoma is mandatory, as these tumors may be part of a multiple endocrine syndrome.

Removal of the diarrheogenic islet cell tumor is followed by prompt resolution of the diarrhea and associated metabolic abnormalities. Immediate postoperative care is similar to that for patients with other endocrine tumors of the pancreas. Recurrent diarrhea during long-term postoperative observation requires reinvestigation with liver scan and arteriographic studies. If recurrent disease or hepatic metastases are found, reexploration and excision of the tumors are indicated. These patients have a good response to drug therapy using tubercidin, streptozotocin, and 5-fluorouracil as for a Z-E tumor patient. Symptomatic relief may be achieved with prolonged use of indomethacin.

REFERENCES

Banting, F. G., Best, C. H., Collip, J. B., Campbell, W. R., and Fletcher, A. A.: Pancreatic extracts in the treatment of diabetes mellitus. Can. Med. Assoc. J., 12:141, 1922.

Beaser, S. B.: Surgical management. In Ellenberg, M., and Rilkin, H. (eds.): Diabetes Mellitus Theory and Practice. New York, McGraw-Hill Book Co., 1970, pp. 746–759.

Fox, P. S., Hofmann, J. W., DeCosse, J. J., and Wilson, S. O.: The influence of total gastrectomy on survival in malignant Zollinger-Ellison tumors. Ann. Surg., 180(4):558, 1974.

Galloway, J. A., and Shuman, C. R.: Diabetes and surgery. A study of 667 cases. Am. J. Med., 34:177, 1963.

Gregory, R. A., Tracy, H. J., French, J. M., and Sircus, W.: Extraction of a gastrin-like substance from a pancreatic tumour in a case of Zollinger-Ellison syndrome. Lancet, 1: 1045, 1960.

Jaffe, B. M., Kopen, D. F., DeSchryver-Kecskemet, K., Gingerich, R. L., and Greider, M.: Indomethacin-responsive pancreatic cholera. N. Engl. J. Med., 297(15):817, 1977.

Jaffe, B. M., Kopen, D. F., and Logan, D. W.: Endogenous serotonin in the control of gastric acid secretion. Surgery, 82:156, 1977.

McGavran, W. H., Unger, R. H., Recant, L., et al.: A glucagon-secreting alpha cell carcinoma of the pancreas. N. Engl. J. Med., 274:1408, 1966.

McGuigan, J. E.: Gastric mucosal intracellular localization of gastrin by immunofluorescence. Gastroenterology, 55:315, 1968.

Pearse, A. G.: Common cytochemical ultrastructural characteristics of cells producing polypeptide hormones (the APUD series) and their relevance to thyroid and ultimobranchial C cells and calcitonin. Proc. R. Soc. Biol., 170:71, 1968.

Rossini, A. A., and Hare, J. W.: How to control the blood glucose level in the surgical diabetic patient. Arch. Surg., 111:945, 1976.

Schein, P. S., DeLellis, R. A., Kahn, C. R., Gorden, P., and Kraft, A. R.: Islet cell tumors: Current concepts and management. Ann. Intern. Med., 79:239, 1973.

Thompson, J., Reeder, D. D., Villar, H. V., et al.: Natural history and experience with the diagnosis and treatment of the Zollinger-Ellison syndrome. Surg. Gynecol. Obstet., 140:5, 1975.

Welbourn, R. B.: Current status of the apudomas. Ann. Surg., 185:12, 1977.

Wilder, R. M., Allan, F. N., Power, M. H., and Robertson, H. E.: Carcinoma of the islands of the pancreas, hyperinsulinism and hypoglycemia. J.A.M.A., 89:348, 1927.

Zollinger, R. M., and Ellison, E. H.: Primary peptic ulcerations of the jejunum associated with islet cell tumors of the pancreas. Ann. Surg., 142:709, 1955.

Zollinger, R. M., Martin, E. W., Jr., Carey, L. C., Sparks, J., and Minton, J. P.: Observations on the postoperative tumor growth behavior of certain islet cell tumors. Ann. Surg., 184:525, 1976.

32

Adrenal Gland Disorders

TIMOTHY S. HARRISON

Among the most demanding problems currently faced in preoperative and postoperative surgical care are those associated with disorders of the adrenal gland. These taxing clinical problems are of two major categories. The first is exemplified by the dramatic effects of chronically excessive circulating catecholamines on the circulation of pheochromocytoma patients. The resulting circulatory instability varies from malignant hypertension and hypertensive crises to profound, potentially irreversible hypotension. Cardiac arrhythmias may be prominent in either circumstance. The clinical picture of catecholamine excess seen preoperatively stands in marked contrast to the early postoperative state in pheochromocytoma, in which circulatory systems chronically adapted to excessive catecholamines are suddenly deprived of this overstimulation. Unique pathophysiologic adjustments are necessary preoperatively and postoperatively, and when such adjustments fail to occur or are inadequate, specific circulatory problems arise that require vigorous, properly directed therapy.

The second category of preoperative and postoperative problems seen with adrenal diseases consists of a variety of metabolic defects inflicted by chronic adrenocortical and medullary hormone excess. Specifically, the striated muscular atrophy and truncal obesity seen in Cushing's syndrome, the profound and sustained potassium loss and sodium retention of hyperaldosteronism, and the relentless lipolysis of pheochromocytoma with its associated cachexia are all dramatic examples of metabolic effects of sustained unregulated hormonal overproduction by the adrenal gland.

In marked contrast to the clinical pictures of hormonal overproduction are those of acute and chronic hormonal insufficiency. For example, the salt wasting, hypotension, and volume contraction of adrenocortical insufficiency are the reciprocal to the picture of excessive adrenocortical hormone production. Similarly, the presence of inadequate circulating catecholamines postoperatively, a situation seldom seen as a clinical entity anymore, is nevertheless a striking contrast to the fever, ileus, and leukocytosis associated with catecholamine excess along with the violent hypertension and striking cardiac arrhythmias of pheochromocytoma.

In order to organize our thinking about these problems, we will consider each specific adrenal disorder individually by reviewing the physiologic control of its hormonal secretion, then describing how this physiologic control is distorted by the disease in question. Finally, we will try to apply these insights to the specific problems of preoperative and postoperative care seen in each of the common disorders of the adrenal gland.

THE ADRENAL MEDULLA — PHEOCHROMOCYTOMA

PHYSIOLOGIC CONTROL OF CATECHOLAMINE SECRETION

In normal, uncomplicated living, the adrenal medulla sequentially converts dietary tyrosine or phenylalanine, both essential amino acids, into norepinephrine and epinephrine. Six reactions are required to complete this entire biosynthesis from phenylalanine to epinephrine. The final two steps take place within the cytoplasmic storage granules of the adrenal medulla. Adrenergic nerves elsewhere in the body (peripheral adrenergic nerves) complete this biosynthesis only as far as norepinephrine. The enzyme phenyl-ethanol-amine-N-methyl-transferase (PNMT), responsible for the conversion of norepinephrine to epinephrine, is known to be induced by large quantities of cortisol, and for this reason it is the adrenal medulla that is uniquely situated to methylate large quantities of norepinephrine, thereby forming epinephrine. The brain also has the capacity to synthesize catecholamines, including small amounts of epinephrine, which comprises about 6 per cent of the central nervous system catecholamines. The central nervous system catecholamines are ubiquitously distributed through the entire central nervous system, with particularly high concentrations found in the hypothalamic nuclei. The induction requirement, vis-à-vis steroids or some other mechanism, of this central nervous system PNMT is not known.

At physiologic concentrations of circulating catecholamines, a blood-brain barrier to catecholamines is present, and therefore at these low physiologic concentrations one would not expect catecholamines synthesized in the adrenal medulla and adrenergic nerves to be actively transported into the central nervous system. At high perfusion concentrations of catecholamines, it is known that the blood-brain barrier to circulating catecholamines can be overcome and that in the cat, for example, hypothalamic norepinephrine levels can be raised by 30-minute infusions of norepinephrine 10 μg per minute.

Whether or not the central nervous system can release its catecholamines into the systemic circulation is not known. Possibly this does not happen physiologically, but it is conceivable that in pathologically altered central nervous system conditions, such as cerebral hypoxia or cerebral edema, such release might occur. In fact, there are no data yet that can be used to settle this fundamental point, either for physiologic conditions or in various disease states of the central nervous system.

In physiologic conditions, both tissue and circulating levels of catecholamines are carefully regulated by remarkably sensitive homeostatic mechanisms. The threshold for tissue uptake of catecholamines from the circulation and the activity of the catecholamine's metabolic enzyme catechol-3-O-methyltransferase (COMT) will keep the plasma levels of catecholamines constant through remarkably wide variations in catecholamine release and excretion. Thus, after total adrenalectomy, free epinephrine excretion will fall about 90 per cent, but in spite of this fall, there is frequently no fall in circulating epinephrine levels.

Tissue content of norepinephrine and epinephrine has been thought for years to be regulated, at least in part, by monoamineoxidase, which is the main enzymatic means of terminating catecholamines besides COMT. An equally important means of regulating tissue catecholamine levels is the inhibition of tyrosine hydroxylase, which ordinarily is the rate-limiting reaction in catecholamine biosynthesis, by excessive tissue concentrations of norepinephrine and epinephrine. This end product inhibition of catecholamine synthesis is a delicately controlled feedback mechanism that can maintain stable tissue levels of catecholamine through a wide range of tissue catecholamine production.

ALTERED PHYSIOLOGY OF CATECHOLAMINES IN PHEOCHROMOCYTOMA

In pheochromocytoma, there is relentless unregulated biosynthesis and release of catecholamines by the chromaffin cells of the tumor. All of the enzymes requisite for catecholamine synthesis are present in pheochromocytomas. The only inconsistently appearing enzyme is PNMT. The 30 per cent of pheochromocytomas that produce appreciable quantities of epinephrine are in or near the adrenal gland and are presumed to have adequate quantities of cortisol available to the tumor for the induction of PNMT. When analyzed for catecholamines, pheochromocytomas contain large quantities of norepinephrine and/or epinephrine. There is, therefore, no effective end product inhibition of catecholamine synthesis by the catecholamine in these tumors, and for this reason we think of the entire biosynthetic production of catecholamines as being unregulated in pheochromocytoma. Large, excessive quantities of norepinephrine and/or epinephrine are synthesized in the tumor, released into the circulation, and actively taken up by other adrenergic nerves and by the uninvolved adrenal gland. The quantity of catecholamine being taken up and stored in adrenergically innervated tissues may exceed the capacity of such tissues to regulate their catecholamine synthesis and metabolism, and the result is that these adrenergically innervated tissues are oversaturated with catecholamines when a pheochromocytoma is present. These increased quantities of adrenergically stored catecholamines in pheochromocytoma can be released by conventional reflex stimulation. When such reflex stimuli are applied to most pheochromocytoma patients, not only are catecholamines released, but they also are released in supernormal quantities. These exaggerated reflex responses revert to normal after the pheochromocytoma has been removed.

Many lines of evidence can be cited now in support of the preceding descriptions of the dynamic features of exaggerated catecholamine release, uptake, and secondary release seen in pheochromocytoma. Increased tumor levels of catecholamines and greatly increased concentrations of circulating catecholamines have been documented in pheochromocytoma by many observers. We have measured catecholamine content in the liver in five pheochromocytoma patients and have found the levels significantly elevated in four of these patients when they have been statistically compared with the catecholamine content of liver biopsies taken from five patients undergoing elective cholecystectomy.

When pheochromocytoma patients are submitted to a standard tilt test, the associated norepinephrine release into the urine is greatly exaggerated when compared with the tilt response of normal subjects or the response of hypertensive patients who prove not to have pheochromocytomas. This exaggerated response had reverted to normal when the patients were studied a week postoperatively.

A final piece of evidence supporting the concept of uptake and secondary release from oversaturated tissue stores of catecholamines in pheochromocytoma comes from the demonstration of moderately increased urinary epinephrine excretion in patients whose pheochromocytomas contain only norepinephrine. After removal of such norepinephrine-containing tumors, the excretion of epinephrine has fallen to normal. In these patients it appears certain that norepinephrine is released from the tumor into the circulation and is taken up by adrenergically innervated tissues, including the opposite adrenal gland. In the opposite adrenal gland, this norepinephrine is methylated to epinephrine, and increased quantities of epinephrine are secondarily released into the circulation and excreted in the urine. The fact that epinephrine excretion returns to normal after the removal of a tumor that does not contain epinephrine but only norepinephrine and its precursors supports this concept of methylation of increased quantities of norepinephrine to form epinephrine by the adrenal gland uninvolved with tumor.

PREOPERATIVE MANAGEMENT OF PHEOCHROMOCYTOMA

It is no exaggeration to say that the most crucial management of pheochromocytoma patients is in the preoperative period. It is at this time that contracted blood volumes when present can be corrected most easily; it is also at this time that cardiac arrhythmias can be brought under control. If one waits to accomplish these objectives during the operation, it will often be impossible to reverse serious trends in the pheochromocytoma patient's course.

Elective Pheochromocytoma Excision

Selective Preoperative Adrenergic Receptor Blockade. Modern adrenergic blocking agents have enhanced greatly the safety of elective pheochromocytoma excision. Whereas marked cardiovascular instability with wide swings in blood pressure and frequent cardiac arrhythmias were often seen during pheochromocytoma operations, these unsettling problems are now rare.

Many physicians who have experience with pheochromocytoma believe that all patients with this tumor should receive alpha-adrenergic receptor blockade preoperatively, generally with phenoxybenzamine. This categorical approach ignores two important points relating to alpha-adrenergic receptor blockade in pheochromocytoma. One is that deaths have occurred from irreversible hypotension in pheochromocytoma when overenthusiastic alpha blockade has been used preoperatively. The second ignored point is that prior to the availability of alpha-adrenergic receptor blocking drugs, many patients tolerated surgical excision of their pheochromocytoma with no difficulty. For these reasons, we believe alpha- and beta-adrenergic receptor blockade should be used in carefully selected patients with pheochromocytoma who demonstrate a clear need for protection against the effects of increased levels of circulating catecholamines. The criteria used for alpha and beta receptor blockades are relatively simple and are shown in Tables 32–1 and 32–2. Using this aproach, 60 to 70 per cent of our pheochromocytoma patients are blocked preoperatively. In no instance have we experienced problems with patients that make us wish in retrospect that we had used alpha-adrenergic blockade routinely as a preoperative measure.

Preoperative Management of Pheochromocytoma. Once the diagnosis of pheochromocytoma has been confirmed biochemically by mea-

Table 32–1. INDICATIONS FOR PREOPERATIVE ALPHA-ADRENERGIC RECEPTOR BLOCKADE IN PHEOCHROMOCYTOMA

Blood pressure > 200/130
Frequent severe uncontrolled hypertensive attacks
Pronounced decrease in plasma volume, i.e., hematocrit > 50 vol per cent
Use of beta-adrenergic receptor blockade

Table 32–2. INDICATIONS FOR PREOPERATIVE BETA-ADRENERGIC RECEPTOR BLOCKADE IN PHEOCHROMOCYTOMA

Pulse rate > 130 per minute
Any history of cardiac arrhythmia
Demonstration of persistent ventricular extrasystoles
Tumors secreting predominantly (> 75 per cent) epinephrine

suring excretion of catecholamines and/or their metabolites and after the circulatory status of the pheochromocytoma patient is under suitable control, with adrenergic receptor blockade if necessary, the surgeon is well advised to have as accurate an idea as possible of the number and location of pheochromocytomas present in the patient. The suggestion has been made, generally by internists who do not operate themselves, that with the diagnosis of pheochromocytoma securely established, abdominal exploration can be carried out after appropriate circulatory control has been achieved by adrenergic receptor blockade if necessary. Most surgeons are uncomfortable with this approach. It is more appealing to remove recognized lesions and then explore the remainder of the abdomen. One can then look for unlocalized tumors without the threat of dangerous catecholamine secretion from the recognized tumor that has been removed.

The common localizing techniques in use today are plain abdominal roentgenogram, excretory nephrotomography, retrograde adrenal venography, regional venous sampling, selective and subselective arteriography, iodocholesterol adrenal photoemission scanning, and pheochromocytoma scanning with meta-iodobenzyl guanidine.

Venography and arteriography may have associated hypertensive crises when they are used. For this reason, pheochromocytoma patients should be well blocked prior to angiographic studies, and if blockade is thought not to be necessary, one should be certain that a large-diameter venous line and blood pressure monitoring are available as well as phentolamine and other adrenergic blocking and stimulating agents.

Caval catheterization is particularly helpful in patients with tiny recurrences of pheochromocytoma. Unsuspected multiple tumors can often be appreciated by caval catheterization when the other localization methods mentioned have failed to demonstrate the lesions.

Acute Pheochromocytoma

Infrequently, pheochromocytoma patients are encountered in a violent adrenergic crisis. Their hypertension is out of control, but there is a great deal more out of control than just their blood pressure. Cardiac arrhythmias are prominent, and frequent runs of ventricular tachycardia may be seen. The patient's circulatory status can be extremely precarious. If the patient is deprived of fluid, for example, amounts less than

1000 ml per day, the urine output dwindles, and there is a moderate but definite increase in serum creatinine and blood urea nitrogen. In addition, the blood pressure tends to fall. If such patients are volume-replaced, their threshold for the development of acute pulmonary edema is very low, and often it is impossible to deliver more than 1000 to 1500 ml of fluid daily without development of clear-cut pulmonary edema. Superimposed on these profound circulatory problems one may encounter high fevers, leukocytosis, and intestinal ileus. The picture simulates sepsis, and on occasion, it is difficult to make a clear distinction when the patient has recently been explored or has some other potential source of sepsis. In this situation, it is important to realize that catecholamine excess can produce all of these signs and that one does not need to implicate uncontrolled sepsis as the explanation for this dramatic clinical picture in pheochromocytoma.

The therapeutic approach to these desperately ill pheochromocytoma patients demands considerable judgment and must be highly individualized to the situation presented by each patient. The ideal solution is to control the circulation with intravenous and, later on, intramuscular alpha- and beta-adrenergic receptor blockade. However, this is not always possible, and one may find that conventional doses of intravenous phentolamine and propranolol seem to have little or no effect, and one is still confronted with an unstable patient whose situation has been compounded by ineffective attempts at adrenergic receptor blockade.

The term "acute pheochromocytoma" has been given to this set of conditions. There is a place for emergency operation with removal of the pheochromocytoma when the other measures mentioned have failed. Unlike the situation of elective pheochromocytoma excision in which the mortality rate is practically zero, the outlook for the patient with acute pheochromocytoma is decidedly more serious. Whichever of the two approaches is used, the mortality in acute pheochromocytoma is currently significant.

POSTOPERATIVE MANAGEMENT OF PHEOCHROMOCYTOMA

Prior to the advent of selective adrenergic receptor blockade, the postoperative management of pheochromocytoma posed problems that were often demanding. Cardiovascular collapse occurring just after tumor excision often required massive volume replacement with whole blood and other colloid-rich solutions. Coupled with this approach of aggressive volume replacement was a need for infusion of sympathomimetic drugs, generally norepinephrine or one of its synthetic analogs. With this program, arterial pressure could generally be supported with no great difficulty, and it was usually possible to wean these patients from their pressor support in 48 to 72 hours.

Now that preoperative blockade is used, the postoperative period following pheochromocytoma excision has become far more manageable. Necessary plasma volume expansion occurs preoperatively, and excision of the tumor is not followed by striking hypotension. Almost never is it necessary to support the circulation artificially with adrenergic stimulants. This is not to say that there are no longer any problems seen in the postoperative pheochromocytoma patient. Rather, the problems are of a different sort and are seen with less frequency and intensity.

Postoperative Cardiac Management

If a pheochromocytoma patient has had unstable cardiac rhythms preoperatively, one will generally notice great improvement in the arrhythmias after the tumor has been removed. As a rule, we do not continue propranolol after operation because the source of the cardiac arrhythmias has been removed. Using the same reasoning, if digitalis has been used preoperatively in supporting the circulation of the pheochromocytoma patient, it is probably wise and certainly easy to wean the patient from the digitalis in the first one or two postoperative weeks. Obviously, if the patient has been on long-term digitalis treatment prior to pheochromocytoma excision, this should be considered and digitalis continued as long as there is a clear-cut indication for it on conventional grounds.

Epinephrine Shock

A rare but recognizable postoperative problem in pheochromocytoma is epinephrine shock. This occurs 24 to 72 hours following the excision of tumors containing and releasing massive amounts of catecholamine, predominantly epinephrine. We are aware of only three reported cases of epinephrine shock in pheochromocytoma. The complication is fatal unless treated properly.

Clinically the picture of epinephrine shock is one of relentless progressive hypotension appearing about 36 hours postoperatively. Usually, obvious measures are tried first, which include infusion of sympathomimetic agents. Frequently, rapid digitalization is attempted with short-acting intravenously administered digitalis analogues. None of these measures will meet with any success. Epinephrine shock is treated successfully by large doses of intravenous hydrocortisone. Intravenous hydrocortisone 200 to 300 mg is given in five minutes, and this dose should be repeated two or three times until improvement is seen. After an initial bolus injection, the same amount of steroid can be infused over a two-hour period. The mechanism of this life-saving steroid effect in epinephrine shock is not known. Patients with epinephrine shock are not, so far as is known, suffering from incipient adrenal insufficiency that has been unmasked by the stress of operation. Epinephrine shock has been produced experimentally in dogs, and dramatic protection from death can be achieved by large doses of intravenous steroids in this species.

Postoperative Metabolic Considerations in Pheochromocytoma

Preoccupation with the life-threatening cardiovascular complications of pheochromocytoma has left the metabolic aspects of this disease relatively underemphasized.

The increased levels of circulating catecholamines in pheochromocytoma chronically overstimulate adrenergic receptors, including β receptors, on the hepatic and fat cells of the body. The resulting glycogenolysis and lipolysis can sometimes be great. Elevated levels of blood glucose and of serum triglycerides and fatty acids have been demonstrated in pheochromocytoma patients, reflecting the active dissolution of body fat stores in these patients. In extreme instances, considerable weight loss will occur.

PROLONGED FOLLOW-UP OF PHEOCHROMOCYTOMA PATIENTS AND RECURRENT PHEOCHROMOCYTOMA

Roughly 10 per cent of the pheochromocytoma patients undergoing elective removal of their tumors develop symptomatic recurrences of the pheochromocytoma. Obviously this mandates prolonged follow-up with determination of blood pressures and overnight resting excretion rates of norepinephrine and epinephrine at annual or biennial visits. Computed axial tomography may become a useful noninvasive method for follow-up to detect recurrences.

One aspect of recurrent pheochromocytoma meriting repeated emphasis is that recurrent pheochromocytoma can be an indolent, slow-growing tumor. Years may elapse before the recurrence becomes apparent clinically. In the most extreme case coming under our care, 17 years passed before the patient noted the symptoms of recurrence following his first operation, and an additional four years passed before the patient was troubled enough to have something done about his recurrent disease. Obviously, years of useful living can be achieved with intelligent palliation.

THE ADRENAL CORTEX

PHYSIOLOGIC REGULATION OF ADRENOCORTICAL FUNCTION

Cortisol (Glucocorticoid) Secretion

The level of cortisol in the circulating blood can regulate the release of adrenocorticotropic hormone (ACTH) into the circulation from the anterior lobe of the pituitary gland. The quantity of ACTH reaching the adrenal cortex will, in turn, regulate the release of cortisol by the reticularis of the adrenal cortex.

It is equally well established that the central nervous system contains a corticotropin-releasing factor (CRF) that, when transported to the pituitary gland by the hypophyseal portal veins, will stimulate the release of pituitary ACTH and therefore of cortisol as well. This stimulation of ACTH release by CRF can supervene and override the feedback regulation of ACTH release by circulating cortisol levels mentioned earlier. The degree to which these two controlling systems operate mutually to regulate the physiologic secretion of cortisol is not yet known. It is clear that in abnormal circumstances, notably Cushing's disease, unregulated increases of cortisol release will occur as a result of the persistent and autonomous stimulation of the pituitary by CRF. Of the seven hypothalamic releasing factors recognized today, only the structure of CRF has eluded identification.

Another physiologic regulating influence on cortisol release is an inherent diurnal variation in ACTH release, which accounts for the "sleep-wake" variation in cortisol secretion. Interestingly, this phasic variation of ACTH release is preserved in patients with adrenocortical insufficiency.

Stressful situations of any type, operation included, will cause the central nervous system to stimulate the release of ACTH.

Physiologic Regulation of Aldosterone (Mineralocorticoid) Secretion

The release of aldosterone, an adrenal corticosteroid with strong salt-retaining and potassium-excreting properties mediated by the renal tubule, is stimulated by the quantity of angiotensin II reaching the glomerulosa cells of the adrenal cortex, which make aldosterone. As is widely recognized, the amount of circulating antiotensin II is controlled by a number of factors, the dominant one of which is the production and release of the peptide renin from the juxtaglomerular cells of the kidney tubules. Renin release in turn is influenced by catecholamines acting through a beta-adrenergic receptor mechanism and also by prostaglandin-E2 (PGE_2). The beta-adrenergic stimulation is also mediated by PGE_2 after the beta receptor itself has been activated. Renin enzymatically controls the cleavage of renin substrate, a circulating globulin, to angiotensin I, which is a circulating decapeptide. Angiotensin I is converted to angiotensin II, an octapeptide, by a converting enzyme found in large concentrations in the pulmonary circulation. Aldosterone suppresses the secretion of renin, thus completing the cycle of what has been called a "long loop" feedback control regulating aldosterone release.

There is a component of aldosterone secretion, an estimated 30 per cent, that is controlled by ACTH. There is also a diurnal rhythm of plasma renin activity that can be demonstrated when other factors known to stimulate renin release, i.e., sodium restriction and postural changes, are kept constant.

Anything causing plasma volume contraction, for example, hemorrhage, central blood volume shifts (as in the tilt test), and chronically restricted sodium intake, will stimulate the release of renin and by doing so promote the formation of angiotensin II.

PREOPERATIVE CONSIDERATIONS

Overproduction of Adrenocortical Hormones

Cushing's Disease and Cushing's Syndrome. The chronic overproduction of glucocorticoid hormones results in the often dramatic clinical picture of Cushing's disease, which is associated with CRF overactivity. The overproduction of glucocorticoids (cortisol is the prototype) is also seen in Cushing's syndrome, which is the term used to refer to excessive cortisol secretion from functioning adrenal neoplasms, adenomas, or carcinomas, which produce and autonomously release cortisol independently of any control by CRF and ACTH. Malignant tumors of other organs, conspicuously the lung and kidney, can synthesize and release ACTH, and the profile of Cushing's syndrome is also seen with this ectopic ACTH release. Presumably, the production and release of CRF is suppressed in the ectopic ACTH syndrome, but it has not yet been possible to substantiate this.

In its full presentation, patients with chronic glucocorticoid excess have a puffy, rounded moon face, obesity of the trunk with a prominent "buffalo hump," hirsutism (particularly pronounced in females), and atrophy of the striated muscle mass, particularly apparent as spindly arms and legs. The skin tends to thin and develops a dark and purplish hue, which is particularly noticeable in fractures of the dermis. These dermal fractures develop into large, purplish striae, which are often the tipoff to the presence of the disease. Hypertension is common, and the reason for it is not clear. Osteoporosis is often manifest. Not every patient will show all of these signs, and one is sometimes led to the diagnosis of Cushing's syndrome by relatively subtle changes in one or another of the manifestations of Cushing's disease we have already mentioned.

Obviously, the metabolic abnormalities of Cushing's disease do not improve operative risk, and in fact they probably increase it. Impaired wound healing, diminished native resistance to bacterial infection, and the hazards of general anesthesia in the obese patient are all undesirable and serve to increase the risk of operation in patients with Cushing's syndrome.

In spite of this realization, little effort has been made in reversing or preventing Cushing's syndrome preoperatively in order to improve the patient's situation before operation. Although the principle of preoperative control is well established in the surgical treatment of endocrinologic disease, for example, in hyperthyroidism and pheochromocytoma, for two reasons it has not evolved in preoperative management of Cushing's disease. One reason is that more and more patients tolerate well-directed surgical control of Cushing's disease without major problems, and the second reason is that there simply has not been a convenient and consistently effective drug regimen available that is suitably nontoxic and problem-free. Various agents have been developed that limit glucocorticoid release and have been tried, only to be found inadequate, generally because of their inherent toxicity. Ortho-para-prime DDD (O-p'-DDD) has undergone clinical trials but has proved to be too toxic for sustained clinical use, and there is also an appreciable percentage of patients who escape the effects of O-p'-DDD. Cyproheptadine, an agent that interrupts serotonin synthesis, has been used effectively in patients with Cushing's disease. The mechanism of action is thought to be the interruption of hypothalamic serotoninergic pathways that promote the release of CRF and consequently of ACTH and cortisol. While theoretically extremely appealing, the use of cyproheptadine to date has been effective in only 30 per cent of the patients in whom it has been tried.

Of the variety of other agents inhibiting glucocorticoid activity, the most promising appears to be aminoglutethimide. This drug, by inhibiting the conversion of cholesterol to pregnenolone, inhibits the biosynthesis of all hormonal steroids at that early biosynthetic conversion. Aminoglutethimide is not an easy drug to take, however, since doses must be taken every six hours without fail, and patients often find it inconvenient to awaken to maintain this regimen for an extended period of time.

Dexamethasone suppression does not work for extended periods of time in Cushing's disease even though it is helpful in making the diagnosis of Cushing's disease when used with high doses.

For these reasons, preoperative care of patients with Cushing's disease is directed toward overcoming any glaring electrolyte or fluid abnormalities, correcting anemia that might be present, and ruling out occult sources of sepsis.

Preoperative Considerations in Hyperaldosteronism — Conn's Syndrome

In hyperaldosteronism, the autonomous release of aldosterone will, as mentioned before, eventually result in a low serum potassium level and a high serum sodium level. Because of the salt retention, the plasma volume tends to be high.

The majority of the lesions autonomously secreting aldosterone are solitary glomerulosa cell adenomas. The removal of these adenomas and the surrounding adrenal gland results in resolution of the metabolic defect, i.e., no potassium loss or hypernatremia, and in about 60 per cent of cases results in satisfactory resolution of the hypertension. In patients with glomerulosa cell hyperplasia, improvement of hypertension has not been the rule, and for this reason most centers now recommend against operation in hyperaldosteronism patients with adrenal hyperplasia. Making the distinction preoperatively between adrenal adenoma and adrenal hyperplasia, therefore, has become of paramount concern in managing hyperaldosteronism. To date, the most convenient way to make this distinction between adenoma and hyperplasia has been the use of iodocholesterol adrenal photoscanning. The picture seen with a hyperfunctioning adenoma is the appearance of a solitary "hot spot" on the scan, the remainder of both glands having a somewhat diminished uptake. If one repeats the iodocholesterol scan after suppression of the patient with dexamethasone, only the hot spot of the adenoma remains.

The scanning pattern of adrenal hyperplasia is distinctly different. Generalized uptake in slightly enlarged adrenal glands bilaterally is the rule, and customarily there are no solitary focal hot spots in the gland. When suppressed with dexamethasone, the entire adrenal silhouette fades from view on both sides, giving a clear functional separation of the hyperplasia patients from those with solitary hyperfunctioning aldosterone-secreting adenomas. If one happens to see two or three hyperfunctioning nodules on the adrenal scan, almost without exception these can be suppressed with dexamethasone and represent nodular fragments of adrenal hyperplasia.

Nonoperative management of hyperaldosterone patients with adrenocortical hyperplasia has been successful with spironolactone. This aldosterone antagonist effectively diminishes the metabolic consequences of excessive circulating aldosterone. Although it is possible to manage solitary adenoma patients in aldosteronism with spironolactone therapy, most centers reporting appreciable experience with hyperaldosteronism prefer to have these patients undergo operative removal of the adrenal gland containing the solitary adenoma.

In addition to iodocholesterol scanning, another means of conveniently localizing the aldosterone-secreting adenoma preoperatively is by catheterization of both adrenal veins. Aldosterone content will be conspicuously higher in the gland harboring the solitary adenoma, whereas the aldosterone content from the uninvolved gland will tend to be closer to the mixed venous level sampled at a location away from the adrenal veins.

Preoperative Adrenocortical Insufficiency

Glucocorticoids. We have already alluded briefly to the fact that stress of various kinds, including that associated with operation itself, will stimulate a burst of adrenocortical hormone release. Carrying this insight one step further, it is apparent that latent adrenal insufficiency will, on occasion, first appear postoperatively unless one has recognized adrenocortical insufficiency preoperatively. With any chronically ill patient, one should remember that latent adrenal insufficiency is a possibility. Hyponatremia, excessive urinary sodium excretion, hyperkalemia, and early subtle bronzing of the skin all may alert one of the need to be certain whether or not occult adrenal insufficiency is present.

In patients on prolonged cortisol suppression, either iatrogenically or because of a cortisol-secreting adenoma, delayed return of normal cortisol levels has been seen for periods as long as nine months. When studied in detail, these patients initially have high cortisol and low ACTH levels. Following removal of their autonomous source of excessive cortisol, circulating cortisol levels fall and ACTH remains low. After four months or so, ACTH rises at first to normal, then to levels above normal. Finally, at about eight or nine months postoperatively, serum cortisol and ACTH levels return to normal. Physiologic responses to dexamethasone suppression and metyrapone stimulation can be demonstrated at this point. While it is not desirable to interpose exogenous steroids into this recovery cycle, obviously patients should be watched carefully for any signs of incipient adrenocortical insufficiency.

Formerly, any patient with a history of adrenal steroid therapy, no matter how remote in time or how long or what doses of steroids were used, underwent a so-called complete steroid prep before operation. This greatly overtreated many patients who had never developed unresponsive pituitary ACTH-adrenocortical systems and whose adrenocortical responsiveness clearly would have been adequate to carry them through the period of surgical stress.

It is far better to test such patients preoperatively by taking, for example, an 8 A.M. and 8 P.M. blood sample for cortisol to demonstrate an intact diurnal cortisol variation and also to draw serum cortisol levels just before and 30 minutes after stimulation with either ACTH or its synthetic analogue cosyntropin (Cortrosyn). If a patient demonstrates adrenal responsiveness in these two situations, there is good reason to believe that the adrenal cortices are equal to the demands imposed by operation and those arising in the postoperative recovery phase. For these reasons, an adrenal steroid prep is necessary only when a lack of adrenal responsiveness can be demonstrated.

If impaired adrenocortical responsiveness is demonstrated preoperatively, then one is well advised to give additional steroid support equivalent to 200 mg daily of hydrocortisone and then to taper the dose gradually postoperatively after the first few postoperative days.

Preoperative Mineralocorticoid Deficiency. While hypoaldosteronism is a well recognized clinical entity, including a genetically transmitted form of the disease, there is seldom a situation in which this specific hormonal deficiency will be manifest initially as a preoperative entity. Hyponatremia and hyperkalemia can alert the physician to the possibility of occult hypoaldosteronism; this can be confirmed or excluded by measuring either the plasma content or the urinary excretion rate of aldosterone. If aldosterone deficiency is demonstrated, treatment with a salt-retaining steroid is appropriate and specific; fludrocortisone (Florinef) is a common agent used to correct this hyponatremia and is effective preoperatively.

POSTOPERATIVE CONSIDERATIONS IN ADRENOCORTICAL DISORDERS

Glucocorticoids

Glucocorticoid Excess. The early postoperative period poses few problems attributable to excessive glucocorticoids present preoperatively. Impaired wound healing and a decrease in native resistance to bacterial infection are likely to occur in the early postoperative period, if at all. In fact, the postoperative course of patients with Cushing's syndrome or Cushing's disease is generally trouble-free. If, however, the source of excessive cortisol has not been removed, as in metastatic functioning adrenal carcinoma, then impaired wound healing, wound infections, and often thromboembolic phenomena are more likely to occur.

The physiologic adrenocortical response to operation is a far different matter than the host of problems that might be seen as a consequence of sustained postoperative adrenocortical hormone excess. It is believed that the postoperative adrenocortical response is probably purposeful in meeting metabolic demands of the surgical patient in the early postoperative period. Certainly there is no question that the adrenocortical postoperative response is self-limiting and requires no specific treatment.

As weeks and months pass postoperatively, the Cushing's syndrome patient whose condition has been corrected notices marked improvement in several ways. Truncal obesity subsides, hypertension is improved, and gradually strength and muscle mass return to weakened limbs as the anabolic phase of recovery progresses.

Postoperative Adrenocortical Deficiency. The most striking adrenal insufficiency problems seen in surgical disease are manifested postoperatively. The increased demands of the postoperative period may call attention for the first time to the patient's latent adrenocortical insufficiency. It is obviously essential for the surgeon to be sensitive to these possibilities in the early postoperative period. Hypotension not responsive to volume replacement and pressor drugs, prolonged fever of unexplained origin, and/or hyponatremia only transiently corrected by saline infusion should alert the surgeon to the possibility of adrenal insufficiency.

A particularly treacherous situation can occur in patients with recognized adrenal insufficiency who are being maintained on hydrocortisone doses of 30 to 50 mg daily, which is perfectly adequate for their usual needs. If this dose is not increased on the day of operation and for the first few days postoperatively, adrenal insufficiency is likely to occur in spite of giving conventional doses of cortisone daily. Increased steroids should be given during the preoperative and postoperative period. These should be administered for one or two weeks postoperatively, after which the patient can be weaned from this increased dose.

As emphasized by Hume (1960) and others, adrenocortical insufficiency may become apparent clinically in any of four different patterns. The first of these appears soon after birth and is a consequence of the salt-losing variety of the adrenogenital syndrome. Fever, weight loss, vomiting, hyponatremia, shock, and renal salt loss characterize this dramatic situation.

Chronic adrenocortical insufficiency that may have been present for months or even years is frequently manifested by weakness, weight loss, pigmentation of the skin, hypotension, fatigability, nausea, vomiting, abdominal pain, hypoglycemia, hyponatremia, and hyperkalemia. If, in these patients with "bronze diabetes," abdominal calcifications are seen, tuberculosis should be suspected more strongly as the reason for their adrenal insufficiency. The heart size may be small in chronic adrenal insufficiency, and this may be the tipoff to the diagnosis.

Acute addisonian crisis frequently accompanies acute bacterial infection, particularly meningococcemia, anticoagulant therapy, and occasionally malignant neoplasms. Hemorrhage into previously healthy adrenal glands is almost always the mechanism involved, but occasionally, as in massive thermal burns, adrenal insufficiency may occur without frank hemorrhage. In this latter situation, some other mechanism must exist by which infection suppresses adrenocortical function. Fever, shock, lethargy, nausea, vomiting, coma, and abdominal pain all occur in rapid order. Hypoglycemia, hyponatremia, and hyperkalemia can contribute evidence for the diagnosis, which may be confirmed by demonstrating a low serum cortisol level or, better yet, by demonstrating a strong therapeutic effect of intravenous hydrocortisone while waiting for the serum cortisol level measurement to return from the laboratory.

Semiacute adrenal insufficiency is the fourth clinical pattern that may occur. These patients are well preoperatively, but in the early postoperative period, hemorrhage may take place into the adrenal glands. Anticoagulants or severe infection may be involved. Patients with massive thermal burns may have this type of adrenal insufficiency. The symptoms develop more slowly than those of acute adrenal insufficiency and progress over a period of days rather than hours. Weakness, intestinal ileus, anorexia, nausea, and profound lassitude may characteristically progress to a peak at the end of the first postoperative week.

Massive renal salt wasting with hyponatremia is seen. The response to desoxycorticosterone is both diagnostic and therapeutic.

Postoperative Mineralocorticoid Problems

Mineralocorticoid Excess. Following the removal of a source of autonomous aldosterone secretion such as a solitary aldosterone-secreting adenoma, the postoperative patient exhibits few, if any, problems attributable to the preoperative presence of aldosterone excess. Serum sodium falls, serum potassium usually stays normal without a need for excessive potassium intake, and there is absence of noticeable weight gain due to retention of body water. As stated earlier, resolution of blood pressure is not seen in all patients. About 50 per cent of aldosteronism patients will be persistently hypertensive. However, even these patients are greatly improved by operation, since their metabolic defect of sodium retention and potassium wasting is corrected and their high blood pressure, although still present, is easier to treat effectively with antihypertensive drugs that previously were minimally effective.

Insufficiency of Mineralocorticoids Postoperatively. Specific mineralocorticoid deficiency is rare as an isolated problem in the postoperative period. One reason for this is that cortisol itself has mild salt-retaining properties, and, consequently, mild degrees of mineralocorticoid deficiency will be helped or corrected when cortisol is given.

However, there is a group of patients whose salt-retaining needs are not met by simple replacement or maintenance doses of cortisol. The pattern is often seen after total adrenalectomy when a maintenance steroid dose in the neighborhood of 30 mg hydrocortisone daily is given. Gradually but inexorably, these patients may become hyponatremic and volume-depleted. They frequently have been discharged from the hospital by this time, and when seen in follow-up two or three weeks postoperatively, weakness, hyponatremia, and low blood pressure may be apparent. Their blood glucose will be normal. Rather than treating these patients with higher doses of cortisol, which would put their salt metabolism in order, it is better to give them small doses of Florinef each day in addition to their maintenance doses of cortisol. This regimen restores their sodium and potassium balance to normal and also prevents drug-induced Cushing's syndrome, which would eventually result from excessively high maintenance doses of cortisol.

CONCLUSION

As with most endocrinologic disorders today, diseases of the adrenal cortex and the medulla can now be identified and studied with precision and efficiency.

During preoperative and postoperative care, specific and often life-saving therapy is available for the common problems relating to the adrenal gland. What modern insights cannot provide, however, is the index of suspicion on the part of the surgeon that will lead to specific diagnosis and effective therapy.

REFERENCES

Bigus, S. T., et al.: Cure of Cushing's disease by transsphenoidal removal of a microade-noma from a pituitary gland despite a radiographically normal sella turcica. J. Clin. Endocrinol. Metab., *45*:1251, 1977.

Conn, J. W., et al.: Primary aldosteronism. J. Clin. Endocrinol. Metab., *33*:713, 1971.

Egdahl, R. H., and Chobanian, A. V.: Acute pheochromocytoma. Surg. Clin. North Am., *46*:645, 1966.

Harrison, T. S., et al.: Current evaluation and management of pheochromocytoma. Ann. Surg., *168*:701, 1968.

Hume, D. M.: Pheochromocytoma in the adult and child. Am. J. Surg., *99*:458, 1960.

Krieger, D. T.: Cyproheptadine induced remission of Cushing's disease. N. Engl. J. Med., *293*:893, 1975.

Melby, J. C., et al.: Diagnosis and localization of aldosterone producing adenomas by differential adrenal vein catheterization. N. Engl. J. Med., *277*:1050, 1967.

Scott, H. W., and Liddle, G. W., et al.: Diagnosis and treatment of Cushing's syndrome. Ann. Surg., *155*:696, 1962.

33

The Urology Patient

JOSEPH N. CORRIERE, JR.
LARRY I. LIPSHULTZ

Although physicians are warned in Hippocrates' oath that diseases of the urinary system may require the talents of someone with special training, it was not until the first half of the twentieth century that the wisdom of his message was appreciated. There are axioms concerning certain problems peculiar to the surgical treatment of the urinary tract and the male genital tract that at first glance appear either so obvious that they seem hardly worth mentioning or so obscure that it is difficult to understand why they should be mentioned at all. In this chapter, we will explore these principles and attempt to disperse the mystery surrounding them. No attempt will be made to discuss specific genitourinary diseases that produce signs or symptoms in other organ systems or the total organism or the evaluation of other systems, as they are covered in other sections of this manual. Our remarks will be limited strictly to the preoperative evaluation and postoperative care of patients with surgical diseases of the urinary and male genital tracts.

PREOPERATIVE EVALUATION

HISTORY

Perhaps with no other patient is the problem of referred pain or reflex symptoms so much a prime consideration as when dealing with diseases of the male genitourinary tract. However, a review of the embryology of renal ascent and testicular descent clarifies some of these diagnostic dilemmas. Patients with pain secondary to a renal or ureteral calculus or lumbar disc disease may have a chief complaint of pain in the ipsilateral testicle. A ureteral calculus in the lower third of the right ureter may cause nausea, vomiting, ileus, low-grade fever, right lower quadrant point tenderness, and a leukocytosis (accounting for the higher incidence of appendectomies in patients with recurrent ureteral calculi than in the general population). Irritation of the trigone of the bladder may be perceived as pain at the tip of the penis, and patients with epididymitis or torsion of the testicle commonly experience associated abdominal pain.

Despite these difficulties, a comprehensive history will usually provide a clue to the problem. Patients with surgical renal disease commonly complain of flank pain; those with bladder or prostatic problems commonly complain of urinary frequency, urgency, nocturia, dysuria, and/or incontinence; and those with pain or masses in the scrotum usually have a disease of the scrotal contents. Moreover, one of the rewarding aspects of urology is the excellent group of available diagnostic studies that aid in determining these diseases with satisfying accuracy and minimal discomfort to the patient. Therefore, once it has been determined that the possibility of disease exists in the genitourinary tract, appropriate tests should be performed.

Two symptoms should be emphasized for special consideration: first, dysuria usually indicates that infection is present in the urinary tract, and, therefore, a urine culture is paramount to making a correct diagnosis; second, hematuria is a symptom that cannot be blithely ignored because it may portend serious disease, especially for the older patient. Questions concerning male genital tract function should emphasize the quality of erection and ejaculation as well as the status of paternity.

PHYSICAL EXAMINATION

It is virtually impossible to palpate normal kidneys except in the infant or occasionally in a very thin female. For this reason, if a physician thinks he or she feels a kidney, he or she should suspect that something may be wrong with the organ and should therefore perform appropriate diagnostic studies. Usually, the kidney moves with respiration and can be distinguished from other masses in the upper abdomen; however, this is not always the case. Accurate diagnosis usually depends upon radiographic examinations. Auscultation of the epigastric area for bruits should be performed in patients with hypertension suspected to be of renovascular origin.

In the child, the bladder is an abdominal organ and as such can be easily palpated when distended. However, after the bony pelvis assumes adult proportions, the bladder cannot be felt easily by mere abdominal examination unless it is grossly overdistended. Dullness to percussion over the suprapubic area is sometimes a helpful indication, but a significant amount of urine must be present in the bladder. If pressing over the hypogastric area elicits the feeling in the patient that he must urinate, he may be retaining urine. Again, this is merely an indication that additional studies are necessary.

Bimanual pelvic examination in the dorsal lithotomy position in the awake female or the anesthetized male (with one finger in the rectum) can be used to good advantage to palpate the bladder and approximate its thickness and mobility. This maneuver is necessary in evaluating a patient suspected to have bladder carcinoma.

The female urethra is situated in the submucosal layer of the anterior vaginal wall and should be palpated for masses along its entire course. By milking the urethra antegrade toward the meatus, diverticula may be emptied of their contents. The appearance of blood or pus at the meatus after such a maneuver should make one suspect the presence of urethral lesions.

In the male, the pendulous urethra is palpable along its entire course. Strictures or tumors can often be felt as hard masses in this organ. It is important to examine the urethral meatus for size as well as to evert the opening and inspect the mucosa for distal lesions.

The prostate gland can be palpated by rectal examination. The patient should bend at the waist with his legs spread apart or lie on his side and tuck his knees up to his chest. Either of these positions should separate his buttocks sufficiently to allow the examiner's finger to reach above the proximal part of the gland, and occasionally the seminal vesicles can be felt if they are abnormal. The patient who continually clamps his buttocks together when attempts are made to examine him in the standing position must be examined on his side. If the physician's free hand is used to grasp the patient's iliac crest, it can prevent the patient from drawing away from the examiner's finger by maintaining his pelvis in a constant position. Some physicians prefer the patient to be in the knee-chest or squatting position. The important aspect of all of these positions is to relax the patient's buttocks by having the knees flexed as much as possible.

The prostate should be felt for both size and consistency. Size is described as "flat" when the prostate is not palpated at all, "four plus" when it virtually obstructs the rectum, and "one plus," "two plus," or "three plus" when it is between these extremes. The shape of a normal gland is best thought of as a valley between two hills — the sulcus between the two lateral lobes. It should be remembered that the middle or subcervical lobe cannot be felt on rectal examination because it enlarges anteriorly into the bladder, not posteriorly into the rectum.

What constitutes the normal limits of consistency is difficult to explain. Most important are any irregularities in the above described contours. An irregular mass or a perception of uneven consistency should make the examiner suspicious that the gland contains an abnormality, such as an abscess, calculus, granuloma, or tumor. The finger examination only suggests that pathology exists. A suspected abnormality in the prostate gland can be evaluated accurately by biopsy alone.

Lesions of the penis are usually found by inspection of the organ. The foreskin must be retracted and the entire glans observed. Palpation for plaques or masses of the corporal bodies should also be performed;

most lesions can be diagnosed by inspection and palpation, but other lesions need to be cultured, smeared, or biopsied for a definitive answer.

Proper examination of the scrotal contents necessitates good anatomic knowledge. The following are important points to remember. Mature testicles are egg-shaped structures, at least 4.5 cm in their longest diameter. The long axis of the testicles should lie in the vertical plane when the patient is standing, which is the best position for adequately evaluating the external genitalia of the male. The left testicle usually hangs lower then the right, and the epididymis, a shrimp-shaped structure, lies in close apposition to the testicle in a posterolateral position. The spermatic vessels are anterior to the vas deferens and should be palpated both while the patient is relaxed and while straining in order to evaluate the presence of an inguinal hernia or varicocele.

The testicles should be examined for general consistency and palpated for any irregularities. A fundamental axiom in urology is "any mass in the scrotum that cannot be separated from the testicle must be considered a testicular tumor until proved otherwise." This usually necessitates surgical exploration.

All other masses in the scrotum are usually benign. It is virtually impossible to determine if they are spermatoceles, lipomas, mesotheliomas, or similar masses by palpation alone. Differentiation is needed only if a mass bothers the patient or if there is any hint of neoplasia.

The presence of a hydrocele warrants a separate discussion. It should always be considered a secondary lesion, and the etiology should be sought. Most of the time no cause will be found, but a genitourinary tract infection, inguinal hernia, or testicular neoplasm must be ruled out. Many times the testicle cannot be palpated because of the large size of the hydrocele and its propinquity to the testicle. It is not adequate to transilluminate the scrotum and "see a testicle"; it must be carefully palpated. If the testis cannot be properly evaluated, the hydrocele either can be aspirated with a syringe or the scrotum surgically explored to provide a definitive diagnosis.

DIAGNOSTIC EVALUATION

SCREENING STUDIES

Prior to operation of any type, all patients should undergo two basic studies to evaluate their urinary tract: a serum creatinine concentration and a routine urinalysis. Creatinine is a breakdown product of skeletal muscle and is, for all practical purposes, eliminated by glomerular filtration. In the normally proportioned person, if this value falls within the limits of normal for the age of the patient, renal function can be considered adequate. If muscle wasting is present or if a more accurate determination of renal function is desired, a creatinine clearance test should be performed. The blood urea nitrogen concentration has also been used as a screening test for renal function, but there are so many variables influencing its level (state of hydration, protein metabolism, liver function, and other factors) that it is being used much less today than previously.

The urinalysis is a uniquely important diagnostic study, for it is truly the end result of self-biopsy of an organ system. Indeed, the urinary tract is the only organ system that does biopsy itself every three or four hours, as can be demonstrated in the form of a urine sample. With this sample we can make an initial diagnosis of glomerular disease by protein content, tubular disease by the presence of casts or the ability to concentrate the urine, or neoplasia or infection by the presence of tumor cells, pus cells, or various bacterial, fungal, protozoan, or parasitic organisms.

Although technically not a true screening test, urine culture and sensitivity determination are important to obtain preoperatively if the urinary tract is to undergo operation or instrumentation. It is especially valuable in an elderly patient, in whom urinary retention may occur postoperatively, to document the presence of infection preoperatively. Urinalysis alone is not a reliable source of this information. More important than identifying the exact organism involved is knowing which antibiotic is effective, especially if sepsis occurs.

Patients with known urinary tract infections should be treated prior to operation as well as during the operative and postoperative periods, especially in view of the fact that manipulation of an infected urinary system showers the bloodstream with organisms. This treatment becomes especially important if the patient has implanted prosthetic devices such as heart valves or hip prostheses. In general, in order to prevent resistant overgrowth, we do not like to treat a urinary tract infection in the presence of a foreign body (such as a catheter or stone) until the foreign body is removed. If we do decide to administer preoperative antibiotics in these instances, we are treating potential sepsis and distant infection, not the primary urinary tract infection. For this reason, an antibiotic with an effective bactericidal blood level should be the drug of choice.

Just as the urinalysis is the best screening test for the urinary tract, semen analysis is the best screening test for the male genital tract and should be performed if fertility impairment is suspected. If seminal quality is normal, no further evaluation is necessary. If azoospermia is present, fructose content should be qualitatively determined. Its absence indicates atresia or obstruction of the ejaculatory duct or dysfunction of the seminal vesicle. It does not rule out vasal obstruction.

ANATOMIC STUDIES

In 1929 it was first announced that a substance had been discovered which, when injected intravenously, was excreted by the kidneys in sufficient concentration to allow radiographic visualization of the entire urinary tract. This discovery probably did more than any other since the development of the cystoscope in 1876 to help develop urology into the exacting diagnostic specialty it is today. An intravenous pyelogram done properly, including nephrotomograms, can give the physician detailed anatomic information about the kidneys, ureters, and bladder with a minimum of difficulty or danger to the patient. It alone is the most important tool in the urologist's armamentarium. It should be used as liberally as the internist uses the chest roentgenogram and electrocardiogram. After this study has given the basic anatomic information, it can then be decided if any subsequent studies are necessary for better confirmation of suspected or suggested abnormalities.

If a lesion exists in the renal parenchyma and further definition is needed, the most helpful and least invasive study is ultrasonography. If it reveals the presence of a cyst, the cyst may be punctured, and the fluid may be aspirated and then sent for biochemical and cytologic study. In addition, contrast medium may be injected into the lesion for better radiographic evaluation of the cyst wall. If the ultrasound studies suggest the lesion to be solid, a renal arteriogram may be performed to outline the vasculature of the mass. The arteriogram is also helpful in evaluating congenital or acquired vascular lesions of the kidney, which may be suggested by observation of decreased perfusion of one kidney or occasionally by a mass effect on the urogram or, as seen with renovascular hypertension, a prolonged nephrogram time and unilateral decrease in kidney size.

In the last few years, computerized axial tomography (CAT) scanning has decreased the use of the arteriogram. If the mass has a solid or a complex pattern on ultrasound, a CAT scan should be performed. If a solid lesion is confirmed, rarely will the arteriogram be necessary.

Occasionally, the trained eye can perceive that a renal mass is most likely due to a hypertrophied column of Bertini, a common anomaly. This represents normal functioning renal tissue. In this instance, rather than arteriography, a renal scan using a tubular tagging radioactive agent makes diagnosis more simple, because the "pseudomass" will become as radioactive as the rest of the renal parenchyma. If the lesion is a cyst or tumor, it will not take up the radioactive agent. One word of caution: The renal scan is not to be used as an anatomic study except in this instance. Lesions of less than 2.5 cm cannot be diagnosed properly with radionuclides, and many false positive and false negative results can be obtained under these conditions. The renal scan is really a function study and will be discussed further in the next section.

If a lesion appears to be present in the collecting system of the kidney — either in a calyx or in the renal pelvis — or if a lesion appears to be in the ureter, the appropriate study for further delineation is a retrograde pyeloureterogram. Prior to the development of intravenous pyelography, urologists learned to catheterize the ureteral orifices through an operating cystoscope and to inject radiopaque material into the upper tracts for radiographic definition. After modern-day intravenous contrast media became available, the earlier study became less important and indeed has at times been overused and abused. It gives virtually no information about the renal parenchyma, may produce misinformation if the collecting system is not fully filled or if air bubbles are allowed to enter the contrast medium, and can introduce bacteria or occasionally cause reflex anuria. Properly performed, when its use is truly indicated, it can give valuable information if the entire collecting system is distended with contrast medium and adequate radiographic exposures delineate the defect in question. When a catheter cannot be passed retrograde up the ureter, it may be possible, with fluoroscopic guidance, to puncture the renal pelvis percutaneously and inject contrast medium in an antegrade fashion.

Unfortunately, the static cystogram, aside from the demonstration of gross reflux and traumatic rupture, does not give as accurate a diagnosis of bladder pathology as might be desired. As often as 40 per cent of the time, the static cystogram either suggests that lesions are present in the bladder that do not really exist, or the bladder appears normal when serious pathology is actually present. The voiding cystourethrogram, on the other hand, is a very valuable tool, especially for the pediatric age group. It can delineate virtually all major lesions in the bladder or urethra, except very small bladder tumors.

However, it is the cystourethroscope that first established urology as a specialty, and it is still the definitive tool in the diagnosis of bladder lesions and, most of the time, urethral lesions. It cannot be overemphasized that endoscopy of these organs is mandatory for any patient in whom mucosal lesions are suspected, as may occur with the patient with hematuria and a normal intravenous pyelogram (IVP).

Most urethral lesions can be seen on a voiding cystourethrogram; however, to carry out this study, one must first pass a catheter into the bladder. Occasionally, urethral strictures will be missed or dilated by this maneuver since wide caliber strictures may only be seen if the urethra is fully overdistended to approximately 1 cm (30 French) in a retrograde fashion, such as with a retrograde urethrogram. It should be remembered that usually the urethra only distends to about 0.4 cm (11 French) during voiding. The importance and place of the retrograde urethrogram in the evaluation of the trauma patient will be discussed in detail later.

Although rarely needed, detailed anatomic definition of the vas deferens and seminal vesicles can be performed by an injection of contrast medium into the scrotal vas. Less well developed is an injection technique for evaluation of the testicle, epididymis, and spermatic vessels. If better detail of these structures is required, scrotal exploration is usually necessary.

Two other anatomic studies deserve special mention: urinary cytology to diagnose urinary tract neoplasia and brush biopsy of upper tract lesions. Abnormal cells in the urine are often hard to see and interpret, but when they are definitely present, they may be very helpful in diagnosis. Recently, a technique of passing a small brush up the ureter to dislodge cells from unknown lesions in the upper tract has increased the accuracy of cytologic studies.

Finally, one should not forget the percutaneous needle biopsy technique, which can provide a definitive diagnosis for medical renal disease and prostatic nodules. Endoscopic biopsy of the bladder and incisional biopsy of the testicle are also used to good advantage in diseases of these structures.

PHYSIOLOGIC STUDIES

If the screening studies suggest an abnormality in the function of some area of the urinary or male genital tract, a more detailed investigation of the physiology of that particular area may be necessary.

If renal disease is suspected, an estimation of the glomerular filtration rate (GFR) is indicated and can best be obtained by an endogenous creatinine clearance test. If the intact nephron theory is correct, the GFR reflects total renal parenchymal function, making it the most useful clinical measurement of renal function. Other studies should be considered if specific problems need more careful evaluation.

For example, if a random urine specific gravity is 1.023 or more, concentrating function may be considered intact; however, if it is less than 1.023 and medullary disease is suspected, an overnight concentration test is a worthwhile procedure to determine the extent of disease. Although usually caused by pyelonephritis, any chronic renal disease may affect specific gravity.

Renal plasma flow and, indirectly, tubular function, can be evaluated by injecting phenolsulfonphthalein (PSP) intravenously and measuring its excretion in urine over a specified period of time. Unfortunately, timing and completeness of the urine collection are critical in this study. If the patient cannot cooperate or does not completely empty his or her bladder, a Foley catheter must be inserted to perform the study properly.

The studies described thus far measure the function of both kidneys. Such information is important when operating on the urinary tract or any other organ system in the body. However, when an operation is to be performed on one kidney, it is often imperative to know the individual function of the left and right kidneys.

Until recently, the only way to obtain this assessment was to collect urine separately from each kidney through cytoscopically placed ureteral catheters. As mentioned previously, this carries certain risks, and, if possible, invasive studies should be avoided.

For this reason, since the advent of more accurate external collimation using the gamma camera, many workers have evaluated the use of radioactive agents that measure glomerular filtration, renal blood flow, and renal tubular function in an effort to quantify the individual contribution of the left and right kidneys to total renal function. This information appears to be informative clinically if the study is carefully performed and if ureteral obstruction is not present. Unfortunately, evaluation of the obstructed, hydronephrotic kidney is one of the most common situations in which knowledge of individual renal function is desired. It is hoped that during the next decade newer agents and refinements of computer technology will become a reality and that these problems will be overcome; accurate studies will then be available for virtually every pathologic situation.

In the hypertensive patient who has a possible renovascular lesion demonstrated by arteriography, the peripheral vein renin level, individual renal vein renin levels or a saralasin challenge test can help the surgeon decide whether the vascular lesion is really causing the hypertension. Of course, many people with normal blood pressure have abnormal renal vessels. The diagnostic study provides a demonstration of a physiologic and not merely an anatomic abnormality.

Currently, the only known function of the ureters is to transport urine from the kidneys to the bladder. Because of their inaccessible position, they have been difficult to study, and their efficiency has usually been implied by their anatomic appearance on IVP. Unfortunately, this has led many times to unnecessary surgical procedures. As we now know, just because a ureter is dilated, it is not necessarily obstructed or inefficient in transporting urine.

Fluoroscopic observation of ureteral peristalsis during an IVP examination may help evaluate ureteral function; for a more accurate assessment, however, the Whitaker test is essential. This study is performed by infusing fluid at a given rate into the renal pelvis through a small percutaneous or surgically placed tube while measuring the pressure in the system. If the fluid can be transported to the bladder without exceeding 10 cm of water pressure, ureteral function can be considered adequate.

Recently administering a diuretic during the performance of a radionuclide study (the diuretic renogram) has shown promise as a noninvasive method to provide this information.

The purpose of the bladder is to store urine and periodically empty itself. This function should be under the voluntary control of the patient, and he should remain continent between episodes of micturition. The ability of the bladder to store and empty urine is best measured clinically by a cystometrogram, performed by placing a catheter into the bladder after the patient has voided, measuring the amount of residual urine, and then infusing fluid into the bladder while testing for sensation, motor function, and intravesical pressure. Denervation supersensitivity can also be studied with bethanechol chloride if a neuropathic lesion is suspected. If bladder function is normal, the act of voiding can be evaluated by performing a urinary flow rate study. The patient urinates into an electronic or mechanical urinometer, and the time and speed of urine flow is recorded. If flow is abnormal, then outlet obstruction is probably present. However, if the bladder is not functioning normally, the flow rate will also be low. In this case, a cystometrogram is invaluable in differentiating the two conditions.

During voiding, the striated muscle around the urethra and perineum normally relaxes to decrease the resistance around the bladder outlet. In some patients who demonstrate poor urine flow, the problem is an abnormal increase in activity of this striated muscle during bladder contraction, which creates a physiologic obstruction in the urethra. This can be studied by electromyography of the perineal musculature while a cystometrogram is being performed.

Finally, the actual intraurethral pressures can be measured by performing a urethral pressure profile. Fluid is infused into the urethra, and the pressures generated along its entire length are measured. This study is most applicable for patients with problems of incontinence.

When testicular failure is suspected, serum follicle-stimulating hormone, luteinizing hormone, and testosterone should be measured. When hypogonadism seems obvious or the genitalia are ambiguous, a buccal smear, fluorescent Y chromosome study, or complete chromosome analysis should be considered.

In patients with suspected testicular tumors, performance of a serum human chorionic gonadotrophin, beta subunit assay, and a serum level of alpha-fetoprotein, should be completed. These studies are most helpful when repeated postoperatively to evaluate the completeness of tumor removal as well as to postulate the tumor cell type of metastatic lesions.

SPECIAL PROBLEMS

Hematuria. One of the cardinal sins of omission of the clinician is to ignore the presence of blood in the urine of patients with suspected urologic disease. Virtually every patient with more than 10 red blood cells per high power field determined by urinalysis needs to be evaluated completely. A simple guide, "S^2IT^3," can be used to remember the diseases to be considered and sought. They are: stones, sickle cell disease, infection, tumors, tuberculosis, and trauma. If we consider that one cause of glomerulonephritis is infection (*Streptococcus*) and that vascular lesions create masses (tumors), every etiology will be included. It is also important to remember that patients with hematuria who are receiving anticoagulants *must* also be studied, for in at least 40 per cent of them a lesion will be found.

Trauma. Any patient with significant trauma who has gross or microscopic hematuria must have an IVP. Any patient with a fracture of the 11th or 12th ribs or a lumbar pedicle must have an IVP. Any patient with a fractured pelvis must have an IVP, retrograde urethrogram, and cystogram.

If lower urinary tract injury is suspected, *never* insert a Foley catheter, even if urine output measurement seems important. It is not essential to know the urine output of a patient the minute he or she enters the emergency room. Later, when the patient's condition is stable, a retrograde urethrogram can be performed. If the urethra is intact, a Foley catheter can be inserted safely to perform a cystogram or to measure urine output. The systemic blood pressure will give the physician a good indication of organ perfusion prior to monitoring urine production while determining the status of the lower urinary tract. If the urethra is ruptured, a catheter is *contraindicated*, and a cystostomy or open surgical repair is imperative.

CORRECTING REVERSIBLE PATHOPHYSIOLOGY

When an abnormality is discovered in the urinary tract, an attempt should be made to correct it preoperatively. This is especially important when there is decreased renal function, for these patients have higher morbidity and mortality rates than patients with normal renal function. Every possible attempt should be made to improve the status of a patient in a poor operative risk group to a good operative risk group.

If obstructive uropathy is present, decompression by insertion of a Foley catheter or ureteral catheter may improve renal function. Postobstructive diuresis should be remembered as a real phenomenon in the bilaterally chronically obstructed patient.

The ureters may be rehabilitated by cutaneous diversion by tube or surgery for a period of time prior to reconstruction, and bladder atony may be reversed by a prolonged indwelling urethral catheter or cystostomy drainage.

Finally, the importance of preoperative treatment of urinary tract infection cannot be overemphasized, especially if the patient is to undergo instrumentation. Again, for emphasis, an antibiotic should be chosen that has a good bactericidal blood level to protect the patient against generalized sepsis.

POSTOPERATIVE CARE

GENERAL CONSIDERATIONS

Most of the principles of postoperative care that apply to patients undergoing operation upon any organ system apply to those undergoing operation on the genitourinary tract. However, there are a few unique axioms applicable to this latter group of patients that should be emphasized.

Following most surgical procedures, the most common cause of fever in the immediate postoperative period is pulmonary atelectasis. This is not true for the urology patient whose infected urinary tract has been manipulated intraoperatively. Fever in this type of patient is probably secondary to urinary tract infection with associated sepsis. Secondly, drains are placed surgically as safety valves to prevent urine collections in urology patients who have had their urinary tracts opened. Even though urine does not leak from the drain for the first few postoperative days, it should be moved or removed for at least a week; late leakage is not uncommon. Similarly, there is no reason to use pins in these drains; they should be sutured to the skin to prevent accidental removal.

When a patient with decreased renal function has undergone operation, especially if the procedure has involved incision of the renal parenchyma and/or the only remaining kidney, careful early monitoring of renal output is critical. If there is any question of decreased urine production but fluid replacement is felt to be adequate, administering diuretics to prevent renal failure should be considered. Either an osmotic agent such as mannitol or one of the high-ceiling agents such as ethacrynic acid or furosemide are appropriate drugs for this purpose.

As was stated earlier, if the preoperative urine culture is positive and the urinary tract is to be manipulated during operation, the patient should be started on an antibiotic regimen preoperatively. Antibiotic therapy should also be continued postoperatively for at least 7 to 10 days. The presence of a foreign body in the urinary tract, such as a catheter, stent, or calculus, may make it impossible to sterilize the urine until the foreign body is removed, but the antibiotic may prevent sepsis. This practice is a two-edged sword, however, because during treatment, the foreign body may promote the overgrowth of an organism resistant to the antibiotic being used, and a more virulent infection may result. If the patient has a sterile preoperative urine, prophylactic antibiotics will not affect the final bacteriologic status of the urinary tract. There is little evidence that an indwelling catheter and a closed urinary collecting system need to be "covered with antibiotics" to prevent a urinary tract infection. Similarly, the use of continuous irrigation with an antibiotic solution through a "three-way" catheter will be of little additional help for the first 72 hours of drainage. After this time, the technique may decrease the incidence of infection. If the catheter remains in the bladder for longer than a week, however, resistant organisms will eventually begin to grow in the urine. After the catheter has been removed, a urine culture should be obtained, and if infection is found, it should be treated appropriately.

NEPHRECTOMY

Uncomplicated excision of a kidney either through an extraperitoneal or intraperitoneal approach is usually accompanied by ileus for at least 48 hours. Although a nasogastric tube is not usually necessary, it is very important, despite the presence of bowel sounds, that the patient be given nothing by mouth during this entire 48-hour period. Afterward, oral feeding can promptly progress to solid food. Drains are usually not placed, but if used they should be removed as soon as possible. The patient can be discharged one week after operation and is usually seen two weeks later to examine the wound and to check for a urinary tract infection. Full activity and return to work can be resumed four to six weeks postoperatively. Renal function studies should be repeated if the amount of residual renal function is questionable.

RENOVASCULAR SURGERY

The patient who has had renal surgery for disease of the vascular tree is managed postoperatively in the same manner as described in the previous section. The particular postoperative complication most feared is thrombosis of the operated vessel. If this occurs, flank pain and hypertension may develop. Unfortunately, even immediate reexploration is usually unsuccessful in reversing the process, and nephrectomy commonly results.

Aside from this conventional follow-up care, frequent blood pressure measurements should be taken. If hypertension persists, drug therapy should be instituted. A urogram or renal scan should be performed four to six weeks after operation to evaluate perfusion and to insure that improvement has occurred. Some surgeons repeat an arteriogram to check the anatomic result, but if the kidney perfuses well and the blood pressure has been lowered, this procedure is probably meddlesome and unnecessary.

UPPER URINARY TRACT RECONSTRUCTION

Obstructed and dilated segments in the upper tracts are common pathologic problems that require surgical correction. Examples are congenital ureteropelvic junction obstruction and dilated, refluxing ureters. The usual surgical technique employed is excision of the obstructed area and any redundant tissue in the renal pelvis or ureter together with reanastomosis and tapering of the reconstructed part.

All suture lines must be drained to allow any leaking urine to escape. Some surgeons use indwelling stents in the ureter and nephrostomy tubes in the pelvis to divert the urine from the suture lines. Stents are usually removed 7 to 10 days postoperatively. At the time of their removal or shortly thereafter, radiographic contrast material may be injected through the stent or the diverting nephrostomy tube to confirm that the system is watertight. If it is, the nephrostomy tube may be removed; if not, urinary diversion should be continued.

When the drain has been completely dry for at least 24 hours (after at least seven postoperative days have passed), the drains can be removed. At times removal may occur as late as four or five weeks after operation.

Any temptation to remove the drain at an earlier time (based on the premise that a fistula tract has been formed and will stay open) should be resisted. A collection of urine is sure to result.

Prior to discharge and after all the tubes have been removed, a urine culture should be obtained. If the culture is positive, the patient should be treated with an appropriate antibiotic regimen for two weeks. Reculture should be done on a subsequent two-week postoperative visit when the wound is evaluated. Full activity may be permitted at four to six weeks.

A urogram is usually performed a few months after operation to determine whether the upper urinary tract has improved. At times the pathologic changes are fixed, and the urogram will not appear much different from the preoperative one. Radionuclide evaluation or a Whitaker test are necessary for these patients to demonstrate that drainage has been improved.

SURGERY FOR CALCULUS DISEASE

When the renal pelvis, renal parenchyma, or ureter have been opened to remove a calculus, three problems may be encountered in the postoperative period: sepsis, renal failure, and urine leakage with formation of a urinoma. All of these problems have been discussed in the preceding sections, and the proper timing and selection of antibiotics, fluid replacement, diuretic therapy, and the proper placement and timing of drain removal have been emphasized. Similarly, the use of stents and nephrostomy tubes follows the tenets outlined in the section on upper urinary tract reconstruction.

Partial nephrectomy, however, adds a fourth hazard, postoperative hemorrhage. Some surgeons place indwelling Foley catheters in patients undergoing this procedure in order to detect intrarenal bleeding. However, significant hemorrhage usually will collect in the retroperitoneal space and exit through the drain, or a mass will be felt in the flank. Abnormal bleeding will occur either in the immediate postoperative period or 10 to 14 days later when tissue sloughing takes place. If no drainage of urine or blood occurs, the drain can be removed in a week, and the patient can be cared for as any other patient who has undergone upper urinary reconstruction.

Finally, careful follow-up must include frequent urine culture, wound examination, and excretory urography as outlined before. Many surgeons obtain nephrotomograms of the kidneys without contrast medium prior to patients' discharge if they have had renal calculus surgery in order to insure that all of the stone fragments have been removed.

URETERONEOCYSTOSTOMY

After ureteral reimplantation, the bladder is drained with either a cystostomy tube or Foley catheter, and drains are placed near the suture lines in the bladder in anticipation of urine leakage. Most of these procedures may be done in children and are performed entirely extraperitoneally so that bowel peristalsis usually returns promptly in 24 or 48 hours, and the patient can then be fed solid food.

Occasionally, ureteral stents are placed and brought out through the anterior bladder wall or through the urethra. One stent is removed on the third to seventh day; if the urine output remains the same that day, implying that the anastomosis is conducting urine, the second stent is removed the following day. The cystostomy tube or Foley catheter is removed 24 hours later, and the patient is then observed for urine leakage at the drain sites. In addition, the voiding pattern is carefully monitored to insure that bladder function is normal. Rarely, the bladder may be temporarily denervated by the operation, and catheter drainage must be continued until bladder function resumes. When the surgeon is convinced that the patient is voiding normally and that the suture lines are intact, the drains can be removed and the patient can be discharged. Finally, a urine culture should be obtained when the last tube is removed. If the urinary tract is infected, the patient should be treated with appropriate antibiotics.

Complications unique to this procedure include the above stated voiding difficulty, ureteral obstruction, and disruption of the anastomosis. If obstruction occurs, it is usually secondary to edema, which commonly resolves in a few days without intervention. Of course, if both ureters obstruct, the patient develops anuria and azotemia. If this becomes a problem, catheterization of the new orifices may be attempted, but this is usually unsuccessful. At this point, either a percutaneous or formal nephrostomy should be performed. It is necessary to drain only one kidney to prevent azotemia. However, if it is felt that the obstruction will not be reversed quickly and the other renal unit will be harmed by prolonged obstruction, it may be preferable to divert both kidneys. Disruption of an anastomosis, heralded by increased urine leakage from the drain, will probably have to be managed by nephrostomy or ureteral tube diversion, insuring adequate drainage of the leaking urine and delayed repair.

Two weeks after discharge, the patient's urine should be cultured in the office when the wound is inspected. A urogram and voiding cystourethrogram should be done after three to six months to insure that obstruction or vesicoureteral reflux is not present. Periodically over the next few years, these studies and urine cultures should be repeated to insure a good, long-term operative result.

RECONSTRUCTIVE BLADDER SURGERY

After a bladder has undergone operation for any reason (vesicovaginal fistula, diverticulectomy, partial cystectomy, etc.), it is usually allowed to rest by inserting a Foley catheter or suprapubic cystostomy tube. The tensile strength of wounds is entirely dependent upon sutures for a minimum of five days. After that, healing progresses in an exponential fashion. The bladder is one of the fastest-healing organs in the body, for it can regain virtually 100 per cent of its tensile strength in 14 days. Most drainage tubes are removed between the fifth and seventh days, with drains left in place to evacuate any urine leakage that occurs from suture lines for at least 24 hours after voiding has been restored. The patient may have to be recatheterized for a period of time if a large postoperative leak develops.

Postoperative micturition is best evaluated by recording the time and volume of all voids. Normal function can be assumed if the patient can hold urine for two to three hours and void quantities of at least 200 ml. Recording merely the 24-hour total urine output reveals something about renal function but nothing about bladder function.

If voiding is frequent and in small amounts, the patient first must be checked for retention with urinary "overflow." This may be done by abdominal examination or urethral catheterization. If the bladder is not emptying, either poor detrusor tone or outlet obstruction may be present. Bethanechol chloride in doses of 5 to 10 mg subcutaneously or 50 to 100 mg by mouth (for adults) is administered every six hours to help initiate bladder emptying. Doses lower than this are not pharmacologically active. However, the drug should not be given if obstruction is suspected. There is now some evidence that bethanechol chloride will not help bladder emptying at all because although it increases detrusor contractility, it also causes bladder neck closure.

A cystometrogram may be necessary to determine bladder function. Sometimes prolonged bladder rest by catheter drainage is the only way to restore detrusor tone and function. If obstruction is the problem, it will obviously have to be corrected. If the bladder is emptying, however, the difficulty is usually secondary to irritation from infection or surgery. A positive urine culture requires appropriate treatment. Symptomatic relief may be obtained using anticholinergic drugs such as propantheline (Probanthine). Musculotropic agents can also be used, such as oxybutynin (Ditropan) or hyoscyamine (Cystospaz). If the complaint is mainly dysuria, infection should be strongly suspected. If infection is not present, phenazopyridine (Pyridium), a mucosal anesthetic, will usually give the patient some relief from the distressing symptoms.

After all tubes and drains are removed, a urine culture should be obtained, and if infection is present, it should be treated appropriately. Postoperative care consists of a two-week wound inspection and urine culture, as well as an assessment of the adequacy of voiding. If all is well, little more in the way of follow-up is required. If there is a question about the mechanics of micturition, urodynamic studies may be helpful.

TOTAL CYSTECTOMY

Removal of the entire urinary bladder (as well as the prostate and seminal vesicles) for cancer is one of the most stressful procedures performed on patients with urinary tract disease. Obviously, urinary diversion is necessary in these patients, and that in itself imposes an entirely separate set of problems during the postoperative period. Urinary diversion is discussed in the following section of this chapter.

Most surgeons drain the pelvic cavity with a Foley catheter inserted through the urethra in addition to a suprapubic Penrose drain. The balloon of the Foley catheter should be deflated over the first two days to hold a minimal amount of fluid and to decrease the dead space created by the balloon. Since the catheter is really acting as a drain, when the largest amount of drainage has declined, usually by the third day, it can be removed. The Penrose drain usually remains relatively dry and can be removed by the fifth to seventh day.

The most common postoperative complications related to cystectomy are pelvic hematoma and pelvic abscess. Significant arterial bleeding may require reexploration and ligation of bleeding points. Venous bleeding can usually be managed by applying increased tension on the urethral catheter if the bleeding arises from the periurethral plexus or by reexploration and sponge packing of the pelvis. Lately, vascular embolization of bleeding vessels by a talented arteriographer using fluoroscopic techniques has obviated surgical procedures for postoperative hemorrhage, if such resources are available.

Fever, a urethral discharge, and pelvic tenderness usually herald a pelvic abscess. This is commonly a late complication, occurring weeks to months after operation. A urethrogram may show a cavity where the bladder used to be; a urethral catheter acting as a drain may be all that is needed to evacuate the collection. However, most frequently a formal suprapubic incision and drainage are necessary. The pus should be cultured, and appropriate antibiotics should be given. Irrigation with an antibiotic solution may be necessary.

When one realizes how close the bladder and prostate are to the rectum, it should come as no surprise that one of the most important axioms to observe in the postoperative care of these patients is that rectal manipulation should *never* be performed for the first few months after operation for fear of rectal perforation. This means obtaining no rectal temperatures, giving no enemas, and performing no rectal examination (except by experienced personnel for important diagnostic reasons such as fecal impaction or pelvic abscess). Most of the follow-up care for these patients is directed toward evaluation of the urinary diversion and continued assessment of the primary disease after the wound has healed and bowel function has returned to normal.

URINARY DIVERSION

Although at times the urine is diverted temporarily from its normal course through the urinary tract by tubes placed in the kidney, ureter, or bladder in order to put an obstructed or operated area at rest, when permanent urinary diversion is performed, it is usually of the tubeless variety. Dilated ureters or a distended bladder may be sutured to the skin (cutaneous ureterostomy, vesicostomy), and an external collecting device may be placed over the stoma. If the ureters are of a normal length and diameter, they usually do not reach the skin and have such a tenuous blood supply that distal slough and stomal stenosis are common. For this reason, an isolated loop of bowel, usually either distal ileum or colon, is interposed as a conduit between the ureters and the skin (cutaneous ureteroileostomy or ureterocolostomy), and an appliance is placed over the bowel stoma. The continuity of the gastrointestinal tract is then restored by an ileoileostomy or a colocolostomy.

Whether a bowel anastomosis is made or not, a nasogastric tube should be used for at least three days postoperatively until bowel function returns to normal. Intravenous fluid replacement during this time should be carefully monitored by obtaining serum electrolyte levels, for if renal function is marginal, any postobstructive diuresis or bowel absorption of urine constituents may upset homeostasis.

The most important immediate postoperative complication is disruption or obstruction of the diversion. If ureteral stents are used, disruption or obstruction may not be apparent until they are removed, usually five to seven days after operation. The first signs of these complications are heralded by a sharp decrease in urine output. For this reason, for the first few postoperative days, hourly or two-hourly urine outputs should be carefully monitored. At the first sign of decreasing output, the conduit should be catheterized. If this increases urine flow, either the stoma is obstructed or ileus is present in the conduit. A few days of tube drainage may be necessary to allow adequate urinary output. If catheterizing the stoma does not help, then an immediate excretory urogram and retrograde conduit injection of contrast medium ("loopogram") should be performed. If obstruction occurs in the first three postoperative days, immediate surgical repair can be attempted; if it occurs later than three days, higher tube diversion and delayed repair may be necessary. Small leaks may close without operative intervention.

The other difficulties that occur in these patients are usually related to their primary disease. Pyelonephritis is the most common complication. Wound care should be the same as with any abdominal incision. Special attention, however, must be directed at securing a good fit of the appliance to the stoma, because the constant wetness from a leaking appliance will quickly macerate the skin. The help of an enterostomal therapist is invaluable, for the cardinal sin after establishing a stoma of any kind is sending the patient home before he can handle any and all of the problems, real or imagined, that his new way of life will produce.

If all goes well, the patient may be discharged in 7 to 10 days and returns for a wound and stoma check in two weeks. There is little reason to treat these patients with antibiotics, and culturing the conduit is difficult because skin organisms commonly inhabit the stoma. Only urine obtained by a catheter deep within the conduit can be considered appropriate for culture purposes. Under no circumstances should urine from the collecting bag be used for meaningful culture.

Long-term evaluation consists of stoma examination for stenosis and periodic IVP studies for anatomic examination of the upper tracts. For the first six months, dilatation may be present because of the recent operation and can usually be disregarded. After this time and if dilatation is progressive, it may mean that obstruction is present. If a refluxing ureteroenteral anastomosis was performed, a "loopogram" will be helpful in making this diagnosis.

OPEN PROSTATECTOMY

When a patient has a prostatic adenoma removed for benign disease, either through the bladder (transvesical or "suprapubic") or through the prostatic capsule (retropubically or perineally), the most immediate postoperative problem is hemorrhage. If the bladder has been opened, a cystostomy tube is usually placed in the dome. This and a urethral Foley catheter will enable thorough irrigation to evacuate the clots. In time the bleeding should stop. If it does not, traction on the urethral catheter can be applied by pulling on the Foley catheter and taping it to the patient's leg. This draws the Foley balloon against the bladder neck and prostatic fossa to tamponade any open vessels. This technique can also be used in patients without cystostomies, but the physician must be aware that traction will decrease the catheter lumen size and impede clot removal.

If clot retention is a problem, the catheter should be irrigated frequently with a piston-type (Toomey) syringe. If irrigating fluid can be inserted but the bladder cannot be evacuated of fluid, then the Foley catheter should be pushed as far as it will go into the bladder to elevate the catheter eye above the clots and allow the urine and irrigating fluid to drain. If clots continue to be a problem, the water should be removed from the catheter balloon. This will increase the inside diameter of the catheter and will allow larger clots to be evacuated. If this does not work, the Foley catheter should be replaced. The proper catheter size that should be used in any patient in whom clots are a problem is 22 to 28 French.

If active bleeding persists, the patient should be returned to the operating room, the bladder opened, and the prostatic fossa packed with ribbon gauze. The packing can be brought out through a stab wound in the bladder and a cystostomy performed. In a few days, when the bleeding has stopped, this packing can be removed. The patient should be given a narcotic during packing removal, as the procedure is quite painful.

One more comment should be made about prostatectomy bleeding. In the past it was felt that fibrinolysins were commonly released after prostatectomy, especially in patients who had prostatic carcinoma. When a coagulopathy is suspected to be the cause of abnormal prostatectomy bleeding, it is now well recognized as more likely to be due to disseminated intravascular coagulation. All abnormal bleeding should obviously be evaluated hematologically and treated appropriately if a coagulation disorder is diagnosed.

If all goes well, the Foley catheter can be removed when the urine begins to clear, usually two to five days postoperatively. Any drains should be left in place until all suture lines have been shown to be intact and the patient is voiding normally. Each void must be checked for volume, and the patient must be observed for continence. Bladder spasms may be treated with an antispasmodic agent, and a urine culture should be performed when the catheter and/or cystostomy are removed. If infection is present, it should be treated with appropriate antibiotics. Rectal examinations are contraindicated for the first six weeks postoperatively, as prostatic manipulation may induce bleeding. The patient may be discharged from the hospital when he is voiding every two to three hours with a full stream and his urine is grossly clear. He should be cautioned not to exert himself or have intercourse for two to three weeks because bleeding may develop from prostatic trauma or contraction. Full activity and sexual intercourse can be resumed in four to six weeks.

The patient's wound should be checked at two weeks, and his urinary stream should be observed. If the stream has decreased or "sprays," a 24 French urethral sound should be passed to diagnose and obviate meatal or fossa navicularis stenosis, urethral stricture, or bladder neck contracture. A urine culture at this time and again at three months completes the extended postoperative evaluation.

A final word should be said about removal of the entire prostate and seminal vesicles ("radical" prostatectomy) with a urethrovesical anastomosis. This procedure is usually performed only for cancer and has a high rate of incontinence. Little more than the preceding care must be observed, although the timetable may be prolonged, and the follow-up must include screening studies for recurrent neoplasm.

ENDOSCOPIC SURGERY

When a patient has undergone endoscopic surgery of any kind, be it cystourethroscopy, manipulation of a ureteral stone, ureteral catheterization, dilatation of a urethral stricture, litholapaxy, or actual resection of a bladder lesion or enlarged prostate, the postoperative care will depend upon (1) the extent of the manipulation, (2) whether perforation of the bladder or urethra occurred, (3) whether the urinary tract was obstructed or infected, and (4) how well bleeding was controlled. If the operation produced minimal trauma and the urinary tract is intact, uninfected, and not grossly bleeding, any Foley catheter placed into the bladder at the end of the operation should be removed as soon as possible, and a return to normal voiding should be encouraged. In most instances this is usually possible within 24 hours postoperatively. Catheters should only be left in place for a longer time if there is a good reason. It has been shown that after 72 hours, the incidence of bacteriuria in the catheterized bladder begins to rise. Also, the incidence of urethral stricture and epididymitis in the male is directly proportional to the duration of catheterization.

Generally, small perforations or deeply resected areas of the bladder recognized at surgery will seal in three or four days. A cystogram can be obtained to confirm this prior to catheter removal. As previously mentioned, positive preoperative urine cultures should be treated *before* instrumentation, and any urinary tract obstructions should be relieved *prior to or at the time of* endoscopy. If postoperative sepsis occurs, appropriate therapy must include relief of any residual obstruction, which may be a ureter requiring catheterization or even open drainage, or a poorly emptying bladder in need of Foley catheter drainage.

Bleeding from the prostate is managed in much the same way as described in the preceding section on open prostatectomy. Prior to open packing of the prostatic fossa, however, it is worthwhile to return the patient to the cystoscopy suite, and while he is under anesthesia, to remove all the clots and inspect the bladder and urethra for bleeding. Most of the time a small bleeding point can be seen and fulgurated, or clot evacuation alone may allow the fossa to contract and close any open venous sinuses. If this fails to control the hemorrhage, open packing may be required.

PENILE AND URETHRAL SURGERY

The greatest postoperative problem following operation on the penis and urethra is the development of edema and skin necrosis, which may produce separation of suture lines or urinary fistulas. Usually a light compression dressing is applied and kept on the penis for one to five days, depending on the extent of the procedure. The glans should always be visible during this time; at the first sign of ischemia or venous congestion, i.e., a blanched or cyanotic appearance, the dressing should be *immediately* removed.

For the first 12 postoperative hours, an ice bag should be kept on the penis to limit edema as much as possible. After this period, ice is usually ineffective. A rubber glove packed with crushed ice in the fingers can be a good ice bag for the penis, for it can be molded around the organ unlike a flat, unyielding, conventional ice bag.

When the dressing is removed, warm tub baths should be started for 20 to 30 minutes three times a day. The key to soaking is the application of wet heat; nothing need be added to the water. Between soaks, the skin must be kept dry to prevent maceration. A heat lamp may be helpful. The suture lines should be carefully inspected three or four times a day, and any necrotic areas should be debrided to prevent deep infection and further necrosis, particularly if large complicated flaps were used in the repair. Most surgeons are now using absorbable sutures on the penis and urethra. If nonabsorbable sutures are used, they may be removed after 7 to 10 days, depending on the type of operation performed.

If a urethral repair has been done, one must be alert for the development of a urethrocutaneous fistula. The urine is usually diverted from the urethra with a urethral catheter, a perineal urethrostomy, or a suprapubic tube. The urethral catheter is usually removed in five days and the perineal urethrostomy or suprapubic tube in 7 to 10 days. If a voiding cystourethrogram is done prior to or at the time of removal and a fistula is seen, the urethral catheter can be reinserted or the suprapubic tube left in place. The perineal urethrostomy, however, usually cannot be replaced. Many times small fistulas close spontaneously with time, even without continued urinary diversion. We prefer employing the suprapubic tube. It can be left in place for weeks, and the urethrogram can be repeated as necessary while the foreign material (urethral catheter) is kept away from the urethral suture line, thus aiding the healing process and decreasing the incidence of fistulas and strictures.

Antibiotics are not necessary, and pain is usually readily controlled by mild analgesics such as aspirin. The patient can be sent home when the catheter has been removed and when he is able to continue care without nursing assistance. The soaks should be continued for at least two weeks after operation and the wound examined for proper healing after two weeks. If a diversion was employed, a urine culture should be done at the time of tube removal, and the patient should be treated appropriately if there is evidence of infection. Intercourse can usually be resumed four to six weeks postoperatively.

SURGERY OF THE SCROTAL CONTENTS

Edema and intrascrotal hemorrhage are the greatest problems following operation on the scrotum and its contents. The edema can be controlled somewhat by ice bags for the first 12 hours and a compression dressing for the the first three to five days. The scrotum has a rich blood supply, and therefore skin necrosis is usually not a problem. When the dressing is removed, warm tub baths with dry intervals as described in the previous section are important for the first two postoperative weeks.

Scrotal and perineal wounds should be considered potentially contaminated because of their great degree of colonization by skin bacteria. Of course, a good blood supply is what prevents superficial wound infections, but deep abscesses can occur. A word of caution: The skin of the scrotum is very sensitive. Use of pHisohex and ether as skin preparations may cause superficial burns, leading to necrosis and bullous edema, and thus should never be applied to the scrotum. Plain soap is all that is necessary to cleanse this area.

There is little that can be done about postoperative intrascrotal hemorrhage. Blood clots do not evacuate well via a Penrose drain, and the lax tissue of the scrotum may lead to a large hematoma. Consequently, scrupulous hemostasis at the time of operation is the best way to prevent this problem. A compression dressing may help, but if the bleeding becomes excessive, reexploration with clot evacuation, hemostasis, and a compression dressing may be necessary.

If a drain is used, it can be removed on the third to fifth postoperative day. When the patient is up and about, an athletic supporter or a tight pair of undershorts should be worn for support and also to hold any dressings that may be needed to keep wound secretions from appearing on the patient's clothes. So-called scrotal supporters are usually worthless because they do not stay in place, and they give virtually no support. While the patient is in bed, the scrotum should be elevated by a folded towel, or the athletic supporter should be worn.

Finally, antibiotics are unnecessary unless there is an infection. Although most surgeons use absorbable suture material on the scrotum, if nonabsorbable sutures are used they can be removed in five to seven days. The patient may be discharged once all drains are removed and once he can adequately manage nursing procedures at home. He should be warned that prolonged standing may produce scrotal edema and increased discomfort for the first few weeks. If this occurs, tub baths, scrotal support, and bedrest will promptly relieve the condition. Nothing more than aspirin should be required for pain. The wound should be inspected in two weeks, and afterward only if necessary. Full activity can usually be resumed in 5 to 10 days, depending on the extent and nature of the disease treated.

SUMMARY

A few general concepts have been stressed in this chapter: First, excellent diagnostic tools are available to pinpoint accurately lesions in the genitourinary tract. If these tools are judiciously employed, "exploratory surgery" with no idea as to the preoperative pathology should rarely be necessary. Second, referred pain is commonly seen, especially if the patient's problem is acute. Third, if the patient's renal function is improving on catheter drainage, operation should be delayed until function is stabilized. Postoperatively, renal function should be monitored closely, and fluids and diuretics should be administered to insure adequate renal perfusion. Finally, frequent urine cultures are vital in the prevention and treatment of septic complications of urinary tract surgery.

If these guidelines are followed, the bulk of potential postoperative problems can be predicted and generally avoided. Moreover, if complications do develop, effective solutions to them are readily available.

34

The Gynecologic Patient

JOHN J. MIKUTA

PREOPERATIVE CARE

Initial evaluation of the patient begins with an office visit, at which time a complete assessment of the patient's chief complaint, a thorough systemic review, and physical examination are done. Occasionally, symptoms that appear to be gynecologic in nature or related to pelvic reproductive organ functions are in fact the result of pathologic processes in adjacent organ systems, most frequently the intestinal or urinary tracts. Specific information relevant to the reproductive organs must be obtained: menstrual history (onset, frequency, duration, amount, association with pain, degree of disability); obstetrical history (including number of pregnancies, live births, abortions, both spontaneous and induced, complications of pregnancy, labor, and delivery); and a history of previous surgical procedures, particularly those dealing with the pelvic organs, since the results and difficulty or complications of any contemplated procedure may be related to procedures that the patient has previously experienced. Finally, a psychosocial and sexual history should be obtained in order to determine the relationship of the symptoms to possible emotional, social, or other environmental factors.

Weight, height, blood pressure, hematocrit or hemoglobin measurements, and urinary determinations for glucose and protein should be obtained. Microscopic urinalysis should be done as indicated, as should urine culture and antibacterial sensitivity. The physical examination should include evaluation of the eyes, ears, nose, and throat, the heart and lungs, the breasts, the abdominal contents, the extremities, the neurologic state, and finally the pelvic area. The pelvic examination should include careful inspection of the vulva, urethra, Skene's ducts, Bartholin's glands, and the anal orifice. The vagina and cervix are carefully inspected, and cytologic smears are taken from the endocervix and ectocervix. In women over 40 years of age, particularly symptomatic postmenopausal patients, endometrial aspiration cytology and/or biopsy is desirable in order to improve the accuracy of the provisional diagnosis prior to hospital admission. The location of the uterine fundus should always be ascertained prior to aspiration or other invasive manipulation. A vaginoabdominal bimanual examination is then performed to determine the size, shape, and position of the uterus and the size, location, and consistency of the adnexal structures. The examination is repeated with the examining fingers in the rectum and vagina both to confirm the findings of the vaginal examination and to determine the presence or absence of intrinsic lower bowel pathology. Areas of tenderness are noted, as are the fixation of structures, malposition of the uterus, and its relationship to the lower urinary and intestinal tracts.

After the complete evaluation, the gynecologist should then present precise information to the patient, ideally in the presence of her husband or companion. The symptoms and physical findings should be reviewed and, in lay terms, the diagnosis and proposed treatment should be presented. If the patient has known the gynecologist for some time, she may have implicit faith in his or her diagnosis and recommendations. However, the gynecologist should always offer the patient reasonable alternative approaches to the primary suggested management, if such are available, and he or she should also provide the patient with the opportunity to consult with another gynecologist for a "second opinion."

Once the necessity for operation is determined and the patient is satisfied with the diagnosis and therapeutic options, her informed consent should be obtained. While this should be comprehensive and informative, it should be presented in such a way that the patient understands the benefits that are expected to accrue from the proposed operation in addition to the risks that the surgical procedure may present. No result or benefits should ever be "guaranteed." Conditions that may potentially produce bad results should be anticipated and presented honestly. The standard mortality and morbidity rates associated with the specific operation should be discussed. Filmstrips and audiovisual aids are helpful in depicting various operative procedures, and they provide an excellent technique to augment the physician's discussion. A note on the record that the patient has viewed such material, has discussed it with her surgeon, and understands the procedure can provide the basis for adequate informed consent.

If the symptoms or findings are strictly of a gynecologic nature, further preadmission evaluation may be limited to ascertaining the general condition of the patient, associated medical problems, and the need for other preoperative studies. Minor gynecologic procedures, such as dilation and curettage, cervical conization or biopsy, vulvar or vaginal biopsy, and Bartholin's cyst marsupialization, do not generally require extensive patient evaluation unless there is a history of problems that might complicate the induction of anesthesia, such as heart disease, hypertension, asthma, drug allergy, or other factors such as anemia, bleeding tendency, diabetes, or other systemic disease. A hemogram, chest film, and electrocardiogram are usually sufficient. No perineal shave is needed in most instances.

If major surgery is contemplated, more extensive evaluation is indicated. Routine evaluations of hemogram, chest roentgenogram, electrocardiogram, electrolytes, blood urea nitrogen, and creatinine levels as well as liver function tests are desirable. Additional specific studies may be suggested based on abnormalities noted in the prior studies. Intravenous pyelography is not always indicated, but it should be considered if there is a history of recurrent urinary tract infection, urinary incontinence, hypertension, or if the anatomic findings suggest that the lower urinary tract may be closely involved in the pathologic process, such as intraligamentous myoma, cervical myoma, or pelvic abscess. Patients being evaluated for radical surgery for gynecologic malignancy require more comprehensive study of the extent of metastatic disease, and the patient's ability to tolerate extensive and prolonged surgical procedures should be evaluated.

Specific urinary tract studies should be carried out in patients who have symptoms associated with the lower urinary tract. These include urinary incontinence, urinary urgency with or without incontinence, frequency, nocturia, hesitation, and difficulty in starting the stream or incomplete bladder evacuation. For these patients, cystoscopy, cystometry, chain cystourethrography, intravenous pyelography, and urinary culture are all indicated prior to operation. There are significant numbers of patients whose symptoms are caused by infection, calculi, detrusor dyssynergia, or neurologic problems. Vaginal plastic surgery in such patients will only aggravate the existing symptoms. Of all the anatomic areas with which a gynecologist must deal, the urinary tract is the most vexing. A comprehensive approach to the urinary tract, particularly as it may be related to infection, is found in Chapter 33.

While the diagnosis of urinary stress incontinence may be made by taking a careful history and may be confirmed by inspection of the external urethral opening while the patient coughs or strains, the approach to the management of this symptom has, in the past decade, undergone some revision. T. H. Green, utilizing the chain cystourethrogram, has identified two varieties of anatomic change associated with stress incontinence, and since the approaches to each are different, i.e., vaginal plastic procedure versus suprapubic suspension, it is mandatory to specifically identify the type of anatomic change. An excellent review on this subject by Green is found in Buchsbaum and Schmidt's *Gynecologic and Obstetric Urology.*

Careful attention must be paid to the lower intestinal tract and to those areas of the bowel that may lie in the pelvis. Symptoms of constipation, bleeding, and recent changes in bowel habits should not be ascribed to gynecologic findings but should be evaluated by barium enema and proctosigmoidscopy prior to gynecologic surgery. The high incidence of diverticulosis in patients over the age of 50 makes these diagnostic procedures particularly worthwhile in elderly individuals. Additionally, lesions that occur in the left pelvic area may in reality be intestinal in origin, and the gynecologist will be better prepared if he or she recognizes possible intestinal involvement preoperatively.

Occasionally, other special studies may be required. The gynecologist should always be aware of the possibility of fistulous tracts between the gynecologic structures and adjacent organs. Previous operations and radiation therapy are most commonly associated with such lesions. Careful inspection of the vagina, bladder, and perineum may identify such areas, and a vaginogram or fistulogram (a catheter in the fistula with dye injected) can show the relationship of the involved structures.

Other studies may help to enlighten the gynecologist regarding the nature and location of a given lesion. A flat film of the pelvis may show calcifications characteristic of a cystic teratoma (dermoid) or myoma. Ultrasonography is also becoming increasingly valuable in defining pelvic masses, and the computerized axial tomography technique is now a method that may replace many conventional procedures.

All of the procedures discussed here can be performed on an outpatient basis. This is advisable economically, but the patient's age, infirmity, domestic geographic location, and emotional status must be considered in making a decision for outpatient evaluation.

Preoperatively, a complete reevaluation may be wise, especially if there has been a significant lapse of time since the initial evaluation. Occasionally lesions such as functional ovarian cysts may disappear and obviate operation. In addition, the patient should be advised to contact the gynecologist if there is evidence of any problem that would contraindicate either anesthesia or operation, such as upper respiratory infection, urinary tract infection, or any significant changes in the presenting symptoms.

Finally, the gynecologist should freely consult other physicians prior to operation. Such individuals as internists, hematologists, urologists, and general surgeons with whom the gynecologist has a working relationship can add greatly to the accuracy of the preoperative diagnosis and maximize preparation for any possible exigencies that may arise intraoperatively.

In general, the in-hospital preoperative evaluation is usually done by the house officer, and evaluation includes taking a complete history and performing a complete physical examination. In hospitals in which there are no house officers, the attending physician performs these functions. The house officer and gynecologist should review the history and physical examination as well as the preoperative diagnostic studies and should order any other studies felt to be appropriate.

PREOPERATIVE PREPARATION

Preoperatively, special attention should be given to the following areas.

Eradication of Infection. This applies particularly to the urinary tract and the genital tract. Patients with infections should have elective operations postponed until a urine culture shows no growth or until local areas of vaginal breakdown, such as from pessaries, are healed.

Correction of Anemia. If time allows, simple iron-deficiency anemias may be corrected by the use of iron and other hematinic agents. In urgent situations, transfusions of whole blood or packed red blood cells may be used preoperatively to return the hematocrit to acceptable levels.

Preparation of the Bowel. If there is a possibility that the bowel may be involved in the pathologic process, appropriate preparation is recommended. This can be accomplished by mechanical cleansing with cathartics and enemas, in addition to a liquid diet and 0.5 gm of neomycin sulfate and 0.25 gm tetracycline orally every six hours for 48 hours prior to operation.

Prophylactic Antibiotics. The latest evidence suggests that administration of such agents may be useful for premenopausal patients undergoing vaginal hysterectomy. It is recommended that the antibiotics be given approximately one hour preoperatively and then every six hours for a total of 36 hours. The goal is to provide a high antibiotic level in the local tissues at the time of operation and subsequently to avoid the development of infection with resistant organisms.

Low-Dose Heparin. In patients with a history of deep venous thrombosis, especially if embolization had occurred, the use of low-dose prophylactic heparin may be considered. Obesity and varicosities may also be considered as indications for this approach.

Intravenous Lines. A peripheral intravenous line placed just prior to the induction of anesthesia is the usual procedure. When an extensive radical procedure is planned or when the patient is at high risk for excessive blood loss or has cardiovascular problems, it is advisable to place a catheter in one subclavian vein for determination of central venous pressure (CVP). Ideally, this should be done the evening before operation so that a chest film can be obtained to verify accurate catheter placement and rule out possible complications such as hemothorax or pneumothorax. An alternative procedure is to pass the catheter through the jugular vein just prior to the induction of anesthesia in the operating room. The former approach (subclavian) is preferred because it is more comfortable for the patient postoperatively.

Blood Samples. Blood should be drawn for the purposes of typing and crossmatching.

For abdominal operations, the abdomen is shaved from the xyphoid to the mons pubis if a longitudinal incision is to be used and from the umbilicus to the mons pubis if a transverse incision is planned. In obese patients, scrubbing the abdomen and groin several days preoperatively with an antiseptic solution will aid in decreasing bacterial contamination. For major vaginal procedures, preoperative douches and local antibacterial agents have been used with variable results. Thorough, vigorous cleansing of the vagina prior to operation with an acceptable antiseptic solution is probably just as effective.

Finally, cleansing of the lower bowel with enemas prior to operation will help to reduce intestinal distention, making abdominal surgical exposure maximal. With vaginal operations, there is a reduced tendency for fecal contamination of the operative field.

Preoperative evaluation of the patient by the anesthesiologist is important to determine the type of anesthesia best suited for her and for the surgical procedure. The anesthesiologist should inform the patient of his or her recommendations, and meeting with her will simultaneously increase knowledge of her medical status. Preoperative medication to provide some relief of anxiety and reduce secretions in the tracheo-bronchial tree is usually ordered by the anesthesiologist with the concurrence of the gynecologist.

INTRAOPERATIVE CARE

It is best for the gynecologist to see the patient prior to the induction of anesthesia. The peripheral intravenous line should be in place for the forthcoming administration of analgesic and sedative drugs as well as fluids. Additionally, cardiovascular monitoring is essential; blood pressure, pulse rate, and electrocardiogram readings should all be carefully followed.

The patient should be comfortably and properly placed for either lithotomy or supine approaches. Areas of possible external body pressure should be identified and properly padded. For vaginal procedures, the bladder may be catheterized after the patient is scrubbed and draped, but for abdominal procedures the catheter should be inserted and a pelvic examination done while the patient is under anesthesia for final review of the pelvic findings. The vagina is then scrubbed thoroughly with an antiseptic solution.

The surgical team should be familiar with the procedures and familiar with all appropriate equipment. Back-up equipment should be available in case of contamination or mechanical failure. When new procedures are introduced, such as laparoscopy, prior educational and informational classes for the operating room personnel are vital to insure smooth performance of the surgical procedure.

The surgeon should carefully note the preoperative and operative findings. He or she should carry out complete abdominal exploration when celiotomy is performed and should record all findings. The operative procedure should be listed by title, and a detailed operative account should be dictated for entry into the hospital record. The duration of the operation, estimated blood loss, and any unusual circumstances encountered, such as operative injuries, should all be recorded.

Use of suture materials should be specified, and the number, position, and type of drains should be noted.

POSTOPERATIVE CARE

Postoperative care begins in the operating room as soon as the operation is completed. As the patient recovers from anesthesia, she should be observed conscientiously for any cardiovascular and respiratory changes. Dressings are applied to the abdominal wound, and vulvar pads are applied, chiefly to provide a method for ascertaining existence and amount of vaginal bleeding.

The patient is moved from the operating table to her own bed as atraumatically as possible, preferably by roller, and is taken to the recovery area. Here vital signs are carefully monitored every 15 minutes until she is fully awake. The patient should be observed for signs of local excessive bleeding through the vagina or in the abdominal wound area. Urinary output is also measured hourly, especially after major operative procedures.

When the patient is fully awake and oriented to time and place and if her vital signs are stable, she may then be transferred to the gynecologic floor. Postoperative orders will have been written to include further monitoring of vital signs every 30 minutes for the first two hours, every hour for the next six hours, and every two hours for the 24-hour postoperative period. Temperature is taken orally or rectally (depending on the patient's cooperation) every two to four hours. Continued observation of urinary catheter drainage, vaginal bleeding, or bleeding into the abdominal dressing are essential.

Following minor operations, most patients are alert within four to six hours after operation. They may then ambulate with assistance and eat what they desire, provided there is no nausea or vomiting. Pain is usually minimal, although an order for mild analgesics should be written on a standby basis.

A patient who has had major abdominal procedures experiences varying degrees of abdominal pain that are related to the location and length of the incision, duration of the procedure, and the patient's tolerance of pain. Generally, the patient who has had a major vaginal procedure has less upper abdominal discomfort than patients who have undergone abdominal procedures and also has a more rapid return of bowel function. This is in part a reflection of the degree of peritoneal irritation.

Monitoring and Return of Special Functions

Cardiorespiratory Function. Careful observation of the cardiovascular-respiratory system is vital in the immediate postoperative period, especially the first 24 hours. Tachycardia and subsequent hypotension may signal the occurrence of internal bleeding that observation of the usual external bleeding sites, i.e., vagina or abdominal wound, has not previously heralded. Such findings, in addition to abdominal distention and signs of impending or actual shock, should lead the physician to carefully examine the patient generally at first and then give specific attention to the abdominal and pelvic areas. Hemoglobin and hematocrit determinations and blood for transfusion are ordered. When postoperative hemorrhage is suspected, arteriography and isotope studies may help localize the site, but reexploration and religation of the bleeding site is usually necessary.

In patients with cardiac problems that have been recognized prior to operation, the postoperative period must be one of careful monitoring for evidence of fluid overload or impending cardiac failure. The use of intravenous diuretics is helpful in ridding the system of excessive fluid and salt and reducing the cardiac burden. If the cardiac situation is precarious, continuous monitoring in the surgical intensive care unit may be advisable.

The respiratory tract in the early postoperative period, especially when the patient is still under the effects of anesthesia and sedation, must be kept free of obstruction and the lungs kept fully expanded. As sedation subsides, the nursing staff must encourage the patient to perform deep breathing exercises, which are augmented by turning and movement of extremities. An incentive spirometer and deep coughing clear mucus from the tracheobronchial tree. Fever and tachycardia associated with dullness to percussion of the chest and absent or diminished breath sounds are signs of atelectasis and can be overcome by deep breathing and coughing for the majority of patients. At times, endotracheal aspiration may cause expulsion of a mucous plug, as much a function of the gagging and coughing it produces as of the suction. In rare instances, bronchoscopy may be necessary.

There is no more frustrating postoperative complication than the development of pneumonia. This is usually the result of inactivity, stasis, and poor pulmonary toilet. A sputum culture should be obtained and antibiotics begun, pending the outcome of the antibiotic sensitivity studies.

Within 8 to 12 hours after operation, the average patient who has undergone major abdominal or vaginal gynecologic surgery may sit up with assistance on the side of the bed in order to have her chest auscultated, and she should be encouraged to perform full lung expansion. The use of the intermittent positive pressure breathing apparatus has not been fully successful in avoiding pulmonary complications; however, its major value may be to encourage the patient to cough and take deep breaths.

Thromboembolic Complications. The most serious and life-threatening problem postoperatively is the development of phlebothrombosis and pulmonary embolism. In the typical patient, passive and active leg exercises in and out of bed are helpful, as is the use of elastic supportive stockings. Administration of prophylactic low-dose heparin (5000 U every 12 hours starting preoperatively) is advisable for high-risk patients, and it should be continued for about seven days postoperatively. Otherwise, the patient should be observed closely for the development of deep vein thrombosis in the lower extremities; unexplained tachycardia may be the first sign. Careful palpation of the deep calf veins for tenderness and Homans' sign should be done at least twice daily. A diagnosis of deep vein thrombosis is an indication for immediate full-dose heparinization for at least 7 to 10 days. Pulmonary emboli may be manifest by acute chest pain with coughing and hemoptysis or by sudden cardiorespiratory collapse. Evidence of pulmonary embolism should be substantiated as soon as possible by the use of lung scan or arteriography and arterial blood gas determinations. Immediate anticoagulation is essential, and proper supportive measures such as oxygen and digitalization should be instituted if necessary. The cardiothoracic surgery team should be alerted in the event that embolectomy or vena cava ligation is necessary.

Fluid and Electrolyte Replacement. Administration of fluids and electrolytes is begun with a peripheral intravenous line prior to operation. For the average minor operation, approximately 2 liters of five per cent dextrose–balanced salt solution in water is given during and after the operation. However, the primary objective is to have a line available in case of unexpected problems. Furthermore, this fluid replacement makes up for the restricted oral intake for the previous 12 hours.

Patients undergoing major procedures require more comprehensive replacement of fluids and electrolytes. The amounts are based on the duration of the operation, vomiting of significant amounts of gastric content, urinary output, perspiration, and fever. For the average healthy patient undergoing abdominal or vaginal hysterectomy, 3000 ml of fluid is usually given in the first 24 hours and should include 1 liter of 0.9 per cent sodium chloride, which will replace 154 mEq of lost sodium and chloride. Fluid orders thereafter are based on an accurate assessment of the patient's needs, taking all facts into consideration. A daily urinary output of 1200 to 1500 ml is desirable. As the patient is able to take in oral fluids and electrolytes, the intravenous administration of fluids is gradually decreased and may be stopped by the second or third postoperative day.

Patients requiring prolonged intravenous feedings require close evaluation of the serum electrolytes as well as total fluid intake, and the most accurate measurements of fluid and electrolyte losses should be obtained. While fluid orders may be written in ordinary situations for a 24-hour period, the critically ill patient or one who has had an extensive operation may need to have fluid and electrolyte needs determined at intervals of 6 to 12 hours.

Gastrointestinal Functions. With major operations, a certain amount of nausea is normal and may last for 12 to 24 hours. When the nausea has abated, oral alimentation may be started with hot tea, broth, or bouillon. The presence of nausea should be a contraindication to oral intake. As it subsides, cold liquids may be used in the form of ice water, ice chips, or carbonated beverages. Auscultation for peristalsis should be done for the first several days. Adequate peristalsis may take 24 to 72 hours to return, and when it occurs, the patient may have a diet as desired, preferably present in small, appetizing portions. Nausea or vomiting or significant abdominal distention signal poor intestinal activity, possibly even ileus, and all oral intake should be stopped. When flatus is passed, the intestinal tract is well on its way to recovery, and a bowel movement signals return of function. At this point, the patient is usually able to ingest a full diet.

During the second or third postoperative day, the patient may experience fairly severe colicky pain. Measures to provide comfort, such as a hot water bottle or heating pad applied to the abdomen, along with a rectal tube, may greatly relieve the distress, allow the passage of gas, and encourage future intestinal motility. Analgesic agents tend to depress intestinal function, and their use at this time should thus be kept to a minimum. The use of mild laxatives or enemas is helpful but should be given only when there are signs that the intestine is ready to function.

Evidence of ileus, as manifested by distention, minimal or absent peristalsis, nausea, vomiting, and absence of flatus, may be managed by restriction of oral intake and careful observation. A roentgenographic series should be obtained to rule out mechanical bowel obstruction. When nausea and vomiting are persistent, the use of gastric lavage or nasogastric suction is usually successful. In some instances, it may be necessary to advance a Miller-Abbott tube into the small intestine. Adequate fluid and electrolyte replacement during this time is important until the bowel begins to function again.

Mechanical obstruction may at first be masked by bowel inactivity, which is a normal accompaniment of the operation, or it may occur later in the recovery period. The usual signs and symptoms are nausea, vomiting, distention, and peristaltic rushes with high-pitched sounds. Such patients are best managed in a fashion similar to patients with ileus, since many may respond to the conservative treatment of introducing a long gastrointestinal tube. Fluid and electrolyte balance must be maintained as well as adequate hematocrit and serum protein concentrations. Persistence of symptoms of obstruction after a period of observation with the long gastrointestinal tube clamped must be usually dealt with by reexploration and correction of the cause of the obstruction.

Most patients are able to tolerate a full diet after the third postoperative day and should be able to continue this regimen when discharged from the hospital.

Urinary Tract. In patients undergoing minor gynecologic surgery, no indwelling catheter is necessary. However, a standing order for catheterization should always be written following both major and minor cases. In patients undergoing abdominal or vaginal hysterectomy (without vaginoplasty), an indwelling catheter should be left in overnight, and if the patient's condition is stable, it may be removed the next morning. Bladder trauma without laceration, hematuria, or the need to closely monitor the urinary output are indications for leaving the catheter in place. When vaginal plastic surgery has been performed on the anterior wall (cystocele repair), or with vesicourethral suspension (Marshall-Marchetti), the catheter is left in place until return of normal bladder function is imminent. This usually occurs after a minimum of five days.

If bladder catheterization is anticipated for more than one or two days, it is advisable to insert a suprapubic catheter and to utilize urinary antibacterial agents. Suprapubic drainage reduces the incidence of urinary tract infection and allows easy observation of the return of bladder function by simple clamping and allowing normal voiding to occur. Simple unclamping will determine the amount of residual urine. A residual urine of 50 ml or less is considered desirable prior to removing the catheter. If the bladder has been injured and then repaired, a suprapubic tube drain should be left in place for 7 to 10 days to allow the suture line to heal securely before voiding is tested.

Vaginal leakage of urine occurring 7 to 10 days after operation may suggest a ureterovaginal or vesicovaginal fistula. This first admonition here is a "don't." Do *not* perform either speculum or digital examination of the vagina, since such examination may break up adhesions and reduce the chances for spontaneous fistula healing. Instead, a dye solution (indigo-carmine in water) should be inserted via a catheter into the bladder. Appearance of the dye solution very shortly thereafter at the introitus constitutes good evidence of a vesicovaginal fistula. If the dye does not appear quickly, the bladder should be emptied, and an ampule of indigo-carmine dye should be given intravenously. If the dye now appears at the introitus, there is suggestive evidence of a ureterovaginal fistula. An intravenous pyelogram should also be performed, since it may help identify the site of the fistula. A vesicovaginal fistula that appears shortly after operation may have a chance for spontaneous closure if the patient is placed on her abdomen and gentle intermittent suction is applied to the indwelling catheter. Treatment of ureterovaginal fistulas must be individualized, although watchful observation and splinting with a ureteral catheter may be initially considered.

The Wound. Following abdominal celiotomy, the wound may or may not be covered. Esthetically, most patients probably prefer a dressing, but from the standpoint of infection and healing, a dressing is unnecessary. Generally the wound is not redressed for three to five days unless there is evidence of bleeding or infection in which the wound may be the source. Once uncovered, the wound should be inspected daily and palpated for signs of serum collection, hematomas, or pus. Collections should be evacuated by reopening the wound as often as necessary to provide adequate drainage. Drains may be needed occasionally, and local irrigation with peroxide and antiseptic agents may be helpful. Necrotic tissue should always be removed by débridement. As the wound granulates, strips of adhesive tape may be used to encourage approximation of the skin edges to provide a better cosmetic result.

Serosanguineous drainage from the wound should alert the surgeon to beginning wound disruption, which heralds dehiscence or evisceration. Careful inspection with removal of several sutures should be done to ascertain the integrity of the wound. Preparations should be made for the return of the patient to the operating room should dehiscence with actual or pending evisceration be observed.

Sutures or clips are usually removed on the fifth or sixth day. A loose dressing may be kept in place, and the patient may be allowed to bathe the wound gently and to reapply the dressing. Some patients are more comfortable with a binder or elastic girdle, although the routine use of these adjuncts is not necessary.

Ambulation. The patient may sit up with assistance on the night of operation or the following morning. On the first day, the patient should be assisted to a chair at least twice and allowed to sit up for periods of 30 to 40 minutes. These periods should be lengthened each day as long as there are no contraindications. By the third or fourth day, usually free of encumbrances such as catheters and intravenous apparatus, she can ambulate freely on her own. Elderly and debilitated patients may need extra help and encouragement to attain full ambulatory status.

Fever. Postoperative fever is not uncommon. In general, most patients experience a low-grade temperature elevation for the first 24 to 48 hours of 99 or 100°F. Higher temperatures are an indication that the site and etiology of the febrile state should be sought. Cultures from the pulmonary tract, the urinary tract, and the vagina should be obtained and a thorough examination carried out in an effort to localize any infectious process. Also, anaerobic bacterial cultures should always be done, since many gynecologic infections are due to such organisms. Collections in either the abdominal wound or vaginal cuff should be handled by opening and drainage. This may be sufficient if either is the source of the fever. Frequently, antibiotics are used before the correct identification of the fever source or the infecting organism. Ideally, such empiric use of antibiotics should be avoided until identification is complete. Persistent fever after an adequate course of antibiotic therapy may be a sign of pelvic thrombophlebitis. A trial of heparin therapy with a good response provides diagnostic help.

CARE AFTER DISCHARGE FROM THE HOSPITAL

The typical patient who has had an uncomplicated vaginal or abdominal hysterectomy may be discharged to her home by the fifth to seventh day. It is very helpful for the patient to receive a specific outline of "do's" and "don'ts" prior to discharge. This list should be given in addition to the appropriate prescriptions for necessary medications.

While each surgeon has his or her own specific instructions, and each with valid reasons, some general guidelines are provided here:

1. Upon reaching home, the patient is advised to continue a hospital-type routine for about 24 hours.

2. Climbing stairs is permitted during the first week, preferably once or twice daily.

3. The patient is to stay indoors or, weather permitting, remain on a secluded patio or porch for the first week.

4. After one week she may go for outside walks and ride in a car, but she may not drive a car for three or four weeks, particularly if it is a standard shift model.

5. She may bathe as she desires; showers, tub baths, and hair washing are permitted.

6. After bathing, if there is an abdominal wound, the patient should pat it dry and apply a light dressing. If the wound is healed, a large loose linen handkerchief may keep the area from rubbing against the underclothes.

7. The patient may observe a light bloody or brown vaginal discharge for approximately 14 days after going home. Steady bleeding resembling a menstrual period should be reported immediately to the physician.

8. Two weeks following discharge from the hospital, after either abdominal or vaginal hysterectomy, saline douches are begun with one teaspoon of table salt added to a quart of warm water.

9. No heavy housework or carrying large packages from shopping trips should be done for four to six weeks.

10. The first postoperative examination should be scheduled four to six weeks after discharge.

11. The patient may return to work in approximately six weeks.

12. For patients who have had vaginal plastic repair or operation for correction of urinary stress incontinence, straining and lifting heavy objects should be permanently avoided.

13. Sexual relations may be resumed in four to six weeks.

This chapter is not designed to cover all of the detailed aspects of the problems that have been described, since comprehensive information is available in other parts of this text. Also, specialized and intensive preparation of patients for infertility and oncology procedures are not detailed because the management is quite different from the preoperative and postoperative care that is applicable to the most frequent type of gynecologic patient.

REFERENCES

Bolling, D. R., and Plunkett, G. D.: Prophylactic antibiotics for vaginal hysterectomies. Obstet. Gynecol., 41:689, 1973.

deAlvarez, R. R.: Textbook of Gynecology. Philadelphia, Lea and Febiger, 1977, pp. 473–486, 523–535.

Forney, J. P., Morrow, C. P., Townsend, D. E., and DiSaia, P. J.: Impact of cephalosporin prophylaxis on conization-vaginal hysterectomy morbidity. Am. J. Obstet. Gynecol., *125*:100, 1976.

Goosenberg, J., Emich, J. P., Jr., and Schwarz, R. H.: Prophylactic antibiotics in vaginal hysterectomy. Am. J. Obstet. Gynecol., *105*:503, 1969.

Green, T. H., Jr.: Urinary stress incontinence. *In* Buchsbaum, H. J., and Schmidt, J. D.: Gynecologic and Obstetric Urology. Philadelphia, W. B. Saunders Co., 1978, pp. 162–187.

Ledger, W. J., Sweet, R. L., and Headington, J. T.: Prophylactic cephaloridine in the prevention of post-operative pelvic infections in premenopausal women undergoing vaginal hysterectomy, Am. J. Obstet. Gynecol., *115*:766, 1973.

Nelson, J. H., Jr.: Atlas of Radical Pelvic Surgery. New York, Appleton-Century-Crofts, 1977.

Nissen, E. D., and Goldstein, A. J.: A prospective investigation of the etiology of febrile morbidity following abdominal hysterectomy. Am. J. Obstet. Gynecol., *113*:111, 1972.

Sustendal, G. F., and Collins, C. G.: Abdominal wound complications in obstetrical and gynecological surgery. Obstet. Gynecol., *1*:264, 1953.

35

The Patient with Neurologic Dysfunction

WILLIAM F. COLLINS
CHARLES C. DUNCAN

Patients with neurologic dysfunction as a group are frequently considered apart from the general surgical population because of some specialized aspects of medical care and specific operative risks. There is no doubt that many of these patients present unique and complex problems, but once a few basic concepts and principles are understood, the care of these patients follows a logical progression in application of such knowledge. No matter how skilled the surgeon, the outcome of the neurologic surgical patient depends as much on the effectiveness of the surgeon's preoperative and postoperative care as it does on the efficacy of the operative procedures the surgeon performs.

The cause of any alteration in the neurologic function and the neurologic status of the patient, that is, the history and physical examination, are central to the care of the patient with neurologic dysfunction. While loss of motor, sensory, or cranial nerve function characterizes local central nervous system damage, consciousness is the sine qua non of a functioning brain and signifies both adequate perfusion of the nervous system and adequate function of the various body mechanisms that preserve homeostasis. It cannot be overstressed that in both the preoperative and postoperative periods, the surgeon must recognize any signs of an altered state of consciousness. This is the most important index of brain function as a whole and the most important parameter to monitor in determining whether the patient is improving or deteriorating. The state of consciousness is also the most sensitive indicator of the effectiveness of the treatment. Today the surgeon must be especially careful not to forget the patient amongst all of the sophisticated neuroradiologic procedures, computer printouts, and digital displays that have become part of the surgeon's armamentarium. He or she should consider what is happening to the function of the nervous system so that these aids to diagnosis can help answer the appropriate questions. A decision to undertake a diagnostic test involves knowledge of what question the test will answer, whether the answer is really necessary for the treatment being considered, how long the test will take, and whether delay may negate the benefit of possible therapeutic intervention based on the confirmed diagnosis.

The specialized problems of performing either neurosurgical or other surgical procedures on patients with neurologic dysfunction relate to maintenance of blood flow to the nervous system, prevention of new or additional compression of focal areas of the nervous system, prevention of shifts of portions of the nervous system to adjacent compartments of the cranium, and protection of the patient from loss of nervous system function vital to maintain the essential physical and chemical balance.

BLOOD SUPPLY OF THE NERVOUS SYSTEM

The blood flow through an organ is directly related to the arterial pressure and inversely to the vascular resistance. In calculating cerebral blood flow, the added factor of intracranial pressure must be considered, since intracranial pressure is essentially the tissue pressure acting to increase resistance to blood flow. In the brain, perfusion pressure equals arterial pressure minus intracranial pressure. A minimum of 50 to 60 mm Hg intracranial perfusion pressure is required for adequate blood flow. Cerebral blood flow remains relatively constant throughout a wide range of systemic arterial pressure (50 to 150 mm Hg mean arterial pressure) by the mechanism of autoregulation. However, in the face of increased intracranial pressure, the only mechanism to retain adequate cerebral perfusion pressure is an elevation of systemic arterial pressure, which occurs at levels of intracranial pressure at which perfusion of the brain is usually compromised. Other factors to be considered in ascertaining perfusion of the brain are the possibilities of blockage of cervical or intracranial vessels by atherosclerosis or other abnormalities or the presence of arteriovenous shunts in tumors or vascular malformations. In these conditions, arterial pressure to a portion or all of the brain is compromised, and any decrease in systemic arterial pressure may be reflected in a loss of focal or general neurologic function.

Patients with stenotic cerebrovascular lesions have a very small margin of safety. If such an individual becomes hypotensive, whether from decreased blood volume, low cardiac output, or pharmacologically induced hypotension, he or she may sustain profound neurologic deficit. Similarly, hypoxia and hypoglycemia are poorly tolerated. Such patients must maintain adequate blood pressure, oxygenation, and blood glucose levels at all times. In some instances of known blockage of cervical vessels, a carotid endarterectomy to reestablish adequate perfusion pressure may be indicated before a procedure that has a high probability of causing hypotension is undertaken.

INCREASED INTRACRANIAL PRESSURE

The problems of increased intracranial pressure are more frequently encountered in neurosurgical patients than in other surgical patients, but the condition can occur in both and may be precipitated by an inadequate understanding of both its mechanism of production and its mechanism for causing secondary neural injury. A wide variety of intracranial disorders lead to increased intracranial pressure, but they fall mainly into three basic categories: mass lesions, cerebral edema, and obstruction of cerebrospinal fluid (CSF) pathways. A combination of mechanisms, i.e., mass lesions causing edema or obstruction of CSF pathways or both, is common. The mechanisms by which increased intracranial pressure causes secondary injury to the brain also fall into three basic types: altered intracranial perfusion, shift of intracranial contents, and compression of neural tissue. Alteration in vascular supply and compression of neural tissue may also produce major secondary injury to the spinal cord. The intracranial compartment, while not an entirely enclosed box, physically acts like one so that intracranial pressure is related directly to volume. The cerebrospinal fluid and other extracellular fluid of the brain accounts for about 10 per cent of the volume, blood is about 3 per cent, and 87 per cent of the volume consists of cellular structures and intracellular fluid. There are several mechanisms, primarily consisting of alteration in the volume of CSF, extracellular fluid, and blood, which can compensate for relatively rapid changes (over a period of hours or days) in intracranial pressure. More long-term compensation (over months and years) relies mainly on changes in cellular components and skull volume, as may be seen in infants.

The ability of the intracranial contents to sustain moderate increases in volume without alteration in pressure is called compliance, and its loss signifies small increases in intracranial volume, which are reflected by large increases in intracranial pressure. Compliance can be measured by plotting the effect of small increases in volume, usually of fluid injected into the ventricles via ventriculostomy, on intracranial pressure. When intracranial pressure monitoring is being performed, compliance can also be estimated by measuring the height of the ventricular pulse wave. With low compliance, the systolic portion of the wave may reflect 50 to 60% of the systolic-diastolic difference or 20 to 30 mm Hg pressure, an ominous sign.

As previously mentioned, cerebral blood flow is related directly to perfusion pressure and inversely related to vascular resistance. The cerebral blood flow and, in part, the intracranial blood volume are directly porportional to arterial P_{CO_2}, since increased P_{CO_2} decreases central nervous system vascular resistance. Variation in PCO_2 alters not only cerebral blood flow but also intracranial blood volume and, in low compliance states, intracranial pressure. The neurologically injured patient undergoing anesthesia may have respiratory depression so that PCO_2 is elevated, causing dangerous levels of increased intracranial pressure, which can markedly decrease perfusion pressure. The need for both direct measurement of PCO_2 and assisted respiration to maintain levels of PCO_2 between 30 and 35 mm Hg has been recognized by anesthesiologists and neurosurgeons for many years.

In lesions involving vascular damage, particularly those that cause increased intracranial pressure, the capacity for autoregulation is frequently lost or markedly impaired. When this happens, cerebral blood flow passively follows the systemic arterial pressure and may cause levels of increased intracranial pressure that impair cerebral perfusion, or brief episodes of hypotension can be devastating because of the attendant decrease in cerebral blood flow. The most frequent deficits resulting from increased intracranial pressure are a result of ischemia. With inadequate or no blood flow to the brain, irreversible neuronal damage occurs in a matter of minutes.

Another factor that must be considered in cases of low compliance states is the ability of water to pass the blood-brain and blood–spinal fluid barriers. A major factor in the passage of water is the relative osmolarity of the intravascular and extravascular components of the intracranial compartments. Thus, an intravenously administered water load that does not contain electrolytes or other osmotic substances can result in an increase in the volume of extracellular or intracellular fluid compartments of the cranium, followed by increased intracranial pressure. They may also increase the intravascular compartments; thus, the rate of administration must be carefully monitored. Intravenous osmotic agents such as mannitol or urea exert their effect because they are large molecules that are prevented from crossing the blood-brain and blood–spinal fluid barriers. They produce an osmotic gradient between the extravascular and intravascular compartment with water moving up the osmotic gradient and out of the brain. Osmotic diuretics thus decrease brain water, thereby decreasing intracranial pressure and increasing compliance. These general comments about compliance are applicable to all forms of increased intracranial pressure, but they are more specifically related to pressure resulting from mass lesions and edema than pressure caused by blockage of cerebrospinal circulation.

Secondary injury from mass lesions can also be caused by the shift of intracranial contents. The brain acts as a solid fluid, i.e., it retains its shape in normal conditions but flows from high-pressure areas toward low-pressure areas when stressed. There are three clinical patterns seen with such a shift. The most common is a shift beneath the falx cerebri after mass effect in one hemisphere, whether from tumor, hemorrhage, edema, or a combination. This shift can cause altered consciousness and psychomotor retardation because of the propensity of the cingulate gyrus of the frontal lobe not only to herniate beneath the falx but also to compress the opposite cingulate gyrus, both a portion of the limbic system. Even more serious shifts are those of the medial temporal lobe and midbrain through the incisura of the tentorium and the cerebellar tonsils and lower brain stem through the foramen magnum.

The incisura syndrome, signifying shift of the uncal-hippocampus gyrus of the temporal lobe and midbrain, most commonly presents as a triad of decrease in level of consciousness, compression of the third nerve with dilatation of the ipsilateral pupil, followed by decerebrate posturing. Both the shift of the midbrain downward and the compression of the midbrain by one or both medial temporal lobes alters its blood supply, causing infarction and hemorrhage. If continued unabated, irreversible damage results; thus, it is necessary to recognize the syndrome before midbrain compromise, and this is why the pupil is watched carefully in patients with mass lesions or those with the potential for mass lesions.

The foramen magnum syndrome is also identified by a triad of symptoms. There is a decreasing level of consciousness, probably a result of decreased function of the brain stem reticular formation, followed by changes in medulla function, which frequently cause slowing of the pulse and respiratory rate with an elevation in blood pressure, or the Cushing reflex. This may be followed by periodic respirations or Cheyne-Stokes respirations and respiratory arrest. Both the incisural and foramen magnum syndromes can occur suddenly, especially following removal of cerebrospinal fluid by lumbar puncture. Although all three of these syndromes can occur with any type of increased intracranial pressure, they occur more commonly in the presence of mass lesions. The definitive treatment to control the brain shift and increased intracranial pressure is surgical removal of the mass. The use of altered PCO_2, osmotic diuretics, and other agents such as corticosteroids affect only temporary control but may be lifesaving in the acute situation.

Hydrocephalus results if there is an obstruction to the flow of cerebrospinal fluid from the ventricles, where it is formed, to the upper surface of the hemispheres, where it is reabsorbed. Removal of cerebrospinal fluid by ventricular puncture is the safest method for gaining temporary control (hours) of increased intracranial pressure caused by hydrocephalus, while shunting of cerebrospinal fluid to an external site by ventriculostomy drainage can give a longer period of control (days), while shunting of cerebrospinal fluid to the venous system or pleural or abdominal cavities via a pressure regulated valve is necessary to control intracranial pressure for any long period of time. Ventriculostomy to an external reservoir has the advantage of allowing both measurement of increased intracranial pressure and removal of CSF as required to control the intracranial pressure, but it has the disadvantage of a high risk of infection. With careful technique, the incidence of infection is low for ventriculostomies in place less than five days but rises rapidly with longer periods of use. When utilizing external ventriculostomy, a daily examination of the CSF, including daily cultures, is indicated in order to diagnose and treat as early as possible any infection that might occur.

When increased intracranial pressure occurs, there is a vital relationship between intracranial perfusion pressure and intracranial pressure that must be controlled for the preservation of neural tissue. There are shifts of the nervous system caused by focal or generalized increased intracranial pressure that can destroy vital central nervous system function. Both effects can be caused by masses, edema, or blockage of CSF. When intracranial pressure rises to levels of arterial pressure or arterial pressure falls below intracranial pressure, brain perfusion ceases and brain death occurs in minutes. Rapid methods of intracranial pressure reduction include reduction in blood P_{CO_2}, removal of water from the extravascular spaces with osmotic diuretics, and removal of CSF. Although the reduction of P_{CO_2} to 20 mm Hg or less decreases intracranial blood volume and, therefore, intracranial pressure, it does so by increasing vascular resistance and decreasing cerebral blood flow. Therefore, it usually can be used for only brief periods. As soon as P_{CO_2} returns to 25 or 30 mm Hg, other methods for reducing intracranial pressure should be utilized. The osmotic diuretic most commonly used to control intracranial pressure is mannitol, usually in a 20 per cent solution. In an emergency situation, 1.0 to 1.5 gm of mannitol per kg body weight are given intravenously over a 10- to 15-minute period. The effect of increased intravascular volume on intracranial pressure and cardiac function must always be considered. Increased cerebral blood volume itself can cause a decrease in the level of consciousness, and in the patient with low cardiac reserve, it may even precipitate cardiac failure. If osmotic diuretics are used, the patient's neurologic functions should be monitored by frequent evaluation, especially of levels of consciousness. Pulmonary wedge or right atrial pressure should be monitored carefully in those patients in whom poor cardiac reserve is suspected. The diuresis with these solutions in a well-hydrated patient can be rapid and of significant volume so that a urinary catheter should be in place in the unconscious patient or in the patient with possible urethral obstruction in order to prevent bladder rupture. If the suspected cause of a neurologic dysfunction is intracranial hemorrhage, such as occurs after trauma or surgery, the tamponade effect of increased intracranial pressure on damaged blood vessels may be lost when the intracranial pressure is rapidly decreased, precipitating further bleeding. In this situation, the patient may improve significantly for a brief period of time and then acutely deteriorate. For these reasons, when such a patient is treated with an osmotic diuretic, the physician caring for the patient is committed to rapid diagnosis and treatment, for the period of improvement may, in the case of arterial bleeding, be very brief. However, neurologic improvement following decreased intracranial pressure should not allow the attending physician to relax his or her vigil. Other methods of decreasing intracranial pressure include removal of CSF by ventricular puncture or spinal tap and removal of mass lesions. A combination of methods may be required in the patient with rapidly progressing neurologic dysfunction or marked neurologic loss, and use of all methods should be considered for patients with increased intracranial pressure of a level that might cause secondary injury to the nervous system.

DIAGNOSTIC PROCEDURES

A few years ago, the patient suspected of having an intracranial mass lesion initially underwent what was rather unkindly referred to by some as the "worthless triad." This consisted of skull films, an isotope brain scan, and an electroencephalogram. Following these procedures, depending upon their outcome, arteriography, air study, or both might be undertaken. If the patient was too ill for such an elective workup, he or she might go directly to the operating room for surgical treatment based on the history and initial neurologic examination.

The neurologic patient may still undergo what appears to be a maze of diagnostic studies, and a brief listing of them along with the information they provide and their possible complications should help to place them in perspective. Currently, computerized cranial tomography or CT scanning has greatly changed the diagnostic approach to both the emergent and elective neurosurgical patient. Government agencies continue to argue about the cost effectiveness of such equipment; however, the impact of the device is so dramatic for the care of the neurosurgery patient that optimal neurosurgical care cannot be practiced without a scanner. The information produced by the scanner is precise anatomic data regarding most structural intracranial lesions but is less specific regarding the pathologic basis for the anatomic lesion. The capability of the scanner to diagnose intracranial pathology is still at its threshold, and further advances are continually occurring.

In patients with intracranial tumor, abscess, or hemorrhage, the CT scanner is accurate in localizing the process and often accurate in suggesting the diagnosis, especially when iodinated intravenous contrast material for the enhancement of the lesion is used. The CT scanner is also very accurate in making the diagnosis and determining the position and extent of the process in patients with intracranial hemorrhage, either occurring spontaneously or secondary to trauma, provided the hemorrhage has occurred within a few days of the scan. The cause of the hemorrhage other than trauma often requires arteriography. Procedural complications of CT scanning are rare and are usually related to allergic reaction to the iodinated contrast material and, unless precautions are taken, to obstruction of the airway of a patient with decreased mental acuity when placed in the machine in the preferred position with the neck flexed.

Cerebral arteriography provides direct roentgenographic visualization of the cerebrovascular tree from the arterial to the capillary and venous phases of the circulation, as well as evaluation of the cervical, carotid, and vertebral arteries. Most studies are done with femoral catheter techniques because they are considerably safer than the formerly used direct carotid and vertebral punctures. Arteriography demonstrates the shift of vessels, areas of obstruction or stenosis either in cervical or intracranial vessels, neovascularization in tumors and malformations, and arteriovenous shunts. The studies are also helpful in determining the presence or absence of collateral circulation when designing surgical revascularization procedures. The major complications are stroke and adverse reaction to the contrast medium. Patients with arteriosclerotic vascular disease are higher risks for such studies than other patients.

The anatomy of the subclavian and innominate arteries provides another means for angiographic studies. Thus, a right retrograde brachial arteriogram can visualize the right carotid and vertebral circulation in most patients, and a left retrograde brachial arteriogram shows the posterior fossa circulation via the left vertebral artery without direct manipulation of either the carotid or vertebral arteries. Specialized techniques, which include subtraction, magnification, and selective arteriography, frequently provide information important in designing surgical approaches to the intracranial contents.

Air studies provide roentgenographic visualization of the ventricular system and subarachnoid spaces and cisterns by the decrease in radiation absorption of air in these structures. Pneumoencephalography is carried out by an injection of air or oxygen into the lumbar cistern while the patient is in an upright position. The air rises to fill subarachnoid spaces and ventricles. When this procedure is carried out in a fractional manner, i.e., using small amounts of air and with the use of laminography, it yields accurate information regarding the cisterns, ventricles, and their surrounding structures. As long as significant shifts, obstruction, and greatly increased intracranial pressure have been ruled out, this is an exceedingly safe examination, although considerable short-term morbidity, frequently expressed by headache, is almost universally encountered. If shifts, obstruction of CSF flow, or increased pressure is present, the patient may acutely decompensate during air studies. In these instances, ventriculography is safer; it gives information regarding the ventricular system and adjacent structures, but little or no information is generally obtained concerning the basal cisterns and subarachnoid spaces. Ventriculography is performed by placing a twist drill or burr hole through the skull and passing a ventricular needle or catheter into the lateral ventricle. Following this, air, or in some instances positive contrast medium, such as radiopaque substances, is exchanged with the CSF. Risks of this procedure include intracranial hemorrhage, infection, and acute decompensation with shift of the nervous system.

The latter, while not as imminent a danger as with pneumoencephalography, is encountered often enough that the use of ventriculography without prior preparation for surgical removal of mass lesions should not be done.

Depending upon the specific diagnostic questions being asked, other studies may be indicated, such as electroencephalography, isotope brain scans, and xenon cerebral blood flow studies. The first identifies areas of markedly altered cortical function and the presence of seizures, while isotope brain scan can confirm the presence of a breakdown in the blood-brain barrier as seen with stroke, infections, or tumor, and it can be used to define the flow of CSF. Cerebral blood flow study has become more important as methods for correcting inadequate focal and general cerebral perfusion are coming into widespread use.

Diagnostic studies for defining spinal pathology include plain radiographic spine films, laminograms of the spine, myelography, CT scanning, and angiography. Myelography is generally carried out with the water-soluble contrast material metrizamide. Most myelograms are carried out by lumbar puncture, although C1-C2 puncture is preferred in a number of specialized situations such as a spinal block in order to define the upper and lower borders of the lesion. The contrast agent is placed in the spinal canal with fluoroscopic control. Complications include adverse reaction to the contrast medium, direct damage to neural tissue by the needle puncture, and decompensation of spinal cord function by shifting of the spinal canal contents. Metrizamide has been associated with seizures in seizure-prone individuals and headache when the contrast medium spills into the head. For these reasons, patients undergoing such myelography should spend the 24 hours following the procedure with the head elevated. Decompensation usually occurs when spinal fluid is removed below a block, causing the cerebrospinal fluid pressure above the block to force the spinal cord and the lesion to move against the bony ring of the spinal canal, resulting in compression and decreased local blood supply. For these reasons, any myelography done when a compressing lesion of the spinal cord or cauda equina is suspected should be performed only when surgical means for relief of such pressure are immediately available.

FLUID MANAGEMENT

The surgical patient who has neurologic dysfunction or who has undergone intracranial operation has first and foremost the requirements of any surgical patient, that is, maintenance of intravascular volume and electrolyte balance. However, there are three aspects of fluid balance in the neurosurgical patient that frequently cause problems, and they must be considered in designing fluid replacement and maintenance schedules. First is the fluid balance of a patient with breakdown in the blood-brain or blood–spinal fluid barriers by disease, operation, or trauma, since passage of water into extravascular spaces occurs not in relation to the availability of electrolytes but in relation to the relative osmotic pressures in the two spaces. Thus, hypo-osmolar solutions can cause increased intracranial pressure by passage of water into the extracellular (including CSF) spaces and intracellular compartments of the cranium. Correct maintenance of intravascular osmolarity is essential. Fluids such as 5 per cent or 10 per cent dextrose in water, when metabolized, become free water, and although water for insensible loss and urination is necessary, any excess can cause a problem. Monitoring of fluid output and serum osmolarity is required. The second problem, one that is frequently missed, is the syndrome of inappropriate antidiuretic hormone (SIADH), which can occur following head trauma or operation on the central nervous system. In this situation, the stimulus for decreasing the output of ADH, that is, hypo-osmolarity, causes an increase in the output of ADH, resulting in retention of water and, secondarily, the excretion of electrolytes. The excretion of electrolytes is probably secondary to alteration in the aldosterone mechanism caused by the increased blood volume associated with the retained water. The condition was formerly called hyponatremia, since the serum sodium concentration is lowered by dilution with retained water. The actual sodium loss, however, is much less than estimated by such a measurement. Although infusion of 3 per cent hypertonic saline can temporarily improve the altered central nervous system function, the infused sodium chloride is usually excreted and the water is retained, causing further dilution and hypo-osmolarity. Restriction of water intake is the treatment of choice, but occasionally methods to bypass or overcome the ADH mechanisms can be used for patients in an acute condition. These include solute diuretics such as mannitol or drugs that decrease tubular reabsorption of water. The latter often increase excretion of electrolytes, and replacement therapy may be necessary. SIADH can be diagnosed by measuring the osmolarity of the serum and urine; the urine osmolarity is high in the face of hypo-osmolarity of the serum. Also, the sodium excretion in the urine is elevated at the same time that the serum sodium is low.

The third problem is the opposite of SIADH, or diabetes insipidus, in which ADH is deficient. This is most commonly seen following pituitary surgery or injury to or manipulation of the hypothalamus or pituitary stalk. It can, however, be seen as a late complication of previous pituitary surgery or injury. In milder forms, replacement of urinary loss with water is the only treatment required, while in more severe cases, administration of vasopressin is necessary for control. Excessive vasopressin administration is always a danger, since it results in SIADH; thus, a careful balance of water intake and output must be maintained when this drug is used.

SPINAL CORD

When operating on patients with spinal cord disease or when operating on the spinal cord itself, potential problems with blood flow that are similar to those described with intracranial problems must be borne in mind. Major sources of blood supply to the spinal cord must be understood, and possible compression of the spinal cord by masses or disorders of the spinal column must be considered.

Although each spinal root has a radicular artery or arteries accompanying it, the blood supply of the spinal cord originates primarily from three sources: the vertebral arteries at C1 forming the anterior spinal artery; the thyrocervical trunk on the left or a branch from the upper thoracic intercostals, entering the spinal canal in the lower cervical or upper thoracic level, supplying blood to the anterior spinal artery; and the artery of Ademkowitz, arising from the aorta in the lower thoracic or upper lumbar area and entering the canal betweel T8 and L1 on the left side. This anatomic configuration of arterial supply leaves a major area of relatively poor perfusion in the midthoracic area. With diseases of the arteries, particularly of the aorta or thyrocervical trunk, this area of poor perfusion may be much more extensive and the cord much more sensitive to hypotension. The same principles concerning blood supply of the cord must be considered when any surgical procedure is contemplated that may involve the integrity of any of the major arterial trunks entering the spinal canal.

Although the spinal canal is not a closed space, the vertebral bony ring enclosing the spinal cord and cauda equina acts as a compressing force if bony spurs, hypertrophy of ligaments, or any mass lesion is present within the ring. Such compressing force increases vascular resistance, placing the cord in jeopardy to systemic hypotension, and can result in spinal cord infarction. Removal of spinal fluid by lumbar puncture beneath a partial block of the spinal canal can also cause compression by shifting the lesion beneath the vertebral ring.

Disorders of the spinal column that may cause compression of the spinal cord include trauma, degenerative disease, and tumors of the bony canal. In the trauma patient, the stability of the spine is, of course, of utmost importance, and radiographic assessments of such stability are necessary before any manipulation, including the induction of anesthesia, is performed. If airway control is required before a film can be made to determine that there is no dislocation or instability of the cervical spine, extreme caution must be exercised. Many patients, particularly older ones, have evidence of stenosis or narrowing of the cervical spinal canal. The diameter of the canal decreases with neck extension, a position very commonly used while intubating a patient. Therefore, great care must be taken at the time of intubation if the patient has osteoarthritis or stenosis of the cervical canal. The degree of extension the patient can voluntarily tolerate should be ascertained before muscle relaxants or anesthetic agents are given. It is quite possible to produce quadriplegia by extending the neck after using muscle relaxants and anesthetics.

Tumors of the bony canal are most often metastatic, and the patient in whom cancer is suspected and for whom either local pain over the spinal column or radicular pain is reported in the history should always arouse the suspicion of a potential compression lesion. Again, a major neurologic deficit in the spinal cord may result unless care is taken to rule out and control such lesions before manipulation or possible hypotension takes place.

STEROIDS

Since Galicich and French introduced the use of glucocorticoid dexamethasone to the practice of neurosurgery, it has become one of the most commonly used drugs in the surgery of the nervous system. Its use in the treatment of cerebral edema has contributed greatly to the increased survival rate of patients with a wide variety of intracranial lesions. Tumor, infection, or trauma appear to produce edema in different ways, and the pathophysiology of cerebral edema is only partially understood. Accordingly, the response of cerebral edema to steroids also varies with the different etiologies. The edema associated with metastatic tumor, for example, responds quite dramatically to steroids in a matter of hours; however, edema associated with trauma is less likely to do so. The evidence is quite clear that neural tissue pretreated with steroids is protected better than if given following a traumatic insult. Therefore, steroids are usually given preoperatively. There is also presumptive evidence that the earlier steroids are given following an insult, the more effective the drug is likely to be. The effect on edema is visible in terms of hours, and so administration of steroids has little bearing on the acute problem of increased intracranial pressure. While the usual adult dose of dexamethasone is 4 mg every six hours, there is recent evidence to indicate that much higher dosages may be more effective, particularly following trauma. Other glucocorticoids such as methylprednisolone can be used in an equivalent dosage. Acute withdrawal of steroids in patients with central nervous system injuries may cause rebound cerebral edema in addition to producing iatrogenic addisonian crisis, and, therefore, discontinuation should be tapered over a number of days.

SPECIAL SITUATIONS IN NEUROLOGIC AND NEUROSURGICAL PATIENTS

MASKING OF SYMPTOMS

Neurologic or neurosurgical patients are not immune to other disorders and frequently require non-neurosurgical procedures. Patients with altered levels of consciousness or with major loss of spinal cord function may not have the symptoms and signs physicians usually recognize to diagnose concurrent disease. The signs and symptoms of fractured bones and chest or abdominal injuries may be absent and recognized only by obvious deformity of a limb or from roentgenographic studies. An acute abdominal disorder may not manifest tenderness or have associated muscle spasm. All too frequently in a patient with a central nervous system injury, an abdomen may be soft on palpation without evidence of tenderness or reflex spasm despite harboring an injured viscus or organ with perforation or hemorrhage. The presence of peripheral vascular collapse or shock, a rare complication of central nervous system injury except as a terminal event, may be the only indication of abdominal or thoracic injury with blood loss. For this reason, careful examination of the abdomen or thorax, catheterization of the urinary bladder, radiologic studies, thoracentesis, paracentesis, and even surgical exploration may be indicated to determine the source of shock.

VENTRICULAR SHUNTS

Patients with ventriculovenous, ventriculopleural, or venticuloperitoneal shunts, which are usually placed to control hydrocephalus, are subject to a series of potential complications whenever they undergo operative procedures or sustain injuries. Since these shunts connect the cerebral ventricles, other body cavities, or the venous system, usual anatomic barriers are chronically transgressed. For this reason, infections are more likely in this group of patients than in other patients with implanted foreign bodies. Pleural, peritoneal, or bloodstream infection can result in ventriculitis and/or meningitis. Pleural and peritoneal infections that spread to the central nervous system are more obvious than the transient bacteremias that occur with endotracheal intubation, oral surgery, or surgery for abscesses. Such transient bacteremias can lead to serious infection in the patient with a ventriculovenous shunt. The most common organism cultured during these transient bacteremias that result in a shunt infection is *Staphylococcus*, and in order to minimize the risk of infection, patients with shunts should receive prophylactic antibiotics, usually oxacillin, before any manipulation is done and for 24 to 48 hours after any manipulation and/or after evidence of active infection has disappeared.

BASILAR SKULL FRACTURES

Patients who have sustained basilar skull fractures with or without evidence of communication from the outside to the subarachnoid space require cautious management from several standpoints. They are more likely to develop meningitis than the average patient. If anesthesia is required, the patient should not have positive pressure assisted respiration by facial mask, as is given before intubation, for this can drive contaminated material into the subarachnoid space. Suctioning and nasal or gastric intubation must be carefully performed in order to prevent further basilar skull damage or even penetration of the cranial cavity.

PITUITARY DYSFUNCTION

Patients who have a history of pituitary surgery, a diagnosis of pituitary tumor, or who have received high doses of steroids for chronic illness are likely to experience difficulties arising from inadequate steroid production or inadequate steroid reserve during periods of stress. Other inadequate pituitary hormone reserves, such as thyrotropic stimulating hormone, gonadotropic hormones, or growth hormones, play a small role in the patient's response to the stress of acute disease, trauma, or surgical operation. Thyroid deficits and the changes in glucose and fat metabolism with growth hormone deficits, however, assume increased importance during prolonged illness. Problems of water balance, as with inadequate antidiuretic hormone, may become critical if not monitored properly, since dehydration can become extreme in a relatively short period of time. Its treatment is replacement of the lost water and administration of antidiuretic hormone with vasopressin (Pitressin).

Possible glucocorticoid deficiency is a paramount concern in a patient with compromised pituitary function. Failure to recognize this problem can lead to catastrophe. Corticosteroid insufficiency may rapidly progress from mild complaints to total peripheral vascular collapse. The signs and symptoms of corticosteroid insufficiency range from vague malaise to nausea, tachycardia, diarrhea, hypotension, and peripheral vascular collapse. When major stress is encountered, as with trauma, operation, or infection, 100 mg of hydrocortisone or its equivalent in glucocorticoid activity should be given by intravenous drip every six hours until the stress has ended; then the dosage should be slowly tapered to the previous maintenance level.

CONVULSIONS

Patients with irritative cortical foci are more likely to have seizures as a result of stress, elevated temperature, metabolic imbalance, respiratory problems, and a wide variety of drug actions and disease processes. Because of the decreased seizure threshold that commonly occurs in the postoperative patient, it is wise to have blood levels of anticonvulsants drawn in patients with a known predisposition to seizures before a surgical procedure. This allows more accurate use of phenobarbital or other anticonvulsants intravenously to control seizures with less risk of respiratory depression or peripheral vascular collapse. The major problems in these patients are status epilepticus, which should be controlled with anticonvulsants, and respiratory depression, which may result from the obligatory use of high doses of anticonvulsants. The most frequent cause of seizures in these patients, however, is the failure of the physician or surgeon to continue anticonvulsants during diagnostic work-up or in the postoperative period.

SUMMARY

The care of the neurosurgical patient presents a number of distinct features whether he or she is primarily undergoing neurosurgical care or requires some other procedure. The basic principle of care is continued assessment of neurologic status. The more frequently utilized diagnostic procedures and complications have been outlined. If the surgeon keeps these aspects of care in mind, he or she should be able to provide appropriate support and treatment of the neurosurgical patient.

REFERENCES

Allen, M. B., Doetsch, G. S., Grindin, R. A., Haar, F. L., and Yaghmai, F.: A Manual of Neurosurgery. Baltimore, University Park Press, 1978.
Howe, J. R.: Patient Care in Neurosurgery. Boston, Little, Brown and Co., 1977.
Plum, F., and Posner, J. B.: Diagnosis of Stupor and Coma. Contemporary Neurology Series, Vol. 10, 3rd ed. Philadelphia, F. A. Davis Co., 1980.
Youmans, J. R. (ed.): Neurological Surgery, 2nd ed. Philadelphia, W. B. Saunders Co., 1982.

36

The Extremities

GEORGE F. SHELDON
DONALD TRUNKEY

Through evolution, the human primate has developed specialized functions for the upper extremities which provide finite tactile skills for food gathering and protection. The hand has developed into an appendage specialized to allow opposition, grasping, and handling of tools. The function of the lower extremities, however, remains primarily as a means of locomotion and support.

Although infrequently the source of life-threatening acute or chronic illness, the truncal appendages are commonly the source of secondary disease or injury. Moreover, metabolic, traumatic, and neoplastic diseases can produce significant disability by involvement of the extremities.

ESSENTIALS OF DIAGNOSIS

Because the extremities are paired structures, evaluation begins by comparing the appearance, circumference, length, range of motion, and temperature of the limbs. Characteristic positions can be assumed which suggest deviation from normal. The position of function of the upper extremity favors reaching the face and perineum. It provides a comfortable and unfatiguing grip, with the elbow held at 90 degrees, the forearm held neutral between pronation and supination, the wrist extended 30 to 40 degrees, and the fingers curled into a pronated position. The position of function is the ideal to be achieved by immobilization with a splint. In the position of rest or pain of the upper extremity, the wrist is flexed, making it awkward and fatiguing for the hand to grasp. Additionally, in the position of pain the forearm is pronated, and the elbow is extended; this is the position that the arm passively assumes after injury and paralysis.

In the position of function of the lower extremity the thigh is slightly adducted, the knee is flexed, and the ankle is in a neutral position between dorsiflexion and plantar flexion. In the position of pain the lower extremity is flaccid, flexed, and dependent. It is a position assumed after paralysis and below-knee amputation or with rest pain associated with vascular insufficiency.

The function of an extremity is frequently limited by pain, which makes evaluation difficult. However, neurologic examination of the hands and feet provides important information regardless of whether the problem is injury, vascular insufficiency, or neoplasm. Both motor and sensory dysfunction occur with brachial plexus injury, and frequently are manifest as mixed weakness of arm, forearm, and hand musculature. Injury of the median nerve (C5, C6, C7, C8, T1) above the elbow results in paralysis of the muscles of the thenar eminence and inability to oppose the thumb to the other digits. It is associated with sensory loss over the palmar aspect of the thumb, index, and middle fingers and the radial half of the fourth finger.

Radial nerve (C5, C6, C7, C8) injury results in wrist drop and inability to extend the fingers and thumb at the metacarpophalangeal joint. Radial nerve injury in the arm is associated with inability to extend the elbow. It characteristically is associated with anesthesia of the dorsum of the thumb, index and middle fingers, and part of the fourth finger.

Ulnar nerve (C7, C8, T1) injury results in inability to spread or close the fingers or flex the metacarpophalangeal joint, producing a "claw" hand. It is associated with anesthesia over the dorsal and palmar aspects of the little finger and ulnar half of the fourth finger.

The lower extremity is also innervated by three nerves. Injury to the sciatic nerve (L4, L5, S1, S2) results in a combination motor and sensory loss, identified by both peroneal and tibial nerve deficits. Injury to the peroneal nerve (L5, S1) results in loss of sensation over the dorsum of the foot and foot drop. Injury to the tibial nerve (L5, S1) causes loss of plantar flexion of the ankle and toes with sensory loss of the lateral aspect of the foot.

The circulation to the extremities carries oxygen and substrate to the tissue, removes carbon dioxide and lactic acid, and is adversely affected by both chronic and acute disorders. Chronic and acute forms of impaired circulation to the extremities are determined primarily by history and physical examination. The history documents duration of symptoms, character of the pain, and loss of function. On physical examination, the pulses are graded and compared with the opposite extremity. No vascular examination is complete without careful recording of all available pulses in conjunction with capillary filling, appearance, and temperature of the skin (see Chapter 28). We grade the pulses on a scale from 0 to 4, with 0 indicating an absent pulse and 4 a normal one.

Because the objective of pre- and postoperative care of the extremities is preservation of function consistent with survival, modalities useful in maximizing the evaluation and effect of treatment will be emphasized. As the management of extremity problems frequently involves specialists with different orientations, a functional approach is presented to emphasize specific treatment of the skin and soft tissue, the circulation, and the bones.

SKIN AND SOFT TISSUE

The skin is the body's largest organ. It serves as a barrier against infection, functions as a primary immunologic defense, and prevents loss of body fluids. The skin regulates body temperature by serving as the effector organ, with the thalamus functioning as the thermostat. The skin is a crude excretory organ, which disposes of water, salt, urea, and cholesterol. Sensory and tactile functions, particularly in the skin of the hand, are vital. The skin synthesizes vitamin D, which is necessary for calcium homeostasis and bone stability. The skin, by differences in texture, distribution, and pigmentation, helps to determine identity.

Evaluation of pre- and postoperative lesions of the extremity skin begins with the history and physical examination. The length of time a lesion has been present, as well as changes in color, size, and shape, requires precise delineation. Moreover, the presence or absence of pain, as well as other sensory changes, is important to evaluate. When injury to the skin has occurred, knowledge of the wounding agent helps to determine if antibiotics are necessary and the degree of tetanus prophylaxis required.

Inspection and palpation should include five observations that are basic to the evaluation of the protective covering of the extremities. Color changes are frequently caused by disease of the skin, alteration in blood supply, or pigmentation. Changes in mass are caused by cellular proliferation, infiltration, or injury. Free fluid within the dermis appears as a solid mass in contusions or cellulitis. Fluid accumulation in the epidermis or between the epidermis and dermis appears as vesicles. Skin lesions, nevi, keratosis, and melanoma appear as alterations in both texture and color. Diabetes, fatty acid deficiency, and vascular insufficiency cause scanty hair growth, a thin scaly epidermis, and poor nail growth. Moreover, tightness of the skin and subcutaneous tissue occurs in scleroderma and other collagen disorders. Skin temperature is an important barometer of perfusion and reflects sympathetic regulation of vascular tone as well as vascular insufficiency from arteriosclerosis. Gradations of loss of blood supply to the skin may occur in response to cold and appear as blanching, pallor, coolness (Raynaud's syndrome), and gangrene (Raynaud's disease).

Infections of the extremity are common, usually present as skin infections, and often are associated with inadequate blood supply or with a systemic disease such as diabetes mellitus. Moreover, infections occurring in the hands or feet have potential for involving pulp spaces, tendon sheaths, and fascial spaces, resulting in disability and amputation. As most extremity infections are due to hemolytic *Streptococcus* or *Staphylococcus aureus* which produce hyaluronidase, rapid progression of infections occurs along fascial planes. For example, paronychia is a localized infective lesion of the finger or foot treated by removing the portion of the nail that acts as a foreign body. Terminal pulp space infections (felon) are also localized and usually are adequately treated by drainage, antibiotics, and immobilization. Localized cellulitis of the terminal digit may indicate a "collar button" abscess rather than a superficial abscess.

Grave infections of the hands or feet involve tenosynovitis and infection of fascial spaces or bursas, and usually are accompanied by lymphangitis; edema is present on the dorsum of the hand or foot, although the abscess usually is located in the palmar or plantar aspect. The extremity usually assumes the position of rest or pain when deep infection is present. Infections of the feet, unlike infections of the hand, occur primarily in the presence of vascular insufficiency or diabetes mellitus.

Occasionally what appears to be an extremity abscess is in fact necrotizing fasciitis, a life-threatening infection that involves muscles and tendons as well as skin and subcutaneous tissue. Necrotizing fasciitis is similar to *Clostridia* myositis (gas gangrene) but is more commonly due to a synergistic infection of anaerobic streptococci associated with gram-negative bacteria. The infection usually originates in puncture wounds, leg ulcers, and sacral decubiti and commonly occurs in addicts who have used unsterile needles. It spreads along fascial planes, producing edema, skin bullae, crepitus, and erythema. Necrotizing fasciitis, which is associated with intense pain, systemic toxicity, and septic thrombophlebitis, requires urgent extensive debridement in association with massive doses (40 million units daily) of penicillin.

Crush injuries involving the forearm or calf may produce vascular insufficiency because of increasing fascial compartment pressures. Muscle, tendon, bone, and nerve damage may also occur secondary to a burn (Chapter 38) or advancing infection. Moreover, nerve damage may occur even in the presence of seemingly adequate perfusion and pulses unless fasciotomy is performed promptly.

Ulcers that occur in the lower extremities usually involve the full thickness of the skin with a base of indolent granulation tissue and a peripheral zone of erythema. Medial malleolar ulcers are usually associated with postphlebitic syndrome and represent infection in an area of venous hypertension. Chronic skin discoloration results from hemosiderin pigment released following diapedesis of erythrocytes from capillaries in which hydrostatic pressure exceeds the ability to maintain cellular elements within the circulation.

Lateral malleolar ulcers are commonly caused by injury in hypertensive patients. Medial, lateral, and pretibial ulcers all heal with difficulty if the venous circulation is compromised by limited motion.

Aerobic, anaerobic, and fungal cultures are essential to the diagnosis of infection. Examination with Wood's light can be helpful by detecting fluorescence in fungal infections and in ulcers or infections caused by *Pseudomonas aeroginosa* and may help define the margins for eschar debridement. Cytologic smears are diagnostic of herpes simplex, herpes zoster, and varicella, which are increasingly encountered in immunosuppressed patients. Biopsy allows definitive diagnosis of skin lesions and aids in determining the quantity of bacteria present in burned skin.

PREOPERATIVE CARE

Shaving the extremity should be avoided in patients with diabetes mellitus or vascular insufficiency. To lower bacterial concentration at the operative site the skin is prepared with a variety of soaps, alcohol solutions, and iodine. Iodophores and chlorhexidene are preferred because they reduce bacterial count without caustic injury to the epidermis. Preoperative shaving and skin preparation should be done immediately preceding operation because the secondary abrasions may otherwise become a source of preoperative contamination and postoperative infection.

When the integrity of the skin has been violated by the disease or injury, protection of the underlying soft tissue and deep structures assumes priority. Open injuries of the skin, subcutaneous tissue, and muscle require different management than when the skin is intact. The primary objective is to excise devitalized tissue and remove foreign material from the wound. The area surrounding the wound should be cleansed with an organic solvent, the area should be draped, and strict aseptic technique should be used. No caustic solutions, antiseptics, or soaps should be introduced into the wound. The wound should be copiously irrigated with isotonic saline solution and dressed aseptically. Definitive repair of lacerations, tendons, or nerves is then accomplished in the optimal environment of the operating room or after transfer to a center for specialized care. If properly prepared, an open wound of the hand or elsewhere on the extremity can be treated 48 to 72 hours after injury as a primary wound and closed. A wound that is not closed primarily will seldom cause morbidity, although a less cosmetic scar will result.

With the exception of finger flexors severed at the wrist, every structure in the hand can be reconstructed secondarily with as satisfactory a result as a primary repair. Long flexor tendons, if divided at the wrist level, will retract; subsequent shortening of muscle usually cannot be overcome and precludes satisfactory rehabilitation. If gross contamination is not present, at least the skin and soft tissue should be closed in hand injuries.

Following meticulous cleansing, fractures are treated preferably with secondary closure five to seven days after injury. Broad-spectrum antibiotics are usually administered to patients sustaining open fractures and large soft tissue injuries; however, this may result in emergence of opportunistic microorganisms. In patients with multiple injuries, antibiotics should be avoided if post-traumatic pulmonary insufficiency is likely, as pneumonic "super-infection" by antibiotic-resistant bacteria or fungi is usually fatal.

Blunt soft tissue extremity injuries without a break in the skin are more common than fractures. Contusions are treated by cold compresses initially. Sprains and other stretch injuries of ligaments may require early immobilization by splint or cast and require operative repair if total tendinous disruption has occurred. Elastic bandages and elevation aid in recovery and minimize discomfort.

Crush injuries of the extremities may result in death of muscle tissue from direct injury or from ischemia secondary to venous rather than arterial obstruction by a tight fascial compartment. The compartment pressure can be measured by several available methods, the simplest of which is to use an 18-gauge needle connected to a strain gauge. If the compartment pressure exceeds 30 to 40 mm Hg or rises to within 30 mm Hg of the diastolic blood pressure, fasciotomy is indicated. Although measurement of fascial compartment pressure is somewhat useful in anticipating the potential of ischemia prior to irreparable nerve and muscle injury, electromyography is probably a superior method for evaluating impending functional loss.

Crush injury of the extremity and fascial compartment syndromes are associated with myonecrosis and may cause acute renal failure by precipitation of myoglobin in the proximal renal tubules. Patients are in danger of developing renal failure following crush injury, and frequent monitoring of the urine for myoglobin is mandatory. Prophylaxis against myoglobin-induced renal failure after crush injury can be provided by an intravenous infusion of 1000 ml 5 per cent dextrose and water, to which has been added one ampule of sodium bicarbonate and one ampule of sodium mannitol. Because the resultant "cocktail" is hyperosmolar and alkaline, it will promote diuresis and alkalinize the urine, thus preventing myoglobin precipitation. The initial liter of solution is administered at 200 ml per hour until a brisk diuresis is induced, when the rate is reduced to 100 ml per hour. While diuresis is occurring, the urine should be checked frequently for myoglobin.

POSTOPERATIVE CARE

Postoperative care maintains coverage of the extremity by primary closure or restores it through skin grafts. If the wound is greater than 20 cm in diameter, it should be immobilized and elevated for seven to ten days to minimize edema and maximize drainage. Dressings should be simple and nonirritating and should not be soaked in antibiotic solution. If wounds are left open, frequent dressing changes will be painful; fine mesh gauze impregnated with petrolatum and placed directly over the wound will minimize discomfort. If postoperative wounds are contaminated or infected, frequent dressing changes are useful; alternating wet and dry dressings every four to six hours allows the dressing to debride the wound gently by capillarity.

Normally, the skin is bathed in an "acid mantle" (pH 5.7 to 6.4) by sebaceous gland secretions. In many wound infections, the pH will increase to 8 or 9; soaking the dressings in acidic solutions such as half-strength Dakin's or acetic acid solution will restore the acid-wound interface and aid infection control.

If skin has been grafted, immobilization, elevation, and moist dressings during the first 72 hours will facilitate a viable result. Rolling the grafts frequently can disperse the fluid accumulation that prevents adherence of the graft to underlying tissue. A mesh skin graft with a ratio of 1.5:1 or 3.0:1 allows greater surface coverage with less skin and minimizes serum accumulation beneath the graft. Split-thickness grafts lack normal skin appendages (e.g., sebaceous glands, hair follicles). When the graft has healed, replacement of the natural skin oils with vitamin A and D ointment, lanolin, or moisturizing creams is useful. Skin grafts frequently develop pigment changes when exposed to ultraviolet light, which can be avoided by protective clothing or sun screen preparations. Pressure dressings and specially fitted elastic garments (Jobst) will reduce scar formation and edema after extensive injuries. These are particularly useful following lower extremity injuries with impaired lymphatic and venous drainage which often result in chronic ulceration.

CIRCULATION

Disease processes originating in arteries account for two thirds of lower extremity amputations. Pre- and postoperative care is directed at preserving the circulation, preventing infection, and assuring optimal recovery and rehabilitation if amputation is necessary. Degenerative diseases such as arteriosclerosis and diabetes mellitus may be manifested as chronic occlusion or dilatation of blood vessels. Single segment arterial occlusion of the upper extremity rarely causes symptoms severe enough to require operative management. However, a variety of disorders labeled thoracic outlet syndromes are caused by compression of the arterial, venous, or neural structures at the base of the neck. Initial management of these problems includes postural correction and physical therapy, but the first or second rib may require resection if mechanical obstruction persists.

Fractures of the middle third of the humerus may injure the brachial artery and radial nerve and result in limb loss or Volkmann's ischemic contracture. Penetrating injuries from gunshot or knife wounds, or injections associated with drug abuse, can threaten limb integrity or loss by direct trauma to arteries or veins and as a source of infection.

Supracondylar fractures of the distal humerus, particularly if displaced or proximal to the olecranon fossa, are surgical emergencies if brachial artery occlusion and peripheral nerve injury are to be avoided. Dislocations and subluxations of the elbow are usually posterior and occur without fracture, but frequently injure the ulnar nerve. Unlike fractures and dislocations of the elbow, forearm fractures, unless compound and/or crushing, are seldom associated with limb loss secondary to arterial injury.

Venous occlusion of the axillary and subclavian vein are potentially debilitating problems. A typical history includes unusual activity involving the upper extremities, followed by pain and swelling within 24 hours of venous occlusion and associated with edema involving the upper shoulder and forearm regions. Fewer than one third of patients with this disorder have a palpable venous cord. Chronic long-term subclavian vein catheterization for intravenous hyperalimentation or monitoring of central venous pressure can be associated with venous thrombosis in one of four patients. Although less common than peripheral thromophlebitis, axillary subclavian vein thrombosis is associated with residual symtomatology in more than 60 per cent of patients affected. Thrombophlebitis of the arm and forearm is usually caused by injury, frequently from an intravenous cannula or basilic vein. The diagnosis is suspected by evidence of erythema extending to the axilla and pain out of proportion to the physical findings.

Although arterial insufficiency of the upper extremity is uncommon, 75 per cent of lower extremity amputations are performed for ischemia secondary to arteriosclerosis. Claudication of the upper extremity is also infrequent, but the most common manifestation of occlusive arterial vascular disease of the lower extremity is onset of pain after walking 90 to 200 meters, which is relieved by a five-minute rest and is associated with a pulse deficit. Arterial insufficiency is associated with pallor, cyanosis, rubor, and temperature difference between the symptomatic extremity and its opposite member. Atrophy of the skin and subcutaneous tissue occurs in the chronically ischemic extremity. The severity of claudication is directly proportional to the degree of arterial insufficiency. Rest pain, which never occurs proximal to the ankle, frequently occurs at night during sleep when the lower extremity is in a prone position and implies severe ischemia. The pain awakens the patient, who usually must hang his foot over the edge of the bed to gain relief.

Preoperatively the patient with occlusive vascular disease is assessed largely by symptoms and physical examination. Acute arterial occlusion, secondary to thrombosis or embolus, is a dramatic event characterized by abrupt, severe ischemia. Persistence of acute occlusion results in motor and sensory paralysis, muscle infarction, and cutaneous gangrene within six to twelve hours of occurrence, depending on the collateral circulation. The clinical syndrome of acute vascular embarrassment to the extremities is characterized by the "five P's": pain, pallor, pulselessness, paresthesia, and paralysis. Coldness, pain in the extremity, and numbness are early symptoms; motor function loss is an intermediate symptom; and muscle edema with compartment compression usually occurs 24 hours after occlusion. Ischemia following occlusion of the superficial femoral artery or profunda femoral artery is often followed by recovery, but maximum collateral circulation to restore adequate nutrient blood flow to the muscles, skin, and nerves requires two to four months. If paralysis occurs, irreversible neuromuscular ischemia is imminent and immediate operative intervention is mandatory if the limb is to be salvaged. Isolated infarction of a terminal digit of the upper extremity is usually caused by an embolus associated with subacute bacterial endocarditis or direct puncture of an artery for physiologic monitoring or drug abuse.

The arterial blood supply to the upper and lower extremity is occasionally compromised by conditions other than arteriosclerosis. Deep venous thrombosis involving the lower extremity (phlegmasia cerulea dolens) can produce extensive edema with closing pressures in the fascial compartments in excess of the arterial pressure, resulting in arterial thrombosis. Arterial occlusion following venous thrombosis is differentiated from primary arterial occlusion by massive pitting edema and thrombophlebitis. Limb loss from arterial occlusion can also follow thermal injury, particularly if caused by electrical current or complicated by infection.

The status of the arterial circulation must be carefully evaluated in all patients with fractures, dislocations, and subluxations. As a general rule, the closer the fracture is to the trunk, the less likely it is to be associated with injury to an artery or nerve. Fracture-dislocations of the elbow or knee, however, are associated with a high incidence of acute or chronic vascular insufficiency. Fractures of the proximal humerus, in the region of the anatomic neck, may develop avascular necrosis but seldom have secondary complications or require treatment other than immobilization. Fractures of the surgical neck (with a fracture cleft distal to the tuberosities) may produce neurovascular injury if the angulation of the fracture is greater than 45 degrees and the cast does not maintain reduction of the fracture. Fractures of the upper extremity are usually managed satisfactorily by long-arm casts placed in a sling. If closed reduction is inadequate, open reduction is necessary to prevent tendon, nerve, or bone damage.

Although the diagnosis of circulatory abnormalities is primarily by history and physical examination, special tests are occasionally useful. Examination by Doppler ultrasound may detect pulses that are not palpable; quantitation of arterial or venous pressure using a blood pressure cuff in conjunction with the Doppler is useful. However, biplane or uniplane arteriography is the most precise method for determining arterial blood supply to the extremities. New isotope methods for detecting skin and muscle blood flow such as xenon clearance are additional tools for determining perfusion levels, and yield useful information in the selection of amputation site.

PREOPERATIVE CARE

When the arterial blood supply of an extremity is compromised, the ability of the limb to survive is largely determined by skin viability. Moreover, in extremities with established dry gangrene, the level of amputation can be minimized if infection is avoided. In addition to the recommendations described in the previous section, the ischemic limb should be protected from abrasion and supported in a cradle. The limb should rest on a sheepskin and the digits should be separated by lamb's wool pads.

If dry gangrene is present cultures are taken from the ischemic part, and broad-spectrum antibiotics are administered to sterilize the surrounding tissue and lymphatics 12 hours prior to amputation. If "wet" or infected gangrene is present, preamputation antibiotic therapy is based on antibacterial sensitivities. Moreover, if a vascular prosthesis is required, an applied tissue level of antibiotics prior to operation is good practice.

The position of the extremity is important. With arterial insufficiency, dependency aids in providing nutritive blood supply to the extremities. On the other hand, venous insufficiency or edema is treated by elevation. Properly used, heparin is an important, sometimes definitive, tool in the preoperative treatment of arterial and venous occlusive disease. Propagation of blood clot into collateral channels is minimized by *immediate* and continuous administration of heparin after acute arterial occlusion. When patients appear with a viable, but ischemic extremity less than 12 hours after acute occlusion, heparin may prevent limb loss and produce less morbidity and mortality than embolectomy or vascular reconstruction. If deep venous thrombophlebitis is present, treatment by heparin rather than embolectomy is preferred unless phlegmasia cerulea dolens occurs.

The treatment of thrombophlebitis, infections, and ulcers is aided by application of warm Koch-Mason dressings. However, warm compresses are contraindicated if arterial insufficiency is present, as heat increases the metabolic rate of the already ischemic part.

POSTOPERATIVE CARE

Most of the principles of preoperative care and diagnosis are useful for postoperative care of the circulation, particularly monitoring of perfusion, immobilization, and skin protection. However, heparin administration is usually unnecessary if adequate circulatory status can be restored by operation.

Postoperative treatment of vascular disease or injuries involves protecting the extremity by immobilization and proper positioning. If grafts of prosthetic material for arterial reconstruction have been placed across flexion or extension creases such as the knee or hip, pillow splints will prevent postoperative acute angulation of the graft and allow the wound to heal. If the extremity remains ischemic after vascular surgery, elevation should be avoided and a neutral position maintained. If the circulation is relatively normal after operation, exercise will facilitate venous return and reduce edema. In the immediate postoperative period, the sitting position should be avoided because it causes venous hypertension, which accentuates edema, increases the likelihood of pulmonary embolus, and reduces arterial inflow. The optimal postoperative position is supine or walking, unless tendon or bone injury precludes ambulation.

BONES

Fractures of the middle and lower third of the *humerus* should alert the surgeon to the possibility of radial nerve or brachial artery injury complications that require operative management. Supracondylar fractures of the distal humerus in the region of the olecranon fossa are often associated with acute injury to the brachial artery and ulnar nerve. Volkmann's contracture, secondary to an ischemic muscle compartment, commonly occurs following elbow fractures and can also be caused by a constrictive cast. Displaced fractures, subluxations, and posterior dislocations of the elbow also have high incidences of brachial artery and ulnar nerve injury.

Shaft fractures of the *radius*, particularly in children, may injure an epiphyseal plate; roentgenograms of the opposite extremity are required for comparison to determine if the fracture is in the region of a growth center. Forearm fractures are usually stable, with little potential for injuring nerves or arteries unless both the radius and ulna are fractured. Classic wrist fractures, such as the Colles fracture (isolated impacted radial fracture), produce a "silver fork" or bayonet deformity, and they are commonly associated with some permanent deformity. Radial nerve injury from bone fragments of a wrist fracture is uncommon.

With the exception of fractures of both bones of the *forearm* and fracture-dislocations of the elbow, upper extremity fractures are treated with immobilization by a cast that extends past one joint proximal to the fracture. Roentgenograms are obtained with the cast in place and the fingers free from the cast to allow evaluation of neurologic and vascular function that can be compromised by a cast that is too tight.

Unlike upper extremity fractures, lower extremity fractures frequently cause significant soft tissue injury and shock. Initial management priorities are resuscitation, evaluation of the neurovascular bundle, and protection of soft tissue. As with the upper extremity, proximal fractures of the lower extremity have less potential for injury to the neurovascular bundle than distal bone injuries. Subtrochanteric fractures of the femur often have extensive associated soft tissue damage and require immobilization and traction at the site of injury. Traumatic *hip* dislocations, with the head of the femur dislocated posterior to the acetabulum, appears as a shortened, adducted leg that is in internal rotation. Hip dislocations are evaluated by anterior, posterior, transpelvic, and oblique roentgenographic views. Posterior dislocations of the hip are surgical emergencies, since sciatic nerve injuries and unsuspected fractures of the head and neck of the femur may be present, and ischemic. Osteoporosis can occur if fracture reduction is delayed.

Fractures of the shaft of the *femur*, the largest bone, should alert the surgeon to the extent of the violence of the injury. Shaft fractures of the femur characteristically assume a flexed position in external rotation with abduction, shortening, and overriding of the fracture. Shock and death will occur if immobilization and systemic resuscitation are not vigorously implemented. Moreover, the sciatic nerve and superficial femoral artery may be injured.

Fractures and dislocations of the *knee* frequently cause popliteal artery and nerve injury by either anterior or posterior displacement of the supracondylar femur fracture fragment. The popliteal artery is injured when it is displaced by the fracture or dislocation. The adventitia and media of the artery stretch, but the inelastic intima tears, with subsequent dissection and thrombosis of the artery. Because pulses may be present even when total transection of the popliteal artery has occurred, reduction of the fracture-dislocation must always be followed by a femoral-popliteal arteriogram to assess the artery. Limb loss and malpractice suits frequently follow inadequate assessment of popliteal artery injury associated with supracondylar femur fractures or knee dislocations. Moreover, monitoring of pulses, skin appearance, and temperature is difficult when the leg is enclosed by a cast.

Fractures of the *tibia* or *fibula* distal to the tibial tuberosity are infrequently complicated by neural or vascular injury. If a particularly violent injury occurs, however, a disruption of the peroneal or posterior tibial artery or nerve may occur. Arteriography is mandatory if limb loss from ischemia is likely, regardless of the fracture. If one nutrient vessel (posterior tibial, anterior tibial, peroneal artery) is uninjured and viability of the limb is assured, treatment by reduction and immobilization of the fracture is adequate.

PREOPERATIVE CARE

Every suspected fracture of a major bone should be splinted before the patient is moved from the site of injury. When battlefield immobilization of fractures by the Thomas splint was introduced in World War I, the mortality from shock and sepsis from compound femur fractures was reduced from 80 per cent to 15.6 per cent. Immobilization minimizes discomfort, reduces blood and fluid loss in the fracture site, avoids soft tissue trauma, and prevents conversion of a closed to an open fracture during transportation.

A splint does not reduce a fracture but maintains reduction and prevents movement. Plaster or inflatable plastic splints can be molded to the individual needs of the injury and are preferable to prefabricated rigid immobilization devices. Fractures of large bones, those nearest the trunk, are associated with considerable hemorrhage from the fracture site and soft tissue injury. Although fractures of large bones are more likely to be associated with shock, small fractures may produce greater disability. Resuscitation with crystalloid and blood transfusion proceeds while appropriate roentgenographic evaluation is performed. The volume of fluid loss can be estimated by measuring the circumference and length of the extremity over the fracture site by using the following formula after making comparable measurement of the uninjured opposite limb:

$$V = \frac{C^2L}{4}$$

where V = the volume of the extremity, C = the circumference, and L = length. The volume of fluid loss is the difference between the volume of the injured and uninjured limb.

If the fracture is associated with other injuries, it usually assumes a lower treatment priority. If an open fracture is present, the trauma team must concur if antibiotics are to be used, common practice in open fracture management. Moreover, operative stabilization of long bone fractures performed at the same operation when other injuries are treated will prevent early and late respiratory complications.

Immediate evaluation of a fracture includes careful examination and recording of pulses and nerve function distal to the fracture site. Following reduction and careful immobilization, evaluation and recording of the pulses should be repeated. Nerve and motor function are frequently evaluated with difficulty after injury. The best examination possible should be done with clear documentation that the ability to perform an optimal examination is limited. Particular care should be taken to determine if the fracture is closed or open. If an open fracture (break in the skin) is present, a dry sterile dressing is applied, and broad-spectrum antibiotics are administered.

Although some fractures assume characteristic positions, the absence of a deformity does not exclude a fracture. Moreover, manipulation of the injured extremity to ascertain the presence of a fracture is contraindicated. It should be emphasized that the force required to produce a single fracture may result in other injuries or additional fractures. Calcaneal fractures, for example, frequently occur in conjunction with compression fractures of the lumbar spine.

POSTOPERATIVE CARE

Regardless of whether fractures are treated by closed or open reduction, certain principles of care are required. Immobilization by cast, splint, internal fixation, or traction should reduce pain. If pain persists or increases after reduction, inadequate reduction or immobilization should be suspected. The cast or traction requires frequent adjustment. Elevation of the injured limb minimizes edema and discomfort. Frequent evaluation of the temperature, capillary filling, and sensation of the digits distal to the fracture should be performed. Bivalving of casts will aid in reduction of edema but when done should result in division of both the plaster and underlying padding.

After resuscitation and initial reduction of a fracture, frequent evaluation by physical examination and roentgenography should be performed to confirm that the fracture is maintained in reduction.

Rehabilitation is greatly facilitated by physical therapy soon after injury. Early contact with the physical therapist is useful for training the patient how to use ambulatory aids such as canes, crutches, and extremity prostheses. Moreover, early range of motion exercises will lessen the likelihood of "frozen" joints that may heal optimally but with significant loss of function. Impacted, stable fractures, particularly of the hand and upper extremity, cause minimal permanent disability if early physical therapy is prescribed; healing of the fracture is enhanced by motion if the fracture is stable.

SUMMARY

The extremities are functional units that are usually not the primary location of disease or the first priority for treatment after injury. However, extremity diseases and injuries account for more hospital bed-days, loss of work, and permanent disability than disease or injury of other organ systems.

Pre- and postoperative care begins with functional assessment. Optimal therapy usually includes immobilization and splinting, protection of the integrity of skin, avoidance of infection, protection of the circulation, and early rehabilitation. The success of optimal pre- and postoperative care is measured by the degree of function salvaged, consistent with survival.

MAXIMS OF EXTREMITY CARE

1. Grade function, size, pulses, and roentgenograms by comparison with the opposite extremity.

2. Immobilize all injured or operated extremities, remembering that splints do not reduce fractures but maintain reduction.

3. The condition of skin and soft tissue will frequently determine the success of treatment.

4. Primary closure of incompletely cleansed or contaminated wounds is a common cause of amputation.

5. A wound that is closed secondarily seldom becomes infected or causes disability.

6. The extremities are frequently the obvious, but not the only, manifestation of injury or illness.

7. If circulation is marginal, maintain the extremity in a neutral or dependent position.

8. If the extremity is edematous and arterial circulation is adequate, elevation is useful.

9. Deformity may not be associated with injury of the part.

10. A small injury may cause a large disability.

11. Early active movements and ambulation prevent muscle wasting and pulmonary embolism and hasten recovery.

12. Successful treatment is measured by survival and usefulness of the extremity.

REFERENCES

Aids to the investigation of peripheral nerve injuries. Medical Research Council, War Memorandum No. 7. London, Her Majesty's Stationery Office.

Committee on Trauma, American College of Surgeons: The Management of Fractures and Soft Tissue Injuries. Philadelphia, W. B. Saunders Co., 1965.

Defore, W. W., Mattox, K. L., and Dang, M. H., et al.: Necrotizing fasciitis. JACEP, 6:62–65, 1977.

Ger, R.: Surgical management of ulcerative lesions of the leg. In Current Problems in Surgery. Chicago, Year Book Medical Publishers, Inc., March, 1972.

Gerlock, A. F.: The use of pedal venous pressure as a guide in evaluating the patency of venous repairs. J. Trauma, 17:108–110, 1977.

Kirk, P., and Wilson, R. F.: Amputations following trauma. *In* Walt, A. J., and Rolent, F. (eds.): Management of Trauma Pitfalls and Practice. Philadelphia, Lea & Febiger, 1975, pp. 270–284.

Legerwood, A. M., and Lucas, C. E.: Massive thigh injuries with vascular disruption: Role of porcine skin grafting of exposed arterial vein grafts. Arch. Surg., *107*:201, 1973.

Patman, R. D., and Thompson, J. E.: Fasciotomy in peripheral vascular surgery. Arch. Surg., *101*:663, 1970.

Peltier, L. F.: Some complications of fractures. *In* Current Problems in Surgery. Chicago, Year Book Medical Publishers, Inc., May, 1967.

Rich, N.: Vascular trauma. Surg. Clin. North Am., 53:1367–1392, 1973.

Rich, N., Baugh, J., and Hughes, C.: Significance of complications associated with vascular repairs performed in Vietnam. Arch. Surg., *100*:646, 1970.

Whitesides, T. E., Haney, T. C., Harada, H., et al.: Tissue pressure as a determinant for the need for fasciotomy. Orthop. Rev., *4*:37–39, 1975.

IV

Special Patient Problems

37

The Patient with Multiple Injuries

B. EISEMAN, M.D.
HENRY CLEVELAND, M.D.

Proper care following multiple injury is best achieved by performing the right operation in the right manner at the right time, but efficient preoperative and postoperative care may mean the difference between death or survival even given utopian circumstances. Elsewhere in this volume, management of specific types of trauma and organ failure are detailed. If those chapters serve as instructions for playing single instruments, this chapter serves as the score for conducting the clinical symphony orchestra.

COMMUNICATIONS

The starting gun in the race for survival following severe injury goes off at the moment of injury, when hypovolemia, poor organ perfusion, and inadequate ventilation may commence. The first objective is to get such a casualty into the evacuation system with the least delay. A central communications center must be notified of the location of the patient and the nature of his or her injuries. The "911 system," whereby any telephone can be used to contact a central dispatcher communicating via radio or telephone with ambulance units, is now almost universally available. Its 24-hour demand for availability of personnel and communication is expensive and is the first of many points where centralization, not diffusion, of responsibility and authority for casualty care in a community is important.

Details of communication equipment, essential personnel, and operation of such 911 communication centers have been detailed elsewhere (Penterman, 1976).

TRANSPORT

Proper transport of a casualty to a trauma center requires (1) modern ambulances, (2) equipment prepositioned for early response and pick-up, and (3) personnel ready to respond who are trained to evaluate injuries and initiate appropriate resuscitation.

Long, low, converted hearses no longer are acceptable for transporting the seriously injured. The best vehicles consist of a 1½ ton truck chassis fitted with a modular ambulance unit high and broad enough to allow Emergency Medical Technicians (EMTs) to provide active care of the casualty en route (Fig. 37–1). Supplies on board should include stretchers styled for easy extraction of a casualty from cramped indoor quarters, inflatable splints, and radio and telemetry monitoring devices that allow free communication between the EMT team in the field and consultant physicians in the hospital trauma center (American College of Surgeons, 1977).

Prepositioning of expertly staffed ambulances should insure that response time from notification to arrival at the scene is no more than four minutes.

The extensive experience with helicopter casualty pick-up during the Vietnam War is applicable to transporting peacetime injured civilians. These systems now can operate in an independent and cost-effective manner in community hospitals (Cleveland et al., 1976). Contrary to previous belief, helicopter ambulances are also effective for short distance pick-ups (under 15 miles) and in urban and suburban environments (Fig. 37–2).

Ambulance teams (ground or airborne) should consist of drivers plus professional EMTs. Basic training to qualify as an EMT is 80 hours of initial study and 500 hours of practice. Qualification for a paramedic requires additional training. To maintain skills and a sense of professionalism, the EMT must regard his or her vocation as a career, not a temporary exciting hobby. Compensation must also reflect this philosophy.

THE TRAUMA CENTER

Management of the severely (and multiply) injured patient requires immediate care by a team ready around the clock in a well-equipped hospital emergency department. It is, therefore, expensive, and society cannot afford the luxury of many hospitals to be so equipped and staffed. For an emergency department thus to qualify, it should have a minimum of 35,000 patient visits per year, 15 per cent of which should involve some type of trauma. Criteria for qualification as a trauma center have been detailed elsewhere (American College of Surgeons, 1976). The requirements start with extensive equipment, supplies, personnel, and space commitments in the emergency department but also include

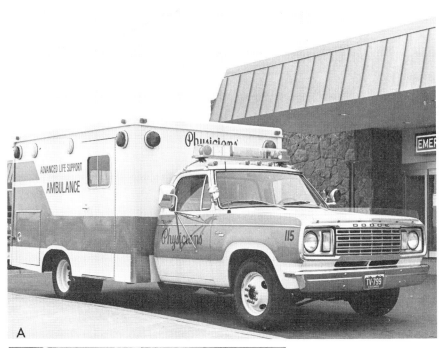

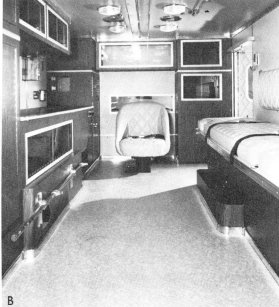

Figure 37–1. Wheeled ambulance. A, exterior; B, interior.

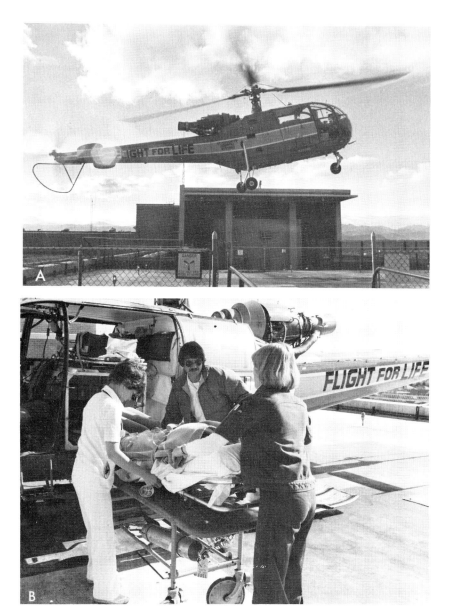

Figure 37–2. Helicopter ambulance: *A*, landing pad (roof of hospital), *B*, removing patient.

equally expensive around-the-clock coverage in the clinical laboratory, blood bank, radiology department, operating rooms, and intensive care units.

EMERGENCY DEPARTMENT CARE

Emergency medicine is emerging as a service specialty. Expertise of its practitioners lies in the early recognition and early care of all acute diseases, including severe multiple trauma. The interface at which the Emergency Medicine Specialist (EMS) bows out and the surgeon takes over is debatable and depends on local availability, but transfer of responsibility should occur no longer than 10 to 20 minutes after the casualty's arrival in the hospital emergency department. With proper communication, this time interval can and should be shortened.

The severely injured patient should be met at the emergency department entrance by a team already alerted by radio as to the EMT's assessment of the patient from the field (Fig. 37–3). The initial team ideally should consist of persons specifically designated and trained in advance to perform the following duties: (1) a team leader (surgeon or EMS trained in trauma); (2) an airway physician (anesthesiologist, surgeon, or skilled EMS) able to insert an endotracheal tube and provide appropriate assisted respiration; (3) an emergency department nurse, EMT, or physician able to insert an intravenous catheter; (4) a nurse or EMT to insert a urinary catheter and nasogastric tube and splint extremities as indicated; (5) a laboratory technician to draw blood and take it to the laboratory and blood bank; (6) a circulating nurse; (7) a recorder; (8) a physician to perform a complete physical examination; (9) a hospital

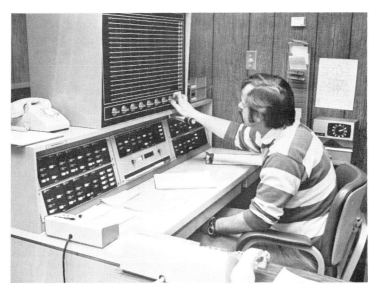

Figure 37–3. Emergency department communications center for helicopter and wheeled ambulance.

employee to take responsibility for listing and safekeeping of the patient's clothes and valuables; and (10) a person to notify the family and start the hospital record.

Even busy emergency departments cannot afford a separate person for each of the preceding duties, but optimal initial care usually requires a team of four to six trained persons to share these duties, all of which demand almost simultaneous attention.

A room adjacent to the emergency department entrance should be devoted to treatment of the seriously injured. It should be convertible to an emergency operating room for the case that occasionally requires immediate thoracotomy or laparotomy. It should have operating lights, suction, oxygen, mechanical respirators, hooks or stands for intravenous solutions, and monitoring equipment and supplies for tracheal intubation, tracheostomy, and tube thoracostomy. Details of its design, equipment, and supplies are described elsewhere (American College of Surgeons, 1970; Carter, 1976).

Resuscitation begins with establishing an airway by clearing the upper respiratory tract, positioning, endotracheal or nasotracheal intubation, or cricothyroidotomy (Brantigan and Grow, 1976). Tracheostomy may be necessary.

Restoration of the depleted vascular space should start with the intravenous administration of Ringer's lactated solution through two or more large cannulae in the extremities. Within 20 to 45 minutes, typed and cross-matched blood should be substituted. Use of unmatched O negative blood, albumin, or plasma substitutes seldom is indicated. However, necessary transfusion should not be withheld for fear of giving uncrossmatched O negative or type-specific uncrossmatched blood.

The initial physical examination must be complete, including rectal examination and visualization and palpation of the entire body for evidence of injury. Priorities in management of the multiply injured patient must be established so that life-threatening injuries are handled first. Concern for the obvious area of injury (for example, an open long bone fracture) must not divert attention from other more potentially lethal injuries.

Initial treatment will depend on the specific injuries, but a convenient guideline includes insertion of six types of tubes: (1) an endotracheal tube, (2) a nasogastric tube, (3) a thoracostomy tube, (4) two or more intravenous catheters, (5) a urinary bladder catheter, and (6) a paracentesis or peritoneal lavage catheter. All six are not always required.

Patients with complicating closed head injuries, respiratory depression, and possible airway obstruction may require intubation and hyperventilation to avoid cerebral hypoxia, which contributes to brain swelling. Large doses of steroids are advocated by some.

Tube thoracostomy with underwater drainage is indicated if the patient does not respond to cardiopulmonary resuscitation and there is suspicion of pneumothorax or hemothorax.

Peritoneal lavage is rarely indicated in the initial evaluation but may be useful when evidence of intraperitoneal bleeding is masked by head or other severe injuries. Five hundred to 1000 ml of physiologic saline or Ringer's lactate should be infused into the peritoneal cavity through a lower midline abdominal catheter. Effluent should then be drained by gravity. A "positive tap" requires erythrocyte concentrations greater than 100,000 cells per mm^3.

Roentgenograms obtained in the emergency department depend on the nature of the injury. Chest films are frequently required to confirm physical findings of hemothorax or pneumothorax or widening of the mediastinum associated with thoracic aortic injury. Following head injury, a cross-table lateral film of the cervical spine should be taken along with films of the head to exclude the possibility of an insidious cervical or cranial fracture.

Following gunshot injuries, the bullet should be localized to give some idea of what organs might have been injured from the point of entrance to the final position of the missile. Supine or erect films of the abdomen may demonstrate intraperitoneal air, an almost certain sign of hollow viscus rupture in a closed injury. Roentgenograms of bones for evidence of fracture takes low priority. Any bone thought to be fractured on physical examination should be splinted as though broken; so, incidentally, should severe soft tissue extremity injuries.

Abdominal or thoracic injury associated with hematuria requires an intravenous pyelogram to exclude renal damage. This can be obtained in the emergency department during initial resuscitation with a single film four minutes after injection of the radiopaque dye.

Indications for specialized studies such as arteriography are beyond the scope of this summary but are helpful when confirmation and localization of major arterial or venous injury are desired.

Laboratory studies in the emergency department need not be extensive. Type and cross-match of blood, arterial blood gases, serial hematocrits, and microscopic examination of the urine for blood are the most important initial studies. Urine output through an indwelling catheter is a good indicator of renal perfusion.

Central venous pressure (CVP) monitoring is most readily obtained via subclavian vein puncture (Knopp and Dailey, 1977) but is associated with a higher complication rate (hemothorax, pneumothorax) than when the catheter is inserted via the jugular vein or a vein at the antecubital space. A CVP monitor should be used in the elderly patient, in whom fluid overload is particularly dangerous and left heart failure can be confused with overhydration or overtransfusion. If doubt exists, a Swan-Ganz catheter floated into the pulmonary artery with a balloon provides more accurate measurement of left heart pressure. This is seldom required immediately following injury.

Broad-spectrum antibiotics (clindamycin, kanamycin, cephalosporins, and others) should be started as soon as possible following injury. They are all but worthless if begun in the postoperative period.

St. Anthony Hospital Systems
Emergency Room Nurses Notes

Time	BP	P	R	T	CVP	Time	Site	#	IV Solutions	Type	By	amt. inf.	amt. disc.	Procedures	Time	Size	By	Time	Urine	Emesis	NG OG	R. chest	L. chest	Suc.	Other
														R. Subclav.											
														L. Subclav.											
														R. Jugular											
														L. Jugular											
														R. Cutdown											
														L. Cutdown											
														R. Chest tube											
														L. Chest tube											
														Abd. Tap											
														Intubations											
														Trach.											
														Open Chest			Total					Total Intake:		
														NG/OG			By Mouth:							
														Ewald			Time	Amt.	Time	Amt.				
														Foley											
														Rectal								Total Output:		
														Pelvic			Totals:							
														Pelvic											
														Scrub			Pupils:							
														Soak			Time	Equal	Right	Left	React	By		
														Suture											

SAC   SAN

Prior to Transport:

Totals: WB: PC:
Albumin: IV Solutions:

Allergies:
☐ EKG Time:
☐ Oxygen time Started: At: /LPM   Time: ☐ Monitor Rhythm: Age: WT: Last Tetanus: LMP:
☐ Cannula
X-RAYS: ☐ Portable   ☐ Mask   At: /LPM   Time: At: /LPM   Time: At: /LPM
☐ Stretcher   ☐ to X-ray   ☐ Both   ☐ T-Piece   ☐ Bag   ☐ O₂   ☐ Other: ☐ Monitor
X-Rays Ordered: ☐ Wheelchair   ☐ RN/LPN/EMT/Other: /LPM
LAB: ☐ CBC   ☐ UA   ☐ RPR   ☐ Lytes   ☐ 6/60   ☐ ENSYMES   Time to X-Ray: Time Returned:
ABG time: Site   Time   Site   Time   Site
☐ T & X   Units   ☐ WB   ☐ PC   ☐ T & Hold
Others:

Doctors Called: Time Called   Doctor Returning Call: Time Arrived

MEDICATION	Time	Dose	Route	Site	By	Effect/Reaction	Ordered By

Responsiveness Scale (EMV):

Eye Opening	Best Motor Response	Verbal Response
4 Spontaneous	6 Obeys	5 Oriented
3 To Speech	5 Localizes	4 Conf. Conversation
2 To Pain	4 Withdraws	3 Innoprop. Words
1 Nil	3 Abn. Flexion	2 Innoprop. Sounds
	2 Extends	1 Nil
	1 Nil	

TIME				TIME				TIME		
E				E				E		
M				M				M		
V				V				V		
TOTAL				TOTAL				TOTAL		

Religion:

Admit Doctor: _____ Valuables: _____ Ticket #: _____ ER Doctor: _____

Room #: _____ (Call for Orders) Relatives Notified ☐ Present ☐ NSG. Manager ☐

Admitting Diagnosis: _____ ER Nurse: _____ Report Called: _____

To NSG. Unit Via: Stretcher ☐ W/C ☐ Carried ☐ RN/LPN/EMT/Other: ☐ O₂ ☐ /LPM ☐ Monitor

Condition In Transport: Remains Same ☐ Improved ☐ Worsened ☐ Changed ☐

Explain:

NURSES NOTES:

Figure 37–4. Emergency department chart for the severely injured patient.

689

Lacking other indications, they can be stopped three to five days following injury (Jones, 1977).

A compact emergency department record is essential for recording the physical findings, laboratory data, and course of the severely injured patient. Diagrams of the body are useful for quick reference in the case of multiple injury. Fill-in tables for monitored vital signs and administered fluids, blood, and other drugs are helpful in this fast-moving situation. Figure 37–4 illustrates such an emergency department chart designed for recording the findings and course of the severely injured patient.

TIMING OF OPERATION

Timing of the proper moment when resuscitation in the emergency department should stop and operation should begin requires mature judgment. In the presence of continued massive bleeding, this may be after the first flood of multiple transfusions when the patient first begins to respond and receives adequate peripheral organ perfusion.

Laboratory studies should not supplant clinical judgment. When the time comes in the resuscitation period to operate, the surgical team, the anesthesiologist, and the operating room must be ready.

POSTOPERATIVE CARE

The cards are stacked against an uneventful postoperative course for the severely injured patient. Without the benefit of unhurried preoperative preparation or evaluation of underlying diseases, he or she has usually suffered serious metabolic insults both by direct injury to vital organs and by varying periods of shock. The operation may involve several organs, may be difficult technically, and may leave the patient at risk for continued bleeding and bacterial infection. Postoperative care often may involve familiarity or expertise with skills mentioned in every chapter of this manual (Table 37–1).

Table 37–1. LABORATORY PROCEDURES IMPORTANT IN THE POSTOPERATIVE CARE OF THE SEVERELY INJURED PATIENT

Determination of blood and fluid loss via tubes, drains, catheters, and into dressings
Urine output
Volume and type of fluid administered
Continuous EKG recording
Arterial blood pressure (cannulated artery)
Central venous pressure
Insertion of Swan-Ganz catheter for pulmonary wedge pressure
Arterial blood PO_2, PCO_2, and pH
Cardiac output (thermodilution)
Core body temperature

It is not by chance that intensive care units developed from shock wards spawned from experience with the care of combat casualties. The trauma surgeon must be "the intensivist," familiar both with the subtleties of metabolic response to injury and the knowledge and ability to reoperate when indicated.

Blood Volume Replacement. A common problem following operation involves blood loss and its adequate replacement. Typically the patient has received large volumes of blood, intravenous crystalloid solutions, and numerous drugs that complicate interpretation of monitored signs of hypovolemia. The operation presumably established hemostasis, but an early postoperative decision must be made as to whether intravascular volume has been adequately restored. A first approximation can be made by comparing known past and continuing blood loss with that already replaced.

The clinical decision is whether (1) to temporize while the patient recovers from the recent physical and pharmacologic insults, (2) to give more blood, (3) to correct a bleeding diathesis, or (4) to reoperate to achieve more secure hemostasis.

In the immediate postoperative one to four hours, it is usually permissible to temporize while awaiting metabolic unloading of the administered drugs and recovery from the extensive fluid shifts consequent to injury. This is a good time to check for a bleeding diathesis. Initial screening should include prothrombin time, partial thromboplastin time, and platelet count. If these are normal, there is only a slight chance of a clotting abnormality in an otherwise healthy person. The usual clotting defect is related to consumption and washout of platelets.

External blood loss must be continually quantified. This includes recording the volume of blood obtained from the nasogastric tube, chest tubes, sumps, and catheters. Of more difficulty is quantifying blood losses in or beneath bulky dressings that can absorb large volumes of blood. Large dressings seldom will tamponade bleeding by external pressure and compound the surgeon's inexorable tendency to underestimate continued bleeding, knowing its consequent reflection on his failure to achieve hemostasis during operation. A 4 in × 4 in dressing can hold 10 ml blood, and the usual soaked abdominal pad can absorb 100 ml. Dressing changes obviously multiply this loss and must be meticulously recorded.

Clinical signs of continued bleeding are those of hypovolemia despite apparent adequate replacement. Hypovolemia should be recognized by the prodromes of shock plus decreased urine output, hypotension, tachycardia, decreased central venous pressure, and decreasing serial hematocrits. Mechanical devices to measure plasma volume by isotope or dye dilution techniques are not routinely used clinically.

A review of 70 patients who during a five-year period required reoperation following trauma (Driver et al., 1978) demonstrated that 15 per cent were reexplored for bleeding, most during the first 24 hours.

Table 37–2. POSTOPERATIVE DIFFERENTIATION OF
HYPOVOLEMIA VS. CARDIAC FAILURE

	HYPOVOLEMIA	LEFT HEART FAILURE
Clinical "shock"	+	+
Arterial blood pressure	↓	↓
Pulse	↑	↑
Respiratory rate	↑	↑
Urine output	↓	↓
Arterial Po_2	↓	↓
Central venous pressure	↓	↑
Swan-Ganz pulmonary artery wedge pressure	↓	↑
Cardiac output	↑	↓
Hematocrits	↓	±

Seven of the 18 patients so explored had undergone their excessive blood loss from drains or sump catheters. Patients with associated major pelvic fractures are particularly difficult to assess. There is inevitable major blood loss (over 1000 ml) into the intraperitoneal pelvic soft tissues, and normally there is little that can be done surgically to stop such seepage.

Heart Failure. The elderly patient with preexisting heart disease presents a special problem in the postinjury period. Massive blood loss, hypovolemia, increased cardiac work, hypoxia, and then massive intravenous infusions and transfusions put an obviously heavy burden on the already diseased heart. The clinical decision is whether decreased cardiac output is caused (1) by hypovolemia, to be treated by more blood transfusions; or (2) by cardiac failure, best treated oppositely (Table 37–2). The Swan-Ganz catheter, which mirrors left atrial pressure (Chap. 20) is of particular importance under these circumstances. Elevated left atrial pressure (LAP) suggests heart failure. As detailed in Chapter 20, essentials in the management of such points include maintenance of good myocardial oxygenation with packed red blood cell transfusions to correct anemia, elevated Fio_2 or mechanical respirators to maintain high (over 70 mm Hg) arterial Po_2, diuretics, cautious administration of intravenous sodium solutions, correction of electrolyte abnormalities, correction of arrhythmias, and digitalization.

Hypothermia. Massive amounts of blood may have to be administered through two or more large-bore catheters within the first 30 to 45 minutes in resuscitating the severely injured patient. Currently there is no way to warm refrigerated blood to 37°C when administered this quickly. The patient stripped of clothing for examination and treatment and suffering partial paralysis of the temperature regulatory mechanisms by shock and drugs gets cold in the preoperative and intraoperative period and may proceed in the postoperative period to thermoregulatory decompensation. This patient cannot rewarm himself or herself and is in essence a poikilotherm.

Hypothermia is usually overlooked by those not familiar with the treatment of the massively injured. Neurologic depression and unconsciousness, bleeding diathesis, hypotension as measured in the extremities, bradycardia, low cardiac output, decreased or absent urine output, acidosis, and blood gas abnormalities, all secondary to hypothermia, present a confusing array of signs, each of which can be ascribed to some other cause, but each is usually a manifestation of generalized hypothermia.

The massively injured patient receiving large volumes of cold blood should have a thermoprobe inserted high into the rectum or into the esophagus for measurement of core temperature.

Treatment requires external warming with hot water blankets and bags or extracorporeal pumping through a blood warmer as used in cardiopulmonary bypass.

Respiration. The problem of postinjury adult respiratory distress syndrome (ARDS), which gained prominence in managing Vietnam War casualties, has been covered in detail elsewhere in this volume (Chap. 14). Etiologic factors include the following: (1) direct lung contusion; (2) overinfusion of fluid, electrolytes (sodium in particular), and protein, which may pool within the alveoli and prolong oxygen exchange; (3) left ventricular failure; (4) increased pulmonary vascular permeability; and (5) microemboli from transfused blood.

During postoperative days, the effects of the following must be added: (6) oxygen toxicity; (7) sepsis; and (8) fat embolism.

Several of these factors are often simultaneously operative.

Diagnostic signs include rales or pulmonary edema, dyspnea, hypoxia, and roentgenographic pulmonary infiltrates.

Fundamentals of treatment include (1) endotracheal intubation; (2) mechanical volume respiration; (3) positive end-expiratory pressure (PEEP); (4) minimal concentration of inspired oxygen (FiO_2) required to maintain the arterial PO_2 above 60 mm Hg after the initial period of resuscitation; (5) minimal intravenous fluid, electrolyte, and protein (plasma, albumin, and other sources) required to avoid cardiovascular collapse; and (6) diuretics.

Intelligent and dedicated treatment now permits an exellent prognosis for early onset ARDS.

Late onset of ARDS (five or more days following injury) carries a far graver prognosis and is usually associated with intraperitoneal sepsis (Walker and Eiseman, 1975).

Sepsis. Open injuries are all contaminated. The surgeon's task is to avoid establishment of infection. Factors at his or her disposal are (1) wound coverage with dressings to avoid additional contamination; (2)

avoidance of prolonged hypotension and depression of the immune response; (3) early wound irrigation and débridement; (4) broad-spectrum antibiotics starting at the earliest possible moment following injury; (5) performing all the required operations properly; and (6) proper (often open) management of soft tissue wounds.

Despite adherence to these utopian directions, penetrating or even severe blunt soft tissue injury is associated with infection in 10 to 21 per cent of cases (Polk et al., 1976).

Multiple Organ Failure. Improved technology in respiratory and other organ support maintains life in injured patients who previously would have died from failure of a single organ system. This technology-created syndrome of failure of two or more vital organ systems has variously been termed multiple organ failure (MOF) or sequential systems failure (Eiseman et al., 1977; Baue, 1975). Characteristically it begins after three or more relatively tranquil postoperative days when resuscitation and convalescence seemed to be progressing normally. Early signs include decreased renal, hepatic, and respiratory function. Such patients usually are already being supported by a mechanical respirator. Preexisting disease such as emphysema, heart disease, or cirrhosis may dictate which major organ is first to fail, but once triggered, the additional metabolic burden thrown on other organs starts the disastrous MOF cascade, which may also include stress bleeding, clotting system failure, late onset ARDS, jaundice and liver coma, and acute renal failure. Each organ failure must be treated by its specific method of organ support as outlined elsewhere in this manual. Cumulatively, these may require prolonged use of a complex array of expensive mechanical devices. Approximately 75 per cent of such patients in MOF will die.

There is a strong positive correlation (75 per cent) between MOF and undrained pus even though the failing organs are not themselves sites of infection.

Symptomatic treatment includes individual organ support, but ultimate success usually depends upon locating and draining the septic focus. Small intraperitoneal accumulations of pus are still difficult to localize either by physical examination or by newer techniques such as ultrasound, isotope studies, and CAT scans. None is reliable in localizing an abscess less than 2 cm in diameter. Reoperation on these desperately ill patients in MOF to drain pus may be necessary, even if definitive evidence of its location is lacking.

MISCELLANEOUS PROBLEMS

Fat Embolism. This problem is usually associated with long bone fracture and is manifested by confusion, fever, petechiae, and respiratory insufficiency 12 to 36 hours after injury. Its treatment is symptomatic with mechanical ventilatory support.

Delirium Tremens. Severe injury can unmask a variety of preexisting psychiatric disorders or drug dependencies. These may both confuse the clinical picture and themselves be associated with morbidity and mortality.

Nutrition. The severely injured patient is in a hypermetabolic state. If bacterial sepsis intervenes, this is significantly multiplied. When such infection intervenes, the injured patient may require intravenous supplementation of calories, vitamins, and proteins to keep him or her in positive balance and to facilitate optimal recovery.

CONCLUSION

1. Preoperative care of the severely injured patient is designed (a) to correct by first aid measures life-threatening mechanical problems such as airway obstruction, ventilation, and bleeding; (b) to restore blood volume toward acceptable normality as quickly as possible; (c) to transport the patient as quickly as possible to a hospital facility staffed, equipped, and organized for care of the acutely injured patient; and (d) to choose the optimal moment for operative achievement of hemostasis and organ repair.

2. Postoperative care of the injured patient includes an understanding of the entire spectrum of mechanical and metabolic organ failure and organ support. It requires sophisticated monitoring in a well-staffed intensive care unit. Improvements in individual organ support have placed these patients at particular risk for MOF, which carries a 75 per cent mortality. Management of the severely injured patient frequently requires availability of all the monitoring and support devices described in this manual plus the knowledge, experience, and wisdom essential for their proper use.

REFERENCES

American College of Surgeons, Committee on Trauma: Guidelines for design and function of a hospital emergency department. Chicago, 1970.

American College of Surgeons, Committee on Trauma: Optimal hospital resources for care of the seriously injured. Bull. Am. Coll. Surg., 61(9):15–19, 1976.

American College of Surgeons, Committee on Trauma: Essential equipment for ambulances. Bull. Am. Coll. Surg., 62(9):7–12, 1977.

Baue, A. E.: Multiple, progressive or sequential systems failure. Arch. Surg., 110(7):779–781, 1975.

Brantigan, C. O., and Grow, J. B.: Cricothyroidotomy: Elective use in respiratory problems requiring tracheotomy. J. Thorac. Cardiovasc. Surg., 71(1):72–81, 1976.

Carter, J. H.: Planning and operation of the emergency room. *In* Eckert, C. (ed.): Emergency Room Care, 3rd ed. Boston, Little, Brown, 1976, pp. 13–29.

Cleveland, H. C., Bigelow, D. B., Dracon, D., and Dusty, F.: A civilian air emergency service: A report of its development, technical aspects and experience. J. Trauma, 16(6):452–463, 1976.

Driver, T., Kelly, G., and Eiseman, B.: Reoperation following abdominal trauma. Am. J. Surg., 135:747, 1978.

Eiseman, B., Beart, R., and Norton, L.: Multiple organ failure. Surg. Gynecol. Obstet., 144(3):323–326, 1977.

Jones, R. C.: Antibiotics in trauma. J. Surg. Pract., 6(5):26–31, 1977.

Knopp, R., and Dailey, R. H.: Central venous cannulation and pressure monitoring. J. Am. Coll. Emerg. Phys., 6(8):358–366, 1977.

Penterman, D. G.: Telecommunications. *In* Jelenko, D., and Frey, C. F. (eds.): Emergency Medical Services: An Overview. Bowie, MD, Robert J. Brady Co., 1976, pp. 97–116.

Polk, H. C., Fry, D., and Flint, L. W.: Dissemination and causes of infection. Surg. Clin. North Am., 56(4):817–829, 1976.

Walker, L., and Eiseman, B.: The changing pattern of post-traumatic respiratory distress syndrome. Ann. Surg., 181(5):693–697, 1975.

38

The Burn Patient

BASIL A. PRUITT, JR.
RICHARD C. TREAT

The early care of severely burned patients can be divided conveniently into two phases, with emphasis placed on maintenance of life and organ function in the resuscitation period and on wound closure and prevention of infection thereafter. The preoperative and postoperative care of burn patients is similar to that of other critically injured patients; however, certain burn specific modifications influence general care as well as preparation for and performance of operative therapy, and postoperative care influences subsequent burn management depending upon the operation performed. The current renaissance of excisional therapy emphasizes the importance of physiologically based treatment of the burn patient and requires awareness on the part of the attending surgeon of the pathophysiologic consequences of thermal injury.

RESUSCITATION

Thermal energy of sufficient intensity and duration causes coagulation necrosis of tissue, which, in areas of cell death and injury, is associated with increased capillary permeability and extravasation of the fluid components of the blood. This process is manifested clinically as edema, the duration and extent of which reflect the magnitude of the capillary "leak" and the resulting decrease in plasma and circulating blood volume. Fluids are given in proportion to the extent of burn* to minimize and replace this deficit in plasma volume and to preserve organ function. The many formulas used to predict or estimate the fluid

---

*Extent of burn is most easily estimated using any of several surface area charts or the Rule of Nines which describes the percentage of body surface represented by anatomical areas, i.e., each upper limb 9%, anterior and posterior trunk each 18%, each lower limb 18%, head and neck 9%, and genitalia and perineum 1%.

needs for postburn resuscitation have all been reported to be effective in the vast majority of burn patients.

FLUID THERAPY

The majority of fluid resuscitation formulas are based on replacement of 2 ml of fluid per kg body weight per percentage of body surface burn, but recently advanced modifications have recommended either 4 ml of balanced salt solution per kg body weight per percentage of burn or less than 2 ml of hypertonic salt solution per kg body weight per percentage of burn, respectively. The effectiveness of more rapid infusion of larger volumes of fluid during the period of maximum capillary permeability is questionable and may further accentuate edema formation. Additionally, laboratory and clinical studies have confirmed clinically satisfactory resuscitation using lesser volumes than 4 ml per kg per percentage of burn, even when the fluid volume approximates one-half the volume requirements estimated by the Brooke formula. Pulmonary edema is uncommon during the resuscitation period and most often occurs during the edema resorption phase when the blood volume is at its greatest, and the resuscitation fluid load is being reprocessed through the circulation, a natural sequence that justifies parsimony of infusion.

The goal of resuscitation is the preservation of vital organ function at the least immediate or delayed physiologic cost. The fluid volume and salt dosage to be infused should be calculated to avoid the side effects and complications noted above. Laboratory and clinical studies have led us to revise the Brooke formula to minimize salt loading and to limit the volume of fluid infused by taking advantage of the time course of vascular permeability changes. During the first 24 hours postburn only lactated Ringer's solution is infused, with the amount necessary estimated according to the formula in Table 38–1. One should plan to administer one-half of the first 24-hour fluid ration in the first eight hours postburn (not eight hours postadmission), which is the period of greatest vascular permeability and most rapid edema formation. As outlined in Table 38–1, the estimates of fluid needs are also age-related. The greater volume of fluid required per kg body weight for resuscitation of the burned child compared with the burned adult is related to the greater surface area per unit body mass of pediatric patients and the relatively greater volume of salt-containing edema fluid, which forms as a consequence of a burn of the same size in relation to body weight. Other formulas may be utilized to estimate resuscitation needs, provided one adjusts the rate of infusion according to the patient's response and avoids excessive volume and/or electrolyte administration.

Recent echocardiographic studies in burn patients during resuscitation have identified hypercontractility of the left ventricle with no

Table 38–1. ESTIMATION OF POSTBURN RESUSCITATION NEEDS

FIRST 24 HOURS
Adults: Lactated Ringer's — 2 ml/kg body wt/% burn
Children: Lactated Ringer's — 3 ml/kg body wt/% burn

SECOND 24 HOURS
Adults and children: Colloid-containing fluid* — 0.3–0.5 ml/kg body wt/% burn
Glucose in water — to maintain urinary output

CLINICAL GUIDES TO RESUSCITATION
Hourly urinary output:
   Adult: 30–50 ml/hr
   Child < 30 kg: 1 ml/kg body wt/hr
General condition
Vital signs
CVP or PCWP cannula only on specific indication

*Plasma, or albumin in physiologic saline solution

evidence of myocardial depression even in those patients with diminished cardiac output; the etiology of the cardiac output depression was an intravascular volume deficit. The cardiac output in some of those study patients appeared to be supported better in the last half of the first postburn day by colloid-containing fluids; accordingly, such fluids should be given to those patients with extensive burns who show evidence of persistently impaired tissue perfusion.

During the second 24 hours, colloid-containing and electrolyte-free fluids are infused to replace any persistent plasma volume deficit and to replenish metabolic losses. The plasma volume deficit that exists at the end of the first postburn day can be measured by radioisotope dilution techniques or estimated as being between 0.3 and 0.5 ml per kg of body weight per percentage of burn (0.3 ml per kg per percentage of burn for those patients with 30 to 50 per cent of the body surface burned, increasing to 0.5 ml per kg per percentage of burn for those patients with burns of over 70 per cent of the total body surface). The measured or estimated plasma volume deficit should be replaced using either plasma, or albumin diluted to physiologic concentration with saline. During the second 24 hours postburn, when cardiac output has been restored and plasma volume restitution is under way, one should make planned attempts to reduce the volume of fluids being infused. In patients deemed clinically to be resuscitated adequately, the infusion rate should be reduced arbitrarily by 25 per cent and maintained at that reduced level for one hour. During that hour, if urinary output remains at satisfactory levels, the lesser infusion rate should be maintained for the succeeding two hours, after which the patient's response to a similar stepwise reduction of infusion rate should be assessed. Both early and late complications of resuscitation can be minimized by such titration of infusion volume and hourly urinary output to prevent excessive fluid loading.

The efficacy of resuscitation is monitored most readily by the hourly urinary output, which should be 30 to 50 ml per hr in the adult and 1 ml per kg body weight per hour for children of less than 30 kg body weight. Therefore, an indwelling urethral catheter should be inserted and connected to a closed drainage system in any patient with a burn of 20 per cent or more of the total body surface. Monitoring of the vital signs and general condition is also helpful, although a blood pressure obtained in an increasingly edematous limb, using a sphygmomanometer, is of uncertain reliability. If the measurement of blood pressure is necessary, an intra-arterial line should be inserted to obtain an accurate measurement of arterial pressure. Restlessness and anxiety frequently are early signs of hypovolemia or hypoxemia, and if those conditions are confirmed, the fluid administration rate should be increased, or oxygen-enriched air should be supplied, or both. Central venous and pulmonary capillary wedge pressure catheters (the latter are preferred) are reserved for use in those patients with preexisting heart disease or those who fail to respond to resuscitation in the anticipated manner.

In patients with conventional thermal injury receiving timely fluid therapy, oliguria during the resuscitation period is rarely due to acute renal failure, and its occurrence should prompt more rapid infusion of fluid, not the administration of a diuretic and restriction of fluid infusion. Renal failure occurs with greatest frequency in burn patients with high concentrations of hemochromogens in their urine (those with high-voltage electric injury or those with crush injury) and in those with extensive burns who remain oliguric despite having received more than their estimated fluid needs. A diuretic of either the osmotic or loop type (the former is generally preferred) should be administered to hasten clearance of urinary pigment, to obtain an adequate urinary output, and to prevent renal failure in such patients. After a diuretic has been given, the urinary output is no longer effective for monitoring resuscitation adequacy, and other indices must be used.

Red cell destruction occurs in burn patients in direct proportion to the extent of full-thickness injury. Reported losses of red cell mass vary considerably, but most investigators have measured 10 to 15 per cent reductions following extensive thermal injury. There may also be additional losses of varying magnitude following resuscitation, depending upon the type and duration of wound care required. During the resuscitation period, when plasma leaks from the capillaries, the administration of whole blood or packed cells is avoided, since their infusion would further elevate an already increased hematocrit and would exert adverse rheologic effects on the microcirculation. Burn patients with significant hemorrhage secondary to associated injury or those with preexisting anemia represent obvious exceptions, and they should be given transfusions of packed red cells.

PAIN MEDICATION

Analgesic medication in the immediate postburn period must always be given intravenously, in small doses as often as necessary. Administration of analgesic medication by the intramuscular or subcutaneous routes during a time of impaired tissue perfusion and edema formation is frequently ineffective, and the lack of pain relief may prompt repeated and multiple administrations of narcotic medications in the subcutaneous or muscular tissue. As resuscitation proceeds and tissue perfusion improves, the multiple previously administered doses may be mobilized from the site of injection and absorbed simultaneously, causing profound respiratory depression. This sequence of events must be considered in any burn patient received in transfer who experiences unexpected respiratory depression of rapid onset, and a narcotic antagonist should be administered.

TETANUS PROPHYLAXIS

Tetanus prophylaxis is dictated by the patient's prior tetanus immunization status, as outlined in the American College of Surgeons' Committee on Trauma Guidelines. A booster dose of toxoid should be administered to those patients who have undergone prior active immunization and have not had a toxoid booster within the preceding five years.

INHALATION INJURY

Respiratory tract injury resulting from the inhalation of heated gases or products of incomplete combustion is a frequent complication of thermal injury. The presence of an inhalation injury significantly increases the mortality and morbidity associated with a given burn and presents a special hazard to the patient undergoing an operative procedure. Early diagnosis and initiation of therapy are important for planning the treatment course and increasing survival in burn victims.

Clinically, there are two types of inhalation injuries. Heat inhalation injuries result from breathing hot gases and usually affect only the upper respiratory tree. The clinical manifestation of this injury is the accumulation of supraglottic edema, which may proceed to cause complete airway obstruction. The inhalation of toxic products of incomplete combustion, on the other hand, primarily causes damage to the small airways and alveoli, often leading to respiratory insufficiency.

The patient's history and physical examination, combined with laboratory and clinical studies, are utilized to diagnose and differentiate inhalation injuries. Respiratory tract damage should be suspected in those patients burned in a closed space, those with facial burns, or those with impaired mental function, such as intoxication or head injury, at time of injury. The signs and symptoms indicative of inhalation injury first appear at varying times postburn, depending upon the severity of the injury, and it may be more than 24 hours before they are evident. The production of carbonaceous sputum indicates that the patient has inhaled soot and is likely to have some degree of inhalation injury. Hoarseness or stridor are commonly noted in patients with hot gas inhalation and are usually indicative of some degree of airway compromise. Wheezing, rales, bronchorrhea, hemoptysis, and coughing are symptoms often reflecting pathologic changes in the small airways and alveoli.

Early significant deterioration in arterial oxygen levels is associated with severe inhalation injury. The alveolar-arterial oxygen gradient should be calculated and monitored regularly, since an increase in this gradient is usually associated with progressive disease. In patients suspected of having inhalation injury, daily chest roentgenograms should be obtained. Progressive change with the appearance of compensatory emphysema and generalized patchy infiltrates may occur if bronchopneumonia develops later. These chest roentgenographic changes may occur prior to significant deterioration of arterial blood gas levels.

Airway findings associated with inhalation injuries can be divided into an extramucosal category, including the presence of carbonaceous material and bronchorrhea, and a mucosal category, including edema, vesicle formation, erythema, hemorrhage, ulceration, or ischemia, and all can be identified by direct examination using the fiberoptic bronchoscope. Edema causing obliteration of the pyriform sinuses, significant supraglottic edema, or massive swelling of the epiglottis may be present to such a degree as to compromise the airway. In this situation, establishment of an artificial airway, preferably by nasotracheal intubation, is mandatory to prevent airway obstruction. An endotracheal tube of appropriate size should be placed over the bronchoscope and should be inserted in the course of the endoscopic examination, if such is deemed necessary. Edema of lesser degree, which limits upper airway diameter but does not threaten patency, should be treated by inhalation of nebulized racemic epinephrine (0.5 ml of a 2.25 per cent solution diluted to 2.0 ml in normal saline) every two to four hours. Such treatment limits further swelling of glottic tissues and, in our experience, has reduced the need for endotracheal intubation.

The use of [133]xenon perfusion ventilation lung scanning to establish the diagnosis of inhalation injury was first reported from the U.S. Army Institute of Surgical Research in 1972. Ten μC of [133]xenon dissolved in isotonic solution are injected into the venous system, volatilized at the pulmonary capillary–alveolus interface, and exhaled via the lungs. Criteria for an abnormal scan include uneven or delayed (more than 90 seconds) clearing of the isotope. Falsely positive scans are associated with pathologic conditions such as chronic obstructive pulmonary disease, bronchitis, bronchiectasis, viral pneumonia, asthma, and other diseases resulting in decreased air movement in the small airways of the lungs. This simple technique does not require patient cooperation and has an 86 per cent accuracy in the diagnosis of inhalation injuries. Although a positive scan indicates parenchymal lung damage, it does not quantify the severity of the inhalation injury. Moreover, the accuracy of the test is influenced by minute ventilation; therefore, marked hyperventilation may result in a falsely negative test. Accordingly, the ^{133}xenon lung scan should be performed during the first three postburn days before the marked increase in postburn hyperventilation occurs.

Frequent, sequential evaluation of patients who may have inhalation injury is mandatory. Routine evaluations by the respiratory therapist or nurse should include observation of the onset of hoarseness or facial edema. Auscultation of the trachea to discern turbulent air flow and of the lungs to listen for decreased breath sounds, wheezing, or rales must also be undertaken. A diagnosis made by history, physical examination, clinical studies, or laboratory tests should be followed by initiation of treatment.

Successful management of the injury depends at least in part on accurate differentiation between heat and chemical injuries. In patients with heat injuries, therapy includes the utilization of humidified oxygen and elevation of the head and neck (elevation should of course be keyed to the volume replacement status of the individual patient). Continuous monitoring of airway patency and early intervention to establish an artificial airway in the presence of progressive accumulation of edema of the upper respiratory tract are essential in the care of these patients. The management of patients suspected of having chemical irritation injuries should include the use of humidified oxygen, the use of incentive spirometry, or, if that is not possible, intermittent positive pressure breathing (IPPB), and frequent performance of chest percussion and postural drainage.

Patients with severe inhalation injury often develop major complications such as pulmonary edema, pneumonia, and respiratory insufficiency despite aggressive treatment. Bronchopneumonia is a frequent complication of inhalation injury, and its causes are multiple. Treatment follows established principles as described earlier. The use of assisted mechanical ventilation is necessary in those patients with inhalation injury who develop respiratory insufficiency. High tidal volumes (15 cc per kg body weight or higher) and frequently the addition of positive end-expiratory pressure may be necessary to combat generalized progressive atelectasis with widespread alveolar collapse in such patients. Deterioration of pulmonary function, coupled with the extreme metabolic demands of burn patients, often induces strikingly high minute ventilation volumes in the range of 25 to 30 liters. Although unusual, minute volumes of up to 40 liters have been required at times to maintain acceptable arterial blood gas levels.

Prophylactic systemic administration of steroids has been recommended for patients with inhalation injury, but studies at this Institute have shown such treatment to have no beneficial effect, and more recent studies by others have identified an increase in septic complications following such treatment. Steroid therapy may be of use in the treatment of inhalation injury patients with intractable bronchospasm as in the case of asthmatics.

The performance of elective operations such as burn wound excision in patients with undiagnosed inhalation injury who receive a general anesthetic and a large-volume intraoperative infusion of blood and other fluids may result in rapid pulmonary deterioration and ultimately death. The performance of a [133]xenon scan may be particularly helpful to identify this group of patients who do not appear to have an inhalation injury by usual clinical criteria but in whom occult respiratory damage is present. Burn victims requiring life-saving operations who are either known or suspected of having inhalation injuries should receive exceptionally frequent monitoring of their pulmonary function both during and following operative procedures. Prolonged assisted mechanical ventilatory support should be anticipated for this group of patients. The anesthesiologist should receive specific notification of this condition and of the possible intraoperative need for mechanical ventilation with high minute volumes and/or positive end-expiratory pressure.

ESCHAROTOMY

Patients who suffer circumferential burns of the extremities require special consideration because the ensuing pathophysiologic events may lead to vascular compromise in these extremities. The physician who treats burn patients, even if he or she is just attempting to stabilize them in the acute resuscitation period prior to transport to a burn center, must be aware of the various techniques of monitoring vascular competence in these patients and must be able to perform emergency escharotomy and occasionally even fasciotomy.

The denaturation and coagulation of protein in the skin results in the formation of unyielding eschar in patients with circumferential third-degree burns. The combination of unyielding eschar and edema formation results in a gradual increase in the tissue pressure. A cycle is therefore established, with increasing tissue pressure further limiting venous flow, which in turn increases capillary leakage and causes a further increase in tissue pressure. Ultimately, such vascular compromise may result in tissue ischemia. The consequence of that ischemia is distal tissue necrosis, which may lead to fibrotic contracture formation.

The adequacy of perfusion in the extremities of burn patients can be assessed in several ways. For years, clinical evaluation was all that was possible and still may be utilized when more sophisticated methods are not available. Cyanosis of unburned skin, impaired capillary refilling, and progressive neurologic change are signs of vascular inadequacy, but all may be difficult to evaluate in a burned limb because of the surface injury itself. The Doppler ultrasonic flowmeter is the instrument most frequently used to determine blood flow adequacy. The examiner should be able to characterize the Doppler tone as normal, abnormal, or absent. In the upper extremity, flow evaluations are performed in the brachial, radial, ulnar, palmar arch, and digital arteries. In the lower extremities, the popliteal, dorsalis pedis, posterior tibial, and digital arteries are evaluated. Surgical decompression is indicated if pulsatile arterial flow is absent or if progressive diminution of the pulse signal is identified by repeated examinations.

The need for escharotomy in extremities that have not received circumferential third-degree burns is rare, since unyielding eschar does not surround these extremities. Prophylactic escharotomy is never indicated, and in our Institute only approximately 20 per cent of extremities with circumferential third-degree burns ultimately require surgical decompression. No accurate predictive criteria are available to determine which extremities will require surgical decompression. Documentation of cardiovascular stability prior to escharotomy is important, since inadequate perfusion may be secondary to shock. Fluid resuscitation, not escharotomy, is needed to improve the circulatory status in the hypovolemic patient.

The escharotomy should be performed on the midmedial or midlateral aspect of the extremity, and on the arm the incision should be anterior to the medial condyle of the elbow to avoid ulnar nerve injury. The escharotomy is carried out over the full length of the compressive third-degree burn and is specifically extended across involved joints, since failure to do this may even result in extremity banding with accentuation of the circulatory compromise. The depth of incision should be limited to that which will permit the incised wound margins to separate, i.e., through the eschar and the underlying superficial fascia. Incision into the deep subcutaneous tissue is not required and will unnecessarily increase blood loss. Escharotomy is performed as a bedside procedure without the use of anesthesia since the eschar is insensate. A scalpel or electrocautery may be used to perform the escharotomy, and success is determined by the return of arterial flow, which is usually documented using the Doppler ultrasonic flowmeter. On the upper extremity, the incision should be extended distally beyond the wrist. If adequate return of vascular flow does not occur following the escharotomy, fasciotomy should be performed. Fasciotomy is rarely required in patients with burns involving only the skin and subcutaneous tissue but may be necessary in burn patients with edema of tissue beneath the investing fascia, i.e., those with high-voltage electrical injury, those with associated mechanical trauma, and those with deep burns involving muscle. Fasciotomy is best performed in the operating room using an anesthetic of choice.

Complications of escharotomy include bleeding and infection. Hemorrhage following this procedure may be controlled with the use of electrocautery or suture ligation. Minor generalized oozing can usually be managed with the application of gauze sponges to the incision for a short period of time. Infection with subsequent invasion and even systemic sepsis can occur in escharotomy wounds. This can best be prevented by the repeated application to the escharotomy incision of the antimicrobial agent used for topical treatment of the burn wound.

Burned fingers are particularly susceptible to ischemia because of the presence of thin skin, minimal soft tissue, absence of venae comitantes, negligible collateral circulation, and frequent thrombosis of dorsal veins secondary to the burn. Finger escharotomy is indicated in patients requiring extremity escharotomy who also have third-degree burns of the fingers with significant edema but is of no value in patients with charred fingers. Intrinsic muscle necrosis is also a threat in patients with severe extremity burns involving both dorsal and palmar surfaces of the hand and may even occur in patients who have undergone extremity escharotomy. Therefore, if the fingers remain in the intrinsic minus position (metacarpophalangeal joints in hyperextension and interphalangeal joints in flexion) following extremity and finger escharotomy, intrinsic muscle ischemia should be suspected, and an intrinsic muscle fasciotomy should be performed. This is easily accomplished following exposure of the intrinsic muscles through small incisions in the first web space and distally between each of the metacarpals.

FLUID AND ELECTROLYTE MANAGEMENT POSTRESUSCITATION

Following resuscitation, fluid management of the burn patient is predicated upon providing enough electrolyte-free water to permit excretion of the salt load infused during resuscitation and replacing evaporative water loss in an amount that permits the patient to return to preburn weight by the eighth to tenth postburn day. As previously noted, pulmonary edema occurs most frequently during the edema resorption diuretic phase. This complication is most commonly encountered in those patients with preexisting heart disease, in those of either extreme of age, and in those who required excessive infusions to achieve hemodynamic stability during resuscitation. Pulmonary edema may occur later in the postburn period if maintenance fluids are not adjusted to take into account (1) the reduction of evaporative water loss when significant areas of the burn are either grafted or placed in occlusive dressings or (2) the volume of saline infused beneath donor sites to improve the quality of autograft harvest. The symptoms and signs of pulmonary edema in burn patients are the same as in other patients, and treatment is similarly keyed to the severity of pulmonary and cardiac derangements. Fluid balance and clinical indices of cardiac and pulmonary function must be monitored, and a daily chest roentgenogram must be obtained to insure early diagnosis of pulmonary edema. The "offloading" of fluid in burn patients with pulmonary edema is enhanced by the evaporative water losses from the burn wound as described below.

Dehydration is the most common disturbance of fluid balance in burn patients following resuscitation. Inadequate replacement of transeschar evaporative water loss is the usual cause of this complication. The burn wound has the characteristics of a free water surface, since thermal injury destroys the epidermal water vapor barrier of the skin. Evaporative water loss in burn patients is directly related to the extent of burn and can be estimated according to the following formula: Evaporative loss (milliliters per hour) = (25 + percentage of body surface burned) × total body surface area in square meters. This formula estimates evaporative water loss at the lower end of the range of observed losses, and the replacement fluids administered should be adjusted on the basis of daily determinations of serum osmolality, serum sodium concentration, and body weight.

Alterations of serum sodium concentration are the most common electrolyte abnormalities occurring in burn patients, with hypernatremia more frequent than hyponatremia, except in those patients treated with 0.5 per cent silver nitrate dressings. The causes of hypernatremia include osmotic diuresis, sepsis, a diabetes insipidus–like osmotic regulatory defect (rare), and inadequate evaporative water loss replacement, the latter having been implicated as the etiology in 61 per cent of the cases of hypernatremia identified at this Institute during an 18-month period. In all patients with hypernatremia, the underlying cause should be identified and corrected, water losses should be determined by careful review of intake and output records, and the measured or calculated deficit should be replaced with electrolyte-free water.

Hyponatremia occurs most commonly as a result of transeschar leeching of sodium in the adult burn patient being treated with 0.5 per cent silver nitrate soaks and as a result of rapid or excessive infusion of electrolyte-free fluid in the burned child. In a review of burn patients treated at this Institute, McManus et al. identified hyponatremia (a serum sodium of 125 mEq per l or less) as the cause of seizures in 42 per cent of burned children who had seizures during their postburn courses of treatment. The occurrence of hyponatremia during resuscitation can be reduced by combining the electrolyte-free fluids and electrolyte-containing fluids prior to administration or by careful regulation of the volume, rate, and salt concentration of the fluids administered. Transeschar salt loss is generally modest in patients treated by the exposure technique, but up to 300 mEq of sodium per day have been recovered from the dressings of burn patients treated by the occlusive technique. These transeschar losses of sodium can be markedly accentuated by 0.5 per cent silver nitrate soak therapy, which may produce profound hyponatremia.* Advocates of 0.5 per cent silver nitrate topical treatment recommend that 10 gm sodium chloride and 30 to 50 ml molar sodium lactate be given daily to patients with burns of up to 50 per cent of the total body surface and that 15 to 30 gm of sodium chloride and 50 to 80 ml of molar sodium lactate be given daily to patients with more extensive burns. Daily measurement of the serum sodium level and careful review of intake and output records are necessary to determine the actual dosage required for any given patient.

Generally, mild hyponatremia may also be present in the early stages of sepsis, presumably as a result of disproportionate reduction in renal free water clearance relative to glomerular filtration rate. In such patients, the septic focus should be identified and treated in addition to correcting the electrolyte deficit. Hyponatremia may also occur as a manifestation of the "sick cell" syndrome which is attributed to a cellular energy deficit rendering the cell unable to excrete sodium. Postburn increases in intraerythrocytic sodium concentration can be corrected or prevented by administration of sufficient calories, and some investigators have reported the sick cell syndrome to be correctable by intravenous administration of insulin and 50 per cent glucose or by blood transfusion.

Disturbances of potassium balance are also encountered in the burn patient, and hypokalemia is the most common disturbance following resuscitation. Hyperkalemia of modest degree occurs frequently during the initial 48 hours postburn as a result of hemolysis and tissue destruction. The serum potassium elevation may be exaggerated during the resuscitation period if acidosis supervenes due to inadequate resuscitation or if acute renal failure occurs. Potassium salts should be omitted from the resuscitation fluids, and if the serum potassium level rises sufficiently to cause cardiac dysfunction, ion exchange resins or glucose and insulin should be administered.

Following resuscitation, renal potassium losses are elevated above normal, and total potassium loss can be increased by the renal effect of mafenide (Sulfamylon) or the leeching effect of 0.5 per cent silver nitrate soaks. In Sulfamylon-treated patients, renal potassium losses of over 200 mEq per day have been measured, and in patients treated with 0.5 per cent silver nitrate soaks, transeschar potassium losses of up to 275 mEq per square meter of burn surface per day have been measured. Daily monitoring of serum potassium levels and urinary potassium losses is necessary, and measured potassium losses should be replaced in order

---

*Chloride loss parallels sodium loss, and if it is unreplaced, hypochloremic alkalosis may result.

to maintain adequate serum levels, especially in those patients requiring digitalis therapy.

Mild hypocalcemia is identified frequently in burn patients, but it seldom causes clinical symptoms requiring treatment. Transeschar calcium leeching of significant degree may occur in patients treated with 0.5 per cent silver nitrate soaks and may require treatment with intravenously administered calcium salts. Documented complications due to postinjury depression of serum zinc or magnesium levels are rare. Commonly employed nutritional regimens appear to provide adequate amounts of zinc and magnesium, and specific supplementation of such constituents is rarely necessary.

WOUND CARE

TOPICAL ANTIMICROBIAL THERAPY

Following resuscitation, care of the burn patient is focused on the burn wound itself, and treatment goals include prevention of infection, preservation of tissue, maintenance of function, and timely wound closure. Thermal destruction of the skin and variable amounts of underlying subcutaneous tissue render the burn wound highly susceptible to infection because the eschar serves as a rich pabulum for microbial proliferation, and the avascularity of the wound limits the effectiveness of both host defense mechanisms and systemically administered antibiotics. Prior to the development of effective antimicrobial topical agents in the mid-1960s, infection in and through the burn wound with microbial densities in excess of 10^5 per gm of tissue in the eschar and adjacent tissues was present in 60 per cent of all burn patients who expired. Effective topical chemotherapy has significantly reduced this complication of thermal injury, and several topical agents of verified effectiveness are currently available. The topical agents do not sterilize the burn wound but do limit the proliferation of microorganisms to a density below that associated with wound invasion. Each available topical agent has advantages and limitations, and the agents should be employed with flexibility to meet specific wound care needs of individual patients (Table 38–2).

Conventional burn wound care entails once daily cleansing with débridement of eschar to the point of pain or bleeding. To avoid impairment of gastrointestinal function and to maintain nutrition, general anesthesia is not employed for daily débridement. Intravenous analgesics can be administered prior to débridement to minimize patient discomfort. In those patients unable to tolerate such procedures, subanesthetic doses of ketamine have been successfully utilized to avoid the gastrointestinal impairment associated with other anesthetic gases. The topical antimicrobial agent of choice is applied following débridement,

Table 38–2. Topical Antimicrobial Burn Wound Agents

	Mafenide Acetate Cream (Sulfamylon)	Silver Nitrate Soaks	Silver Sulfadiazine Cream (Silvadene)
Form of treatment	Exposure	Occlusive dressings	Exposure or single layer dressing
Concentration of active agent	11.1%	0.5%	1.0%
Advantages	Diffuses through eschar Compatible with treatment of associated injuries Wound visible Broad gram-negative antimicrobial activity Joint motion unimpeded	Pain-free on application Absence of hypersensitivity Broad gram-negative antimicrobial activity Decreases wound heat loss	Pain-free on application Wound visible if exposure treatment employed Compatible with treatment of associated injuries Joint motion unimpeded
Limitations	Exaggerates postburn hyperventilation Postapplication pain in second-degree burns Delayed eschar separation Hypersensitivity reactions	Does not penetrate eschar Losses of Na^+, K^+, Ca^{++}, and Cl^- through eschar Dressings impair joint motion Stains unburned skin and environment Methemoglobinemia (rare)	Limited eschar penetration Neutropenia due to bone marrow suppression Hypersensitivity (rare) Resistance of some *Pseudomonas* sp. and many *Enterobacter cloacae* Eschar separation delayed

and topical creams are reapplied, or 0.5 per cent silver nitrate dressings are changed every 12 hours.

Burn Wound Biopsy

Since none of the currently available topical agents sterilizes the burn wound, any patient may escape from microbial control and develop burn wound infection. The patients at greatest risk for this complication are those with burns involving more than 30 per cent of the body surface and those of either extreme of age, particularly burned children. At the time of daily cleansing, the entire burn wound must be examined for the clinical signs of burn wound infection in Table 38–3. Identification of such wound changes necessitates biopsy of the burn wound to confirm or exclude that diagnosis. Using a scalpel, a 500 mg lenticular-shaped specimen is excised from that area of the wound suspected of harboring infection. The specimen must include underlying and/or adjacent un-burned subcutaneous tissue. One-half of the specimen is submitted to the microbiology laboratory for quantitative culture, and the other half is placed in 10 per cent formalin and sent to the pathology laboratory for processing by rapid, but not frozen, technique.

A report of 10^5 or more organisms per gm of tissue on quantitative culture is consistent with, but not diagnostic of, invasive burn wound sepsis, since microbial proliferation in the subeschar space may occur just prior to spontaneous eschar separation in the absence of invasive infection. The pathologist examines the tissue prepared for histologic study and looks for signs of invasive sepsis, the most important of which is the presence of microorganisms in unburned tissue. Histologic confirmation of invasive burn wound infection necessitates therapeutic intervention. If a nonabsorbable topical agent is being used, it should be replaced by Sulfamylon burn cream. A change in topical agent is also warranted if rapid progression of bacteria or fungi through the eschar and microbial proliferation in the subeschar space are noted on serially obtained biopsy specimens.

Table 38–3. Clinical Signs of Burn Wound Infection

Accelerated eschar separation
Marked subeschar suppuration
Focal black, dark brown, or violaceous discoloration of the eschar
Degeneration of wound granulation tissue with neoeschar formation
Conversion of partial-thickness burn to full-thickness necrosis
Hemorrhage into subcutaneous tissue
Edema, hemorrhagic discoloration, or superficial ulceration of
  unburned skin at wound margins
Ecthyma gangrenosum
Vesicular lesions in healed or healing partial-thickness burn

Patients with confirmed burn wound invasion should be given systemic antibiotics to which the offending organism is sensitive and should also receive general supportive measures as indicated. In those patients in whom the invasion is focal or even multifocal, an antibiotic solution to which the invading organism is sensitive should be injected subeschar, as described by Baxter et al. (1973). Recent studies indicate that the effectiveness of subeschar antibiotic infusions in the treatment of such infection is related to the physical properties of the antibiotic (i.e., its tissue diffusibility) to a much greater extent than to in vitro activity of the antibiotic against the causative organism. The tissue beneath foci of *Pseudomonas* invasion should therefore be injected twice each day with a solution of 10 gm of carbenicillin dissolved in 150 ml of saline. A No. 20 spinal needle is used for these injections to minimize the number of injection sites. The sodium content of the antibiotic solution must be considered in planning electrolyte replacement for these patients. If the invasive process is generalized, consideration should be given to surgical excision and débridement following an immediate subeschar antibiotic infusion beneath all infected tissue and a second such infusion six hours later. The excised wound should be covered immediately with a biologic dressing. If the invasive infection extends beneath the investing fascia on a limb, the infected muscle must be debrided, and amputation may be required. Generalized burn wound sepsis is almost invariably fatal, and all treatments for this complication are attended by a small salvage.

Nonbacterial Infections

Improved control of the bacterial population of the burn wound has resulted in a relative increase in the incidence of fungal and viral infections in burn patients, although the occurrence of clinically significant fungal or viral infections in the total population at risk remains small. The previously detailed principles of burn wound biopsy and treatment also apply to fungal burn wound infections, but excisional therapy is inappropriate in the treatment of viral wound infections. *Candida* species are the most frequent nonbacterial organisms recovered from the burn wound, but they are seldom invasive. In the severely compromised host, invasive candidal infections may occur, and those, as well as invasive infections caused by the true fungi, necessitate excisional therapy and the systemic administration of the antifungal agents amphotericin B and/or 5-fluorocytosine. Invasive infection with systemic spread of *Herpesvirus hominis* requires treatment with systemically administered adenine arabinoside in a dosage of up to 20 mg per kg per day. The dose and duration of therapy are guided by the severity of the disease.

WOUND CLOSURE

When wound care proceeds uneventfully and the eschar has separated, wound bed maturity determines subsequent care. Those wounds with a bright red, finely granular bed of granulation tissue can be closed immediately with cutaneous autografts. Immature wounds should be covered with a biologic dressing to maintain control of wound microorganisms and to hasten the maturation of granulation tissue. If the eschar separates, leaving behind significant amounts of tenacious, nonviable dermis, those areas should be treated with occlusive dressings soaked in an antimicrobial solution and changed three times a day to hasten débridement. The lesser effectiveness of microbial control of such dressings dictates that they be applied to no more than 20 per cent of the total body surface at a given time.

BIOLOGIC DRESSINGS

Biologic dressings available for use in burn care today include cutaneous allograft, cutaneous xenografts from a variety of species (porcine xenograft in various forms is presently available from several commercial sources), and amnion. Fresh, frozen, and lyophilized forms of cutaneous allograft and xenograft have all been used, but the fresh viable form of each is generally preferred. In addition to promoting granulation tissue development and reducing microbial density of the burn wound, the biologic dressings decrease blood, protein, and evaporative water losses from the wound, diminish wound pain, facilitate joint motion, and improve the rapidity and quality of healing of some second-degree burns. In addition to being used for temporary coverage of burn wounds between the time of eschar separation and definitive grafting, the biologic dressings can be used for immediate coverage of superficial second-degree burns, for immediate coverage of excised wound beds, and for temporary coverage of traumatic, ulcerative, or incisional wounds. Viable cutaneous allograft is the preferred biologic dressing and the material against which all other materials used for temporary wound closure must be judged. The greater effectiveness of cutaneous allograft may be related to the fact that allograft success is associated with direct graft-to-recipient vascular connection, while adherence of the other biologic dressings appears to occur without such direct vascular connection.

Cutaneous allografts are preferentially harvested from cadavers in the operating room following conventional preparation of the donor sites. The grafts are taken at a thickness of .0012 to .0015 of an inch and can be stored in the nonfreezing compartment of a refrigerator in a sterile Petri dish to which penicillin solution may be added if desired.

The grafts so stored remain useful for up to 14 days but deteriorate with time; they function best when used immediately after harvest. To avoid possible transmission of disease, patients who expire with hepatitis, syphilis, significant cutaneous infection, or cutaneous malignancies are excluded as donors.

Cutaneous allografts are applied as a ward procedure to wounds of 5 per cent or more of the total body surface from which the eschar has separated but which are not ready for autografting, or they are applied to more mature wounds for which autograft skin is unavailable because of paucity of donor sites. These grafts are inspected daily; if adherent and vascularized, they are left in place for up to five days, at which time they should be changed. Removal of cutaneous allografts that have been left in place for longer periods of time requires either rejection with potentially adverse systemic effects or surgical excision attended by considerable blood loss. Grafts that are nonadherent or beneath which suppuration occurs should be removed and replaced with fresh allografts (focal subgraft collections of purulent material may be evacuated if of limited extent). Initially such grafts may need to be replaced daily, but as the underlying wound matures, the need for change decreases in frequency. If the patient becomes clinically toxic following application of biologic dressings, all such grafts should be removed, and topical antimicrobial therapy should be resumed. General adherence of the biologic dressings indicates wound readiness for autografting, which will be attended by a predictably excellent result.

AUTOGRAFTING

Following this program of wound preparation, the burns are definitively closed by autografting. Wounds ready for autografting are characterized by absence of nonviable tissue, a bright red, firm, finely granular bed of granulation tissue, absence of peripheral inflammation, firm adhesion of cutaneous allografts, and a wound bacterial count of less than 10^5 per gm of tissue. Wounds with exuberant or edematous granulation tissue should be treated with dry compression dressings for 24 to 48 hours prior to grafting and may need débridement at the time of grafting. Quantitative culture has been used by some to confirm readiness for grafting, but in our experience this is generally unnecessary, and clinical appraisal of the wound is reliable.

Area coverage to reduce the extent of burn takes priority in patients who have burns of more than 50 per cent of the total body surface. Functional areas take priority in patients with less extensive burns, with face, hand, foot, neck, and joint area burns closed before burns of other areas. The presence of beta-hemolytic streptococci on the burn wound may result in such rapid postoperative lysis of freshly applied grafts that graft destruction will have occurred before the diagnosis can be made.

To avoid this complication, prophylactic penicillin is given in the perioperative period. In patients who are allergic to penicillin, some other antistreptococcal medication, such as erythromycin, should be employed.

As part of the preoperative preparation of any burn patient, the anesthesiologist should be reminded not to use succinylcholine as an intraoperative muscle relaxant. A significant number of burn patients will respond to administration of succinylcholine by increasing their serum potassium levels by 10 per cent or more. This elevation in serum potassium is rapid, may be sustained for as long as seven minutes, and, if of sufficient magnitude, may cause cardiac irregularities. Although this reaction to succinylcholine most commonly occurs when it is administered to patients between the 10th and 60th postburn days, it is best omitted from the anesthetic management of any burn patient.

The postoperative care of skin grafts is dictated by the graft type and its location. Sheet grafts, which are preferred for coverage of well-prepared wounds in patients with sufficient donor sites, are left exposed if at all possible. The grafts are inspected every two to three hours, with subgraft collections of serum or blood expressed by rolling a cotton-tipped applicator from the site of the collection to the periphery of the graft or by using a scalpel to make a small incision over such collections and expressing their contents, or by needle aspiration of serum collections. The adherence of the graft, which increases with time, reduces the frequency with which such graft care is required.

In patients with limited donor sites and extensive burns, mesh grafts are commonly employed, and these should be kept covered by occlusive dressings moistened with an antimicrobial solution (in grafted areas of limited extent, saline may be used) to prevent desiccation of the exposed granulation tissue and the development of wound infection. At the time of initial dressing change, following autograft application, the innermost layer of the dressing (the fine mesh gauze applied directly over the graft) should be left in place if the grafts appear to be taking satsifactorily. After the third postgraft day, the entire dressing should be changed, and the grafts should be inspected in detail on a daily basis. If occlusive dressings are required for graft coverage, they should be firmly compressive to prevent avulsion of the grafts by movement of the dressing, and the limb should be immobilized by including a joint above and a joint below the graft site within the dressing.

Although poor nutritional status and certain specific metabolic defects may on rare occasions be the cause of graft failure or poor graft take, infection, inadequate wound preparation, and graft motion are the overwhelmingly predominant causes of graft failure. The risk of graft-lysing infection can be reduced by prophylactic antistreptococcal antibiotic therapy as noted earlier, and loss of grafts due to inadequate blood supply or infection by other inhabitants of the burn wound can be minimized by adequate pregraft débridement and preparation as previously described. Motion is a particular risk in small children and agitated adult patients, and such patients who require grafting, particularly of circumferential wounds of the limbs, have optimal graft take when the grafted limb is suspended in skeletal traction and left exposed during the postoperative period. All grafts treated by the exposure method should be protected from abrasion against the bed clothes by the use of bed cradles or other devices to prevent graft avulsion.

Postoperative care of donor sites begins in the operating room, where the donor sites are covered with a single layer of fine mesh gauze trimmed to size, and hemostasis is achieved by the application of warm moist laparotomy pads. When the patient returns to the ward, the laparotomy pads are removed and the donor site is dried by exposure to a heat lamp. Thereafter, the donor site should be kept dry by use of heat lamps following any wetting of the donor site dressings in the course of maintaining patient hygiene. If the donor site becomes infected or if suppuration occurs beneath the donor site dressing, the fine mesh gauze should be removed following application of warm, wet soaks, and topical antimicrobial therapy should be instituted.

BURN WOUND EXCISION

Burn wound excision as a means of reducing the risk of burn wound and systemic infection, limiting the duration and severity of pathophysiologic change, and shortening the hospital stay is currently enjoying a renaissance. Scalpel excision of the burn wound to the level of the investing fascia has been a frequently employed treatment for full-thickness burns of 20 per cent or less of the total body surface. Scalpel excision has also been used, though much less commonly, in the treatment of invasive burn wound sepsis and in attempts to salvage patients with massive burns, but the patient salvage in either instance has been meager. More recently, tangential and what is termed sequential excision have been used in the treatment of both partial-thickness and full-thickness burns with variable success. Tangential excision is specifically employed in the treatment of deep partial-thickness burns, particularly burns of the hand, while sequential excision has been used to treat full-thickness burns or burns of variable depth.

All forms of excision are associated with surprisingly great blood loss; in the case of tangential excision, loss can be reduced by the topical application of a solution of thrombin and epinephrine. Scalpel excision of areas of intermixed partial and full-thickness burns also results in the sacrifice of viable skin. The excised wound bed is also susceptible to infection by bacteria from adjacent, unexcised burn, and such wounds must be covered with a biologic dressing or autograft skin at the time of excision. The pulmonary effects of general anesthesia and the stress of operation further limit the usefulness of excision in patients with inhalation injury or other limitations of pulmonary reserve. Lastly, the uncertainty of graft take on the wound bed produced by tangential or sequential excision is a limiting factor in patients with massive burns and limited donor sites.

These adverse effects of burn wound excision and our observation that scalpel excision appears to benefit only those patients with burns from 40 to 60 per cent of the total body surface have defined more explicitly those situations in which these procedures are most useful. Scalpel excision to the level of the investing fascia is best employed in the treatment of patients will full-thickness burns of limited extent, patients requiring debridement of high-voltage electrical injury, and patients with burn wound sepsis. Tangential excision is best employed in the treatment of deep, partial-thickness, dorsal hand burns in which the injury does not involve the extensor tendons. Sequential excision is best employed in the staged excision of extensive burns with excision limited to 20 per cent of the total body surface at a single sitting or in the removal of persistent eschar later in the postburn course. Following excision, the excised wound bed must be covered with a biologic dressing or cutaneous autografts and thereafter must be treated by one of the techniques described earlier.

TREATMENT OF FRACTURES AND OSSEOUS INJURY IN BURN PATIENTS

Thermal injury may directly involve bone (most commonly seen in patients with high-voltage electrical injury or prolonged contact burns) or may destroy overlying soft tissue, resulting in desiccation of exposed periosteum, cortex, or both. The soft tissue defect should be closed to the periphery of the exposed cortex before undertaking decortication, which is then best achieved by using a bone chisel or rotary power tool, rather than by placing multiple drill holes in the cortex. Following the development of an adequate bed of granulation tissue, the wound is closed in the usual manner.

Associated skeletal trauma complicates the care of the burn patient in that long bone fractures limit one's options in positioning the patient and frequently necessitate use of mesh or air fluidized beds. Plaster fixation of long bone fractures underlying burn wounds heightens the risk of burn wound infection by precluding the use of topical antimicrobial agents and promoting rapid bacterial proliferation and consequently should not be employed. Similarly, internal fixation is seldom attempted because of the invariable microbial contamination of the wound at the time of operation and the frequent occurrence of bacteremia and septicemia, which can result in hematogenous seeding of the implanted foreign body. External compression devices, such as the Charnley clamp, can be used to advantage in the treatment of unstable joint injuries or long bone fractures that are not amenable to skeletal traction. The pin–soft tissue interface of external compression or skeletal traction devices should be cleansed daily, and a gauze sponge saturated with an antiseptic solution should be wrapped around the pin and fixed gently against the soft tissue. Significant bone infection as a complication of the use of these devices is infrequent, although focal cortical dissolution at the pin sites and pin tract infections are common. Hematogenous infection of a fracture hematoma may serve as a source of systemic infection, and that possibility should be investigated in a septic burn patient with associated fractures in whom no other source of infection can be identified. Although amputation may be necessary in such a situation, the infected hematoma should be drained initially.

GASTROINTESTINAL COMPLICATIONS

The gastrointestinal effects of burn injury range from ileus, which occurs in the immediate postburn period in nearly all patients with burns of 25 per cent or more of the total body surface, to acute upper gastrointestinal tract ulceration, acalculous cholecystitis, and obstruction of the duodenum by the superior mesenteric artery later in the postburn course. In patients with ileus, a nasogastric tube should be inserted and connected to suction to prevent gastric dilatation and aspiration. The nasogastric tube should be removed as soon as gastrointestinal motility returns in order to minimize associated pulmonary complications and mechanical trauma to the nasopharyngeal, esophageal, and gastric mucosa. Ileus is a common accompaniment of sepsis, and tube decompression of the stomach may therefore have to be reinstituted later in the postburn treatment course.

CURLING'S ULCER

Acute ulceration of the upper gastrointestinal tract is the most frequent life-threatening enteric complication of burn patients, and the incidence is related to the extent of the burn. Although the precise etiology of Curling's ulcer remains undefined, early disturbances of gastric and duodenal mucosal blood flow, bile reflux, gastric acid production, and sepsis appear to be contributing factors.

The correlation of gastric acid production with progression and severity of mucosal disease emphasizes the importance of antacid prophylaxis in preventing the development of clinically significant complications of postburn stress ulceration. A controlled trial of antacid prophylaxis carried out at this Institute confirmed a significant reduction in the incidence of bleeding and perforation in the group of burn patients who were given prophylactic antacid. The protective effect of such treatment was evident even in those patients predisposed to severe mucosal disease and clinical complications because of disruption of their gastric mucosal barrier as assessed by the lithium flux technique. The results of that trial have prompted us to employ antacid prophylaxis in all patients with burns of over 35 per cent of the total body surface. Immediately postburn, following insertion of a nasogastric tube and evacuation of the gastric contents, sufficient antacid should be instilled via the nasogastric tube to produce a pH of 5 or above in the gastric aspirate when sampled one hour later. To maintain such an intragastric environment, a similar amount of antacid is instilled on an hourly basis until gastrointestinal motility is restored and the tube is withdrawn. Similar doses of antacid are given by mouth thereafter until the burn wounds have healed or have been grafted. Several cases of intestinal obstruction secondary to inspissated antacid compounds have been reported, but maintenance of adequate hydration and use of the minimum volume of antacid to effect adequate buffering should minimze the occurrence of this complication.

A more recent clinical study has shown the H_2-antagonist cimetidine to be as effective as antacid prophylaxis in reducing the clinical complications of Curling's ulcer. Cimetidine was given in a dosage of 400 mg every four hours, intravenously when an intravenous line was in place and orally when the patient was receiving no intravenous fluids. After the tenth postburn day, the cimetidine dosage interval was increased to six hours. The absence of·side effects of cimetidine treatment, the elimination of the risk of medication bezoar formation, and the fact that cimetidine can be administered parenterally all favor its preferential use in burn patients for stress ulcer prophylaxis.

If prophylactic therapy is ineffective and perforation of a Curling's ulcer should occur, operative intervention is necessary. In a group of 212 burn patients with Curling's ulcer, hemorrhage was the most frequent complication, and bleeding was considered massive in 43 per cent. Distention and pain are both uncommon symptoms, the latter usually associated with perforation or massive, exsanguinating hemorrhage. Conservative, nonoperative treatment should be employed initially but should not be prolonged unduly, since it will deplete further the limited physiologic reserves of severely burned patients. In burned children with bleeding from a Curling's ulcer, blood volume replacement prior to surgical intervention should be limited to 60 per cent of the estimated blood volume because of the higher mortality observed in children receiving greater transfusion volumes. If stress ulcer bleeding is not controlled by nonoperative means, surgical treatment is necessary.

ACALCULOUS CHOLECYSTITIS

Laboratory evidence of nonspecific hepatic dysfunction occurs in approximately 60 per cent of extensively burned patients. The occurrence of jaundice in burn patients is an ominous sign and a frequent reflection of sepsis or hypoxia. Jaundice may also be caused by acute acalculous cholecystitis, and its occurrence in association with right upper quadrant pain should suggest that diagnosis. Prior to the widespread use of topical antimicrobial therapy, hematogenous infection of the gallbladder as part of generalized systemic infection secondary to burn wound invasion was the most frequent form of acalculous cholecystitis. At the present time, inflammation of the gallbladder without direct microbial infection of that organ is more common, with dehydration, biliary and gastrointestinal stasis, and hemolysis considered to be contributory factors. Abdominal examination of the burn patient suspected of having an inflamed gallbladder is difficult because of accompanying ileus, burns of the abdominal wall, and patient obtundation. If a tender, distended gallbladder is palpated on abdominal examination or identified by ultrasound scanning, cholecystectomy should be performed.

SUPERIOR MESENTERIC ARTERY SYNDROME

Burn patients of asthenic habitus who sustain significant weight loss during their course of therapy may develop the superior mesenteric artery syndrome. This usually partial obstruction of the duodenum is characterized by large volumes of gastric aspirate and postprandial abdominal distention or projectile vomiting. Roentgenologic examination of the upper gastrointestinal tract should be performed in such patients to identify the radiographic signs characteristic of this disease — dilatation of the proximal duodenum, obstruction of the duodenum at the level of the superior mesenteric vessels, and what appears fluoroscopically to be retrograde peristalsis. At the time of fluoroscopy, the patient should be examined in several positions to identify that position, usually the left lateral decubitus, which permits passage of contrast material beyond the partially occluding mesenteric vessels.

Initial treatment of the superior mesenteric artery syndrome should always be nonoperative, and duodenojejunostomy should be reserved for those patients in whom nonoperative treatment is ineffective or cannot be employed because of other concurrent complications. A nasogastric tube should be inserted, and gastric drainage should be maintained until the obstruction is relieved and the volume of gastric aspirate falls below 30 ml per hour. During and following meals, the patient should be placed in the position that permits passage of the contrast material (as identified at the time of the roentgenographic examination) in order to facilitate passage of duodenal contents beyond the site of the superior mesenteric vessels. If there is a position in which the patient can be placed to permit passage of duodenal contents, the enteral route of nutrition can be employed. If adequate nutrition cannot be maintained by such means, parenteral nutrition is essential to prevent further weight loss and to promote weight gain.

SEPSIS

The heavy microbial contamination of the burn wound and the severe disruption of host defense mechanisms by burn injury make sepsis the most frequently encountered complication in burn patients. As previously noted, effective topical antimicrobial therapy has reduced the occurrence of burn wound infection, but that reduction has served to emphasize the importance of other septic complications. Pulmonary infection is presently the most frequent septic process in burn patients and may be of either the hematogenous type (one-third of cases) or bronchopneumonic type (two-thirds of cases).

Hematogenous pneumonia results from the blood-borne spread of organisms from a distant septic focus such as an infected burn wound, a site of suppurative thrombophlebitis, an occult visceral perforation, or an inapparent soft tissue infection. This form of pneumonia may be first diagnosed by identifying solitary or multiple but discrete nodular infiltrates on the chest roentgenogram of a septic burn patient. Randomly distributed multiple infiltrates may be evident on subsequent chest roentgenograms, and these may coalesce into broad areas of infiltration, difficult to distinguish from the roentgenographic picture of bronchopneumonia, if the primary site of infection remains untreated. Hematogenous pneumonia occurs relatively late in the postburn course, i.e., late in the second postburn week and beyond, and is associated with a high mortality but, because of its secondary nature, is less commonly a principal cause of death than bronchopneumonia. Such roentgenographic findings demand that a primary source of infection be sought and controlled to prevent further blood-borne microbial dissemination and that appropriate systemic antibiotic therapy be instituted. Airborne pneumonia or bronchopneumonia occurs earlier in the postburn period, i.e., early in the second postburn week, and is less commonly fatal than hematogenous pneumonia but is more commonly a principal cause of death. The diagnosis and treatment of bronchopneumonia are the same in the burn patient as they are for other surgical patients, with emphasis placed upon ventilatory support and specific antibiotic therapy.

Suppurative thrombophlebitis may occur in any previously cannulated vein, with the incidence increasing as the duration of cannula placement increases. To date, local signs have been present in less than one-half of the burn patients who have had this septic complication. Systemic sepsis or the occurrence of hematogenous pneumonia in a burn patient with no other identifiable focus of infection necessitates exploration of every previously cannulated vein. A cutdown site should be opened, residual ligatures should be removed from the previously cannulated vein, and the vein should be "milked" toward the cutdown site. If pus exudes from the vein, the diagnosis of suppurative thrombophlebitis is confirmed, but if the vein was cannulated percutaneously or if nothing can be extruded from a cutdown site, the vein should be explored at the site where the cannula tip lay. Identification of intraluminal suppuration at that site confirms the diagnosis, but if no suppuration is apparent, intraluminal clot should be extracted, and an excised segment of the inflamed vein should be submitted for culture and histologic examination. Recovery of normal-appearing liquid blood, either from a cutdown site or a surgically explored vein, can be considered a negative result. Diagnosis of suppurative thrombophlebitis necessitates excision of the entire length of vein involved by the septic process. Suppurative thrombophlebitis in central veins has been treated at this Institute by systemic antibiotics administered in maximum doses with the addition of heparin therapy in those patients in whom pulmonary emboli occurred. Persistent sepsis following excision of a vein involved with suppurative thrombophlebitis has occurred in those patients with suppuration in more than one vein, patients in whom a limited excision may cause the surgeon to overlook more proximal sepsis, and those patients in whom acute bacterial endocarditis developed as a consequence of septic emboli from the peripheral vein.

Acute bacterial endocarditis may occur either primarily or secondary to hematogenous seeding from a focus of suppurative thrombophlebitis. This septic complication may involve the valves on either side or both sides of the heart, although right heart involvement is predominant. Staphylococci predominate as the infecting organisms, but gram-negative and mixed flora may also cause these infections. Cardiac murmurs have been recorded in only a small fraction of the patients with acute bacterial endocarditis treated at this Institute; clinical signs are generally unreliable, and premortem diagnosis is difficult. Because of the paucity of clinical signs and the high mortality associated with this complication in burn patients, we consider the diagnosis of acute bacterial endocarditis in any burn patient in whom two or more blood cultures are positive for the same organism (particularly if staphylococci are recovered from the blood culture) and in whom no other source of infection is obvious. Maximal dosage of that antibiotic to which the organism is most sensitive is begun and continued for three weeks if no other source of infection is identified. Signs of valvular insufficiency or failure of antibiotic therapy indicate the necessity for cardiac catheterization studies to determine the need for valve replacement by operative means.

Blood culture–positive septicemia from no obvious source is a common occurrence in patients with extensive burns. Critically ill burn patients may even show a succession of different bacteria in sequential blood cultures or growth of multiple organisms from a single blood culture. If the patient's clinical condition is compatible with the blood culture results and the physician is confident that the positive culture is not the result of faulty technique, sampling from a contaminated indwelling vascular cannula, or contamination of the blood culture needle on passage through the burn wound, then broad-spectrum antibiotic therapy should be instituted using the agent or agents that will be effective against all of the organisms recovered. The dosage and duration of treatment are dictated by the adequacy of the patient's renal function, the side effects of the antibiotics, and the patient's response. The initial choice of antibiotics should be governed by the antibiotic sensitivities of the microbial flora common in the burn unit or hospital at that time as determined by the microbial surveillance program. Therapy should be adjusted as indicated following determination of the sensitivities of the organisms recovered from the patient.

METABOLIC SUPPORT

The metabolic response to thermal injury is one of hypermetabolism, so that the metabolic rate in patients with burns of 40 per cent or more of the body surface approaches two to two and one-half times normal. Recent studies have indicated that this response results from alteration of neurohormonal metabolic regulators, which profoundly affect mechanisms of temperature control in the burn patient. The response is characterized by the previously noted increase in metabolic rate, erosion of body mass, weight loss, and increase in cardiac output and oxygen consumption. Although external heating will not abolish postburn hypermetabolism, a warm ambient environment can reduce by approximately 10 per cent the metabolic rates of these patients. A warm microenvironment, achieved by the use of properly positioned heat reflective blankets and heat lamps or heat shields, should be maintained to reduce cold stress and the total energy needs of such patients. The judicious use of analgesics and narcotics, particularly at the time of wound manipulation, to reduce the stress of painful or noxious stimuli is also indicated. The metabolically deleterious effect of sepsis can be minimized by prevention and prompt control of infections. Planned maintenance of muscle activity by institution of specific physical therapy regimens minimizes muscle wasting associated with bedrest.

Of major importance in the metabolic support of burn patients is provision of sufficient calories and nitrogen to satisfy metabolic needs and to maintain body mass. Calorie and nitrogen requirements for burn patients can be measured or can be estimated for patients with burns of 40 per cent and more of the total body surface as being 2000 to 2200 calories per square meter of body surface per day and 10 to 20 gm of nitrogen per square meter of body surface per day. The gastrointestinal tract is the preferred route for feeding the burn patient, but if ileus, facial burns, or mental obtundation limit oral intake, tube feedings or parenteral alimentation should be instituted as dictated by the individual patient's status.

ELECTRICAL BURNS

High-voltage electricity can cause dangerous cardiac arrhythmias or cardiac arrest. Emergency first aid of these patients includes immediate documentation of the cardiac rhythm and cardiopulmonary resuscitation if necessary. When arrhythmias are noted, cardiac monitoring should be instituted as soon as possible, and appropriate treatment of the arrhythmias should be undertaken as soon as a firm diagnosis has been made.

The heat production associated with injury due to electrical current is proportional to current flow. Since the current density is much higher in extremities than on the trunk owing to the smaller size of the limb, internal thermal coagulation necrosis secondary to heat production is more common in these locations and at entrance and exit sites, which exhibit a higher resistance with increased heat production. Muscle damage may result in excessive fluid accumulation in muscle compartments and a need for fasciotomy if the circulation is compromised.

Other injuries are commonly associated with electrocution. Violent muscular contractions secondary to the electrical current or falls are responsible for a high incidence of associated fractures. Electricity may damage any part of the nervous system, and a careful neurologic examination must be performed and the findings recorded on admission and at regular intervals thereafter. Transient paralyses following electrical injuries have been well documented and are especially common following lightning injuries. Visceral injuries may occur but are unusual following electrical contact. Later sequelae of electrical injury include cataracts and bone sequestra.

Special attention should be directed toward the renal system following electrical injury. Muscle destruction results in the release of hemochromogens into the bloodstream, and these may cause renal damage or acute renal failure. Careful monitoring of the urine for the presence of hemochromogens should be maintained throughout resuscitation. When only slight amounts of these pigments are present in the urine, successful management is usually accomplished by increasing the rate of resuscitation fluid administration and the rate of urine flow. If clearing of the urine does not occur with fluid loading and if severe pigmenturia persists, administration of diuretics is mandatory. Osmotic diuretics, rather than loop diuretics, are generally preferred. Clearing of the pigment from the urine is the goal of treatment. The administration of as much as 300 gm of mannitol in 24 hours may be required in severe cases.

Surgical exploration of the extremities involved in electrical injuries is necessary if there is any indication of deep tissue injury such as stony hardness of muscle compartments noted on palpation. This procedure is usually performed 24 to 36 hours following injury. Proper preoperative preparation is important, because massive débridement and possibly major amputation may be performed at the time of operative exploration. In an extremity with obvious circulatory compromise and no other signs of injury, a preoperative arteriogram may be helpful in defining the extent of vascular damage. Following completion of the débridement, a biologic dressing (preferably cutaneous allograft) is used to cover the operative site. Reexploration at approximately 48-hour intervals is indicated until all devitalized tissue has been removed.

CHEMICAL INJURIES

Tissue damage as a result of exposure to any chemical is dependent upon (1) strength or concentration of the agent, (2) quantity of the agent, and (3) manner and duration of skin contact. Since progressive tissue damage will occur until the offending agent is inactivated by chemical combination with the tissues, eliminated from the body surface, or neutralized, rapid removal of the noxious agent by copious water lavage is imperative. Prompt removal of clothing is also important, since contaminated clothing will allow prolonged contact of the chemical agent with skin despite other treatment. Evaluation for possible inhalation injury or systemic effects following chemical absorption should be undertaken. Subsequent signs of progressive tissue destruction may indicate the need for neutralization of the chemical or surgical intervention to excise tissue containing the offending chemical.

OCULAR INJURIES

Chemical injuries to the eye constitute a special category, since the delicate cornea may be permanently damaged even by seemingly minor chemical injury. Frequent symptoms of ocular chemical irritation include blepharospasm, tearing, rubbing of the eyes, and the occurrence of semidilated pupils. Corneal swelling and clouding may occur early. The later pathologic changes that may develop as a result of this injury are associated with a high incidence of severe vision impairment or blindness. Corneal ulceration, iritis, lens damage, and increased intraocular pressure may occur following severe chemical injuries to the eye, especially those due to strong alkalis. Again, immediate initiation of treatment is of utmost importance to prevent permanent damage to the eye and to maintain normal vision. Prompt irrigation with water is the preferred immediate treatment. As with other chemical injuries, the irrigation should be copious and performed for at least 30 minutes. Cycloplegic eyedrops are instilled to minimize synechia formation. In general, chemically injured eyes should not be patched, and lubricant ointments should be used in an attempt to maintain globe mobility. Ophthalmic antibiotic ointments are also indicated in the treatment of ocular chemical injuries as prophylaxis against secondary infection.

REFERENCES

Agee, R. N., Long, J. M., III, Hunt, J. L., Petroff, P. A., Lull, R. J., Mason, A. D., Jr., and Pruitt, B. A., Jr.: Use of ^{133}xenon in early diagnosis of inhalation injury. J. Trauma, 16:218, 1976.

Baxter, C. R., Curreri, P. W., and Marvin, J. A.: The control of burn wound sepsis by the use of quantitative bacteriologic studies and subeschar clysis with antibiotics. Surg. Clin. North Am., 53:1509, 1973.

Janzekovic, Z.: The burn wound from the surgical point of view. J. Trauma, 15:42, 1975.

Levine, B. A., Sirinek, K. R., and Pruitt, B. A., Jr.: Wound excision to fascia in burn patients. Arch. Surg., 113:403, 1978.

McAlhany, J. C., Jr., Czaja, A. J., and Pruitt, B. A., Jr.: Antacid control of complications from acute gastroduodenal disease after burns. J. Trauma, 16:645, 1976.

McManus, W. F., Hunt, J. L., and Pruitt, B. A., Jr.: Postburn Convulsive Disorders in Children. J. Trauma, 14:396, 1974.

Moncrief, J. A.: Burns. N. Engl. J. Med., 288:444, 1973.

Pruitt, B. A., Jr.: Advances in fluid therapy and the early care of the burn patient. World J. Surg., 2:139, 1978.

Pruitt, B. A., Jr., and Foley, F. D.: The use of biopsies in burn patient care. Surgery, 73:887, 1973.

Pruitt, B. A., Jr. and Silverstein, P.: Methods of resurfacing denuded skin areas. Transplant. Proc., 3:1537, 1971.

Wilmore, D. W.: Nutrition and metabolism following thermal injury. Clin. Plast. Surg., 1:603, 1974.

39

The Cancer Patient

EDWARD M. COPELAND, III
JOHN M. DALY

"The cancer patient" was chosen as a separate topic because of the uniqueness of the problems that often affect patients with malignancies as a group. In a way, cancer is a chronic illness with either death or cure as an eventual end point. During the course of the illness, multiple forms of treatment, including surgery, radiation therapy, chemotherapy, immunotherapy, and rehabilitation therapy, are utilized. The first three treatment modalities can limit food intake and may result in malnutrition. Weight loss is a symptom for patients with many types of malignancies, even though the anatomic site of the cancer may not produce pain while eating, obstruction of the alimentary tract, or malabsorption. Usually, patients will report that their food intake has been curtailed because of anxiety over the symptoms or signs of a malignant process. A common time interval between onset of symptoms and diagnosis is five to six months, and during this period 10 to 20 pounds can be lost easily because of decreased food intake.

Oncology is a rapidly expanding field, and most university training programs now have medical and surgical oncology divisions, immunology divisions, and departments of radiation therapy. Useful treatment modalities, particularly chemotherapy, have been developed that result in prolonged palliation and, given as an adjuvant, can increase the rate of cure. Better techniques of radiation therapy have reduced the complications from radiation burns, and improved equipment has allowed delivery of large doses of radiation to finite areas without extensive damage to neighboring structures. The ability to stimulate the immune system nonspecifically and the discovery of tumor-specific antigens have opened a new research field and broadened treatment possibilities. The importance of rehabilitative medicine and good nutritional care is more widely recognized. Segments of this manual are already devoted to extensive review of the preoperative and postoperative management of diseases of the gastrointestinal, respiratory, endocrine, lymphoid, and urinary tract systems. This chapter will discuss malignant diseases of these areas only briefly and will detail more specifically the management of soft tissue neoplasms such as carcinoma of the breast and malignant melanoma. Also, we hope to outline benefits of treatment programs aimed at ameliorating complications common to many forms of oncologic therapy and to give specific recommendations that might eliminate post-therapy morbidity and mortality. Emphasis is given to integrated therapy, with surgery and radiation therapy used for local and regional control of disease and chemotherapy and immunotherapy used for control of systemic disease.

General axioms are that surgery is the best treatment for macroscopic disease, particularly when localized to the organ of origin, and that radiation therapy is best used to eradicate microscopic disease that may go unnoticed by the surgeon, particularly if the primary malignancy is large and has spread via the lymphatics to regional lymph nodes. When a tumor is small, well-contained within the organ of origin, and manifests no lymphatic spread, radiation therapy, chemotherapy, and immunotherapy usually are not indicated, and operation alone is the treatment of choice. There are obvious exceptions to this rule; for example, small invasive vocal cord lesions may be cured equally as well with radiation therapy as with operation, and the larynx is preserved with the former method of treatment. If the cancer has manifested any potential to spread beyond the confines of the organ of origin, chemotherapy and immunotherapy must be considered, because clinical trials currently under way are indicating that these treatment modalities may reduce the incidence of systemic metastases if they are utilized when the tumor burden is still relatively small.

METASTASES TO REGIONAL LYMPH NODES FROM AN UNKNOWN PRIMARY SITE

Often the physician is asked to evaluate a patient with a mass in an area of regional lymph nodes, such as the neck, axilla, or groin. Usually this mass represents one or more lymph nodes enlarged secondary to an inflammatory process originating in the area draining to the regional lymph nodes. These nodes are often multiple and tender, and the primary area of inflammation is usually obvious. Cat scratch fever or insect bites, however, may obscure a diagnosis. If the mass represents a solitary lymph node or several distinct painless nodes with no obvious etiology, the question of biopsy to diagnose cancer is raised. Biopsy should be avoided until a thorough search for the source of a primary malignancy is made. Excisional biopsy of lymph nodes containing metastatic cancer can release viable cancer cells into the biopsy wound because efferent and afferent lymphatics containing such cells are divided in the process. Also, the node or group of nodes containing metastatic disease may be incised, thus increasing the risk of seeding the wound with cancer cells and violating the surgical principle of en bloc resection of the primary malignancy, regional lymphatic channels, and regional lymph nodes. Once malignant disease is growing free in connective tissue and no longer is contained within the lymphatics or lymph nodes, local eradication of disease surgically becomes quite difficult, because the anatomic limits of dissection that encompass the area containing malignant tissue are no longer clearly defined. For example, if a hematoma occurs in a biopsy wound, the area of ecchymosis can be quite large and represents the extravasation of red blood cells throughout the wound. Common sense dictates that if a red blood cell can migrate to the periphery of an ecchymotic area, then a cancer cell, free in the biopsy wound, can do likewise. When the primary source of cancer is discovered and the oncologic surgeon is asked to operate upon the patient, the area of ecchymosis usually has resolved, and the surgeon has no idea of the potential area seeded with cancer cells secondary to prior incision through lymphatics or into lymph nodes containing metastatic cancer. In this setting, local recurrence rates are greatly increased. If the cancer is radiosensitive, such as squamous cell carcinoma, radiation therapy can lower the recurrence rate, since radiation therapy will eradicate microscopic disease remaining in the skin flaps or outside the margins of dissection. Malignant melanoma is much less radiosensitive, and once this disease is free within the connective tissue of the wound, eradication by any modality of treatment can be quite difficult. Local recurrence of malignant melanoma has resulted in major amputation for palliation alone, because regional disease became bulky, painful, and ulcerated.

Regional lymph node metastasis should always be suspected, especially in an adult, when an unexplained mass appears in the cervical, axillary, or inguinal area, and a thorough search for the primary source should be instituted before biopsy is undertaken. In the head and neck region, the oral cavity, pharynx, and larynx should be thoroughly investigated. If the mass is in the axilla or groin, the skin of the corresponding extremity and portion of the trunk should be examined, and the patient should be queried as to previous removal of skin lesions, particularly moles. If a primary lesion is discovered, then possibly en bloc resection can be accomplished and the incidence of regional recurrence minimized. Occasionally, nodal metastases to one of the areas in question, particularly the supraclavicular area, are from a distant primary source such as the lung, stomach, adrenal gland, or ovary, and such sites should not be overlooked in the search for the primary site. If no primary tumor can be found and the nodal enlargement is not inflammatory in origin, then lymph node biopsy is indicated for diagnosis. The majority of patients with Hodgkin's disease and lymphoma are diagnosed in this manner.

THE BREAST

Carcinoma of the breast has been reported to occur in as many as 7 per cent of women living in this country. Women with family histories of breast cancer constitute an even higher risk group. Because of the prevalence of this disease, every physician should know how to examine the breast physically and should be familiar with current policies for treatment for both benign and malignant diseases of the breast. Each woman 21 years of age or older should be taught breast self-examination and should have a breast examination done at least annually by a competent physician. This examination usually can be done by the gynecologist at the time of the patient's annual gynecologic evaluation. At age 35, women with family histories of breast cancer should have a mammogram done to serve as a baseline examination to compare with any subsequent mammogram required because of a palpable abnormality. These women in high-risk groups should have physical examinations every six months. However, routine, yearly mammograms are usually unwarranted. If a palpable breast abnormality is identified in a woman who is between the ages of 21 and 35 years, a mammogram should be obtained. Not only is the mammogram obtained to evaluate the palpable mass, but it is also useful to rule out any subclinical abnormality in the other breast.

Fibrocystic disease is often painful just before and during menstrual flow, and cysts may fluctuate in size during the menstrual cycle. The palpable mass may be cystic and have distinct borders or may be diffuse with no three-dimensional characteristics. Fibroadenomas classically are painless, ovoid, small, firm, movable, and constant in size during the menstrual cycle. Carcinoma is firm to hard and painless and has indistinct borders but usually is three-dimensional and does not fluctuate in size with the menstrual cycle. Carcinoma may be fixed to the overlying skin, to the pectoralis major muscle fascia, or to Cooper's ligaments, resulting in skin dimpling, especially when the patient raises her arms directly above her head.

Nipple discharge can be a helpful diagnostic aid. By pressing on the lactiferous ducts in the various quadrants of the breast, the area of abnormality can be localized. Clear, turbid, or greenish discharge is indicative of fibrocystic disease. Bloody discharge most commonly results from an intraductal papilloma, a benign condition, but it must be considered a positive sign of intraductal carcinoma until proved otherwise. Confirmation of the diagnosis is usually obtained by excising that portion of the breast containing the duct from which the bleeding arises. Often the duct can be cannulated with a small probe, and the area of breast tissue surrounding the probe is excised. Bloody nipple discharge may accompany lactation during the third trimester of pregnancy and immediately postpartum. This bleeding, however, soon ceases, and biopsy is usually unnecessary.

Aspiration of cystic lesions with a 22- to 25-gauge needle may be done as an office procedure. A Papanicolaou smear should be obtained of the fluid removed from the breast of a woman in a high-risk category, and a suspicious Papanicolaou smear or a bloody aspirate requires an open biopsy of the area containing the cyst.

Patients with solid lesions suspected to be malignant should have thorough physical examinations with particular emphasis on the ipsilateral axilla and supraclavicular area. Mammogram, skeletal roentgenologic survey, chest roentgenogram, and liver function tests should be obtained. Those patients who have suspicious skeletal surveys of clinically palpable metastatic disease in the axilla or supraclavicular region should have isotopic bone scans, since this technique has proved to be most sensitive for detecting skeletal metastases. Patients with abnormal liver function tests should undergo liver scans. If no evidence of distant metastases is identified, a treatment plan based on the anatomic location of the lesion, its physical characteristics, and evidence of regional metastases is instituted, often in consultation with a radiation therapist and a medical oncologist. As a rule, open or needle biopsy of the suspicious lesion and frozen section examination are done under general anesthesia and immediately prior to a mastectomy. Excisional biopsy under local anesthesia, particularly as an office procedure, can be quite difficult because the lesion may be deeper in the breast than initially anticipated. Needle biopsy under local anesthesia is much easier to do, but the lesion must be 1.5 cm or larger to consistently obtain an adequate needle biopsy specimen. Both of these office procedures are acceptable for diagnosis, but the planned mastectomy should be done within 48 to 72 hours of biopsy and before any hematoma initiated by the biopsy has had time to disseminate throughout the tissues and produce a large ecchymotic area in the breast that potentially contains viable cancer cells.

Many patients who have had biopsies done elsewhere are referred to the M. D. Anderson Hospital for definitive therapy. These patients are classified as having "disturbed breasts." The chest wall recurrence rate after mastectomy for such patients was 25 per cent until a protocol of preoperative radiation therapy was instituted. Radiation therapy has apparently eradicated those viable cancer cells that remained in the skin flaps, for now the local recurrence rate for "disturbed breasts" is only 4 per cent. Because of this experience with other physicians' patients who have had biopsies done several days prior to mastectomy, this technique is only used sparingly in our institution.

Circumscribed carcinomas smaller than 4 cm in diameter, limited to the lateral aspect of the breast, and without fixation to the skin or pectoral fascia can usually be treated by operation alone if no lymph node metastases are found in the pathologic specimen. If lymph node metastases are present or if the carcinoma is medially or centrally located, a combination of operation and postoperative radiation therapy is used to insure control of local chest wall disease. The type of surgical procedure recommended and the areas to receive radiation therapy depend upon the location of the primary lesion in the breast. Lesions in the lateral aspect of the breast drain primarily via the axillary lymphatic channels, and disease can be cleared from the chest wall by a modified radical mastectomy. Inclusive in the definition of this operation is the removal of the pectoralis minor muscle, since the apex of the axilla is less accessible with this muscle in place. Laterally located cancers with axillary lymph node metastases may be associated with internal mammary or supraclavicular lymph node metastases as often as 25 to 30 per cent of the time; consequently, radiation therapy is used for these latter two areas (so-called peripheral lymphatic radiation therapy). Medially located cancers can be associated with internal mammary node metastases 30 per cent of the time, and if axillary metastases are also present, the highest incidence of internal mammary node involvement reported is 50 per cent. If no axillary metastases are present clinically, medial cancers are treated by modified radical mastectomy and peripheral lymphatic radiation therapy. Chest wall radiation therapy is also added when greater than 20 per cent of recovered axillary lymph nodes contain cancer, since metastatic disease coursing to the axilla through the subdermal lymphatics from the medially located primary site may remain in the skin flaps, particularly when many lymph nodes contain cancer.

Lesions located in the central portion of the breast and/or medially located lesions with clinically palpable axillary lymph node metastases smaller than 2.0 cm in size are treated by radical mastectomy and peripheral lymphatic and chest wall radiation therapy. It is these cancers that are most likely to metastasize through lymphatics coursing along the neurovascular bundle medial to the pectoralis minor muscle. This bundle is preserved during modified radical mastectomy in order to maintain innervation of the pectoralis major muscle and prevent its atrophy following mastectomy. In a radical mastectomy, the neurovascular bundle, associated lymph channels, and areolar tissue are removed with the specimen, and an adequate surgical extirpation of regional disease is thereby better insured.

The responsibility of the surgeon and radiation therapist is to provide the patient with the best chance for local control of chest wall disease with minimal morbidity. Usually, radiation therapy sterilizes lymph nodes 1 cm in size or smaller. Complete surgical dissection of the axilla and axillary radiation therapy should not be used together for treatment of axillary metastases because the subsequent incidence of lymphedema of the arm is greatly increased. Major lymphatic channels are removed surgically, and remaining collateral channels may be destroyed by radiation therapy. If axillary metastases are multiple, large, or matted, a mastectomy is done in conjunction with a dissection of the lateral axilla. The medial limit of the dissection is the lateral border of the pectoralis muscles (an "extended simple mastectomy"), and radiation therapy is applied to the axilla, chest wall, and peripheral lymphatics. In this way, the primary cancer and large lymph nodes (greater than 1 cm in size), which are unlikely to be sterilized by radiation therapy, are removed surgically. The metastatic cancer in smaller, centrally located axillary lymph nodes, often intertwined around axillary structures and not adequately removed surgically, are usually destroyed by radiation therapy.

Carcinomas larger than 4 cm in diameter and associated with minimal clinical axillary disease are often best treated by preoperative radiation therapy and either a radical, modified radical, or extended simple mastectomy, depending upon the location of the lesion and the amount of radiation therapy delivered to the apical axilla.

Patients with distant metastases, which include supraclavicular node metastases, are treated primarily with chemotherapy, but local chest wall control of the cancer often is best obtained by a limited surgical procedure, possibly combined with radiation therapy. A similar approach is taken with inflammatory breast carcinoma and with large, fixed, or ulcerated lesions, although operation is used less frequently in these circumstances. The choice of procedure should be individualized.

Current clinical trials indicate that chemotherapy given "prophylactically," i.e., to patients with axillary metastases but no distant metastases, prolongs the disease-free interval and may increase the survival rate. Our choice of treatment is 5-fluorouracil (5-FU), doxorubicin (Adriamycin), and cyclophosphamide (Cytoxan). In order to recommend such therapy rationally, the pathologic status of the axillary lymph nodes must be known, a step that requires the surgical removal of at least a portion of the nodes. "Lumpectomy" (tylectomy), axillary sampling and radiation therapy are satisfactory treatments if the cancer is small, if axillary lymph nodes are clinically negative, if the breast is small enough to allow uniform radiation treatment, and if the radiation therapist is experienced with this type of treatment. If the therapist is not so experienced, the results of primary radiation therapy for carcinoma of the breast can be disastrous. The breast can become painful, fibrotic, edematous, and ulcerated. A reasonable approach to laterally located small cancers with no clinical axillary disease is to combine a quadrant dissection of the breast with a limited axillary dissection and postoperative radiation therapy. In this way, the breast is preserved, and the status of at least a sample of the axillary lymph nodes is known. The results of this approach are currently under evaluation, and it is not as yet recommended as standard treatment. Estrogen and progesterone receptor activities should be obtained on the pathologic specimen whenever possible to aid the medical oncologist in the plan for treatment if breast cancer should recur.

Minimal breast cancer, that is, invasive breast cancer smaller than 5 mm in diameter or in situ intraductal or lobular breast cancer, is seldom associated with lymph node metastases. An extended simple mastectomy is done for in situ breast cancer regardless of the location of the lesion in the breast; however, invasive carcinoma below the basement membrane is treated as described in the initial part of this section regardless of how small the invasive lesion is. In situ intraductal carcinoma may be multicentric, but the incidence of bilaterality is not as frequent as it is for in situ or invasive lobular carcinoma, often reported to be as high as 50 per cent. Mirror image biopsy of the opposite breast should be done for lobular carcinoma, in situ or invasive, but not necessarily for intraductal carcinoma.

The site of biopsy incisions should be removed with the definitive pathologic specimen; therefore, some thought should be given to the position of biopsy incisions. Ideally, a mastectomy should be done via a transverse or oblique incision. Cosmetically, these incisions are more pleasing, and breast reconstruction is easier. Sixty per cent of recurrent breast cancers occur within two years of mastectomy. If the proper local treatment for breast cancer has been done initially, local chest wall recurrence rates should be almost zero. Nevertheless, breast reconstruction should be delayed for women with invasive breast cancer until two years have elapsed and should be discouraged for women who have had axillary lymph node metastases. The major criticism of breast reconstruction is the potential for delay in diagnosing local chest wall recurrence. By the time local recurrence is diagnosed, it might be quite extensive. If there is a place for immediate breast reconstruction, it would be following the treatment of in situ breast cancer, but experience with this procedure to date is too limited for it to be recommended as standard therapy. The cancer surgeon should plan the ablative operative procedure with eventual plastic reconstruction in mind but should not compromise the opportunity for local control of disease in order to preserve cosmetic appearance. When indicated, a transverse or oblique incision is made, and the pectoralis major muscle should be left in place. Skin flaps are made in the natural plane between the subcutaneous tissue and the investing fascia of the breast. Skin grafts are seldom needed. If postoperative radiation therapy, particularly to the chest wall, is planned, primary wound healing is necessary, and extremely thin skin flaps often slough, delaying further therapy.

Following breast biopsy for benign conditions, meticulous hemostasis is achieved, and the breast tissue is reapproximated. A drain is not used routinely. After mastectomy, two suction catheters are employed and are not removed until drainage is less than 20 ml per day. A pressure dressing is applied in the operating room and is not removed for four days. If the patient has had radiation therapy preoperatively, no pressure dressing is used. Patient reevaluation is done every three months for two

years and then every six months for life, since these patients by definition are at high risk for development of cancer of the other breast.

MELANOMA

Skin lesions, particularly moles than change color, grow noticeably, itch, scale, ulcerate, or even begin to disappear should be biopsied, preferably by excision. Treatment of malignant melanoma is based on the depth of skin invasion, location on the body, and areas of metastatic spread. Punch biopsy is satisfactory, but excisional biopsy to include a small amount of subcutaneous fat is preferable in order for the pathologist to define the depth of invasion. Interpretation of a frozen section preparation can be very misleading, and a diagnosis should await the interpretation of the permanent histologic sections. Excisional biopsy does not increase the metastatic tendency of a melanoma.

Thin malignant melanomas that have not penetrated through the papillary dermis (Clark's level 1 and 2) seldom metastasize or recur locally and have a 95 per cent chance for cure by adequate initial local excision. Five per cent of these patients may have regional lymph node metastases or local recurrence; thus, long-term follow-up is necessary. Usually, adequate local excision can be obtained by widely excising the biopsy scar with margins sufficient to allow primary closure of the wound. Some lesions, particularly the superficial spreading type, may be too large for excision and primary closure, and skin grafting may be necessary; similarly, skin grafts may be needed in areas of the body where skin is not easily mobilized, such as the sole of the foot.

Thick lesions that have penetrated to the reticular dermis (level 3), into the reticular dermis (level 4), or through it and into the subcutaneous fat (level 5) have a proportionally greater malignant potential that is directly proportional to the depth of invasion and to the location on the body (head and neck greater than trunk greater than extremity). All regional node-bearing areas and the area between the primary melanoma and the regional lymph nodes should be carefully evaluated to detect clinical regional lymph node metastases or in-transit metastases coursing to the regional lymph nodes via the intradermal or subdermal lymphatics. In-transit metastases seldom are found unless stasis occurs in the regional lymphatics secondary to multiple lymph node metastases or previous resection of the regional lymph nodes. Patients are considered to have stage 1 disease if no regional or distant metastases are identified clinically, stage 2 if regional, satellite metastases exist only within a 3 cm radius of the primary melanoma, stage 3A if in-transit metastases exist, 3B if regional lymph node metastases exist, 3AB if both types of metastases are identified, and stage 4 if metastases distant to the regional lymph nodes are found.

Surgical treatment of all thick melanomas must be directed at eradication of the primary disease, the areas of potential in-transit metastases, and the regional lymph node–bearing areas. Treatment should also be practical. For example, a thick melanoma in the middle of the trunk may metastasize potentially to the axillary, inguinal, or even the supraclavicular lymph node areas, and prophylactic dissection of each of these locations is impractical. Prophylactic lymph node dissection as treatment for stage 1 thick melanomas is controversial. The incidence of subclinical lymph node metastases is between 20 per cent and 40 per cent in patients with thick melanomas. Some investigators believe that patients with resected subclinical lymph node metastases have similar prognoses to patients with stage 1 disease and pathologically negative lymph nodes, whereas other investigators believe that subclinical lymph node metastases represent stage 3 disease and that the prognoses of both groups of patients coincide. If the latter philosophy is correct, then between 60 per cent and 80 per cent of patients with clinically negative regional lymph nodes are receiving lymph node dissections unnecessarily, and those patients with regional metastases might have waited until the lymph nodes became clinically positive before undergoing lymph node dissection, since their prognoses would be no better if these metastatic deposits had been removed when they were subclinical. We maintain somewhat of a "middle of the road" philosophy concerning prophylactic lymph node dissection and do a regional lymph node dissection in continuity with a wide excision of the primary melanoma and intervening lymphatic channels if the area of lymph node drainage can be predicted accurately, and the lesion is greater than 1.5 mm in depth. For example, a melanoma lying directly over the primary lymph node–bearing area or very close to it, such as at the junction of the proximal one-third and distal two-thirds of the anterior thigh, would receive such treatment. If the area of regional lymph node drainage cannot be predicted accurately, as is so often true with melanomas of the trunk, which may drain to two or more nodal groups, then wide local excision alone is done. The long axis of the wide excisional wound is directed at a potential regional lymph node–bearing area in order to remove the lymphatic channels coursing to at least one potential metastatic site. Primary closure of these wounds usually can be accomplished, since the wounds are longitudinal and not circular. Utilizing this treatment program, local recurrence rates have been only 2 to 3 per cent for melanomas of the trunk. Patients are then reexamined every three months for at least two years. The direction of spread in patients with stage 3A or 3B melanoma is obvious, and these patients should have regional node dissections in continuity with the primary lesion if possible. If six months or more have elapsed between excision of the primary site and appearance of the lymph node metastases, then disease has probably cleared the intervening lymphatic channels, and only regional node dissection is indicated.

A thick melanoma, greater than 1.5 mm in depth, on the extremity not adjacent to the axilla or groin presents a special problem because the tissue intervening between the primary and the regional nodes cannot be excised in continuity with practicality. The incidence of "trapped" in-transit metastases can be as high as 20 per cent if the primary lesion and regional lymph nodes are excised simultaneously. We have lowered this incidence to 2 per cent for patients with stage 1 melanomas of the extremity by doing isolated limb perfusions with phenylalanine mustard in conjunction with a limited excision of the primary lesion. If the regional lymph nodes are negative clinically, they are not dissected, and the excision site of the primary lesion usually can be closed primarily. If the capability to do isolated limb perfusions is unavailable and regional lymph node dissection is indicated because of clinically positive lymph nodes, an interval of two to four weeks should elapse between excision of the primary lesion and regional lymph node dissection in order for malignant cells to advance from the intervening lymphatic channels. There is no actual proof that this waiting period lowers the incidence of in-transit metastases, but theoretically it is logical. If the regional lymph nodes are clinically negative, the primary melanoma should be excised, and the patient should be re-evaluated every three months for at least two years. In the past, regional lymph nodes were dissected only if the lymph nodes became positive clinically. Evidence is mounting that the risk:benefit ratio for discontinuous lymph node dissection for lesions with a measured depth of invasion between 1.5 mm and 4.0 mm favors the patient. In other words, the risk of trapping in-transit metastases within the limb is overcome by the survival benefit afforded the patient.

Isolated limb perfusion with phenylalanine mustard, actinomycin-D, and nitrogen mustard has been quite beneficial in increasing survival rates and providing adequate local control for patients with stage 2 and 3A disease as well as 3B disease if the primary lesion is intact or recently excised. Perfusion is the treatment of choice for patients in these categories. Prophylactic perfusion for patients with stage 1 disease appears to improve 10-year survival rates and to lower the incidence of regional recurrence. Unfortunately, no randomized control studies have been done, and comparisons with historical control studies are sometimes difficult to interpret.

Malignant melanoma responds poorly to radiation therapy; initial surgical procedures should be designed to eradicate local disease totally by en bloc dissection, if possible. Lymph node biopsy should be avoided. If lymph nodes are enlarged palpably in the area of regional node drainage, then dissection is justified without biopsy unless there is another reason for lymphadenopathy, such as nearby BCG scarification. In this latter instance, lymphadenopathy will regress as the scarification wounds heal.

Recent clinical trials indicate that the interval between the discovery of malignant melanoma and recurrent disease is lengthened by treatment with chemoimmunotherapy utilizing dimethyl triazenoimidazole carboxamide (DTIC) and BCG by scarification. Both modalities of treatment are recommended for patients with stages 3A, 3B, 3AB, and 4 disease. BCG scarification alone is recommended for patients who have stage 2 melanomas, thick stage 1 melanomas of the trunk, and melanomas that are at level 5 in depth.

Actual depth of invasion can be measured in millimeters and correlated with survival rates. Melanomas less than 0.76 mm in depth seldom metastasize or recur locally. These lesions correspond prognostically to those within level 1 and 2 invasion. In some areas of the body where the skin is either thick (back) or thin (breast), the level of invasion may not correlate with the measured thickness of the lesion. For example, a melanoma of the back may be 1.5 mm in depth but only invade the superficial papillary dermis. It should be treated as a thick melanoma (i.e., as if it were level 3). Conversely, a melanoma of the skin of the female breast may be level 3 in invasion but less than 0.76 mm in depth. This lesion usually can be treated as a thin melanoma (i.e., as if it were level 2). If an inconsistency in the treatment plan exists between level and measured depth of invasion, the latter usually should dictate treatment.

GASTROINTESTINAL TRACT

Patients with gastrointestinal cancers share certain characteristics and symptomatology, such as melena and weight loss, and will be discussed as a group. Important treatment suggestions used by our team will be outlined here with no attempt to provide an overall management program for gastrointestinal cancers.

ESOPHAGUS AND STOMACH

The major problem for patients with carcinoma of the esophagus and stomach is malnutrition. It should be identified and properly treated preoperatively. In nutritionally healthy patients, an attempt should be made to resect the cancer if not for cure, then for palliation. If a patient can ingest adequate rations of nutrients by mouth, the quality of remaining life is improved, and the opportunity for further palliative therapy, such as chemotherapy and radiation therapy, is increased. In properly selected patients, surgical palliation for carcinoma of the esophagus should include bypass by colon interposition. Patients with esophagogastric lesions and small liver metastases should have palliative esophagogastrectomies, if possible. If the lesion is unresectable, a feeding gastrostomy should be placed below the cancer. For patients with large gastric or esophagogastric lesions, the risk of a major postoperative complication resulting from palliative resection must be evaluated together with the anatomic and physiologic realities of accomplishing such a resection. The surgeon must keep life expectancy and quality of remaining life constantly in mind while deciding between palliative resection, bypass, or neither.

PANCREAS

Ultrasonography and computerized axial tomography are relatively new useful aids for diagnosing pancreatic cancer. The danger of bile peritonitis after percutaneous transhepatic cholangiography for the patient with obstructive jaundice is much less now that radiologists are using smaller needles (22 to 23 gauge). In the past, this procedure was done immediately prior to exploratory laparotomy so that any bile leakage from the punctured liver surface could be stopped subsequently by suturing the puncture wound. Now, percutaneous transhepatic cholangiography is done as a routine study without preoperative preparation; nevertheless, the possibility of bile leakage must not be forgotten. Radiologists have also mastered the technique of percutaneous transabdominal pancreatic biopsy. The procedure can yield a diagnosis for the unresectable patient and can sometimes eliminate the need for intraoperative biopsy for resectable patients.

If no evidence of distant or regional metastases from carcinoma of the pancreas can be identified, the patient is a candidate for pancreaticoduodenectomy. Our practice has been to nutritionally prepare the patient preoperatively with intravenous hyperalimentation unless deteriorating liver function secondary to biliary obstruction necessitates immediate biliary decompression. Otherwise, biliary decompression followed at a later date by a pancreaticoduodenectomy is not recommended because the adhesions secondary to the decompressive procedure make the definitive operation more difficult. Also, percutaneous decompression can be accomplished preoperatively by leaving a catheter in the biliary tree at the time of transhepatic cholangiography. We have not found yet that the elevated serum bilirubin and alkaline phosphatase levels in well-nourished patients with normal hepatocellular function increase the postoperative morbidity or mortality following pancreaticoduodenectomy. A histopathologic diagnosis of pancreatic carcinoma is desirable before pancreaticoduodenectomy and can be obtained by transduodenal biopsy or direct needle biopsy of the pancreas. Pancreatic fistulas have not occurred if the biopsy needle avoided the major pancreatic ducts. If the portal or superior mesenteric vein is invaded, the patient should have a biliary and/or gastric bypass. Resection and reconstruction of these major venous structures in continuity with the pancreas and duodenum by most surgeons have only increased the morbidity and mortality of the procedure without increasing the survival rate or the quality of remaining life. If the pancreatic duct is obstructed by carcinoma of the head of the pancreas, the body and tail may be quite hard, making the definition of the medial border of the pancreatic cancer nearest the superior mesenteric vein difficult to determine. Under these circumstances, the distal major pancreatic duct can be decompressed by inserting a 22-gauge needle into it and extracting the pancreatic fluid. The body and tail of the pancreas will become more pliable, and determination of the relationship of the pancreatic tumor to the superior mesenteric vein will be easier.

A surgeon should not operate upon a jaundiced patient unless he or she is prepared to treat definitively whatever pathologic process is discovered. Nevertheless, a resectable carcinoma of the pancreas is sometimes found at operation by a surgeon who may not wish to do the definitive procedure, and there may not be a surgeon immediately available who can do it. When this situation occurs, the surgeon should do a simple biliary bypass, refrain from mobilizing the duodenum and pancreas, and not biopsy the pancreas unless the lesion is easily accessible. Often patients who have undergone each of these procedures are referred to our institution postoperatively as candidates for pancreaticoduodenectomy. The dissection planes have been destroyed by the previous wide and unnecessary pancreatic mobilization, and if any pancreatitis surrounds the biopsy site, dissection in this area may be very difficult and hazardous, particularly if the biopsy was posterior and adjacent to the vena cava.

LIVER

Advances in anesthesia, blood transfusion, and surgical techniques have made major hepatic resection feasible. Patients with primary hepatoma or certain solitary metastases such as carcinoma of the colon or breast should be evaluated for possible curative resection. If liver function tests indicate any degree of hepatocellular malfunction in the uninvolved liver, the patient is a borderline candidate for a major resection, and any other minor contraindications such as advanced age or multiple organ system disease dictate against resection. Isotopic hepatic scanning is the most cost effective test for screening patients for liver disease, but its sensitivity is limited. Arteriography will better define small deposits of metastatic cancer and also will outline the arterial blood supply to the liver. The variations in origin of the right and left hepatic arteries must be known preoperatively, particularly if hepatic artery ligation or infusion is contemplated as an alternative procedure to resection. The venous phase of the arteriogram will often identify the portal system. Cancer in the portal vein is a contraindication to major resection. Inferior vena cavography with identification of the hepatic veins will aid in evaluating the invasion of malignant disease into these structures, another contraindication to resection. Computerized axial tomography and ultrasonography are also sensitive tests that identify small metastatic deposits, and these tests are much better than arteriography for detecting disease in the lateral segment of the left hepatic lobe.

At exploration, solitary metastases or metastatic disease limited to one hepatic lobe (particularly metastatic carcinoid) should be considered for resectability either by wedge excision or lobectomy. If the cancer is unresectable, hepatic arterial devascularization or chemotherapeutic infusion or both may be done. The infusion catheter is inserted through the right gastroepiploic artery into the common hepatic artery via the gastroduodenal artery. This route is circuitous but reduces the hazard of hemorrhage if the catheter gets dislodged from the vascular tree. Once in place, the catheter is injected with fluorescein dye to insure that both hepatic lobes are being infused and that other structures supplied by branches of the celiac axis will receive little drug. Immediately postoperatively the catheter is attached in an infusion pump. Chemotherapeutic infusion, usually with 5-FU, is begun when the patient has recovered from the surgical procedure. To insure that the catheter has not been dislodged from the common hepatic artery during this interval, a liver scan is obtained by injecting macroaggregates of radioiodine-labeled serum albumin directly into the catheter. Most investigators have reported a slight but significant improvement in the length of survival (measured in months) for patients undergoing chemotherapy by direct hepatic infusion when compared with systemic treatment. This slight improvement, however, does not warrant a major abdominal surgical procedure in order to insert an infusion catheter. If the patient is not a candidate for resection as shown by preoperative tests, then chemotherapy is administered systemically or by percutaneous catheterization of the hepatic artery via a proximal brachial or femoral artery.

After surgical excision of the hepatic lobe, dependent external drainage of the hepatic bed is important and can be accomplished by using soft sump-type drains constructed from two No. 18 French red rubber catheters inside a large Penrose drain. These sump drains are placed in the area of the resected hepatic bed and exit through the posterior flank. The gallbladder is removed, but the biliary tract is not decompressed. If the patient has received proper nutritional care preoperatively, if sound judgment has been used in determining candidacy for major resection, and if technical errors are avoided (such as obstructing the blood flow from the remnant of the middle hepatic vein), postoperative care is relatively uncomplicated.

COLON

Preoperative preparation and technical procedures for colon surgery have become routine in most institutions. Good surgical judgment is necessary when operating upon any part of the colon, but it is most important when dealing with carcinoma of the rectum and rectosigmoid colon. The surgical oncologist should provide the patient with the best opportunity for cure and local control of disease combined with the least chance of postoperative morbidity, mortality, and loss of function. Sphincter-saving procedures are now taught in most surgical residency programs, but these operations should not be done if the chance for local control is the least bit jeopardized. A properly constructed and functioning sigmoid colostomy is acceptable to almost every patient. Malignant lesions within 6 cm of the dentate line that invade through the muscularis mucosa should be removed by abdominoperineal resection. Large lesions in the 6 to 10 cm range that have obviously invaded the pericolic fat or have lymph node metastases should also be considered for removal by abdominoperineal resection, particularly for men. A pelvic recurrence in the male can be a more difficult problem to treat than in the female because the recurrent cancer has easier access to the urinary tract. For example, a suture line recurrence is usually much easier to ablate surgically by dissecting the colon from the posterior wall of the vagina (or including a portion of the vagina in the specimen) than is dissection of a similar lesion from the prostate. The posterior approach (Kratsky) to colon resections and anastomoses is seldom used; the wide female pelvis makes low anterior resection and anastomosis easy, but low lesions in men with narrow pelves are usually treated by abdominoperineal resection, particularly if the disease has penetrated through the bowel wall.

Carcinoma in situ within a colonic polyp can be treated by total surgical removal of the polyp. This can be accomplished by local excision of most villous or adenomatous polyps in the distal colon. If total removal is not insured by local excision, then colon resection is indicated. Our group does sphincter-saving procedures most frequently for invasive carcinoma limited to the muscularis mucosa or to the stalk of a pedunculated adenomatous polyp.

Adjunctive Treatment. Radiation therapy is used as an adjunct to surgery for patients with cancer of the rectum or rectosigmoid that has metastasized to regional lymph nodes or invaded the pericolic fat. Our preference is to close the perineal floor primarily following abdomino-perineal resection and to use radiation therapy postoperatively. Radiation enteritis in that portion of the small bowel adherent to the pelvic peritoneal closure is a potential problem that can be partially solved by interposing the omentum between the pelvic floor and small bowel. To gain enough length to reach into the pelvic floor, the omentum usually must be detached from the right half of the transverse colon. The best integration of radiation therapy and operation may be to split the course of radiation therapy, dividing the dose between the preoperative and postoperative periods. In this way, the small bowel that does become fixed by adhesions in the pelvis postoperatively will receive a radiation dose that should not result in radiation enteritis and potential stricture. Preoperative radiation therapy is particularly valuable for reducing the size of bulky rectal cancers. These lesions become more easily removed especially from the prostate, and the incidence of local recurrence for patients with Duke's C lesions appears reduced. Low anterior resection followed by postoperative radiation therapy for cancer in the distal colon is under evaluation and may result in local control equal to that obtained by abdominoperineal resection followed by radiation therapy, but long-term results of such treatment are not yet available. Certainly, if a low anterior anastomosis is done and metastatic disease in the lymph nodes is discovered in the histopathologic specimen, adjunctive radiation therapy should be considered.

Radiation therapy in conjunction with resection of a portion of the abdominal colon, pancreas, or stomach for carcinoma has not been of any predictable value as adjunctive treatment. Radiation therapy for gastric lymphoma may be quite beneficial, particularly if the lymphomatous involvement is diffuse.

Results of combination chemotherapy have been promising as treatment for metastatic carcinoma of gastrointestinal tract origin. Also, a recent study at our Institution indicated that 5-FU and BCG by scarification increased the disease-free interval when used adjunctively with surgery for patients with rectal and rectosigmoid carcinoma metastatic to regional lymph nodes. This study gives promise that immunotherapy might have a place in the treatment of·gastrointestinal cancers.

ADULT SOFT TISSUE SARCOMAS

Soft tissue sarcomas in adults can grow to a large size without detectable metastases; however, prognosis does correlate with the size of the malignancy and the degree of pleomorphism. Traditionally, soft tissue sarcomas have been treated surgically. This included amputation if the lesion was on the extremity. Local recurrence rates ranged from 18 per cent to 30 per cent after radical amputation. Local recurrence rates after radiation therapy alone were reported as high as 66 per cent. Currently, postoperative radiation therapy combined with an adequate local surgical excision is the treatment used for soft tissue sarcomas of the trunk and extremities. Emphasis is placed on preservation of limb function. For such therapy, patients should be 16 years of age or older and should have no evidence of distant metastases. Rates of local recurrence and distant metastases using this combined approach have been 22 per cent and 32 per cent, respectively, and both percentages compare favorably with those obtained for patients treated by operation alone. Radiation necrosis has occurred in only two patients in the M. D. Anderson Hospital series; otherwise, limb function has been preserved for more than 100 patients with primary lesions of the extremities or trunk. Ideally, the surgeon and radiation therapist should plan their approach jointly. The entire operative site should be irradiated to minimize local recurrence. Thus, the location and length of the scar and stab wounds for drain sites should be planned to fit easily within a logical radiation field.

A large primary sarcoma of the extremity that cannot be removed by conservative excision requires amputation of the extremity. At M. D. Anderson Hospital, however, several such patients have been treated preoperatively with 6000 rads in six weeks followed by conservative excision five to six weeks later. Although healing has been delayed, to date local recurrence rate has been acceptable, and limb function has been preserved. Nevertheless, results of this treatment are too preliminary to recommend preoperative radiation therapy followed by local excision as the treatment of choice for all large soft tissue sarcomas of the extremity.

The use of Adriamycin alone or in combination with other chemotherapeutic drugs has greatly increased the potential for partial or complete remissions in patients with metastatic soft tissue sarcomas. The current drug regimen used for metastatic sarcoma is Adriamycin, cyclophosphamide, and DTIC. Randomized prospective trials utilizing Adriamycin in combination with several other drugs as adjunctive chemotherapy in an attempt to reduce the incidence of distant metastases are under way, but it is too early to evaluate the results of these treatment programs.

CANCER, NUTRITION, AND IMMUNITY

Malnutrition in our institution is defined as a recent unintentional loss of 10 per cent or more of body weight, a serum albumin level of less than 3.4 gm per cent, and a negative reaction to a battery of recall skin test antigens. Malnutrition depresses established delayed hypersensitivity reaction (T cell immunity), whereas humoral immunity (B cell immunity) is affected less severely. Short courses of chemotherapy can limit the cellular immune response to a primary antigen but has less effect on the established delayed hypersensitivity response (the response to an antigen to which the patient has been sensitized previously). Thus, if a malnourished patient receives chemotherapy, primary and established cellular immunity can be depressed, and the patient becomes more vulnerable to infection. Also, leukocytes are depressed during most chemotherapy, and this further lowers the patient's resistance to most microorganisms. Nutritional repletion will restore the established delayed cutaneous hypersensitivity reaction, a very important line of defense in adults who usually have previous immunity to most common microorganisms, such as the influenza viruses and *Candida* species. Similarly, if immunotherapy is to be effective, nutritional restoration is necessary so that the body's immunologic mechanisms can function optimally.

In a group of malnourished cancer patients treated with chemotherapy, our team demonstrated that previously negative reactions to a battery of skin test antigens (dermatophytin, dermatophytin-O, strepto-kinase-streptodornase [Varidase], purified protein derivative [PPD], and mumps) would convert to positive reactions during nutritional repletion with intravenous hyperalimentation (IVH) in an average period of 11.4 to 18 days of nutritional therapy. Tumor response to chemotherapy occurred most often in those patients whose skin tests were positive, and conversion of skin test reactivity to positive occurred before clinical regression of metastatic disease. Those malnourished surgical patients whose skin tests converted to positive during treatment with IVH preoperatively had an uncomplicated postoperative recovery period, whereas 50 per cent of the patients whose skin tests remained negative died after operation, usually from sepsis. In patients receiving radiation therapy, conversion of skin tests to positive reactivity was difficult to achieve even though nutritional repletion with IVH was adequate. The majority of these patients were receiving radiation therapy to large segments of bone marrow or blood (i.e., the pelvis, heart, or mediastinum) or to the thymus. Possibly radiation therapy to these areas reduced the number or efficacy of circulating T-lymphocytes that are responsible for delayed hypersensitivity reactions. Although skin test reactivity remained negative, there were no complications secondary to radiation therapy, again indicating the benefits of good nutritional status during treatment.

Cachexia is harmful to cancer patients because the malnourished patient has a much narrower safe therapeutic margin for most chemotherapy and radiation therapy. The cancericidal doses of these agents may be much closer to the lethal dose for normal tissues in the malnourished patient than in the well-nourished one. Similarly, in the undernourished patient, the increased risk of complications secondary to malnutrition can limit the tolerable dose of chemotherapy or radiation therapy, and the patient may not be classified as a reasonable candidate for treatment even though he or she has a potentially responsive malignant lesion.

Absorption of nutriments via a functional gastrointestinal tract is the best means of obtaining adequate nutrition. For some patients, such as those with pharyngeal malignancies, restoration of good nutritional status may be obtained by nasogastric intubation with a small feeding tube. Gastrostomy and jejunostomy feeding tubes may be used for patients with obstructing carcinomas of the esophagus, stomach, or pancreas. However, delivery of adequate foodstuffs to the gut does not always result in rapid nutritional restoration of the starving patient, because malnutrition may lead to malabsorption, and a vicious cycle therby ensues. Nutritional rehabilitation via the gastrointestinal tract can be time-consuming, and the operative insertion of feeding tubes can impose on the patient an acute surgical stress that further delays nutritional repletion. Similarly, nutritional replenishment via the gut may not be rapid enough to achieve adequate nutritional restoration before the patient must undergo oncologic therapy. Under these circumstances, the use of intravenous hyperalimentation may be indicated.

Any cancer patient who has a lesion that is potentially responsive to oncologic therapy and who cannot be nutritionally rehabilitated and maintained by enteral means should be considered a candidate for IVH. In a large group of surgery patients who received IVH both preoperatively and postoperatively, increase in strength and weight gain, a significant rise in serum albumin concentration, and a return of immunocompetence were much easier to accomplish with IVH preoperatively rather than postoperatively. Because these patients had so few surgical complications, we recommend that measures to correct malnutrition be instituted before operation instead of waiting until a catastrophic postoperative complication such as an anastomotic breakdown, pelvic abscess, or fistula has occurred.

Nutritional repletion of malnourished cancer patients has resulted in a return of immunocompetence, a reduction in sepsis, proper wound healing, and an apparent increase in tumor response to chemotherapy. Methods of restoring and maintaining adequate nutrition should be added to the treatment plan for each patient with cancer. When enteral alimentation fails or is inadequate, IVH should be utilized. By combining both methods of treatment optimal nutritional and antineoplastic results can be expected for the malnourished cancer patient.

REFERENCES

Breslow, A., and Macht, S. D.: Optimal size of resection margin for thin cutaneous melanoma. Surg. Gynecol. Obstet., *145*:691, 1977.

Copeland, E. M., and Dudrick, S. J.: Nutritional aspects of cancer. Curr. Probl. Cancer, *1*:1, 1976.

Copeland, E. M., MacFadyen, B. V., Jr., and Dudrick, S. J.: Effect of intravenous hyperalimentation on established delayed hypersensitivity in the cancer patient. Ann. Surg., *184*:60, 1976.

Copeland, E. M., MacFadyen, B. V., Jr., Lanzotti, V., and Dudrick, S. J.: Intravenous hyperalimentation as an adjunct to cancer chemotherapy. Am. J. Surg., *129*:167, 1975.

Copeland, E. M., and McBride, C. M.: Axillary metastasis from an unknown primary site. Ann. Surg., *178*:25, 1973.

Copeland, E. M., Miller, L. D., and Jones, R. S.: Prognostic factors in carcinoma of the colon and rectum. Am. J. Surg., *116*:875, 1968.

Copeland, E. M., Souchon, E. A., MacFadyen, B. V., Jr., Rapp, M. A., and Dudrick, S. J.: Intravenous hyperalimentation as an adjunct to radiation therapy. Cancer, *39*:609, 1977.

Fletcher, G. H., Lindberg, R. D., Tapley, N., Guillamondegui, O. M., Byers, R. M., Perez, C. A., and Gunderson, J. J.: Emerging roles of radiation therapy in four selected areas: Soft tissue sarcoma, salivary glands, prostate, rectal and sigmoid carcinoma. Curr. Probl. Cancer, *1*:40, 1976.

Frazier, T. G., Copeland, E. M., Gallager, S. H., Paulus, D. D., and White, E. C.: Prognosis and treatment in minimal breast cancer. Am. J. Surg., *133*:697, 1977.

Goldstein, H. M., Zornoza, J., Wallace, S., Anderson, J. H., Bree, P. L., Samuels, B. I., and Lukeman, J.: Percutaneous fine needle aspiration biopsy of pancreatic and other abdominal masses. Radiology, *123*:319, 1977.

Rittenhouse, M. D., and Copeland, E. M.: Carcinoma *in situ* of the distal colon and rectum. Surg. Gynecol. Obstet., *146*:225, 1978.

Sugarbaker, E. V., and McBride, C. M.: Melanoma of the trunk: The results of surgical excision and anatomic guidelines for predicting nodal metastasis. Surgery, *80*:22, 1976.

Veronesi, U., et al.: Inefficiency of immediate node dissection in stage 1 melanoma of the limbs. N. Eng. J. Med., *297*:627, 1977.

40

Physiologic Support Systems

LOUIS R. M. DEL GUERCIO
JOSEPH D. COHN

In the management of the critically ill or injured patient, a surgeon today is faced with a bewildering multitude of laboratory data and clinical measurements. It is the purpose of this chapter to describe methods for the organization and display of this mass of data so that it is transformed into information upon which diagnostic and therapeutic decisions can be based. The process by which data becomes information in the brain of the beholder, through comprehension and logical inference, is expedited if the facts are displayed in a systematic array based upon what is known about organ failures and common physiologic aberrations.

In any physiologic support system, the highest order of importance is placed on the precision, accuracy, and reproducibility of the directly measured variables. These are the fundamental building blocks that form the structure of all subsequent calculations. Errors of sample handling or careless instrument calibration cannot be tolerated and require constant vigilance. Clinical measurements such as patient temperature, height, weight, and fractional inspired oxygen concentration (FIO_2) must also be conscientiously obtained, checked, and recorded. The zero level, the horizontal projection of the tricuspid valve on the chest wall, is an important consideration in all right heart pressure recordings. If any of the directly measured variables are unsound, the information derived will be worse than useless.

Derived physiologic variables are the next step upward in the logical order. Mathematical ratios of measured variables are used as an expression of physiologic principles. For example, vascular resistance is defined as the ratio of blood pressure to blood flow, which is the application of Poiseuille's law of physics to circulatory dynamics. Since

748

resistance to flow is the sum of the influence of vasomotor nerves, hormonal substances, and metabolic products on the state of terminal arterioles and anatomic arteriovenous anastamoses in the vascular beds, this derived variable is of some broad clinical utility. When high flow states exist in the presence of low mean blood pressure, causes of lost vasomotor tone, such as sepsis, should be sought.

Starling's law of the heart, "the energy set free at each contraction of the heart is a simple function of the length of the fibers composing its muscular walls," can also be expressed in terms of derived variables. The energy of contraction is described as the left ventricular stroke work (LVSW), the product of the stroke index, the mean aortic blood pressure, and the specific gravity of mercury. The myocardial fiber length is expressed as the filling pressure of the left ventricle (the greater the pressure, the greater the stretch). This pressure in the left atrium is recorded from a flow-directed balloon-tipped catheter (Swan-Ganz) inserted in a branch of the pulmonary artery. With the balloon temporarily inflated, the manometer registers the pressure (PAw) transmitted back through the pulmonary vein and capillaries to the catheter tip. The Starling relationship, displayed on a graph (Fig. 40–1, right lower quadrant) with LVSW on the ordinate and PAw on the abscissa, was originally shown by Sarnoff (1955) to be a good measure of myocardial contractility. Myocardial contractility is simply the state of health or vigor of the heart muscle. It is depressed, of course, in myocardial infarction but also on occasion following burns, sepsis, and traumatic shock. The Sarnoff ventricular function curve is of value to the surgeon because the response to and need for a fluid volume expansion, in terms of cardiac work, can be predicted. With increased venous return, the index moves upward and to the right, along a curve parallel to the shaded area representing the normal range. Beyond a filling pressure of 15 mm Hg it can be seen that very little improvement in LVSW is likely unless some therapeutic agent is added to improve contractility. Another way of viewing this physiologic relationship is that the cardiac output and its four determinants, i.e., preload, contractility, afterload, and pulse rate (Braunwald, 1971), are all represented on the ventricular function diagram. Cardiac output, pulse rate, and blood pressure (afterload) are recorded along the ordinate and left ventricular filling pressure (preload) on the abscissa. The function plotted thus defines myocardial contractility.

Other clinically useful derived variables provide estimates of the efficiency of oxygen uptake in the lungs and of oxygen transport and release at the capillary level. Pulmonary failure is a frequent problem in critically ill surgical patients, and an early and sensitive measure of this is the venoarterial admixture (Qs/Qt) or the percentage of the right heart output that is not exposed during transit to ventilated alveoli. This so-called pulmonary shunt is calculated using the following directly measured variables: FIO_2, arterial blood gases, mixed venous blood

Automated Physiologic Profile

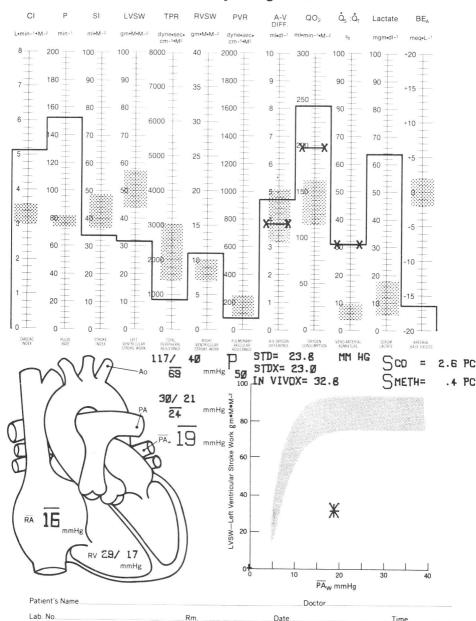

Figure 40–1. Physiologic variables in a 50 year old man with postoperative septic shock. The hyperdynamic state with high cardiac index, low total peripheral vascular resistance and wide pulse pressure is shown. Severe contractile failure of the heart is evident on the ventricular function diagram in the lower right. Adult respiratory distress syndrome has produced severe venoarterial admixture as well as pulmonary hypertension. Standard P50 is reduced, indicating increased oxyhemoglobin affinity. This, combined with other septic factors limiting oxygen extraction, resulted in oxygen consumption insufficient to meet increased metabolic requirements. Although oxygen consumption is increased over that predicted for the basal resting state, oxygen debt is shown by the elevated lactate and severe metabolic acidosis. If the P50 were normal the oxygen consumption would be 245 ml/min/M² instead of 200 ml/min/M².

gases (sampled from the Swan-Ganz catheter with the balloon deflated), and hemoglobin concentration. Assessment of pulmonary function relying on arterial blood gases alone, as is sometimes done in the form of the alveolar-arterial oxygen tension gradient, (A-aDO$_2$) can be misleading. For example, a fall in cardiac output resulting in a reduction of mixed venous oxygen content will produce an increase in the A-aDO$_2$ even though there is no increase in pulmonary shunting. The clinician, mistakenly interpreting the increased hypoxemia as a need for more PEEP, might be trapped by a therapeutic vicious cycle when more PEEP further reduces the cardiac output. The reverse can also occur in the clinical setting when the mixed venous oxygen content increases owing to the septic hyperdynamic state. In the calculation of venoarterial admixture, the oxygenation of blood going into the lung is just as important as that coming out. This illustrates the danger of relying on isolated individual variables for monitoring and the need for an information system that emphasizes the relationships between cardiac, pulmonary, and oxygen transport functions.

One such system is based upon the premise that a graphic display is more readily scanned and comprehended than columns of figures. Physicians, in particular, are better at pattern recognition than they are at number assimilation. The information array in its bar-chart format is shown in Figure 40–1 and is called the automated physiologic profile. A minicomputer is commercially available that uses a built-in microprocessor to calculate and automatically record the derived variables on the report form with preprinted scales, legends, and zones of normal function.* Other methods of data reduction can also be used for subsequent display on the physiologic profile format. A programmable calculator with attached alphanumeric X-Y plotter is presently in use at several institutions. The 1848-step program, in assembly language, is stored on standard magnetic tape cassettes so that the calculator can be used for other purposes. Other centers have published similar programs designed for use with each of the two popular brands of advanced model hand-held calculators (Civetta, 1977; Shabot et al., 1977). The numbers as they appear sequentially on the display can be recorded on the profile sheet by hand. Even less expensive is the practice of sharing computer facilities between hospitals using low-cost facsimile transcribers to send the measured data from the patient over ordinary voice-quality telephone lines and return the completed physiologic profile sheet from the computer center a few minutes later.

In clinical practice, the access for arterial and mixed venous pressure measurements and blood sampling can utilize percutaneous techniques or peripheral cutdowns. The fact that these are bedside techniques does not obviate the need for strict glove, mask, and cap sterile precautions. Special Seldinger-type catheter introducers for the Swan-Ganz catheter are used when the subclavian or internal jugular vein route is chosen.

---

*Life Sciences Inc., Greenwich, Conn.

When the catheter tip reaches the superior vena cava, the balloon is inflated, which results in the catheter being pulled along with the blood flow into the pulmonary artery. Pressures are recorded from each heart chamber as well as the "wedge position" in the pulmonary artery as described earlier. Adequacy of the ulnar collateral circulation to the fingers is always confirmed by means of the Allen test before the radial artery is cannulated.

Cardiac output determinations are made with either the thermal dilution or the indocyanine green dye dilution technique. The former is more simple but requires an expensive thermistor-tipped catheter. The dye dilution technique requires calibration of the densitometer with incremental amounts of the dye in the patient's blood. The calculation of the calibration factor is automated by the minicomputer. The dye dilution method, recorded across the entire heart and lungs rather than the right heart alone as with thermal dilution, permits mathematical analysis of the shape of the time-concentration curve as well as the area. The area of the curve is inversely proportional to cardiac output, but the shape yields information regarding mixing volume in the heart and lungs as well as ejection fraction. As heart failure develops, the cardiac output may be maintained for a time, but the residual volume in the ventricle after each beat increases in proportion to the amount of blood ejected.

When the pulmonary and radial arterial catheters have been secured with sterile dressings, blood samples are obtained simultaneously from each for blood gas analysis and hemoglobin, hematocrit, lactate, oxygen saturation, and carboxyhemoglobin saturation determinations. Semiautomated spectrophotometric and polarographic instruments permit these blood analyses in the intensive care unit. These values are then fed into the minicomputer through the keyboard.

A patient whose physiologic profile is shown in Figure 40–1 will serve as a good example of the need for this problem-oriented approach to monitoring. On morning rounds five days after a gastric resection, this 50-year-old man was found to be febrile, weak, and dyspneic. Blood pressure was 120/60 mm Hg, but his pulse was rapid at a rate of 150. There were no localizing abdominal signs, but the patient was obviously in grave trouble. A Swan-Ganz catheter and radial arterial cannula were used to obtain an automated physiologic profile.

The directly measured variables associated with hemodynamic function were a cardiac index of 5.16 l per min per m^2 with a pulmonary wedge pressure (PAw) of 19 mm Hg. Considered as isolated variables, these would suggest more than adequate blood flow and venous return, but when correlated with others, they revealed severe left ventricular failure.

The stroke index was low because of the fast pulse, and this multiplied by the decreased mean arterial blood pressure produced a value for left ventricular stroke work that was about 60 per cent of normal. The magnitude of the myocardial contractile failure is revealed in the ventricular function diagram, so that in spite of the high total blood flow, the first clinical problem to be corrected is cardiac failure. The patient had no prior history of cardiac disease, and the ECG was normal, but the heart was obviously in failure, and myocardial depressant factors have been demonstrated in many critical syndromes. The wide pulse pressure and low total peripheral vascular resistance are suggestive of a loss of vasomotor tone associated with sepsis. Vasopressors are not indicated, however, because they would simply increase afterload and stroke work without improving contractility. Immediate inotropic therapy is needed, and a wide variety of agents are available: rapid-acting digitalis drugs, dopamine, high-dose glucose-insulin-potassium infusions, glucagon infusions, or even intra-aortic balloon pumping. Sequential use of the physiologic profile with ventricular function curves allows titration of the dose of the inotropic agent, which is essential. Before any diagnosis is confirmed regarding the presence of septic shock or its cause, the problem of myocardial contractile failure requires prompt attention because survival is dependent on maintenance of the high cardiac output.

Factors associated with pulmonary function in this patient are also alarming. While breathing 100 per cent oxygen via an endotracheal tube, his partial pressure of arterial oxygen (PaO_2) is 112 mm Hg with a separately measured oxygen saturation (SaO_2) of 96.8 per cent. The normal PaO_2 under these conditions should be more than 500 mm Hg. This wide A-aDO_2 implies extensive venoarterial admixture, which is an early sign of respiratory distress syndrome. The chest roentgenogram at this point was normal. The calculated pulmonary shunt (Qs/Qt) of 30 per cent was partially due to the high concentration of inspired oxygen, which of itself causes shunting. The physiologic profile program can calculate shunt at any FIO_2.

Ordinarily, when cardiac output increases, as in exercise, the pulmonary vascular resistance falls, and pulmonary artery pressure remains stable. In this patient with a blood flow almost 60 per cent greater than normal, the pulmonary vascular resistance has not decreased much, and the pulmonary artery pressure is elevated to 30/21 mm Hg (normal = 25/8 mm Hg). The rise in diastolic pressure in particular is consistent with pulmonary vasoconstriction, which is often associated with such factors as hypoxia, alveolar collapse, and excessive airway pressures. Pulmonary constriction increases right ventricular afterload. In this unfortunate patient, the combination of the increased load on the right ventricle and the myocardial depressant factors have already resulted in right ventricular failure as evidenced by the high right ventricular end-diastolic pressure of 17 mm Hg. Thus, the second critical problem revealed by the physiologic profile is the adult respiratory distress syndroem (ARDS). Immediate treatment with a volume-cycled respirator and PEEP is needed in order to increase functional residual capacity (FRC) of the lungs and to take over the work of breathing, which in such patients may represent a large portion of their metabolic demands. But the optimal level of PEEP is critical and can be determined only by combined assessment of cardiac, pulmonary, and oxygen transport functions. These also indicate how much fluid volume expansion may be necessary for the maintenance of adequate cardiac output at a given PEEP setting. Since the objective of PEEP in respiratory support is to improve the delivery of oxygen to the tissues and since oxygen transport is the product of arterial oxygen content and the cardiac output, excessive PEEP may result in a net reduction in oxygen delivery even though the blood gases improve.

Attention is now directed to the derived variables representative of oxygen transport in this patient. Oxygen consumption ($\dot{V}O_2$) is estimated by multiplying the cardiac output by the arteriovenous oxygen content difference (a-$\bar{v}CDO_2$), an application of the Fick principle. In this case, greater than normal quantities of oxygen are being consumed, but the normal values shown refer only to the basal resting state. A number of factors are at work here in raising oxygen needs. For every degree Centigrade of fever, there is approximately a 15 per cent increase in oxygen requirements. Circulating endogenous catecholamines also increase the metabolic rate, as does the increased work of breathing owing to reduced pulmonary compliance.

Oxygen requirements are increased in other critical states, such as severe burns, in which the heat of vaporization of the tremendous quantities of body water lost through the burn eschar increases energy expenditure. In this exemplary patient, there is insufficient oxygen utilization confirmed by the hypoxic acidosis (base deficit) and very high serum lactate. Lactic acid is the end product of anaerobic metabolism, whereas the end products of normal cellular respiration in the presence of sufficient cellular oxygen are CO_2 and water. This unsteady state will result in death before many hours pass unless normal cellular respiration is restored. But, patients do not die *of* lacticacidemia, they die *with* it. When oxygen is available to the mitochondria, the excess lactate is readily metabolized in the liver. Although it would be easy to correct the acidosis with intravenous sodium bicarbonate, that would reverse the beneficial shift to the right of the oxyhemoglobin dissociation curve, which allows release of oxygen at the capillary level at higher oxygen tensions. These higher oxygen tensions result in better diffusion of oxygen out to the cells. When the PO_2 at the venous end of the capillary is less than 20 mm Hg, there is insufficient pressure to supply the cells on the periphery of the cylinder of cells surrounding each capillary. When the pH falls below 7.15, some bicarbonate should be used, however, because at that low level the cardiovascular response to catecholamines may be reduced.

The mixed venous oxygen saturation ($S\bar{v}O_2$) in this patient was 71 per cent (normal is 75 per cent), and the a-$\bar{v}CDO_2$ was not increased. Why was more oxygen not being extracted from that available in the arterial blood flow? This inappropriate oxygen extraction is one of the fundamental problems of septic shock. There is some evidence that tissue utilization of oxygen can be improved in septic shock following pharmacologic doses of adrenocortical steroids; in this case, the physiologic profile would show increased a-$\bar{v}CDO_2$ and $\dot{V}O_2$ with reduction of hypoxic acidosis.

One final physiologic aberration of clinical importance is revealed by the computerized data analysis. Use of the Hill equation, which closely approximates the sigmoidal oxyhemoglobin dissociation curve, combined with correction factors for temperature, pH, and base excess, permits prediction of the oxygen saturation at any given PO_2. When the predicted saturation does not coincide with that measured spectrophotometrically under clinical conditions, shifts in the dissociation curve exclusive of the Bohr effect can be calculated. The magnitude and direction of these shifts are reported as the P50, the oxygen tension at standard pH and temperature that produces 50 per cent oxygen saturation. The normal P50 is approximately 27 mm Hg, but it may be increased in chronic hypoxia or anemia. This effect is mediated through an increase in red cell 2,3 diphosphoglycerate, the most important regulator of oxyhemoglobin affinity. P50 abnormalities are also seen in patients with cirrhosis of the liver, hemoglobinopathies, thyrotoxicosis, burns, carbon monoxide poisoning, pancreatitis, phosphate depletion, septic shock, and following massive transfusion with blood stored for longer than seven days. In the last two conditions, which produce a low P50, adrenalcortical steroids in large doses may restore oxyhemoglobin affinity to normal.

In the patient under study, the P50 is low, 23.8 mm Hg. Because of his fever and severe acidosis, the Bohr effect has shifted his in vivo P50 up to 32.8. But since the Bohr effect is additive, if his standard P50 had been normal, oxygen unloading to the tissues would have been much better. The magnitude of the difference in a-$\bar{v}CDO_2$ and $\dot{V}O_2$ caused by the low standard P50 is shown by the lines with the x's on the bar chart. Oxygen consumption is only about 80 per cent of what it would have been had oxyhemoglobin affinity been normal.

Physiologic support of this patient was based upon complex relationships between organ systems displayed on one integrated report form within a few minutes of the diagnostic intervention. Drainage of his subhepatic abscess and appropriate antibiotics were certainly just as important as the physiologic assessment and titration of support regimens, but it is unlikely that he would have survived in the absence of either approach.

Although the automated physiologic profile has had its widest application in postoperative and post-traumatic critical states, it is likely that more lives can be saved when this approach is used to evaluate the elderly or high-risk patient prior to operation. The national overall operative mortality rate in patients over the age of 65 is 4.88 per cent!

Many of these deaths are related to a cardiorespiratory reserve insufficient to overcome the stress of anesthesia and operation or the increased metabolic demands of the recovery period. Subtle but significant abnormalities not detected by the electrocardiograph or the five senses of the skilled clinician are often revealed by the physiologic profile. Delay of operation to allow physiologic fine-tuning, choice of a lesser procedure, or a change to a different therapeutic modality are alternatives when surgical risk is found to be excessive. If even only one patient is saved from death or weeks of intensive care, the costs of the physiologic support system are recouped.

REFERENCES

Braunwald, E.: On the difference between the heart's output and its contractile state. Circulation, *43*:171, 1971.

Civetta, J. M.: Cardiopulmonary calculations: A rapid, simple and inexpensive technique. Intensive Care Med., *3*:209, 1977.

Cohn, J. D., Engler, P. E., and Del Guercio, L. R. M.: The automated physiologic profile. Crit. Care Med., *3*:51, 1975.

Del Guercio, L. R. M., and Cohn, J. D.: Monitoring operative risk in the elderly. J.A.M.A., *243*:1350, 1980.

Gudwin, A. L., Goldstein, C. R., Cohn, J. D., et al.: Estimation of ventricular mixing volume for prediction of operative mortality in the elderly. Ann. Surg., *168*:183, 1968.

Harken, A. H.: The surgical significance of the oxyhemoglobin dissociation curve. Surg. Gynecol. Obstet., *144*:935, 1977.

Powers, S. R., and Dutton, R. E.: Correlation of positive end-expiratory pressure with cardiovascular performance. Crit. Care Med., *3*:64, 1975.

Sarnoff, S. J.: Myocardial contractility as described by ventricular function curves. Physiol. Rev., *35*:107, 1955.

Shabot, M. M., Shoemaker, W. C., and State, D.: Rapid bedside computation of cardiorespiratory variables with a programmable calculator. Crit. Care Med., *5*:105, 1977.

Swan, H. J. C., Ganz, W., Forrester, J., et al.: Catheterization of the heart in man with use of a flow-directed balloon-tipped catheter. N. Engl. J. Med., *283*:447, 1970.

Appendix

RICHARD E. WARD
HENRY T. RANDALL

The following is a compilation of normal values, various formulas, and other miscellaneous information that can be useful in the solution of clinical problems related to the care of the surgical patient.

NORMAL BLOOD, PLASMA, AND SERUM VALUES

For some procedures, the values may vary depending on the method of analysis used. The range of normal includes both normal biologic variation and the error inherent in the laboratory method of determining a particular value. In many instances, the ranges will be the mean (average) value in humans, plus or minus two standard deviations of the mean, and thus will encompass 95 per cent of the total distribution of values found in groups of presumably well persons of various ages and of both sexes.

Good biochemical and clinicopathologic laboratory procedures should include not only frequent checking of methods against meticulously prepared standards, including serum pools, but also the routine of repeating the determination on any blood or other specimen in which an abnormal value has been found. Additional specimens should be obtained for analysis whenever needed to check an abnormal value. Serious deviation from normal should be reported at once as an emergency to permit immediate action in treatment. Emergency reporting levels are suggested in the tables for a number of procedures.

It is wise for the surgeon to determine from each laboratory to which he or she may send specimens what the normal range is for that laboratory for each commonly used test. It is also important to consult with the clinical pathologist or clinical biochemist in charge of the laboratory when wide fluctuation in reported values or abnormal values that do not apparently fit the clinical picture are found. Repeating the determinations and reexamining the patient will usually solve the problem. Additional tests may be recommended that will assist in clarifying more obscure difficulties.

BLOOD, PLASMA, OR SERUM VALUES

DETERMINATION	REFERENCE RANGE	MATERIAL ANALYZED	MINIMAL ML. OF BLOOD REQUIRED	NOTE	METHOD
Acetoacetate plus acetone	0.3–2.0 mg per 100 ml	Serum	2		Behre; J. Lab. Clin. Med., 13:770, 1928 (modified)
Aldolase	1.3–8.2 mU per mol	Serum	2	Use fresh, unhemolyzed serum	Beisenherz et al.: Z. Naturforsch, 8b:555, 1953
Alpha amino nitrogen	3.0–5.5 mg per 100 ml	Plasma	5	Collect with heparin	Szentirmai et al.: Clin. Chim. Acta, 7:459, 1962
Ammonia	80–110 μg per 100 ml	Blood	2	Collect in heparinized tube; deliver immediately packed in ice	Seligson, Hirahara: J. Lab. Clin. Med., 49:962, 1957
Amylase	4–25 U per ml	Serum	3		Huggins, Russell: Ann. Surg., 128;668, 1948
Ascorbic acid	0.4–1.5 mg per 100 ml	Blood	7	Collect in heparin	Roe, Kuether: J. Biol., 147:399, 1943
Barbiturate	0 Coma level: phenobarbital, approximately 10 mg per 100 ml; most other drugs, 1–3 mg per 100 ml	Serum	5		Goldbaum: Anal. Chem., 24:1604, 1952
Bilirubin (van den Bergh test)	One minute: 0.4 mg per 100 ml; direct: 0.4 mg per 100 ml; total: 0.7 mg per 100 ml; indirect is total minus direct.	Serum	3		Malloy, Evelyn: J. Biol. Chem., 119:481, 1937
Blood volume	8.5–9.0 per cent of body weight in kg				Isotope dilution technique with ^{131}I albumin
Bromide	0	Serum	3		Adapted from Wuth: J.A.M.A., 82:2013, 1927
Bromsulfalein (BSP)	Less than 5 per cent retention	Serum	3	Inject intravenously 5 mg of dye per kg of body weight; draw blood 45 min later	Goebler: Am. J. Clin. Pathol., 15:452, 1945

Test	Normal Value	Specimen	ml	Notes	Reference
Calcium	8.5–10.5 mg per 100 ml	Serum	3	BSP dye interferes (slightly higher in children)	Bett, Fraser: Clin. Chim. Acta, 4:346, 1959 Kessler, Wolfman: Clin. Chem., 10:686, 1964 (modified)
Carbon dioxide content	24–30 mEq per l, 20–26 mEq per l in infants (as HCO_3)	Serum	3	Draw without stasis under oil or in heparinized syringe	Van Slyke, Neill: J. Biol. Chem., 61:523, 1924 Tech Auto Analyzer Method
Carbon monoxide	Symptoms with over 20 per cent saturation	Blood	5	Fill tube to top; tightly stopper; use anticoagulant	Bruchner, Desmond: Clin. Chim. Acta, 3:173, 1958
Carotenoids	0.08–0.40 µg per ml	Serum	3	Vitamin A may be done on same specimen	Natelson: Microtechniques of Clinical Chemistry, 2nd ed., 1961, p. 454
Ceruloplasmin	27–37 mg per 100 ml	Serum	2		Ravin: J. Lab. Clin. Med., 58:161, 1961
Chloride	100–106 mEq per l	Serum	1		Modification of Schales; J. Biol. Chem., 140:879, 1941 Tech Auto Analyzer Method
Cholinesterase (pseudocholinesterase)	0.5 pH U or more per hr 0.7 pH U or more per hr for packed cells	Serum Packed cells	1		Michel: J. Lab. Clin. Med., 34:1564, 1949.
Copper	Total: 100–200 µg per 100 ml	Serum	3		MGH Methodology, atomic absorption
Creatine phosphokinase (CPK)	Females 5–35 mU per ml; males 5–55 mU per ml	Serum	3	Immediately separate and freeze serum	Rosalki: J. Lab. Clin. Med., 69:696, 1967 (modified)
Creatine	0.6–1.5 mg per 100 ml	Serum	1		Fabriny and Ertingshausen: Clin. Chem., 17:696, 1971
Cryoglobulins	0	Serum	8	Collect and transport at 37°C	Barr et al.: Ann. Intern. Med., 32:6, 1950 (modified)
Cryoprecipitable proteins	0	Serum Citrate Heparin plasma	10 5 10		
Doriden (glutethimide)	0	Serum	5		Rieder, Servas: Am. J. Clin. Pathol., 44:520, 1965

BLOOD, PLASMA, OR SERUM VALUES *Continued*

DETERMINATION	REFERENCE RANGE	MATERIAL ANALYZED	MINIMAL ML OF BLOOD REQUIRED	NOTE	METHOD
Ethanol	0.3–0.4 per cent, marked intoxication; 0.4–0.5 per cent, alcoholic stupor; 0.5 per cent or over, alcoholic coma	Blood	2	Collect in oxalate and refrigerate	Natelson: Microtechniques of Clinical Chemistry, 2nd ed., 1961, p. 208
Gastrin	0–200 pg per ml	Plasma	4	Heparinized sample	Dent et al.: Ann. Surg., 176:360, 1972
Glucose	Fasting; 70–110 mg per 100 ml	Plasma	2	Collect with EDTA-fluoride mixture	Suguira and Huano: Clin. Chim. Acta, 75:387, 1977 Stein in Bergmeyer: Methods of Enzyme Analysis, 1965, p. 117
Iron	50–150 µg per 100 ml (higher in males)	Serum	5	Shows diurnal variation; higher in A.M.	Tech Auto Analyzer Method (modified)
Iron-binding capacity	250–410 µg per 100 ml	Serum	5		Scalata, Moore: Clin. Chem., 8:360, 1962 Tech Auto Analyzer Method
Lactic acid	0.6–1.8 mEq per l	Blood	2	Collect with oxalate fluoride mixture; deliver immediately packed in ice	Hadjivassiliou, Rieder: Clin. Chim. Acta, 19:357, 1968
Lactic dehydrogenase	60–120 U per ml	Serum	2	Unsuitable if hemolyzed	Wacker et al.: N. Engl. J. Med., 255:449, 1956
Lead	50 µg per 100 ml or less	Blood	2	Collect with oxalate fluoride mixture	Berman: Atom. Absorp. Newsletter 3:9, 1964 (modified)
Lipase	2 U per ml or less	Serum	3		Comfort, Osterberg: J. Lab. Clin. Med., 20:271, 1934
Lipids	120–220 mg per 100 ml	Serum	2	Fasting	Tech Auto Analyzer Method

			(ml)		
Cholesterol esters	60–75 per cent of cholesterol	Serum	2	Fasting	Creech, Sewell: Anal. Biochem., 3:119, 1962. Tech Auto Analyzer Method
Phospholipids	9–16 mg per 100 ml as lipid phosphorus	Serum	5	Fasting	Fiske, SubbaRow: J. Biol. Chem., 66:2, 1925
Total fatty acids	190–420 mg per 100 ml	Serum	10	Fasting	Stoddard, Drury; J. Biol. Chem., 84:741, 1929
Total lipids	450–1000 mg per 100 ml	Serum	5	Fasting	Freedman: Clin. Chim. Acta, 19:291, 1968
Triglycerides	40–150 mg per 100 ml	Serum	2	Fasting	Tech Auto Analyzer Method
Lipoprotein electrophoresis (LEP)	Distinct beta band; negligible chylomicron and pre-beta bands	Serum	2	Fasting; do not freeze serum	Lees, Hatch: J. Lab. Clin. Med., 61:518, 1963
Lithium	Toxic level 2 mEq per l	Serum	1		Flame photometry
Magnesium	1.5–2.0 mEq per l	Serum	1		Willis: Clin. Chem., 11:251, 1965 (modified)
Methanol	0	Blood	5	May be fatal at 115 mg per 100 ml; collect in oxalate	Natelson: Microtechniques of Clinical Chemistry, 2nd ed., 1961, p. 298
5' Nucleotidase	0.3–3.2 Bodansky U	Serum	1		Rieder, Otero: Clin. Chem., 8:727, 1969
Osmolality	280–295 mOsm per kg water	Serum	5		Crawford, Nicosia: J. Lab. Clin. Med., 40:907, 1952
Oxygen saturation (arterial)	96–100 per cent	Arterial blood	3	Deliver in sealed heparinized syringe packed in ice	Gordy, Drabkin: J. Biol. Chem., 227:285, 1957
Pco_2	35–45 mm Hg	Arterial blood	2	Collect and deliver in sealed heparinized syringe	By CO_2 electrode
pH	7.35–7.45	Arterial blood	2	Collect without stasis in sealed heparinized syringe; deliver packed in ice	Glass electrode
Po_2	75–100 mm Hg (dependent on age) while breathing room air; Above 500 mm Hg while on 100 per cent O_2	Arterial blood	2		Oxygen electrode

BLOOD, PLASMA, OR SERUM VALUES *Continued*

DETERMINATION	REFERENCE RANGE	MATERIAL ANALYZED	MINIMAL ML BLOOD REQUIRED	NOTE	METHOD
Phenylalanine	0–2 mg per 100 ml	Serum	0.4		Cullay et al.: Clin. Chem., 8:266, 1962 (modified)
Phenytoin (Dilantin)	Therapeutic level, 10–15 μg per mol	Serum	3		Gas liquid chromatography
Phosphatase (acid)	Males, total: 0.13–0.63 sigma U per ml Females, total: 0.01–0.56 sigma U per ml Prostate: 0–0.7 Fishman-Lerner U per 100 ml	Serum	1	Must always be drawn just before analysis or stored as frozen serum; avoid hemolysis	Bessey et al.: J. Biol. Chem., 164:321, 1946
Phosphate (alkaline)	13–39 IU per l; infants and adolescents, up to 104 IU per l	Serum	1	BSP dye interferes For Bodansky U, multiply by 0.15 up to 90 U; 0.13 up to 256 U	Bessey et al.: J. Biol. Chem., 164:321, 1945
Phosphorus (inorganic)	3.0–4.5 mg per 100 ml (infants in 1st year up to 6.0 mg per 100 ml)	Serum	2	Obtain blood in fasting state; serum must be separated promptly from cells	Fiske, SubbaRow: J. Biol. Chem., 66:375, 1925 Adapter for Tech Auto Analyzer Method
Potassium	3.5–5.0 mEq per l	Serum	2	Serum must be separated promptly from cells (within 1 hr)	Flame photometry
Primidone (Mysoline)	Therapeutic level 4–12 μg per ml	Serum	3		Gas liquid chromatography
Protein: Total	6.0–8.4 gm per 100 ml	Serum	1	Patient should be fasting; avoid BSP dye	Refractometry (American Optical Co.)
Albumin	3.5–5.0 gm per 100 ml	Serum	1		Doumas et al.: Clin. Chim. Acta, 31:87, 1971
Globulin	2.3–3.5 gm per 100 ml			Globulin equals total protein minus albumin	Gornall et al.: J. Biol. Chem., 177:751, 1949 (modified)
Paper electrophoresis	Percentage of total protein	Serum	1	Quantification by densitometry	Kunkel, Tiselius: J. Gen. Physiol., 35:89, 1951 Durrum: J. Am. Chem. Soc., 72:2943, 1950

Albumin globulin:
  Alpha₁
  Alpha₂
  Beta
  Gamma
	52–68
	4.2–7.2
	6.8–12
	9.3–15
	13–23				

Pyruvic acid	0–0.11 mEq per l	Blood	2	Collect with oxalate fluoride; deliver immediately packed in ice	Hadjivassiliou, Rieder: Clin. Chim. Acta, *19*:357, 1968
Quinidine	Therapeutic: 1.5–3 µg per ml Toxic: 5–6 µg per ml	Serum	1		Fluorometry after extraction
Salicylate	0 Therapeutic: 20–25 mg per 100 ml 25–30 mg per 100 ml to age 10 yrs 3 hrs post dose Toxic: Over 30 mg per 100 ml; over 20 mg per 100 ml after age 60	Plasma	5	Collect in heparin or oxalate	Keller: Am. J. Clin. Pathol., *17*:415, 1947
Sodium	135–145 mEq per l	Serum	2		Flame photometry
Sulfate	0.5–1.5 mg per 100 ml	Serum	3	Avoid hemolysis	Letonoff, Reinhold: J. Biol. Chem., *114*:147, 1936
Sulfonamide	0	Blood or serum	2	Value given as unconjugated	Bratton, Marshall: J. Biol. Chem., *128*:537, 1939
Thymol: Flocculation	Up to 1 + in 24 hrs	Serum	1	Checked with phosphate buffer of higher molarity to rule out false-positive reaction	Maclagen: Nature, *154*:670, 1944
Turbidity	0–4 U				
Transaminase (SGOT)	10–40 U per ml	Serum	1		Karmen et al.: J. Clin. Invest., *34*:126, 1955
Urea nitrogen (BUN)	8–25 mg per 100 ml	Blood or serum	1	Urea = BUN $\times$ 2.14 Use oxalate as anticoagulant	Bretaudiere et al.: Clin. Chem., 22:1614, 1976 Weatherburn: Anal. Chem., 39:901, 1967
Uric acid	3.0–7.0 mg per 100 ml	Serum	1	Serum must be separated from cells at once and refrigerated	Praetorius: Scand. J. Clin. Lab. Invest., *1*:22, 1949
Vitamin A	0.15–0.6 µg per ml	Serum	3		Natelson: Microtechniques of Clinical Chemistry, 2nd ed., 1961, p. 451
Vitamin A tolerance test	Rise to twice fasting level in 3 to 5 hrs	Serum	3	Samples taken fasting and at intervals up to 8 hrs after test dose	Josephs: Bull. Johns Hopkins Hosp., 65:112, 1939

(From normal reference values. N. Engl. J. Med., 298(1):34–45, 1978.)

URINE VALUES

DETERMINATION	REFERENCE RANGE	MINIMAL QUANTITY REQUIRED	NOTE	METHOD
Acetone plus acetoacetate (quantitative)	0	2 ml	Keep cold	Behre: J. Lab. Clin. Med., 13:770, 1928
Alpha amino nitrogen	64–199 mg per day; not over 1.5 per cent of total nitrogen	24-hr specimen	Preserve with thymol; refrigerate	Hamilton, Van Slyke: J. Biol. Chem., 150:231, 1943
Amylase	24–76 U per ml	24-hr specimen		Huggins, Russell: Ann. Surg., 128:668, 1948
Calcium	150 mg per day or less	24-hr specimen	Collect in special bottle with 10 ml of concentrated HCl	Atomic absorption
Catecholamines	Epinephrine: under 20 μg per day, norepinephrine: under 100 μg per day	24-hr specimen	Should be collected with 12 ml of concentrated HCl (pH should be between 2.0 and 3.0)	DuToit: WADC Tech. Report No. 59–175, 1959
Chorionic gonadotropin	0	1st morning voiding		Immunologic technique
Copper	0–100	24-hr specimen	Specific gravity should be at least 1.015	MGH Methodology Atomic Absorption
Coproporphyrin	50–250 μg per day Children under 80 lb, 0–75 μg per day	24-hr specimen	Collect with 5 gm of sodium carbonate	Schwartz: J. Lab. Clin. Med., 37:843, 1951 With Scand. J. Clin. Lab. Invest., 7:193, 1955
Homogentisic acid	0	Freshly voided sample or 24-hr sample kept cold	Must be refrigerated if not determined at once; test also measures gentisic acid and may be positive in patients on high doses of salicylates	Neuberger: Biochem. J., 41:431, 1947
5-Hydroxyindole acetic acid	2–9 mg per 24 hrs (women lower than men)	24-hr specimen	Collect in special bottle with 10 ml of concentrated HCl	Sjoerdsman et al.: J.A.M.A., 159:397, 1955
Lead	0.08 μg per ml or 120 μg or less per 24 hrs	24-hr specimen		Willis: Anal. Chem., 34:614, 1962 (modified)

Test	Normal Value	Specimen	Notes	Reference
Phenolsulfonphthalein (PSP)	At least 25 per cent excreted by 15 min; 40 per cent by 30 min; 60 per cent by 120 min	Total output of urine collected 15, 30, and 120 min after injection	Inject 1 ml (6 mg) intravenously; BSP interferes	Chapman: N. Engl. J. Med., 214:16, 1936
Phenylpyruvic acid	0	Freshly voided unless quantification needed		Penrose, Quastel: Biochem. J., 31:266,1937
Phosphorus (inorganic)	Varies with intake; average 1 gm per day	24-hr specimen	Collect in special bottle with 10 ml of concentrated HCl	Tech Auto Analyzer Method
Porphobilinogen	0	10 ml	Use freshly voided urine	Watson, Schwartz: Proc. Soc. Exp. Biol. Med., 47:393, 1941
Creatine	Under 100 mg per day or less than 6 per cent of creatinine. In pregnancy, up to 12 per cent, in children under 1 yr, may equal creatinine, in older children, up to 30 per cent of creatinine	24-hr specimen	Also order creatinine	Folin: Laboratory for Manual Biology and Chemistry, 5th ed., 1933, p. 163
Creatinine	15–25 mg per kg of body weight per day	24-hr specimen		Folin: Laboratory Manual for Biology and Chemistry, 5th ed., 1933, p. 163
Creatinine clearance	150–180 l per day (104–125 ml per min) per 1.73 m^2 of body surface	24-hr specimen	Order serum creatinine also	Brod, Sirota: J. Clin. Invest., 27:645, 1948
Cystine or cysteine	0	10 ml	Qualitative	Hawk et al.: Practical Physiology and Chemistry, 13th ed., 1954, p. 141
Follicle-stimulating hormone:		24-hr specimen		Radioimmunoassay
Folicular phase	5–20 IU per 24 hrs			
Midcycle	15–60 IU per 24 hrs			
Luteal phase	5–15 IU per 24 hrs			
Menopausal	50–100 IU per 24 hrs			
Men	5–25 IU per 24 hrs			
Hemoglobin and myoglobin	0	Freshly voided sample	Chemical examination with benzidine	Spectroscopy
Protein:				
Quantitative	<150 mg per 24 hrs	24-hr specimen		Meulmans: Clin. Chim. Acta, 5:757, 1951
Electrophoresis				See blood protein

URINE VALUES *Continued*

DETERMINATION	REFERENCE RANGE			MINIMAL QUANTITY REQUIRED	NOTE	METHOD
Steroids:						
17-ketosteroids (per day)	Age	Males	Females	24-hr specimen	Not valid if patient is receiving meprobamate	Vestergaard: Acta Endocrinol., 8:193, 1951. Normal values taken from Hamburger: Acta Endocrinol., 1:19, 1948
	10	1–4 mg	1–4 mg			
	20	6–21	4–16			
	30	8–26	4–14			
	50	5–18	3–9			
	70	2–10	1–7			
17-hydroxysteroids	3–8 mg per day (women lower than men)			24-hr specimen	Keep cold; chlorpromazine and related drugs interfere with assay	Epstein: Clin. Chim. Acta, 7:735, 1962
Sugar:						
Quantitative glucose Identification of reducing substances	0			24-hr or other timed specimen 50 ml	Collect with toluene; refrigerate; use freshly voided urine; no preservatives	Stein, in Bergmeyer: Methods of Enzyme Analysis, 1965
Fructose	0			50 ml	Use freshly voided urine; also quantify total reducing substances	Roe et al.: J. Biol. Chem., 178:839, 1948
Pentose	0			50 ml	Use freshly voided urine	Roe, Rice: J. Biol. Chem., 173:507, 1948
Titratable acidity	20–40 mEq per day			24-hr sample	Collect with toluene; refrigerate	Henderson, Palmer: J. Biol. Chem., 17:305, 1914
Urobilinogen	Up to 1.0 Ehrlich U			2-hr sample (1–3 P.M.)		Watson et al.: Am. J. Clin. Pathol. 15:605, 1944
Uroporphyrin	0			See Coproporphyrin		Schwartz et al.: Proc. Soc. Exp. Biol. Med., 79:463, 1952
Vanillylmandelic acid (VMA)	Up to 9 mg per 24 hrs			24-hr specimen	Collect as for catecholamines	Pisano et al.: Clin. Chim. Acta, 7:285, 1962

(From normal reference values. N. Engl. J. Med., 298(1):34–45, 1978.)

Cerebrospinal Fluid Values

Determination	Reference Range	Minimal ml Required	Note	Method
Bilirubin	0	2		See Blood, bilirubin (adapted)
Cell count	0–5 mononuclear cells	0.5		
Chloride	120–130 mEq per l	0.5	20 mEq per l higher than serum; obtain serum for comparison	See Blood, chloride
Colloidal gold	0000000000-0001222111	0.1		Wuth, Faupel: Bull. Johns Hopkins Hosp., 40:297, 1927
Albumin	Mean 21 mg per 100 ml Range ± 1 SD 11.4–38.4 ± 2 SD 6–71	2.5		Mancini et al.: Immunochemistry, 2:235, 1965
IgG	Mean 3.5 mg per 100 ml Range ± 1 SD 2.0–5.9 ± 2 SD 1–10			
IgG:Albumin Ratio	Range ± 1 SD 0.0094–0.25 ± 2 SD 0.05–0.53			
Glucose	50–75 mg per 100 ml	0.5	20 mg per 100 ml less than blood; compare with blood	See Blood, glucose
Pressure (initial)	70–180 mm H_2O			
Protein: Lumbar	15–45 mg per 100 ml	1		Meulmans: Clin. Chim. Acta, 5:757, 1960
Cisternal	15–25 mg per 100 ml	1		
Ventricular	5–15 mg per 100 ml	1		

(From normal reference values. N. Engl. J. Med., 298(1):34–45, 1978.)

HEMATOLOGIC VALUES

DETERMINATION	REFERENCE RANGE	MATERIAL ANALYZED	MINIMAL ML OF BLOOD REQUIRED	NOTE	METHOD
Coagulation factors:					
Factor I (fibrinogen)	0.15–0.35 gm per 100 ml	Plasma	4.5	Collect in Vacutainer containing sodium citrate	Ratnoff, Menzies: J. Lab. Clin. Med., 37:316, 1951
Factor II (prothrombin)	60–140 per cent	Plasma	4.5	Collect in plastic tubes with 3.8 per cent sodium citrate	Owren, Aas: Scand. J. Clin. Lab. Invest., 3:201, 1951
Factor V (accelerator globulin)	60–140 per cent	Plasma	4.5	Collect as in Factor II determination	Lewis, Ware: Proc. Soc. Exp. Biol. Med., 84:640, 1953
Factor VII-X (proconvertin-Stuart)	70–130 per cent	Plasma	4.5	Collect as in Factor II determination	Same as Factor II
Factor VIII (antihemophilic globulin)	50–200 per cent	Plasma	4.5	Collect as in Factor II determination	Tocantins, Kazal: Blood Coagulation, Hemorrhage, and Thrombosis, 2nd ed., 1964
Factor IX (plasma thromboplastic cofactor)	60–140 per cent	Plasma	4.5	Collect as in Factor II determination	Tocantins, Kazal: Blood Coagulation, Hemorrhage, and Thrombosis, 2nd ed., 1964
Factor X (Stuart factor)	70–130 per cent	Plasma	4.5	Collect as in Factor II determination	Bachman et al.: Thromb. Diath. Haemorrh., 2:29, 1958
Factor XI (plasma thromboplastic antecedent)	60–140 per cent	Plasma	4.5	Collect as in Factor II determination	Tocantins, Kazal: Blood Coagulation, Hemorrhage, and Thrombosis, 2nd ed., 1964
Factor XII (Hageman factor)	60–140 per cent	Plasma	4.5	Collect as in Factor II determination	Tocantins, Kazal: Blood Coagulation, Hemorrhage, and Thrombosis, 2nd ed., 1964
Coagulation screening tests:					
Bleeding time	3–8 min				
Clotting time (glass)	Below 15 min	Whole blood	6	Collect in 3 glass tubes (10 × 74 mm)	Mielke: Blood, 34:204, 1969 Lee, White in Cartwright: Diagnostic Laboratory Hematology, 3rd ed., 1966, p. 152
Prothrombin time	Less than 2—see deviation from control	Plasma	4.5	Collect in Vacutainer containing 3.8 per cent sodium citrate	Colman et al.: Am. J. Clin. Pathol., 64:108, 1975
Partial thromboplastin time (activated)	25–37 sec	Plasma	4.5	Collect in Vacutainer containing 3.8 per cent sodium citrate	Babson: Am. J. Clin. Pathol., 62:856, 1974

Test	Normal value	Specimen	Instructions		Reference
Whole-blood clot lysis	No clot lysis in 24 hrs	Whole blood	Collect in sterile tube and incubate at 37°C	2.0	Page, Culver; Syllabus, Laboratory Examination and Clinical Diagnosis, 1960, p. 207
Fibrinolytic studies:					
Euglobulin lysis	No lysis in 2 hrs	Plasma	Collect as in Factor II determination	4.5	Sherry et al.: J. Clin. Invest., 38:810, 1959
Fibrinogen split products:					
Method I: latex agglutination (Thrombo-Wellcotest)	Negative reaction at greater than 1:4 dilution	Serum	Collect in special tube containing thrombin and epsilon amino acid	4.5	Carvalho: Am. J. Clin. Pathol., 62:107, 1974
Method II: Staphylococcal clumping	Positive reaction at greater than 1:16 dilution	Serum	Collect as in Method I	4.5	Carvalho: Am. J. Clin. Pathol., 62:107, 1974
Thrombin time	Less than 5 sec deviation from control	Plasma	Collect as in Factor II determination	4.5	Stefanini, Dameshek: Hemorrh. Discord, 1962, p. 492
"Complete" blood count:		Blood	Use EDTA as anticoagulant; the seven listed tests are performed automatically on the Coulter counter Model S, which directly determines cell counts, hemoglobin (as the cyanmethemoglobin derivative), and MCV and computes hematocrit, MCH, and MCHC	1	
Hematocrit	Males: 42–50 per cent / Females: 40–48 per cent				
Hemoglobin	Males: 13–16 gm per 100 ml / Females: 12–15 gm per 100 ml				
Leukocyte count	4800–10,800 per mm^3				
Erythrocyte count	4.2–5.9 million per mm^3				
Mean corpuscular volume (MCV)	80–90 cu μ^3				
Mean corpuscular hemoglobin (MCH)	33–38 per cent				
Mean corpuscular hemoglobin concentration (MCHC)	% Hb/cell or gHb/dl RBC / Adults and children: 31–36				
Erythrocyte sedimentation rate	Males: 1–13 mm per hr / Females: 1–20 mm per hr	Blood	Use EDTA as anticoagulant	5	Modified Westergren method / Gambino et al.: Am. J. Clin. Pathol., 35:173, 1965
Erythrocyte enzymes:					
Glucose 6-phosphate dehydrogenase	12.1 ± 2.1 IU/gm Hb	Blood	Use special anticoagulant (ACD solution)	9	Beck: J. Biol. Chem., 232:251, 1958
6-Phosphogluconate dehydrogenase	8.8 ± 0.8 IU/gm Hb	Blood	Use special anticoagulant (ACD solution)	9	Beutler: Red Cell Metabolism, 2nd ed., 1975, p. 66
Glutathione reductase	10.4 ± 1.5 IU/gm Hb	Blood	Use special anticoagulant (ACD solution)	9	Beutler: Red Cell Metabolism, 2nd ed., 1975, p. 69

Hematologic Values *Continued*

Determination	Reference range	Material analyzed	Minimal ml of blood required	Note	Method
Pyruvate kinase	15.0 ± 2.01 IU/gm Hb	Blood	8	Use special anticoagulant (ACD solution)	Beutler: Red Cell Metabolism, 2nd ed., 1975, p. 60
Folic acid	6–15 ng per ml	Serum	1		Baker et al.: Clin. Chem., 5:275, 1959; Goulian, Beck: Am. J. Clin. Pathol., 46:390, 1966
Haptoglobin	100–300 mg per 100 ml	Serum	1		Behring Diagnostic Reagent Kit
Hemoglobin studies: Electrophoresis for abnormal hemoglobin		Blood	5	Collect with anticoagulant	Singer: Am. J. Med., 18:633, 1955
Electrophoresis for A₂ hemoglobin	2.0–3.0 per cent	Blood	5	Use oxalate as anticoagulant	Kunkel et al.: J. Clin. Invest., 36:1615, 1957
Fetal hemoglobin (alkali resistant)	Less than 2 per cent	Blood	5	Collect with anticoagulant	Miale: Laboratory Medicine—Hematology, 2nd ed., 1962, p. 845
Methemoglobin and sulfhemoglobin	0	Blood	5	Use heparin as anticoagulant	Michel, Harris: J. Clin. Lab. Clin. Med., 25:445, 1940
Serum hemoglobin	2–3 mg per 100 ml	Serum	2		Hunter et al.: Am. J. Clin. Pathol., 20:429, 1950
Thermolabile hemoglobin	Negative	Blood	1	Any anticoagulant	Dacie et al.: Br. J. Haematol., 10:388, 1964
Lupus anticoagulant	Absent	Plasma	4.5	Collect as in Factor II determination	Margolius et al.: Medicine, 40:145, 1961
Lupus erythematosus (LE) preparation: Method I	Negative	Blood	5	Use heparin as anticoagulant	Hargraves et al.: Proc. Staff Meet. Mayo Clin., 24:234, 1949
Method II	Negative	Blood	5	Use defibrinated blood	Barnes et al.: J. Invest. Dermatol., 14:397, 1950

Test	Normal value	Specimen	mL	Special handling	Reference
Leukocyte alkaline phosphatase:				Special handling of blood necessary	
Quantitative method	15–40 mg phosphorus liberated per hr per 10^{10}	Isolated blood leukocytes	20		Valentine, Beck: J. Lab. Med., 38:39, 1951
Histochemical method	Males: 95.1 ± 32.5 units; Females (off contraceptive pill): 110.6 ± 38.8 units	Blood smear			Kaplow: Am. J. Clin. Pathol., 39:439, 1963
Muramidase	Serum, 74 ± 16 μg per ml; Urine, 0–2 μg per ml	Serum; Urine	1; 1		Osserman, Lawlor: J. Exp. Med., 124:921, 1966
Osmotic fragility of erythrocytes	Increased if hemolysis occurs in over 0.5 per cent NaCl; decreased if hemolysis is incomplete in 0.3 per cent NaCl	Blood	5	Use heparin as anticoagulant	Beutler, in Williams et al. (eds.): Hematology, 1972, p. 1375
Peroxide hemolysis	<10 per cent	Blood	6	Use EDTA as anticoagulant	Gordon et al.: Am. J. Dis. Child., 90:669, 1955
Platelet count	200,000–350,000 per mm^3	Blood	0.5	Use EDTA as anticoagulant; counts are performed on Coulter counter Model B; when counts are low, results are confirmed by hand counting	Hand count: Brecher et al.: Am. J. Clin. Pathol., 23:15, 1955
Platelet function tests:					
Clot retraction	50–100 per cent at 2 hrs	Plasma	4.5	Collect as in Factor II determination	Benthaus: Thromb. Diath. Haemorrh., 3:311, 1959
Platelet aggregation	Full response to ADP, 1-epinephrine, and collagen	Plasma	18	Collect as in Factor II determination	Born: Nature, 194:927, 1962
Platelet Factor 3	33–57 sec	Plasma	4.5	Collect as in Factor II determination	Rabiner, Hrodek: J. Clin. Invest., 47:901, 1968
Reticulocyte count	0.5–1.5 per cent of red cells	Blood	0.1		Brecher: Am. J. Clin. Pathol., 19:895, 1949
Vitamin B_{12}	150–450 pg per ml	Serum	12		Difco Manual, 9th ed., 1953, p. 221 (modified)

(From normal reference values. N. Engl. J. Med., 298(1):34–45, 1978.)

SPECIAL ENDOCRINE TESTS — AUTOANTIBODIES

DETERMINATION	REFERENCE RANGE	MATERIAL ANALYZED	MINIMAL ML. REQUIRED	NOTE	METHOD
Thyroid, colloid, and microsomal antigens	Absent	Serum	2	Low titers in some elderly normal women	Doniach et al.: Protocol of Autoimmunity Laboratory, Middlesex Medical School, London
Stomach parietal cells	Absent	Serum	2		Doniach et al.: Protocol of Autoimmunity Laboratory, Middlesex Medical School, London
Smooth muscle	Absent	Serum	2		Doniach et al.: Clin. Exp. Immunol., 1:237, 1966
Kidney mitochondria	Absent	Serum	2		
Rabbit renal collecting ducts	Absent	Serum	2		Forbes et al.: Clin. Exp. Immunol., 26:426, 1976
Cytoplasm of ova, theca cells, testicular interstitial cells	Absent	Serum	2		Forbes et al.: Clin. Exp. Immunol., 26:436, 1976
Skeletal muscle	Absent	Serum	2		Osserman, Weiner: Ann. NY Acad. Sci., 124:730, 1965

(From normal reference values. N. Engl. J. Med., 298(1):34–45, 1978.)

Special Endocrine Tests — Steroid Hormones

Determination	Reference Range	Material Analyzed	Minimal ml Required	Note	Method
Aldosterone	Excretion, 5–19 µg per 24 hrs	24-hr urine	5	Keep specimen cold	Bayard et al.: J. Clin. Endocrinol., 31:507, 1970
	Supine, 48 ± 29 pg per ml	Serum or EDTA plasma	3	Fasting, at rest, 210 mEq sodium diet	Poulson et al.: Clin. Immunol. Immunopathol., 2:373, 1974
	Upright, 2 hr, 65 ± 23 mg per ml			Upright, 2 hr, 210 mEq sodium diet	
	Supine, 107 ± 45 pg per ml			Fasting, at rest, 110 mEq sodium diet	
	Upright, 2 hr, 239 ± 123 pg per ml			Upright, 2 hr, 110 mEq sodium diet	
	Supine, 175 ± 75 pg per ml			Fasting, at rest, 10 mEq sodium diet	
	Upright, 2 hr, 532 ± 228 pg per ml			Upright, 2 hr, 10 mEq sodium diet	
Cortisol	8 A.M., 5–25 µg per 100 ml; 8 P.M., below 10 µg per 100 ml;	Plasma	1	Fasting	Murphy: J. Clin. Endocrinol., 27:973, 1967
			1	At rest	
	4-hr ACTH test; 30–45 µg per 100 ml		1	20 U ACTH IV per 4 hrs	
	Overnight suppression test, below 5 µg per 100 ml;		1	8 A.M. sample after dexamethasone midnight; keep specimen cold	
	excretion; 20–70 µg per 24 hrs	Urine	2		
11-Deoxycortisol	Responsive; over 7.5 µg per 100 ml	Plasma	2	8 A.M. sample, preceded by 4.5 gm of metyrapone PO per 24 hrs or by single dose of 2.5 gm PO at midnight	Kilman: Adv. Tracer Method, 4:277, 1968
Testosterone	Adult male, 300–1100 ng per 100 ml; adolescent male, over 100 ng per 100 ml; female, 25–90 ng per 100 ml	Plasma	2	A.M. sample	Chen et al.: Clin. Chem., 17:581, 1971
Unbound testosterone	Adult male, 3.06–24.0 ng per 100 ml; adult female, 0.09–1.28 ng per 100 ml	Plasma	2	A.M. sample	Forest et al.: Steroids, 12:323, 1968

(From normal reference values. N. Engl. J. Med., 298(1):34–45, 1978.)

SPECIAL ENDOCRINE TESTS — POLYPEPTIDE HORMONES

DETERMINATION	REFERENCE RANGE	MATERIAL ANALYZED	MINIMAL ML REQUIRED	NOTE	METHOD
Adrenocorticotropin (ACTH)	15–70 pg per ml	Plasma	5	Place specimen on ice and send promptly to laboratory	Ratcliffe, Edwards: Radioimmunoassay Methods, Edinburgh, Churchill-Livingstone, 1971
Calcitonin	Undetectable in normals, >100 pg per ml in medullary carcinoma	Plasma	5	Test done only on known or suspected cases of medullary carcinoma of the thyroid	Deftos et al.: Metabolism, 20:1129, 1971 Deftos et al.: Metabolism, 20:428, 1971
Growth hormone	Below 5 ng per ml; children, over 10 ng per ml; males, below 5 ng per ml; females, up to 30 ng per ml; males, below 5 ng per ml; females, below 10 ng per ml	Plasma	1	Fasting, at rest After exercise	Glick et al.: Nature, 199:784, 1963
Insulin	6–26 µU per ml Below 20 µU per ml Up to 150 µU per ml	Serum or plasma	1	Fasting During hypoglycemia After glucose load	Morgan, Lazarow: Proc. Soc. Exp. Biol. Med., 110:29, 1962
Luteinizing hormone	Males, 6–18 mU per ml Females, 5–22 mU per ml; 30–250 mU per ml	Serum or plasma	2	Pre- or postovulatory midcycle peak	Odell et al.: J. Clin. Invest., 46:248, 1967
Parathyroid	<10 µl equiv per ml	Plasma	5	Keep blood on ice, or plasma must be frozen if it is to be sent any distance	Segre et al.: J. Clin. Invest., 51:3163, 1972
Prolactin	2–15 ng per ml	Serum	2	A.M. sample	Sinha et al.: J. Clin. Endocrinol. Metab., 36:509, 1973

SPECIAL ENDOCRINE TESTS — POLYPEPTIDE HORMONES *Continued*

DETERMINATION	REFERENCE RANGE	MATERIAL ANALYZED	MINIMAL ML REQUIRED	NOTE	METHOD
Renin activity	Supine, 1.1 ± 0.8 ng per ml per hr	Plasma	4	EDTA tubes on ice; normal diet	Haber et al.: J. Clin. Endocrinol. Metab., 29:1349, 1969
	Upright, 1.9 ± 1.7 ng per ml per hr				
	Supine, 2.7 ± 1.8 ng per ml per hr			Low sodium diet	
	Upright, 6.6 ± 2.5 ng per ml per hr				
	Diuretics, 10.0 ± 3.7 ng per ml per hr			Low sodium diet	

(From normal reference values. N. Engl. J. Med., 298(1):34–45, 1978.)

SPECIAL ENDOCRINE TESTS — THYROID HORMONES

DETERMINATION	REFERENCE RANGE	MATERIAL ANALYZED	MINIMAL ML REQUIRED	NOTE	METHOD
Thyroid-stimulating hormone (TSH)	0.5–3.5 µU per ml	Serum	2		Ridgway et al.: J. Clin. Invest., 52:2785, 1973
Thyroxine-binding globulin capacity	15–25 µg T₄ per 100 ml	Serum	2		Levy et al.: J. Clin. Endocrinol. Metab., 32:372, 1971
Total tri-iodothyronine by radioimmunoassay (T₃)	70–190 ng per 100 ml	Serum	2		Larsen et al.: J. Clin. Invest., 51:1939, 1972
Total thyroxine by RIA (T₄)	4–12 µg per 100 ml	Serum	1		Chopra: J. Clin. Endocrinol. Metab., 34:938, 1972
T₃ resin uptake	25–35 per cent	Serum	2		Taybearn et al.: J. Nucl. Med., 8:739, 1967
Free thyroxine index (FT₄I)	1–4 ng per 100 ml	Serum	2		Sarin, Anderson: Arch. Intern. Med., 126:631, 1970

(From normal reference values. N. Engl. J. Med., 298(1):34–45, 1978.)

MISCELLANEOUS VALUES

DETERMINATION	REFERENCE RANGE	MINIMAL QUANTITY REQUIRED	NOTE	METHOD
Ascorbic acid load test	0.2–2.0 mg per hr in control sample 24–49 mg per hr after loading	Urine — approximate 1½-hr sample Urine — 2 timed samples of about 2 hrs each	Administer 500 mg of ascorbic acid orally	Harvard Fatigue Labs, Laboratory Manual, 1945
Carcinoembryonic antigen (CEA)	0–2.5 ng per ml, 97 per cent healthy nonsmokers	20 ml EDTA plasma	Must be sent on ice	Hansen et al.: J. Clin. Res., 19:143, 1971
Chylous fluid			Use fresh specimen	Todd et al.: Clinical Diagnosis, 12th ed., 1953, p.624
Duodenal drainage			pH should be in proper range with minimal amount of gastric juice	
pH	5.5–7.5		1 ml	
Amylase	Over 1200 U per total sample	1 ml		Huggins, Russell: Ann. Surg., 128:668, 1948
Trypsin	Values from 35 to 160 per cent "normal"	1 ml		Anderson, Early: Am. J. Dis. Child, 63:891, 1942
Viscosity	3 min or less	4 ml	Run ice cold in 340 sec viscosimeter	
Gastric analysis	Basal: Females, 2.0 ± 1.8 mEq per hr Males, 3.0 ± 2.0 mEq per hr Maximal (after histalog or gastrin): Females, 16 ± 5 mEq per hr Males, 23 ± 5 mEq per hr			Marks: Gastroenterology, 41:599, 1961
Immunologic tests: Alpha-fetoglobulin Alpha 1-antitrypsin Antinuclear antibodies	Abnormal if present 200–400 mg per 100 ml Positive if detected with serum diluted 1:10	5 ml of clotted blood 10 ml of blood 10 ml clotted blood	Send to laboratory promptly	
Anti-DNA antibodies Bence Jones protein Complement, total hemolytic	Less than 15 units per ml Abnormal if present 150–250 U per ml	10 ml 100 ml of urine 10 ml	Must be sent on ice	Pincus: Arthritis Rheum., 14:623, 1971 Hook, Muschel: Proc. Soc. Exp. Biol. Med., 117:292, 1964

C3	55–120 mg per 100 ml	10 ml	
C4	20–50 mg per 100 ml	10 ml	
Immunoglobulins:			Barth: Serum Proteins and Dysproteinemias, Sunderman, 1964, p. 102
IgG	1140 mg per 100 ml Range, 540–1663 mg		
IgA	214 mg per 100 ml Range, 66–344 mg		
IgM	168 mg per 100 ml Range, 39–290 mg		
Viscosity	1.4–1.8	5 ml of serum	Expressed as the relative viscosity of serum compared to water
Iontophoresis	Children, 0–40 mEq sodium per l; adults, 0–60 mEq sodium per l		Value given in terms of sodium Gibson, Cooke: Pediatrics, 23:545, 1959
Stool fat	Less than 5 gm in 24 hrs or less than 4 per cent of measured fat intake in 3-day period	24-hr or 3-day specimen, preferably with markers	Van de Kramer et al.: J. Biol. Chem., 177:347, 1949
Stool nitrogen	Less than 2 gm per day or 10 per cent of urinary nitrogen	24-hr or 3-day specimen	Peters, Van Slyke: Quantitative Clinical Chemistry, Vol. 2 (Methods), 1932, p. 353
Synovial fluid:			
Glucose	Not less than 20 mg per 100 ml lower than simultaneously drawn blood sugar	1 ml of fresh fluid	Collect with oxalate-fluoride mixture See Blood, glucose
Mucin	Type 1 or 2	1 ml of fresh fluid	Grades as: Type 1—tight clump Type 2—soft clump Type 3—soft clump that breaks up Type 4—cloudy, no clump
D-Xylose soft clump absorption	5–8 per 5 hrs in urine 40 mg per 100 ml in blood 2 hrs after ingestion 25 gm of D-xylose	5-hr collection of urine 5 ml of blood	For directions see Benson et al.: N. Engl. J. Med., 256:335, 1957 Roe, Rice: J. Biol. Chem., 173:507, 1948

(From normal reference values. N. Engl. J. Med., 298(1):34–45, 1978.)

CENTIGRADE TO FAHRENHEIT TEMPERATURES

F°	C°	F°	C°	F°	C°	F°	C°
90 =	32.2	95 =	35.0	100 =	37.8	105 =	40.6
91 =	32.8	96 =	35.6	101 =	38.3	106 =	41.1
92 =	33.3	97 =	36.1	102 =	38.9	107 =	41.7
93 =	33.9	98 =	36.7	103 =	39.4	108 =	42.2
94 =	34.4	99 =	37.2	104 =	40.0	109 =	42.8

FEET AND INCHES TO CENTIMETERS
(1 cm = 0.39 in; 1 in = 2.54 cm)

Ft	In	Cm	Ft	In	Cm	Ft	In	Cm	Ft	In	Cm	Ft	In	Cm
0	6	15.2	2	4	71.1	3	4	101.6	4	4	132.0	5	4	162.6
1	0	30.5	2	5	73.6	3	5	104.1	4	5	134.6	5	5	165.1
1	6	45.7	2	6	76.1	3	6	106.6	4	6	137.1	5	6	167.6
1	7	48.3	2	7	78.7	3	7	109.2	4	7	139.6	5	7	170.2
1	8	50.8	2	8	81.2	3	8	111.7	4	8	142.2	5	8	172.7
1	9	53.3	2	9	83.8	3	9	114.2	4	9	144.7	5	9	175.3
1	10	55.9	2	10	86.3	3	10	116.8	4	10	147.3	5	10	177.8
1	11	58.4	2	11	88.8	3	11	119.3	4	11	149.8	5	11	180.3
2	0	61.0	3	0	91.4	4	0	121.9	5	0	152.4	6	0	182.9
2	1	63.5	3	1	93.9	4	1	124.4	5	1	154.9	6	1	185.4
2	2	66.0	3	2	96.4	4	2	127.0	5	2	157.5	6	2	188.0
2	3	68.6	3	3	99.0	4	3	129.5	5	3	160.0	6	3	190.5

ESTIMATION OF SURFACE AREA OF THE BODY

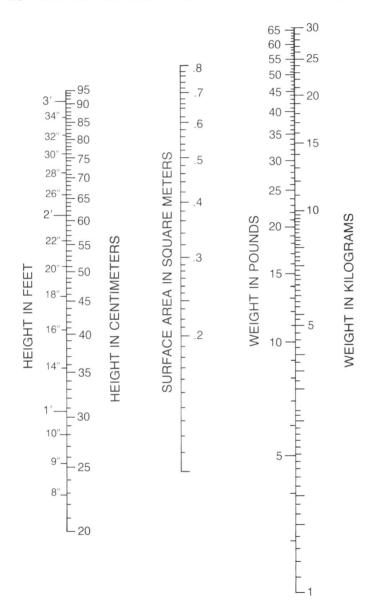

Surface Area.Sq Cm $= Wt.^{0.426} \times Ht.^{0.725} \times 71.84$

(Copyright 1920 by W. M. Boothby and R. B. Sandiford, Mayo Clinic.)

ESTIMATION OF SURFACE AREA OF THE BODY

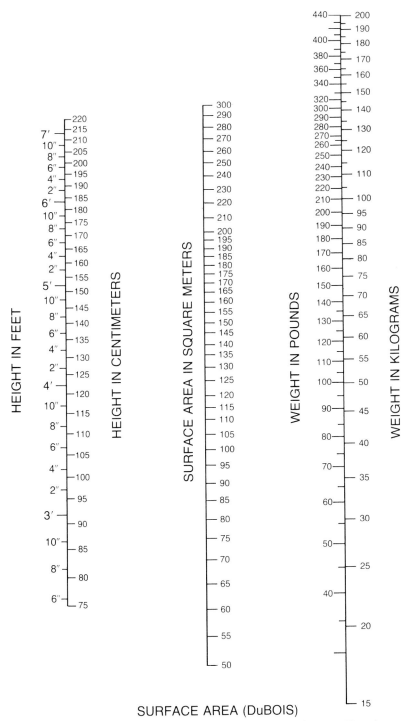

SURFACE AREA (DuBOIS)

(Copyright 1920 by W. M. Boothby and R. B. Sandiford, Mayo Clinic.)

Pounds to Kilograms
(1 kg = 2.2 lb; 1 lb = 0.45 kg)

Lb	Kg	Lb	Kg	Lb	Kg	Lb	Kg	Lb	Kg
5	2.3	50	22.7	95	43.1	140	63.5	185	83.9
10	4.5	55	25.0	100	45.4	145	65.8	190	86.2
15	6.8	60	27.2	105	47.6	150	68.0	195	88.5
20	9.1	65	29.5	110	49.9	155	70.3	200	90.7
25	11.3	70	31.7	115	52.2	160	72.6	205	93.0
30	13.6	75	34.0	120	54.4	165	74.8	210	95.3
35	15.9	80	36.3	125	56.7	170	77.1	215	97.5
40	18.1	85	38.6	130	58.9	175	79.4	220	99.8
45	20.4	90	40.8	135	61.2	180	81.6		

Average Electrolyte Content of Oral and Gastrointestinal Secretions

Secretion	Na (mEq/l)	K (mEq/l)	Ca (mEq/l)	Cl (mEq/l)
Resting saliva	44	20.4	6.5	
Overnight gastric	49	11.6	3.6	
Gastric	66.5	13.7		100.6
Gastric	136	5.3		98
Small bowel	111.3	4.6		104.2
Ileostomy (recent)·	129.4	11.2		116.2
Ileostomy (adapted)	46	3.0		21.4
Bile	148.9	4.98		100.6
Pancreas	141.1	4.6		76.6

(From Surgery, Principles and Practice, 3rd ed. Moyer, C. A., Rhoads, J. E., Allen, J. G., Harkins, H. N. J. B. Lippincott Co., 1965, p. 82.

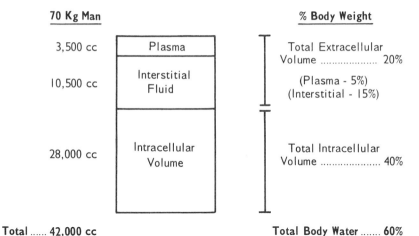

70 Kg Man   **% Body Weight**

3,500 cc	Plasma	Total Extracellular Volume 20%
10,500 cc	Interstitial Fluid	(Plasma - 5%) (Interstitial - 15%)
28,000 cc	Intracellular Volume	Total Intracellular Volume 40%

Total ...... 42,000 cc   **Total Body Water 60%**

Functional compartments of body units. (Supplied by G. Tom Shires, M.D.)

PLASMA — 154 mEq/l / 154 mEq/l

CATIONS		ANIONS	
Na^+	142	Cl^-	103
		HCO_3^-	27
		SO_4^{--}	3
		PO_4^{---}	
K^+	4		
Ca^{++}	5	Organic Acids	5
Mg^{++}	3	Protein	16

INTERSTITIAL FLUID — 153 mEq/l / 153 mEq/l

CATIONS		ANIONS	
Na^+	144	Cl^-	114
		HCO_3^-	30
K^+	4	SO_4^{--}	3
		PO_4^{---}	
Ca^{++}	3	Organic Acids	5
Mg^{++}	2	Proteins	1

INTRACELLULAR FLUID — 200 mEq/l / 200 mEq/l

CATIONS		ANIONS	
K^+	150	$HPO_4^{\equiv}$	150
		SO_4^{--}	
		HCO_3^-	10
Mg^{++}	40	Protein	40
Na^+	10		

Chemical composition of body fluid compartments. (Supplied by G. Tom Shires, M.D.)

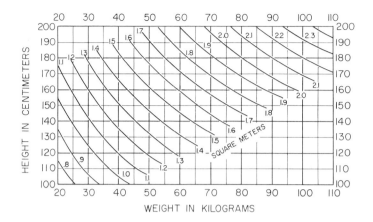

Electrolyte Concentrations of Several Commonly Used Parenteral Solutions

Solution	Gm/l	meq/l Cations	meq/l Anions
Ammonium chloride 0.9%	9.0	167 NH₄	167 Cl
Ammonium chloride 2.14%	21.4	400 NH₄	400 Cl
Potassium chloride 0.3%	3.0	40 K	40 Cl
Sodium bicarbonate 1.5%	15.0	178 Na	178 mM bicarbonate
Sodium chloride 0.45%	4.5	77 Na	77 Cl
Sodium chloride 0.9%	9.0	154 Na	154 Cl
Sodium chloride 5.0%	50.0	850 Na	850 Cl
Sodium lactate 1/6 molar	19.0	167 Na	167 mM lactate
Ringer's USP	8.6 NaCl 0.3 KCl 0.33 CaCl₂ (2 H₂O)	147 Na 4 K 4.5 Ca	155.5 Cl
Lactated Ringer's USP (Hartmann's)	6.0 NaCl 0.3 KCl 0.2 CaCl₂ (2 H₂O) 3.1 Na Lactate	130 Na 4 K 2.7 Ca	109.7 Cl 27 mM lactate
Lactated potassic saline NF (Darrow's)	4.0 NaCl 2.6 KCl 5.9 Na Lactate	122 Na 35 K	104 Cl 50 mM lactate

(From the American Society of Hospital Pharmacists: American Hospital Formulary Service, Section 40:00, Electrolyte, Caloric, and Water Balance. January, 1980.)

EVALUATION OF VARIOUS ORGAN SYSTEMS

PULMONARY FUNCTION TESTS

Vital Capacity.   Two formulas give vital capacity in cubic centimeters of air.

Males: $(-38 \times$ age) + (121 $\times$ height in inches) $-$ 2100. $\pm$ 970 cc
Females: $(-22 \times$ age) + (110 $\times$ height in inches) $-$ 2980. $\pm$ 790 cc

Alternate formula:

Males: $[27.63 - (0.122 \times$ age in years$)] \times$ height in cm
Females: $[21.78 - (0.101 \times$ age in years$)] \times$ height in cm

Pulmonary Ventilation.   Clinical and fluoroscopic evaluation of reasons for hypoventilation consist of measurements of rate, tidal volume, and minute volume, plus basal oxygen consumption.
   Rate (basal conditions).   11 to 14/min (adult).
   Tidal volume (basal conditions).   450 to 600 ml (adult).
   Minute volume (basal conditions).   SA = surface area in square meters. SD = standard deviation. The result is expressed in liters/minute.

Age Range	Males	Females
16–34	3.6 × SA (SD 0.3 × SA)	3.2 × SA (SD 0.4 × SA)
35–49	3.1 × SA (SD 0.5 × SA)	3.2 × SA (SD 0.4 × SA)
50–69	3.9 × SA (SD 0.45 × SA)	3.4 × SA (SD 0.4 × SA)

Basal oxygen consumption.   135 to 145 ml/min/square meter $\pm$ 10%.
   DISTRIBUTION.   Clinical and radiologic evidence of uneven expansion of lungs, changes in breath sounds, percussion notes, and radiolucent areas.
   Pulmonary Circulation.   Clinical, electrocardiographic, and radiologic means provide evidence of pulmonary hypertension or congestion, circulation times, and venous pressure.
   Abnormalities of pulmonary vascular markings can be determined by radiography. Pulmonary bruits and lung scanning with albumin microaggregates may indicate abnormalities.
   Alveolar-Capillary Diffusion.   There are no specific tests. See Comroe for discussion.*
   Arterial O_2, CO_2, and pH.   Look for cyanosis and for increased RBC mass and hemoglobin; measure changes in respiration rate and pulse on breathing oxygen. Measure blood gases and pH (normal values for blood oxygen, arterial pH, and serum carbon dioxide are given on pages 759 and 761).

---

*Comroe, J. H., et al.: The Lung: Clinical Physiology and Pulmonary Function Tests, 2nd ed. Chicago, Year Book Medical Pub., 1963.

Mechanical Factors in Breathing. All tests are to be performed before and after administration of bronchodilator drugs.

Maximum expiratory and inspiratory flow rates (normal, > 200 l/min at peak).

Maximum voluntary ventilation (maximum breathing capacity), which depends highly on patient cooperation. Normal values:

Males: [86.5 − (0.522 × age in years)] × SA in square meters
Females: [71.3 − (0.474 × age in years)] × SA in square meters

Forced expiratory volume (timed vital capacity). Normal values are 75 to 83% of vital capacity in 1 sec; 97% of vital capacity in 3 sec.

Analysis of spirogram. A high-speed record of single maximum inspiration and expiration and pattern during maximum voluntary ventilation test may show significant changes.

CIRCULATORY FUNCTION TESTS

Blood Volume. "Normal" blood volume depends upon the method of determinations and also on patient age, sex, body habitus, and history of recent change in body weight. Blood volume determinations are most useful in comparing sequential changes in the same patient. Plasma volume determinations using either I^{131}-labeled albumin (RISA) or Evans Blue dye with multiple sampling points on the dilution curve are more accurate than single sample determinations and are considerably more accurate than whole blood counting of an isotope, which is large vessel hematocrit–dependent. Cr^{51}-tagged red blood cell dilution measurements with timed samples are quite accurate when utilized with hematocrit determinations. Tourniquets seriously alter measurement accuracy by concentrating both red blood cells and plasma protein, with its label, in the vein distal to the occlusion. A false low value for blood volume and a high value for hematocrit result.

The mixing time of radioactively labeled albumin or red blood cells and of dyes is prolonged in shock, and caution must be used in interpreting results obtained.

For a discussion of blood volume measurements and nomograms for predicting normal values, see Dagher et al.: Advances in Surgery, Vol. 1, Chicago, Year Book Medical Pub., 1965, pp. 69–108.

Approximate values for normal blood volumes as measured by the sum of Cr^{51}-tagged RBC and I^{131} RISA are as shown in the following table:

AGE	BLOOD VOLUME AS % OF BODY WEIGHT	AGE	BLOOD VOLUME AS % OF BODY WEIGHT
Females: 20–40	7.0%	Males: 20–40	8.0%
40–60	6.5	40–60	7.5
Over 60	6.0	Over 60	7.0

Obese patients will have a smaller blood volume in terms of body weight, and thin or very muscular patients will have a somewhat higher value.

Cardiac Output. Cardiac output is measured either by the direct Fick method, measuring oxygen consumption in ml/minute and dividing by the arterial mixed central venous oxygen difference in ml/l, or by the dilution method, using a rapid central venous injection of an indicator dye and measuring changes in concentration of the dye during its initial circulation by continuous sampling of arterial blood. Cardiac output in the normal-sized, resting, healthy male averages almost exactly 6.0 l/min. Cardiac output falls slowly with age and may be 7 to 10% lower in females. Cardiac output is increased by exercise, mild anoxia, fever, anxiety, pulmonary disease, anemia, hyperthyroidism, and arteriovenous shunts. It usually rises significantly following trauma and with infection. It is low in myocardial infarction, severe valvular disease, and in traumatic, hemorrhagic, and sometimes septic shock. A failure to respond by increasing cardiac output following major surgery and with infection may herald a fatal outcome; a fall in output is often followed by death.

Cardiac output is usually expressed as the cardiac index, which is the cardiac output in l per min divided by the body surface area (m^2). The cardiac index of healthy young adults averages 3.52; that of 45-year-old healthy patients averges 3.0. A cardiac index of 2.8 has been used as a baseline in surgical studies, relating cardiac index to response to surgery.

Central Venous Pressure. Central venous pressure measurements are determined at the level of the right atrium by the insertion of a venous catheter through a peripheral vein, either arm, or external jugular, in the superior vena cava. The required catheter length from the point of insertion should be measured on the body surface, following the known course of the veins, prior to insertion of the catheter. The catheter is then attached to a simple water manometer or to a strain gauge transducer. The level of the right atrium is approximated externally at the midaxillary line. An infusion set is connected to permit flushing of the catheter and filling of the manometer with saline or other intravenous fluids, but this must be excluded when pressures are measured. Intrathoracic position of the catheter tip is indicated by changes of several millimeters of water pressure with each respiration and by a sharp and immediate rise with the Valsalva maneuver.

Excessive catheter length is to be avoided to prevent the catheter tip's entering the heart or passing below the diaphragm. Catheters may be filled with a dilute heparin solution in saline between measurements if a slow infusion is contraindicated. It is better to use other venous channels for blood replacement and other parenteral fluids to avoid interruption of therapy with each venous pressure measurement.

Normal central venous pressure is from 6 to 16 cm of saline or 5 to 12 mm of Hg. If the central venous pressure is less than 6 or 7 cm of saline, hypotension is likely to be due to decreased blood volume, whereas if the pressure is 15 cm or more of saline, hypotension is unlikely to be due to a volume defect, and blood and fluid replacement are not ordinarily indicated.

RENAL FUNCTION TESTS

Urinalysis along with determination of protein, sugar, and osmolality are useful in assessing renal function and aiding in diagnosing renal disease.

Blood urea nitrogen, serum creatinine, and creatinine clearance are the most often used indicators of renal function. Elevated BUN and elevated creatinine in the absence of muscle destruction indicate decreased renal function.

Renal clearance of various indicators is useful in assessing overall function by eliminating abnormally high serum levels of urea or creatinine for reasons other than decreased renal function from consideration.

$$Cx = \frac{UxV}{Px}$$

Cx = Clearance of x (ml/min)
Ux = Concentration of x in urine (mg/ml)
 V = Volume of urine in 1 min (ml/min)
Px = Concentration of x in plasma (mg/ml)

Clearance Tests. The values shown have been corrected to 1.73 sq m of body surface area.

Glomerular filtration (GFR):

Inulin clearance
Mannitol clearance   } Males, 110 to 150 ml/min
Endogenous creatinine clearance   Females, 105 to 132 ml/min

Renal plasma flow (RPF):

Para-amino hippurate (PAH)   } Males, 560 to 830 ml/min
Diodrast   Females, 490 to 700 ml/min

Filtration fraction (FF)
   $\frac{GFR}{RPF}$ } Males, 17 to 21%
                Females, 17 to 23%

Maximal PAH excretory capacity (Tm_{PAH}) 80 to 90 mg/min

Phenolsulfonphthalein excretion (PSP). Urine excretion following intravenous injection:

> 25 per cent in 15 min
> 40 per cent in 30 min
> 55 per cent in 2 hrs

Concentration in 24 hours. Dry day, specific gravity 1.025; wet day, specific gravity 1.003.

GASTRIC ANALYSIS TESTS

Basal acid output:

Males   4 mEq/hr   > 15 mEq/hr suggests Zollinger-Ellison syndrome
Females   6 mEq/hr

Maximal stimulated acid output:

Males   30 mEq/hr
Females   40 mEq/hr

Serum gastrin:

Normal < 200 pg/ml
300–400 suspicious of gastrinoma
> 400 in patient with hyperacidity without retained antral
mucosa after Bilroth II is strongly suspicious of gastrinoma.

In the work-up of gastrinoma, calcium and secretin infusion tests are useful. Infusion of 4 mg/kg/hr of calcium over 4 hrs will cause a marked rise in serum gastrin over the basal level compared with normal patients or those with duodenal ulcer disease.

Infusion of secretin 1 mg/kg/hr will cause an increase in serum gastrin in Zollinger-Ellison syndrome in contrast to a decrease in normal patients with duodenal ulcers.

GASTROINTESTINAL ABSORPTION TESTS

d-Xylose Absorption Test.   After an 8-hour fast, 10 ml/kg body weight of 5 per cent d-xylose is given by mouth. Nothing further is given by mouth until the test is completed. All urine voided in the next 5 hours is pooled, and blood samples are taken at 0, 60, and 120 min. Normal urinary excretion is 16 to 33% of ingested xylose, average 26 per cent, and normal blood levels of 25 to 40 mg/100 ml are found at one and two hours.

Fat Absorption Tests. I^{131} triolein, 2 to 5 microcuries is given by mouth, with neutral fat carrier. Normally, 90 to 95% of the radioactivity is absorbed from the intestine; 10% of the total dose is present in the total blood volume at 4 to 6 hours after ingestion.

TOTAL FAT.   Normally, 90 to 95% of total ingested fat is absorbed, and stool contains less than 10% of dietary fat with intake of 50 to 200 gm of fat a day.

Vitamin A Absorption Test.   A fasting blood specimen is obtained, and then 200,000 units of vitamin A are given by mouth. Serum vitamin A levels should rise to twice fasting levels in 3 to 5 hours.

Vitamin B_{12} Absorption Test.   One microcurie of CO^{57}-labeled vitamin B_{12} is given in 5 μg vitamin B_{12} by mouth. Plasma activity is 1% of the total dose per liter of plasma at 8 hours. Following 1 mg vitamin B_{12} intramuscularly (flushing dose), 15 to 20% of the administered dose appears in the urine in 24 hours.

LIVER FUNCTION TESTS

Hepatic functions are assessed routinely by measurement of excretory and metabolic function.

Serum bilirubin elevation is an indication of excretory dysfunction. Bilirubin may be divided into direct-reacting (bilirubin conjugated to glucuronic acid) or indirect-reacting types (bilirubin bound to plasma protein).

Urine bilirubin and urine and fecal urobilinogen are also useful indicators of excretory dysfunction. Alkaline phosphatase is a measure of hepatic excretory function and is most commonly elevated in obstructive jaundice, although elevation may also be seen with metastatic deposits in the liver, during pregnancy, and with osteoblastic disorders of bones.

The measurement of serum transaminases (SGOT, SGPT) is indicative of hepatocellular destruction, although OT is also elevated in severe cardiac or skeletal muscle destruction.

Bromsulfalein. Less than 5% remaining in serum 45 min after intravenous injection of 5 mg/kg body weight. Not valid in the presence of jaundice.

Cephalin Cholesterol Flocculation. 0 to 2+ in 48 hours.

Galactose Tolerance. Excretion in the urine of not more than 3.0 gm galactose during 5 hrs after ingestion of 40 gm.

Hippuric Acid. Excretion of 3.0 to 3.5 gm hippuric acid in the urine in 4 hrs after ingestion of 6.0 gm sodium benzoate; or excretion of 0.7 gm hippuric acid in the urine in 1 hr after intravenous administration of 1.77 gm sodium benzoate.

Thymol Turbidity. 0 to 50 units.

Other tests of importance include direct and total serum bilirubin, alkaline phosphatase, and SGOT.

GLUCOSE TOLERANCE TESTS

The patient should be on a 300 gm/day carbohydrate diet for 3 days preceding a glucose tolerance test. Values are given for true glucose.

Oral. After 100 gm glucose, or 1.75 gm/kg, blood glucose level should not be above 160 mg/ml at 1 hr, 140 mg/ml at 90 min, and 120 mg/ml after 120 min.

Intravenous. Blood glucose does not exceed 200 mg/ml after infusion of 0.5 gm glucose/kg in 30 min. Blood glucose falls below the initial level by 2 hrs and returns to preinfusion levels by 3 to 4 hrs.

THYROID FUNCTION TESTS

Assessment of thyroid function has progressed with the availability of radionuclides of iodine, and basal metabolic rate (BMR) is no longer precise enough. Protein-bound iodine (PBI) and butanol extractable iodine (BEI) are no longer used because of sensitivity to contamination by extravenous iodine.

Tri-iodothyronine (T_3) adsorption and thyroxine (T_4) levels, along with radio-nuclide uptake and imaging, are the usual diagnostic tests.

Radioactive iodine uptake is 20 to 50% of a dose in 24 hrs. Radioactive iodine excretion is 30 to 70% of an administered dose in 24 hrs.

PARATHYROID FUNCTION TESTS

Serum calcium and phosphate are most often used as indicators of parathyroid function. They are inversely related, and the product of the two is normally between 30 and 40.

More sophisticated diagnostic tests based upon decreased tubular reabsorption of phosphate by parathormone have been useful in identifying patients with hyperparathyroidism but are not diagnostic. Glucocorticoid suppression is also useful but is not diagnostic. In conjunction with elevated serum calcium, the radioimmunoassay for parathyroid hormone (PTH) has become the most useful test for diagnosis of hyperparathyroidism.

ADRENAL FUNCTION TESTS

Adrenocortical Inhibition Test.   0.5 mg of either Δ-1,9-α-fluorocortisone or 16-methyl-α-hydrocortisone every 6 hrs reduces the excretion of 17-OH corticoids from 4 to 20 mg/24 hrs to less than 2.0 mg/24 hrs.

Corticotropin (ACTH) Response Test (Eosinophil Response Test — Thorn).   4 hrs after administration of 25 USP units of ACTH intramuscularly, the decrease in eosinophil count should be more than 50% of the original count.

Plasma 16-Hydroxycorticoids.   After an 8-hr infusion of 25 USP units of ACTH, plasma 17-hydroxycorticoids rise from a normal level of 5 to 25 μg/100 ml to 35 to 55 μg/100 ml.

Urinary Steroids.   After an 8-hr infusion of 25 USP units of ACTH, urinary 17-hydroxycorticoids rise 200 to 400%, and urinary 17-ketosteroids rise by 50 to 100% above the control level.

NOMENCLATURE AND EQUIVALENT VALUES IN ACID-BASE BALANCE

Equivalents and Milliequivalents (Eq and mEq).   An equivalent is the amount (in grams) of an ion that will react with or be equivalent to 1 gm of hydrogen ions, and a milliequivalent is 1/1000 of an equivalent. An equivalent of an ion is equal to its gram molecular weight divided by its valence. Thus, sodium has a molecular weight of 23 and a valence of 1, so 1 Eq of $Na^+ = \dfrac{23}{1} = 23$ gm. The gram molecular weight of calcium is 40, and its valence is 2. One Eq of Ca^{++} = 20 gm; 1 mEq = $\dfrac{40}{2}$ = 20 mg. Some molecules behave as ions under biologic conditions. For example, biocarbonate (HCO_3) accepts one electron and has a single negative charge. The molecular weight is 61 $(1 + 12 + 3(16))$. One Eq of $(HCO_3)^-$ = $\dfrac{61}{1}$ = 61 gm. One mEq of $(HCO_3)^-$ = 61 mg.

The table indicates the gram molecular weight, valence, and equivalent weight of common ions in human plasma.

SYMBOL	GRAM MOLECU-LAR WEIGHT	VALENCE	EQUIVALENT WEIGHT
H^+	1	1	1
Na^+	23	1	23
K^+	39	1	39
Ca^{++}	40	2	20
Mg^{++}	24	2	12
Cl^-	35.5	1	35.5
$(HCO_3)^-$	61	1	61
$(SO_4)^{--}$	96	2	48
$(HPO_4)^{--}$	96	2	48

Salts that dissociate virtually completely in water, as do those containing sodium or potassium, ionize into positively charged cations ($^+$) and negative charged anions ($^-$). For example, 1 Eq of NaCl will dissociate into 1 Eq of Na^+ and 1 Eq of Cl^-. In the same fashion, 58.5 mg of NaCl will dissociate into 1 mEq of Na^+ and 1 mEq of Cl^-.

How many mEq of Na^+ and Cl^- are there in 1 l. of 0.9% NaCl?

$$0.9\% = 9.0 \text{ gm/l}$$

The molecular weight of 1 Eq of NaCl is 58.5.

$$\frac{9}{58.5} = 0.154 \text{ Eq}$$

Therefore, there are 154 mEq of Na^+ and 154 mEq of Cl^- in 1 l. of 0.9% NaCl.

How much KCl must be added to 1 l. of 5% glucose in water to have 40 mEq of potassium?

$$1 \text{ mEq of KCl} = 39 + 35.5 = 74.5 \text{ mg}$$
$$40 \text{ mEq} \times 74.5 = 2980 \text{ mg or } 2.98 \text{ gm KCl}$$

Conversion of CO_2 in Volumes % to Milliequivalents. 1 molecular weight of a gas is contained in 22.4 l at 760 mm Hg barometric pressure and 0°C.

$$\frac{CO_2 \text{ in volumes \%}}{2.24} = \text{mEq of } HCO_3/l$$

Moles and Millimoles (M and mM). A mole is 1 gm molecular weight of an ion without regard to valence, and a millimole (mM) is $\frac{1}{1000}$ of a mole. For univalent ions, mole and equivalent are the same; however, with divalent ions, an equivalent is $\frac{1}{2}$ of a mole.

$$1 \text{ mEq } Na^+ = 23 \text{ mg}$$
$$1 \text{ mM of } Na^+ = 23 \text{ mg}$$
$$1 \text{ mEq of } Ca^{++} = 20 \text{ mg}$$
$$1 \text{ mM of } Ca^{++} = 40 \text{ mg}$$

Osmoles and Milliosmoles (Osm and mOsm). Each substance in solution, whether it be extracellular or intracellular, exerts an osmotic effect in proportion to its concentration. Each of several ions produces an independent effect. As in calculating moles, valence is not considered in computing milliosmoles. Hence, 1 mM of NaCl in solution in water to make 1 l. has a milliosmolar effect of 2 mOsm, one each for Na^+ and Cl^-. Sugar, urea, and other undissociated substances have an osmotic effect equal to their molecular weight and concentration only, as they do not dissociate into ions. A milliosmole, therefore, equals

$$\frac{\text{mg of substance or ion per l of solution}}{\text{atomic weight of substance (or ion if dissociated)}}$$

Thus:

$$23 \text{ mg Na per l} = 1 \text{ mOsm per l}$$
$$35.5 \text{ mg Cl per l} = 1 \text{ mOsm per l}$$
$$58.5 \text{ mg NaCl per l} = 2 \text{ mOsm per l}$$
$$60 \text{ mg urea per l} = 1 \text{ mOsm per l}$$
$$180 \text{ mg of glucose per l} = 1 \text{ mOsm per l}$$

The normal milliosmolar tension of extracellular fluid is about 286 mOsm, which includes both ionizable and nonionizable substances. The milliosmolar concentration of 0.9% NaCl is determined as follows:

$$9 \text{ gm NaCl per l} = \frac{9}{58.5} = 0.154 \text{ Eq} =$$

$$\begin{array}{r} 154 \text{ mEq } Na^+ \\ + 154 \text{ mEq } Cl^- \\ \hline 308 \text{ mOsm} \end{array}$$

A 5% glucose in water solution contains 50 gm of glucose per l, whereas an osmolar solution contains 180 gm.

$$\frac{50}{180} = 0.278 \text{ Osm} = 278 \text{ mOsm}$$

The 5% glucose solution is, therefore, hypotonic to plasma.

A 5% solution of glucose in 0.9% NaCl contains 308 mOsm for Na^+ and Cl^- plus 278 mOsm for glucose. The total milliosmolar concentration is 586 mOsm, and this solution is hypertonic to plasma.

Osmolarity and Osmolality. The preceding discussion pertains to the common method of making solutions, that of weight-volume, in which a specific amount in weight of a substance, for example 9 gm of NaCl, is dissolved in distilled water to make a volume of 1 l. This produces a 0.9% solution of NaCl with an osmolarity of 308 mOsm. However, the common method of determining osmotic activity depends on the effect of dissolved substances in depressing the freezing point of water. Such determinations are expressed in terms of the effect on 1 l. of water, rather than 1 l. of solution. This is more important biologically, and, therefore, osmolality rather than osmolarity is discussed and used in this manual.

These differences are quite small at biologic concentrations, because the amounts of electrolytes, urea, glucose, and other substances necessary to produce normal concentrations, when added to 1 l. of water, would increase the volume only very slightly. Much more important is the permeability of cell membranes to various substances in solution and the effect of these substances on the balance between intracellular and extracellular water. Urea, for example, is distributed evenly in cellular and extracellular water; it adds to total osmolality by 16.7 mOsm for each 100 mg per 100 ml increase in concentration but does not affect the hydration of cells except as it acts as an osmotic diuretic and reduces ECF volume. Glucose is relatively slowly permeable through cell membranes, and sodium is normally largely excluded by cells. A rapid infusion of a hypertonic solution, such as 5% glucose in 0.9% saline, will result in a shift of water from cells to extracellular fluid. Excessive water administration, usually as 5% glucose solution, in a patient with reduced renal free water clearance will result in reduction of the extracellular osmolality as the glucose is metabolized and in dilutional overhydration of cells and ECF.

Serum sodium, under most circumstances, is an accurate measure of osmolality. Twice the serum sodium will closely approximate plasma osmolality if excessive amounts of glucose or urea are not present.

ACID-BASE TERMINOLOGY

The traditional method of determining the state of acid-base balance was to determine the pH of arterial or arteriolized venous blood and the total CO_2 content of the plasma. Now the partial pressure of CO_2 is most commonly measured directly in whole blood or calculated from pH and CO_2 content.

From these data, H_2CO_3 can easily be determined, as can bicarbonate, and the $\dfrac{BHCO_3}{H_2CO_3}$ ratio can be directly evaluated. Pure states of respiratory acidosis or alkalosis, and metabolic acidosis and alkalosis, rarely exist except transiently in an acute form, because compensation takes place quite rapidly.

Most patients will have a pattern that consists of the effect of the primary alteration and of the compensations that have been made in response to it.

For these reasons, a careful study of all the clinical problems and physiologic mechanisms present is essential to a complete understanding of any clinical problem involving acid-base derangements.

Several different methods of approaching an understanding of acid-base balance have been developed and are in use today. Unfortunately, each has its own specific terminology, and it is necessary to understand not only the terms but also the methods used in arriving at a conclusion in order to interpret the values for clinical use.

Whole Blood Buffer Base. Whole blood buffer base represents the sum of the red cell and plasma buffers, including bicarbonate in both plasma and red cells, hemoglobin, plasma proteins, and phosphate in both red cells and plasma. The total quantity of buffer anions in normal blood with normal hematocrit is about 45 to 50 mEq/l, almost all of it in bicarbonate and hemoglobin.

Whole blood buffer base is not altered by changes in PCO_2 in vitro. It may be calculated from any two of the three components of the Henderson-Hasselbalch equation (pH, PCO_2, and bicarbonate concentration) with the hematocrit or hemoglobin concentration of blood by using a nomogram constructed by Singer and Hastings* and a clinical interpretation diagram described by Singer, which indicates variations in both buffer base, due to changes in fixed acid, and in PCO_2.

One of the popular ways of visualizing acid-base changes has been to plot the plasma bicarbonate concentration against the value for pH. The development of this approach to visualizing acid-base chemistry has been presented by Davenport in successive editions, over 25 years, of a small monograph entitled The ABC of Acid Base Chemistry.† A slight modification of this pH-bicarbonate diagram is taken from Moore (in The Metabolic Care of the Surgical Patient) and reproduced herein (Fig. 8).

Standard Bicarbonate and Base Excess. In the past five years, an ingenious apparatus developed by Astrup and his associates has come into extensive use in the United States. This apparatus permits the measurement of the pH of blood as drawn from the patient and also the pH of the blood when saturated with oxygen and equilibrated with CO_2 at two known partial pressures.

Standard bicarbonate is defined as the concentration of bicarbonate in plasma when whole blood fully saturated with oxygen is equilibrated with carbon dioxide at a PCO_2 of 40 mm Hg at 38°C. Normal values (95% range) are given as 21.3 to 24.8 mEq/l.

Standard bicarbonate does not directly show the amount of fixed acid or base causing a change in the base content of whole blood, because bicarbonate is responsible for only about 75% of buffering at a fixed PCO_2. This is approximated in the Astrup system by multiplying the variation in standard

---

*Singer, R. B., and Hastings, A. B.: An improved clinical method for the estimation of disturbances of the acid-base balance of human blood. Medicine, 27:223, 1948.

†Davenport, H. W.: The ABC of Acid-Base Chemistry, 5th ed. Chicago, University of Chicago Press, 1969.

bicarbonate by 1.20. An exact correction requires knowledge of the hemoglobin concentration of whole blood, as is also the case with whole blood buffer base.

Base excess is the actual buffer base minus the normal buffer base. It may have either a positive or a negative sign. Thus, a negative base excess is a base deficit, representing an increase in fixed acid. The 95% range for normal base excess is stated to be -2.3 to $+2.3$ mEq/l.

The Siggaard Andersen* nomogram is used with the Astrup apparatus in determining standard bicarbonate, buffer base, base excess, and PCO_2. It assumes that the blood is at least 90% saturated with oxygen, and correction factors must be used if this is not so either because venous blood is used or because of arterial blood unsaturation.

The pH of the blood is measured in oxygen at 38°C at two known PCO_2 values, one higher and one lower than PCO_2 of 40 mm. pH values at these PCO_2 values are plotted on the nomogram and connected by a straight line. The PCO_2 of the blood sample is then read at its actual pH. Standard bicarbonate, buffer base, and base excess are read at the points where the line crosses the appropriate scales.

The problems inherent in the use of either the Singer-Hastings, the Davenport, or the Astrup method of interpretation of acid-base derangements are discussed in detail by Schwartz and Relman.† This article should be read carefully by any surgeon who wishes to understand the limitations, as well as the advantages, of some of the newer methods of approach to problems in acid-base balance. In particular, the nature of normal compensation for respiratory acidosis and for respiratory alkalosis must be understood if acid-base changes of an acute nature superimposed on a chronic and compensated respiratory alteration are to be understood and properly treated.

FORMULAS FOR CARDIOPULMONARY FUNCTION

NORMAL VALUES

$FVC = 70$ ml/kg
$AaDO_2 = 30–40$ mm Hg
$Qs/Qt = 0.02–0.03$
Effective compliance $= 100$ ml/cm H_2O (erect)
$\qquad\qquad\qquad\qquad\quad 75$ ml/cm H_2O (supine)
$CaO_2 \geq 12$ ml O_2/100 ml blood

INDICATIONS TO VENTILATE PATIENT

pH < 7.25
$AaDO_2\ 1.0 > 350$
VC < 10 ml/kg
$Qs/Qt > 0.15$

---

*Siggaard Andersen, O.: The Acid-Base Status of the Blood, 3rd ed. Baltimore, Williams and Wilkins Co., 1966.

†Schwartz, W. B., and Relman, A. S.: A critique of the parameters used in the evaluation of acid-base disorders. N. Engl. J. Med., 268:225, 1963.

PULMONARY

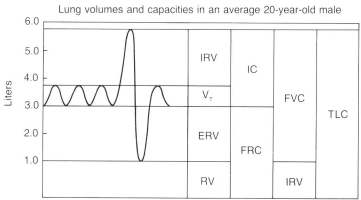

Lung volumes and capacities in an average 20-year-old male

Spirometry in a normal patient. Normally at least 75% of the forced expiratory volume should be exhaled during the first second. The MMFR from 25% to 75% of the forced expiratory volume should be about 4.0 liters per second or about 240 liters per minute.

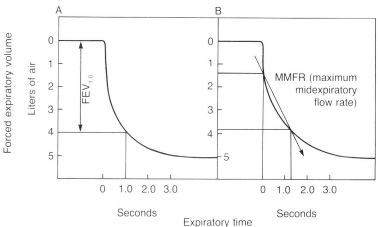

Expiratory time

(From Wilson, R. F. (ed.): Critical Care Manual: Principles and Techniques of Critical Care. Kalamazoo, MI, the Upjohn Co.)

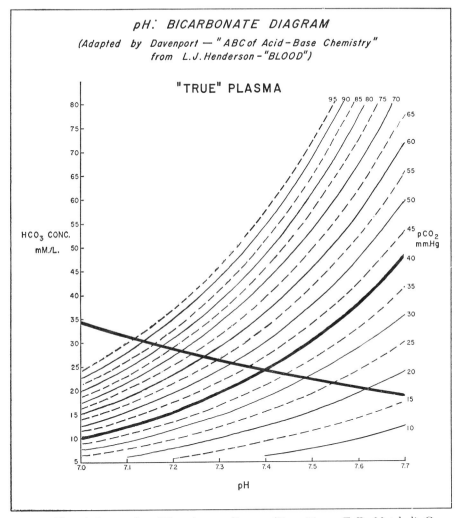

Acid-base balance. The pH-bicarbonate diagram. (From Moore, F. D.: Metabolic Care of the Surgical Patient. Philadelphia, W. B. Saunders Company, 1959.)

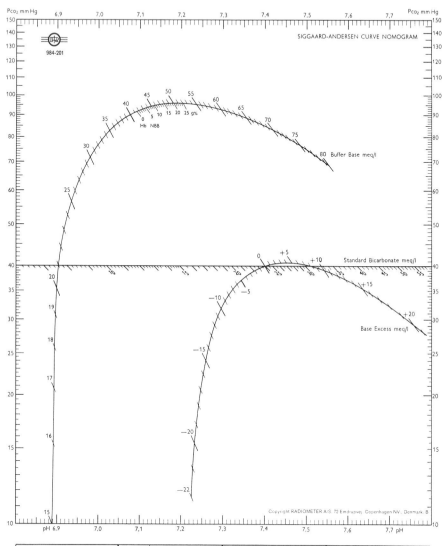

SIGGAARD-ANDERSEN CURVE NOMOGRAM

984-201

Buffer Base meq/l

Standard Bicarbonate meq/l

Base Excess meq/l

Copyright RADIOMETER A/S, 72 Emdrupvej, Copenhagen NV., Denmark. B

Patient's name:		Barometric pressure		mm Hg	READINGS			RESULTS	
		CO₂ percentage	Cylinder No 1:	%	Before equilibration	Actual pH:		Actual Pco₂	mm Hg
Dept:	Sample No.:		Cylinder No 2:	%				Base Excess	meq/l blood
Date:		CO₂ partial pressure	Cylinder No 1:	mm Hg	After equilibration	high Pco₂	pH:	Buffer Base	meq/l blood
Hour of Sampling:			Cylinder No 2:	mm Hg		low Pco₂	pH:	Standard Bicarb.	meq/l plasma
Remarks:		Hemoglobin:		g/100 ml	Readings made by:			Actual Bicarb.	meq/l plasma
		Oxygen Saturation:		percent	Signature:			Total CO₂	meq/l plasma

FORMULAS FOR RESPIRATORY FUNCTION

1. $PAO_2 = Pb - PH_2O - PCO_2 (FIO_2 = 1)$
   PAO_2 = Alveolar O_2 tension
   Pb = Barometric pressure
   PH_2O = Vapor pressure H_2O at given temperature
   PCO_2 = CO_2

2. $AaDO_2 = PAO_2 - PaO_2$
   PaO_2 = Arterial O_2 tension

3. $Qs/Qt = \dfrac{AaDO_2 \times 0.0031}{(AaDO_2 \times 0.0031) + (CaO_2 - CvO_2)}$

   CaO_2 = Arterial O_2 content

   CvO_2 = Mixed venous O_2 content

4. FIO_2 required for PaO_2 100 $= \dfrac{AaDO_2 + 100}{760}$

5. $CaO_2 = 1.34 \times O_2$ saturation $\times$ Hgb (gm/100 ml) $+ O_2$ solubility in blood $\times PaO_2$
   O_2 solubility in blood at 760 mm Hg pressure $= 0.0223$

6. Effective compliance $= \dfrac{TV}{\text{peak airway pressure}}$

VAPOR PRESSURE OF WATER

	TEMP. °C	VAPOR PRESSURE mm Hg
1	0	4.6
2	5	6.5
3	10	9.2
4	15	12.8
5	20	17.5
6	22	19.8
7	24	22.4
8	26	25.2
9	28	28.3
10	30	31.8
11	31	33.7
12	32	35.7
13	33	37.7
14	34	39.9
15	35	42.2
16	36	44.6
17	37	47.1
18	38	49.7
19	39	52.4
20	40	55.3

(From Altman, P. L., and Ditmer, D. S.: Biological Handbooks: Respiration and Circulation. Federation of American Societies for Experimental Biology, 1971.)

Index

Numbers followed by (t) refer to tables; numbers in *italics* refer to illustrations.